Common Medical Problems in the Tropics

in the Tropics

Second Edition

Christopher R. Schull
MB BS (Hons) (Qld), DPH (Eng), FRACP

Consultant Physician,
Thoracic Medicine,
Greenslopes Private Hospital,
Brisbane, Australia

Formerly Specialist Medical Officer (Physician).
Madang and Honorary Senior Lecturer and
Clinical Tutor (Internal Medicine) College of
Allied Health Sciences, Madang, Papua New
Guinea

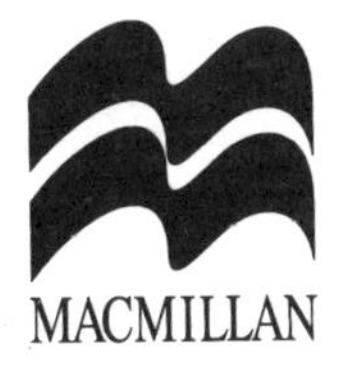

Macmillan Education
Between Towns Road, Oxford OX4 3PP
A division of Macmillan Publishers Limited
Companies and representatives throughout the world

ISBN 0333 67999 7

First published 1987

This edition 1999

www.macmillan-africa.com

TALC, St Albans, UK received assistance in the production of this book as a low cost edition from Community Aid Abroad in Australia

Printed and bound in Malaysia

2007 2006 2005
10 9 8 7 6 5 4

Contents

Important notes about drugs and drug doses

1. *Manufacturer's recommendations.* Always check the drugs you use with the manufacturer's recommendations (these are usually on a leaflet with the drugs) and with your country's treatment guidelines. The author has made every effort to ensure that the drugs and doses recommended in this book are the most appropriate for 'tropical countries' at the time of writing. However, errors and omissions may have occurred, or time and tests may have shown that other drugs or doses are better.

2. *Doses.* Use the doses of drugs given in weight, e.g. mg or g. Where only one size of tablet or one strength of a solution is commonly used, the dose may also be given in brackets as number of tablets or volume of solution. Always use the dose of drug given by weight (and not the number of tablets or volume of solution) until you have checked that the strength of tablets or solution in the book is the same as that in use in your country.

3. *Drug doses and children.*

   All drug doses in this book are for adults.

   Some of the doses of drugs given to adults would be dangerous or even fatal for children.

   For details about children with diseases and especially for the correct doses of drugs for children, you MUST look in a book on child health and children's diseases.

4. *Drug doses and drug choices in all patients.* If your country has a national essential drugs list and/or standard treatment guidelines for drug doses, then you MUST use those drugs and the doses listed in them. The drugs and doses recommended in these lists and guidelines will be the most safe and effective for people in your country.

Foreword

TALC is delighted that a further edition of this most useful book has been developed. At the present time many standard books on tropical health are going out of print and *Common Medical Problems in the Tropics* is now perhaps the only low cost widely available book for doctors and other healthworkers working in developing countries on adult tropical diseases. All those who practise medicine and the patients who receive better treatment thanks to this book owe Dr Chris Schull a very deep sense of gratitude. On their behalf I would like to express my sincere thanks. Dr Schull has not only undertaken a massive re-write but also has been in touch with many experts around the world to make this book up to date. If this was not enough he is accepting no royalties for all his months of work. He and his family have found the financial resources which will bring this book to you at a phenomenally low price. His fellow Australians should be proud he has made such a wealth of knowledge and experience available to some of the most needy populations worldwide.

David C. Morley
Emeritus Professor of Tropical Child Health
Institute of Child Health
University of London

Preface to the First Edition

If you are a health worker in a rural health centre in a tropical or developing country, this book was written specifically for you. If you are a health worker in a small provincial hospital, an urban health centre, or the outpatients' department of a large hospital, this book was written especially for you also. If you are a health worker of any other sort interested in the promotion of good health, prevention of disease and treatment of medical problems of adults in tropical and developing countries, this book was written for you too.

Most of you will be paramedical workers such as Health Extension Officers, Medical Assistants, Nurses and similar workers. Some of you will be Medical Officers working outside a large well-equipped hospital. Most of you will be doing most of the work which most medical 'general practitioners' in the industrialised western countries do. This book was written in the way it is as you usually (1) work without direct or easy contact with a Medical Officer in a well-equipped hospital; (2) cannot easily and quickly get pathology tests done in a reliable laboratory; but you (3) can refer or transfer patients to a Medical Officer in a hospital – if this is needed. An important feature of this book is helping you to make decisions based on clinical findings without waiting for laboratory help. It is very important for you to be able to do this, as experience in a number of countries has taught that even when laboratory services are supposed to be available, they are in fact not available or give very unreliable results which are misleading or even dangerous. Another important feature of this book is helping you to decide if and when a patient of yours should be referred or transferred to a Medical Officer in a hospital.

If you are a Medical Officer and especially if you are a consultant physician (in internal medicine), this book was written in the hope you also could use it – summarise it, expand it, or alter it, to make it specific and more useful for the health workers in the area in which you live and practise medicine. It is hoped you can do this without your having to first do all the groundwork to get basic information together and then make it relevant to the above health workers and the people in tropical and developing countries.

When you read this book, especially if you are a Medical Officer, please remember that some things stated as facts and some explanations given are so stated and so given for the Health Extension Officers, Medical Assistants and Nurses who have only a very short training in the basic medical sciences and pathology. Discussion of controversial subjects and pathophysiological explanations can be found in standard texts and journals.

This book grew out of work and teaching done with Health Extension Officers and Nurses in Papua New Guinea in the 10 years up to 1982, and also time previously spent in Nigeria and other places. The author worked for a year in a rural health centre without hospital facilities in post-war Nigeria and for another year in a rural health centre in Papua New Guinea. After these years, from a new position as consultant physician for an area as well as a hospital, the author regularly visited health centres and their staffs of paramedical workers and discussed with the staff all their patients and also any of their other problems. Also, all the adults with medical problems transferred by the health workers from health centres were received into the author's hospital ward. Also, about half the author's time each day was spent teaching paramedical workers in the half of the hospital ward which was run (with the aid of the trainee paramedical workers and their tutors) as a health centre and not a hospital ward. (All new urban patients were admitted to and managed in the health centre ward, and were transferred to the Medical Officer section of the ward only if transfer to Medical Officer and hospital care became necessary.) (Patients transferred from rural health centres were admitted directly to the Medical Officer section of the ward.) Half of most nights and the majority of most weekends were spent by not only the author but also his wife, devising the management regimes, the indications for transfer or referral of patients and all the other things which went into the preparation of books such as this. These regimens and books were then tried out by the health workers locally and later in all of Papua New Guinea; and then in the light of the usefulness or otherwise of parts of them, modifications were made and new editions of books produced. Many parts of these books, which some Medical Officers said should be removed, were left in because Health Extension Officers and Nurses repeatedly asked for that information and were certain it should not be removed.

This present book is a modification of the final reference book produced for Papua New Guinea *Adult Internal Medicine in Papua New Guinea – A Reference Book for Health Workers in Health Centres and Hospital Outpatients Departments*, 1984, C.R. Schull, published by the Government Printer, Port Moresby, Papua New Guinea. The author was asked to try to make the Papua New Guinea book useful to paramedical workers in other parts of the world. The author realised that he was not knowledgeable enough or experienced enough to do this adequately. It was clear, however, after searching in vain for a similar book for the rest of the world through all available libraries, that no one else had felt qualified or experienced enough to write it; or if they had, they had not been motivated enough to do it. Although there were books for paramedical workers in Child Health, Surgery and Obstetrics and Gyneacology, there were none along these lines in Adult Internal Medicine for senior paramedical workers. Hence this book.

This book is a reference book. It is not meant to be all learned. It is meant to be read during the years of student life when training to be a health worker; and then to be then referred to during working life to help when problems arise. The book is therefore large and has many words to try to explain things as clearly as could be done.

It is hoped that supervising or teaching Medical Officers in each country, who do not have time to prepare all the books needed by paramedical workers, may be able to take the parts from this book which apply to their country, simplify and summarise those parts (and alter or amplify or add to other parts if needed), and produce perhaps two other more useful books.

One book probably needed would be a 'summary' i.e. a book with just those things which the student and health worker must *know*, i.e. be able to recite orally or write, interpret on patients and use in practice to solve the problems of patients and the common health problems of the area. Such a book for Papua New Guinea is *Common Medical Problems of Adults in Papua New Guinea – A Summary*, 1979, C.R. Schull, Kristen Press Inc., Madang, Papua New Guinea.

The other book which is probably needed is a small book that can be carried in the health worker's pocket all the time and which has the details of the management of the common health problems in that area including drug doses (and it is much safer to look these up than to try to remember them and perhaps make a fatal mistake). Of course the health worker must be taught actually to look up the book when he is seeing the patient. Such a book is *Diagnosis and Treatment of Common Health Problems of Adults in Papua New Guinea*, 1980, C.R. Schull, Kristen Press Inc., Madang, Papua New Guinea.

Experience with Health Extension Officers and Nurses has taught that only one part of the book is likely to be consulted at any one time. Experience has also taught that repetition is a good teacher. The above will also partly explain some of the repetition in the book.

After the introductory chapters most chapters are set out using the following plan (modified as needed). At first there is a short description of the anatomy and physiology of the system. Then there is a list of the symptoms and signs which can be caused by abnormal structure or function of that system. This section includes details of how to examine the patient to find these signs. Next there is a section which includes the common conditions and diseases of the system. Finally, there is a section which summarises the cause of and management of the common symptoms and signs caused by disorders and diseases of the system.

Although this is a reference book, the health worker student should become familiar with it before graduating. During student life you should read the following.

1. All of the first *eleven* chapters including diagnosis of disease, management of a patient and control and prevention of disease.
2. All sections of Anatomy, Physiology, Pathology, Symptoms and Signs in chapters which have these discussed.

3. The sections on all the common important diseases in the country in which he is working.

These will include the following in almost all countries:

1. Severe bacterial infections including septicaemia (Chapter 12).
2. Malaria (Chapter 13).
3. Tuberculosis (Chapter 14).
4. Leprosy (Chapter 15).
5. The common infectious diseases which occur almost everywhere (Chapter 16).
6. Any of the other infectious diseases which occur in your area (Chapter 17 and 18).
7. Syphilis, gonorrhoea, and HIV infection and AIDS (Chapter 19).
8. Otitis of various types, the common cold, influenza, acute bronchitis, pneumonia, asthma and chronic bronchitis; and causes of cough, sputum, haemoptysis, shortness of breath and pain in chest (Chapter 20).
9. Anaemia, hyperreactive malarious splenomegaly and, if it occurs in your area, sickle cell anaemia (Chapter 21).
10. Filariasis (Chapter 22).
11. Gastro-enteritis, intestinal parasites and peptic ulcer; and causes of vomiting, haematemesis, diarrhoea and dysentery (Chapter 23).
12. Jaundice, hepatitis, liver abscess, hepatoma and cirrhosis (Chapter 24).
13. Meningitis of all types, cerebral malaria and other types of 'encephalitis', convulsions, epilepsy, paralysis, unconsciousness and headache (Chapter 25).
14. Urinary tract infections, causes of urinary frequency and pain, nephrotic syndrome, chronic kidney failure and causes of proteinuria (Chapter 26).
15. Osteomyelitis and pyomyositis (Chapter 28), acute bacterial arthritis, 'tropical arthritis', tuberculous arthritis and osteoarthrosis (Chapter 29).
16. Foreign bodies in the eye, conjunctivitis, corneal ulcer and iritis (Chapter 31).
17. Tinea, impetigo and scabies and the principles of treatment of all skin conditions (Chapter 32).
18. Snakebite (Chapter 33).
19. Swallowed poisons (Chapter 34).
20. Acute and chronic organic psychoses, schizophrenia, manic-depressive psychoses, acute psychotic reactions, anxiety states and 'acting out' states (Chapter 35).
21. Some important symptoms and signs including fever, generalised oedema, generalised wasting, dehydration, abdominal pain, abdominal tenderness – guarding – rigidity, abdominal masses and abdominal distension.
22. Resuscitation including artificial ventilation (Chapter 37) and treatment of shock (Chapter 27).

Any other diseases which are common in the area in which the health worker is, must be added to this list.

Malnutrition is not only a cause of disease, but also interacts with infection in a number of ways. Malnutrition decreases immunity or resistance to infection. Malnutrition makes any infection present more serious, and makes it less likely for the body to overcome that infection, even when correct treatment of the infection is given. Infection in a person who already has malnutrition makes that malnutrition even worse. As these conditions are even more important for children than adults, and as they are dealt with at length in the books on child health and children's diseases, malnutrition has not been discussed in a separate chapter in this book and the interaction of malnutrition and infection has not been emphasised. This is not meant to indicate that malnutrition and its relation to infection and its prevention and its treatment are not important for adults – they are. For detailed discussions of these, however, see books on child health and children's diseases; but remember that these things apply to adults also.

If the health worker does decide to purchase some other books in adult internal medicine, the first three to consider are:

Edwards, C.R.W. *et al.* (latest edition) *Davidson's Principles and Practice of Medicine*. Edinburgh, Churchill Livingstone.

Lawrence, D.R. (latest edition) *Clinical Pharmacology*. Edinburgh, Churchill Livingstone.

Munro, J. and Edwards, C. (latest edition). *MacLeod's Clinical Examination*. Edinburgh, Churchill Livingstone.

All of these books are available in low-priced editions. The latest edition should, of course, be obtained.

The author is only too well aware of the many imperfections in this book. If the book is to be improved, advice on how to do this is needed from those who use it. If Health Extension Officers, Medical Assistants, Nurses, Tutors and Medical Officers who use this book in any way for any purpose would be kind enough to write to the author and tell him of errors or omissions noted or things which are hard to understand, etc. and also make specific suggestions for improvements, this would greatly help. PLEASE WRITE.

It is hoped that what is in this book will show how health workers using only simple and cheap items (available in most health centres and hospital outpatients departments) are able to manage almost all of the medical health problems of adults safely and effectively.

C.R. Schull
1987

Preface to the Second Edition

I was asked by Professor Morley from TALC, some staff from The Australian College of Tropical Medicine at the James Cook University, Townsville and others, to update the first edition of this book, as apparently no other similar book has recently been published. As I now live and work in Australia, I no longer have constant contact with paramedical workers to make sure what I write is truly relevant to them and what they want. However the first edition of this book has been used by an even greater range of health workers and teaching institutions than I expected. As well as this, situations in one country do still differ very greatly from situations in another country. No book could possibly cover all of the practical aspects needed for all users of this book for all countries. No book could do this for many of the users without including many details not important to them.

I have therefore done my best to retain in the book what paramedical workers have told me they want and I have added what appears to be new and important. Great changes in health have been caused by the epidemic of HIV infection; increasing numbers of people living in cities but still without access to good health services; increase in diseases associated with urban living, such as vascular disease; some diseases, such as leprosy, becoming less of a problem; some diseases, such as tuberculosis, becoming more of a problem; and exciting changes for possible control of some of the helminthic and other diseases which previously could not be controlled. I have tried to alter the text to take account of these developments.

It is still essential that a specialist in internal medicine in each country indicates to paramedical health workers in that country, what they do and do not need to know. They can then delete from this book what is not important in their country and add anything missed out that is important. I am of course happy for such Medical Officers to use this book as a basis for any local literature produced, if an explanation of what has been done is included.

It is also still essential that such a Medical Officer produces a summary of what the paramedical health worker needs to learn and to know. If a photocopy of such booklets as *Diagnosis and Treatment of Common Health Problems in Papua New Guinea* and *Standard Management of Common Medical Problems of Adults in Papua New Guinea*, which I previously wrote, would help as a basis for the production of such local booklets, I would be happy to send these copies on request although they now are out of date.

This book is a reference book to be used throughout training. It is then to be used as a source of information by the health worker when he is working independently and he comes across a problem not covered by his existing knowledge.

In many places I have added explanations of treatment carried out and names of drugs used by Medical Officers in hospitals but not available at health centres. This is so that when patients, who have been referred to hospital, return to the health centre, the paramedical workers will understand about the treatment and drugs the patients has been given. Paramedical workers should not try to learn these sections where such things as 'Drugs used by Medical Officers in hospitals will include …' are written.

To try to save space and time the words 'he, him, his' stand also for 'she, her, hers' where the text could refer either to a man, boy or woman, girl.

Publications of particular value to paramedical workers and Medical Officers include those listed on page 512 at the back of this book.

I would like to thank those few people who did write with suggestions for improvement of the first edition. Most of these suggestions have been included in this second edition. If you have any suggestions for improvement of this second edition, please write.

Sheila Jones, Freelance Editor, has done the difficult and thankless task of editing the whole manuscript – not only for the first edition but also for this second edition. I am grateful for her help and acknowledge how much she has contributed.

Shirley Hamber, Freelance Publisher, who has overseen all the work, could not have been more helpful.

My wife, Judith, has not only helped more than anyone else in the re-writing of this second edition but has in fact been the one who has made it possible.

C.R. Schull
Greenslopes Private Hospital
Newdegate Street
Greenslopes, 4120
Queensland
Australia

Acknowledgements

This book was prepared with the help of many of my friends and colleagues. So many helped in so many ways over so many years it is now no longer possible to record all the people who helped – even in major ways.

Foremost among those who made this book possible were my wife and children. They not only went without many things so that this and the other books for Papua New Guinea could appear; they also gave encouragement and help and my wife did all the typing for the numerous Papua New Guinean drafts and editions.

Many of my colleagues in Papua New Guinea gave encouragement and help. In particular Doctors John and Narelle Stace helped in very many ways and in every way they could. Dr Brother Andrew SSF contributed significantly to the chapter on mental illnesses. Professor George Wyatt made valuable suggestions and Dr Greg Lawrence read the whole of the Papua New Guinean edition and made numerous suggestions for improvement. Papua New Guinean health workers, and in particular Dr Puka Temu and HEO Tutor Mr Mika Kenas gave invaluable guidance. Of course, many of the ideas in the book came from observation of what happened to patients and other situations which arose during health centre work and then discussion of these with the staff involved.

For the International edition, Dr F.J. Wright of Edinburgh kindly and helpfully checked the various chapters with diseases with which the author had not had significant practical experience. Dr C.J. Ellis of Birmingham then read through the text and made many valuable suggestions. Both of these doctors have had vast experience in tropical and developing countries and are internationally recognised authorities in tropical diseases. The author is very grateful to them for their invaluable advice.

Two editors, at first Mrs Jennifer Gamel and later (for the bulk of the work) Mrs Sheila Jones, did a large amount of important work in preparing and improving the text for publication.

As the author did not plan to publish any works for distribution outside Papua New Guinea until he was requested to do so just before he had to leave Papua New Guinea to return to Australia, and as there was no copyright law in Papua New Guinea, no particular record of the origin of diagrams and descriptions of laboratory procedures etc. collected for use of health workers was kept. Most of these which the author did not produce in Madang were obtained from slides or photographs in the Medical Learning Resources Unit of the University of Papua New Guinea in Port Moresby, and most of these were not documented as to origin. If, therefore, there are any parts of the book, and especially any diagrams, which have been inadvertently reproduced without appropriate acknowledgement made, the author apologises for this and would make such acknowledgement if permission for the use of these were granted for any future edition, and the publishers would make the necessary arrangements.

Money to assist in travel for library research and typing of the International text was kindly supplied by the Damian Foundation, Belgium, Boehringer Ingelheim Australia and the World Health Organization, Geneva. Large grants were then given by both the Swedish International Development Agency and the Australian Government's Australian Development Assistance Bureau to Teaching Aids at Low Cost, London, to provide money for the printing and sale of the first edition by Macmillan at a price well below the normal price for a book of this size. The author has and will accept no payment of any kind in a further attempt to keep the price as low as possible. It is only through the generous assistance of the above charitable, company and government bodies, however, that it has been possible to produce and distribute this book.

Despite all the above help, however, the production of this and the other books has been an 'after hours' effort by a clinician who considers himself in no way an academic or an author. Responsibility for errors and omissions, therefore, rests with the author, and not those who helped in so many ways.

To all the people, as well as the above, who helped the author, he gives his thanks. The author knows these people well enough to be certain that if this book helps improve the health of people in tropical and developing countries then those who contributed to the production of this book will be thanked enough.

C.R.S

The author and publishers are grateful to the World Health Organization for permission to reproduce maps showing the distribution of diseases.

The author and publishers wish to thank the following for permission to use copyright material:
World Health Organization for **Figure 19.18** from *WHO Technical Report No. 810*, **Table 14.5** adapted from A.D. Harries and D. Maher (1996) *TB/HIV A Clinical Manual*, **Figure 19.3** from (1991) *WHO Technical Report No. 810* and (1995) *WHO Model Prescribing Information* and **Table 35.2** from (1992) WHO ICD-10: *International Classification of Diseases*, 10th edn.

The author and publishers wish to acknowledge, with thanks, the following photographic sources:
Dr A. Buck p 438 (from A Colour Atlas of Tropical Medicine and Parasitology by W. Peters and H.M. Gilles, Wolfe Medical Publications Ltd)
Dr Rod Hay, School of Hygiene and Tropical Medicine, London p 433 top
Dr D. M. Minter p 144 right (from A Colour Atlas of Tropical Medicine and Parasitology by W. Peters and H.M. Gilles, Wolfe Medical Publications Ltd)
St. Bartholomew's Hospital, Department of Medical Photography pp. 175 right, 176 top (photograph Morris Sydney), 434 (photograph Roy Gray)
TALC pp. 87, 181, 185 top and bottom, 186, 187 left and right, 188, 190, 194
Tropix Photograph Library pp. 142, 144 left
C. James Webb pp. 146 top, 236, 245, 446 right
WHO pp. 146 bottom, 444 (photograph J. Abcede), 445 (photograph D. Deriaz), 446 left (photograph E. Mandelmann), 448 bottom
All other photographs are courtesy of the author.
Cover photographs courtesy of TALC, C. James Webb and the author

The publishers have made every effort to trace the copyright holders, but if they have inadvertently overlooked any, they will be pleased to make the necessary arrangements at the first opportunity.

1

The Purpose of the Health Worker

You (and all of us who are really effective health workers) must have three aims:

1. to promote good health,
2. to prevent disease,
3. to treat disease.

These three aims must be for both

1. individuals and
2. the whole community.

When you treat disease, again you have three aims:

1. to cure the patient, (this is not always possible);
2. to relieve the patient's symptoms (this is almost always possible);
3. to comfort and encourage the patient and his relatives (this is always possible).
   By what you say and what you do, you need to reassure the patient and his relatives that you are also a real person and that you understand his health problems and the worries these cause him. The patient should understand that you will not leave him without all the medical and personal help that you are able to give to him. You need to be optimistic and continue to be optimistic (hopeful and cheerful) about your being able to give good relief of his symptoms, cure him if possible or help him die without distress but in dignity.

It is very easy to spend all your time treating disease and so have no time to prevent disease and promote health. This is not the best way to spend your time. Of course you must treat patients with disease. This helps the patient and his relatives. It also shows the community that you know how to help them and that you do want to help them. It is only when the community discovers this that they will take any notice of your work to prevent disease and promote health. Unless you really do prevent disease and promote good health, your work in treating the sick will not help the community very much. It is no good curing a patient if you do not prevent the patient getting the same disease again when he goes home. His family and friends may also get the disease. So:

1. You must use some of your time to treat patients with disease.
2. You must use some of your time to prevent disease.
3. You must use some of your time to promote good health.

You will often find it difficult to leave your work in the health centre and go out into the community to prevent disease and promote health. But you must do this. You can also do a lot to control and prevent disease in the health centre. When a person comes to you in the health centre and you diagnose his disease, you can give the patient and his family and friends education about how to control and prevent disease, and about other things which would improve their health. Remember two things:

First, when people are well they usually take no notice of health education as they feel they will not get a disease. But when they are sick, the patient and his family and friends will often take notice of health education, as they then know they can get the disease.

Second, most cases of undiagnosed infectious diseases such as leprosy and tuberculosis are in the family and friends of patients with these diseases. Therefore, before you go out of the health centre to look for these sorts of disease in the whole community, first make sure you educate and examine all the family and friends who have come (with the patient) to you in the health centre.

This does not mean you should stay in the health centre all the time. It means you should never miss the chance to control and prevent disease and promote health when a sick person comes to the health centre.

You, the Health Worker, must also remember that what you *do* to treat and prevent disease and promote health will have much more effect than what you *say* about these things. Your effectiveness as a Health Worker will depend on what sort of person you really are and the way you live and work.

2

Some Clinical Definitions

> Do not try to learn these definitions until you have:
> 1. read more about them in later chapters,
> 2. talked about them with your teachers, and
> 3. used the things they are about in your practical work.

Anatomy
Anatomy is the science of the *structure* of the body; or *how the body is made.*

Physiology
Physiology is the science of the normal *function* of the body; or *how the living body works.*

Definition of a disease
In this book the definition of a disease is a short statement about the nature of the disease; or what kind of disease it is.

Frequency
The frequency is how often the disease occurs. There are more accurate terms. These include the following:

Prevalence: This is the *total* number of persons with the disease at a *stated* time in a *stated* population.

Incidence: This is the number of *new* persons developing the disease during a *stated* time in a *stated* population.

A classification of the causes of disease (aetiology)
There are ten common kinds or classifications of disease (congenital, traumatic, inflammatory (four types), neoplastic, degenerative, chemical – induced, malnutrition, psychological, body system failure (especially vascular) and others including unknown). The causes of many of these classifications of diseases are known (see Chapter 4). In fact, some of the classifications are based on the cause of disease. However, there are also causes that are not yet known about. For example, it is said that a patient's disease may be degenerative (or due to the body wearing out); but it is not known why the body, which can repair itself, eventually wears out. The most common causes of disease in tropical and developing countries are infections with organisms, trauma and malnutrition. (See Chapter 4.)

Pathology
The cause of the disease can make changes in the normal anatomy and physiology of the body. These changes are called pathology. See Chapter 3.

Epidemiology
Epidemiology gives the known answers to the questions:

1. *Who* gets a particular disease and *how many* people get it?
2. *When* and *where* do these persons get the disease? and
3. *How* and *why* do they get the disease? (See Chapter 5.)

Symptoms
Symptoms are *what the patient feels.*

The patient *tells* you his symptoms when he talks to you about what he *feels.*

You can usually discover symptoms when you take a *medical history* from the patient. When you take a medical history you must ask about:

1. General information.
2. The patient's symptoms and how long he has had each one. (Record these in the patient's own words.)
3. The history of the present illness (or the story of how the patient went from being well to sick).
4. The specific questions (or specific interrogation) that you must ask to discover if there are also symptoms of a disease of any other system of the

body (as well as those the patient has already talked about).
5. The past history – you ask the patient about the drugs he has taken, treatment he has been given by traditional healers, previous attacks of this illness, other illness, operations, accidents and previous and present pregnancies, etc.
6. The family and contact history – you check if an illness in the family or in one of his contacts could be affecting the patient.

There are three other things you must do when you take a medical history.

1. If the patient may have a mental condition, take the history again from a relative or another witness.
2. Check the patient's outpatient card and any inpatient notes for any history in them.
3. Tell the patient a summary of the history and ask him to correct anything wrong.

Signs

Signs are what you find (see, feel, percuss, hear, etc.) when you examine the patient.

You do the *clinical* or *medical* or *physical* examination to discover all the patient's signs. You must do it systematically (or in a special order) in nine sections, so that you never forget anything.

1. Basic observations. These help you decide if the patient is 'sick' or not. They also help you to look for common diseases (even if the patient does not complain of their symptoms). If you find these diseases while they are still not serious you can treat them and prevent them from getting worse. These observations include: level of consciousness and signs of meningeal irritation; temperature; pulse rate; respiration rate and type of respiration; blood pressure, weight with observations about dehydration, oedema, malnutrition or chronic wasting illness; and colour, especially anaemia.
2. Head and neck including ear, nose, throat, lymph glands and thyroid.
3. Chest, including spine.
4. Abdomen.
5. Skin.
6. Muscles, bones, joints.
7. Ear, nose and throat (if not done before).
8. Any special examinations, if needed.
9. Examination of mental state (psychiatric examination), if needed.

See Chapter 6 page 19.

Course and complications

The course is what usually happens to a person who has the disease. Complications are other things which do not usually happen in the course of the disease. Complications are other clinical conditions which can happen on top of the original clinical condition.

Tests or investigations

You do tests for three reasons:

1. to help you decide between different possible diagnoses,
2. to confirm a diagnosis, and
3. to provide a baseline by which you can judge if the patient is getting better or worse.

There are three groups of tests:

1. Those you can do at the health centre, e.g. haemoglobin, urine tests, lumbar puncture, etc.
2. You take a sample at the health centre, but send it to the hospital laboratory to be examined there, e.g. 'serum tests', malaria smear, sputum smears, etc. (In some large health centres there is a medical laboratory assistant who can do some of these tests at the health centre.)
3. If you cannot do the test or take a sample at the health centre, you must send the patient to the hospital for the test, e.g. X-rays, etc.

See Chapter 6 page 22.

Differential diagnosis

The differential diagnosis (DD) is the list of all the diseases *which could* be causing the patient's main symptoms and signs. See Chapter 6 page 21.

Diagnostic features

In this book diagnostic features are the most typical things about the disease (in a short list). These features are nearly always present if that disease is present.

Provisional diagnosis

The provisional diagnosis (PD) is the disease (or diseases) you think the patient really has. You decide this after eliminating all the other diseases in the differential diagnoses because they do not fit the patient's symptoms and signs as well as the provisional diagnosis does. When you have made a provisional diagnosis, you manage the patient for this disease. See Chapter 6 page 21.

Management

Management is not only the treatment of the patient. A patient who has a disease creates problems for many people. To manage these problems you must do at least these four things:

1. treat the patient;
2. notify or advise certain other people;
3. control the spread of the disease, if necessary;
4. prevent other members of the community from getting the disease and the patient from getting it again.

These things are considered separately below. See also Chapters 7, 8 and 9.

Treatment of the patient

Treatment includes the following nine things:

1. *Decision on outpatient treatment or admission for inpatient treatment.*
2. *Nursing care* of many types including at times, bed rest; special positions; special care of respiratory tract, eyes, bladder, pressure areas etc.; isolation; observations; food; fluids; etc.
3. *Specific treatment* to attempt to *cure* the disease, e.g. drugs, fluids, food, surgery, dressings, plasters, physiotherapy and psychiatric counselling.
4. *Symptomatic treatment,* to attempt to relieve the patient's symptoms and make him *feel* better, e.g. drugs, etc. as in 3 above; nursing care as in 2 above.
5. *Giving an explanation, reassurance and comfort to the patient and relatives.*
6. *Giving health education* about control and prevention of the disease to the patient and to the relatives.
7. *Consultation about the patient with the preventive medicine/administrative Health Officer or hospital Medical Officer* (sometimes). This can be for advice or about transfer of the patient to Medical Officer care or referral of the patient to the next visiting Medical Officer.
8. *Discharging the patient* and giving final health education.
9. *Following up the patient,* if needed.

See Chapter 7.

Indications for consultation, transfer or referral

Some symptoms and signs mean that you should do one of the following three things:

1. Describe the patient's condition to the Health Officer or hospital Medical Officer by telephone or radio, and ask for advice (that is 'consult').
2. Transfer.
   (a) Transfer the patient to the hospital as an emergency case for urgent treatment by a Medical Officer as soon as you can find a plane or car or boat to take him there, i.e. 'urgent transfer'.
   (b) Transfer the patient to the hospital as a non-emergency case using the next available usual transport, i.e. 'non-urgent transfer'.
3. Ask the next Medical Officer who visits the health centre to see the patient, i.e. 'referral'.

See Chapter 7 page 28.

Prognosis

The prognosis is what the likely result of a condition will be (e.g. cause the patient's death, get better quickly, last for a long time, etc.)

See Chapter 6 page 22.

Notification

1. You must notify certain diseases to the Health Officer or Health Department if they occur. Some have to be notified immediately if any new case occurs. Some have to be notified immediately if an epidemic occurs. This second group and another group usually have to be notified monthly if any cases occur.
2. You must notify certain cases to the coroner or (patrol) officer in charge of the station and the police. These include all cases of 'sudden and unnatural death' and cases when you do not know the cause of death, including persons who are 'dead on arrival'. Notify all fights, accidents, alleged poisoning, etc. if the patient is ill.
3. You should notify relatives and friends (and sometimes other people) and advise them of the patient's condition, treatment and probable future.

See Chapter 8.

Control

Control is what you must do to stop the disease spreading. You need to know the epidemiology of the disease so that you can choose the best means of control. These means may include one or more of the methods:

1. inactivating the specific (or causative) agent in the reservoir (usually killing a parasite in the body of the original host);
2. blocking the means of spread of the specific (or causative) agent from the reservoir to susceptible persons;
3. increasing the resistance of the susceptible persons; and
4. giving prophylactic treatment to susceptible persons who are probably infected.

See Chapter 9.

Prevention
Prevention is what you need to do to stop the disease occurring. You need to know the epidemiology of the disease so that you can choose the best means of prevention. The means used for prevention are the same as for control. (See above and Chapter 9.)

Acute
Any condition which comes suddenly and lasts a short time may be called 'acute'. This often means less than one month.

Chronic
Any condition which lasts a long time may be called 'chronic'. It usually starts slowly, but an acute condition may become a chronic condition. This usually means more than one month.

Subacute
A subacute condition is one which is somewhere between acute and chronic.

Lesion
Lesion is a general or non-specific term for a pathological change in a body tissue. It is often used to mean damage to the structure of part of an organ, especially damage caused by an injury or infection.

Syndrome
Syndrome is the name given to a *group of symptoms and/or signs*. When these symptoms and signs *all occur together* this means that a certain pathological process is present. There may be a number of causes of this syndrome.

Curative or clinical medicine
Curative medicine or clinical medicine are terms sometimes used for the processes of seeing a patient, taking a history, doing an examination, doing tests, making a diagnosis and treating the patient.

Note on prefixes and suffixes

Certain words or syllables may be added to the beginning of a word (prefix) or the ending of a word (suffix) to form a new word with a different meaning. Some of the prefixes and suffixes often used in medicine are listed below.

Common prefixes
hypo- less than normal or under.
e.g. hypothermia: temperature less than normal; hypodermic: under the dermis or skin.
hyper- more than normal or above.
e.g. hyperthyroidism: thyroid makes more hormone than normal.
an- without.
e.g. anuric: without urine or no urine made.
exo- outside.
e.g. exophthalmos: eye pushed out.
endo- within or inside (not to the outside).
e.g. endocrine: gland which secretes into the blood.
macro- large.
e.g. macroscopic: large enough to be seen by the naked eye.
micro- small.
e.g. microscopic: so small can be seen only with the aid of a microscope.

Common suffixes
-aemia or -emia refers to the blood.
e.g. anaemia: without normal amount of blood.
-uria refers to the urine.
e.g. haematuria: blood in the urine.
-pathy disease.
e.g. encephalopathy: disease of the brain .
-itis inflammation of.
e.g. conjunctivitis: inflammation of conjunctivae.
-oma tumour of organ.
e.g. meningioma: tumour of meninges.

SI units

The International System of Units (SI) is based on the units; metre, kilogram, second, ampere, kelvin, candela and mole. It is already used by many countries as their only legal system.

Names and symbols for basic SI units

Physical quantity	*Name of SI unit*	*Symbol for SI unit*
length	metre	m
mass	kilogram	kg
time	second	s
thermodynamic temperature	kelvin	K
amount of substance	mole	mol

Prefixes for SI units

Prefixes can be used to show decimal fractions or multiples of the basic (or derived) SI units.

Fraction	*Prefix*	*Symbol*
$\frac{1}{10}$ or 10^{-1}	deci	d
$\frac{1}{100}$ or 10^{-2}	centi	c
$\frac{1}{1\,000}$ or 10^{-3}	milli	m
$\frac{1}{1\,000\,000}$ or 10^{-6}	micro	μ

Multiple	*Prefix*	*Symbol*
$\times$ 10 or 10^1	deca	da
$\times$ 100 or 10^2	hecto	h
$\times$ 1 000 or 10^3	kilo	k
$\times$ 1 000 000 or 10^6	mega	M

Length

The SI unit of length is the metre (m).

1 micron (μ) (obsolete) = 10^{-6} m = 1 μm.
1 inch (in) = 2.54 cm = 0.254 m.
1 foot (ft) = 0.3048 m.
1 yard (yd) = 0.9144 m.

Volume

The SI unit of volume is the cubic metre (m^3); but since this is inconveniently large for most measurements in medicine, the litre (l) has been kept as an alternative to the cubic decimetre (dm^3).

1 m^3 = 1000 l.
1 fluid ounce (oz) = 28.41 ml.
1 pint = 20 fluid oz. = 568 ml.
1 gallon = 4.55 l.

Mass

The SI unit of mass is the kilogram (kg).

1 kg = 1000 grams (g).
1 grain = 64.8 mg.
1 ounce (oz) = 28.35 g.
1 pound (lb) = 16 oz = 453.6 g.
1 ton = 2240 lb = 1016 kg.
1 tonne = 1000 kg = 0.984 ton.

Amount of substance

Where the molecular weight of a substance is known, its amount should usually be expressed in terms of the mole (mol). One mole of a substance is that amount of the substance which contains the same number of particles (whether atoms, molecules, ions or radicals) as 12 g of carbon 12. In short, 1 mole is the particle weight (such as atomic weight or molecular weight) expressed in grams.

The 'equivalent' is now not used. It was used to express the amount of an ionised substance; it is the number of moles multiplied by the valency.
Thus 10 mol Na^+ = 10 equiv.;
but 10 mol Ca^{++} = 20 equiv.

Concentration and osmotic pressure

Concentrations of substances in biological fluids should be expressed in molar terms if the molecular weight is known and in terms of mass if not. Thus plasma glucose is expressed as mmol/l while plasma albumin is expressed as g/l. In each case the reference unit of volume is the litre. A special exception is haemoglobin whose concentration in blood is expressed as g/dl.

Osmotic pressure is expressed as osmolarity (moles per litre of solution) or osmolality (moles per kilogram of water).

Pressure

The SI unit of pressure is the pascal (Pa); this is the pressure exerted by 1 newton acting on an area of a square metre (1 Pa = 1 N m^{-2}).

1 cmH_2O = 98.1 Pa.
1 mmHg = 1 torr = 133.3 Pa = 0.1333 kPa.
1 kPa = 7.50 mmHg = 10.1 cmH_2O.
1 normal atmosphere = 760 mmHg = 101.3 kPa.

Temperature

The SI temperature scale is the kelvin scale (K) but this is inconvenient to use in medicine and the Celsius (formerly 'centigrade') scale (°C) has been retained.

Degree Celsius = K – 273.15.

Conversion from the Fahrenheit scale to the Celsius scale can be carried out with either of these formulae:

$9/5\ C = F - 32$

$9/5\ (C + 40) = F + 40$

Where F is the temperature in degrees Fahrenheit and C is the temperature in degrees Celsius.

Time

1 hour (h) = 60 minutes (min) = 3600 seconds (s).

The use of hertz (Hz) for frequency to replace cycles per second is recommended provided it is not used for the timing of discontinuous events, i.e. not, for example, for the frequency of passing urine or the dispensing of doses of medicine. It should not be used for frequency of rotation.

Abbreviations

The following abbreviations are in common use in some places and are sometimes used in this book.

b.d.	Two times each day.
BP	Blood pressure.
C°	Temperature in degrees Celsius or Centigrade.
IMI	Intramuscular injection.
IM	Intramuscularly.
IVI	Intravenous injection.
IV	Intravenously.
nocte	At night; each night.
oral	By mouth.
PR	Pulse rate.
p.r.n.	If needed; if necessary.
q.d.s.	As for q.i.d. (see below) but should be used only for things which are taken (swallowed).
q.i.d.	Four times each day (e.g. before morning meal, in the middle of the day, before evening meal and at night before going to sleep).
RR	Respiration rate.
SCI	Subcutaneous injection (into the fat under the skin).
stat	Immediately, straight away.
T°	Temperature.
t.d.s.	As for t.i.d. (see below) but should be used only for things which are taken (swallowed).
t.i.d.	Three times a day (e.g. before morning meal, before evening meal and at night before going to sleep; *or* before morning meal, in the middle of the day and before evening meal).
>	Greater than; more than.
<	Smaller than; less than.

3

Pathology

The normal human body is made in a certain way. This is called its structure or its *anatomy*. The normal human body works in a certain way. This is called its normal function or *physiology*. Many things can damage the normal anatomy of the body or upset the normal physiology of the body and cause changes in the anatomy and/or the physiology. These are called *pathological changes*.

> Pathology (or pathological change) is the change in the normal anatomy and physiology made by the cause of disease.

The pathological changes (and sometimes the causes of them) show themselves as the symptoms, the signs and the abnormal tests of disease.

When a part of the body is attacked by things which may damage it (see Chapter 4 page 11) this can cause many different types of pathological change. Three very important pathological changes are:

1. death of part or all of the body,
2. inflammatory reaction (or inflammation), and
3. neoplasm (or 'cancer' formation).

Inflammation

Inflammation is the change which happens in a tissue when it is injured, if the injury does not completely destroy the tissue.

Some causes of inflammation are:

1. trauma,
2. infection,
3. chemicals,
4. allergy (see Chapter 4 page 11).

There are two main types of inflammation:

1. acute,
2. chronic.

The type and amount of inflammation depends on the cause. Acute serious injury or infection with some organisms causes acute inflammation. Chronic mild injury or infection with other organisms (especially those which cause leprosy and tuberculosis) causes chronic inflammation.

Acute inflammation

In acute inflammation more blood flows to the area. This is because the blood vessels become wider. Fluid (containing white blood cells, antibodies and other proteins from inside the blood vessels) goes through the capillary walls into the tissues of the area. Then some or all of the following processes happen, depending on the cause of the inflammation.

- Fluid dilutes the cause, e.g. a chemical.
- White blood cells try to digest the cause, e.g. dirt in a wound.
- Proteins make a wall around the area to limit the spread of bacteria, e.g. tuberculosis (see Chapter 14, page 75 and Chapter 10 page 37).
- Antibodies attach themselves to bacteria or viruses and destroy them or make it easier for white cells to digest them.
- Immune white cells attach themselves to bacteria or viruses and destroy them.
- Pus, made of dead cells and tissue, is formed in the area.

Some of the symptoms and signs of acute inflammation are:

1. swelling,
2. redness or shininess,
3. heat,
4. pain and tenderness,
5. loss of function,
6. sometimes, fluid or pus in the area.

Chronic inflammation

Chronic inflammation can happen because of a chronic mild injury or infection by some types of organisms or because an acute inflammation has been in the area for a long time and the body has not quite been able to destroy the cause.

In chronic inflammation the blood vessels become only a little wider and fluid, protein and cells escape only slowly into the area. However, the structural body cells normally present in the area are slowly killed and replaced by fibrous tissue. As the fibrous tissue gets older, it shrinks and causes scarring. The tissue in the area of the chronic inflammation is slowly destroyed. Pus may be made if many white cells are killed.

Symptoms and signs of chronic inflammation in an area include:

1. swelling, but not usually very much,
2. redness is not usual,
3. heat, but only slight,
4. pain and tenderness but not usually very much,
5. loss of function is usual,
6. there can be fluid or pus.

Chronic inflammation will stop if the cause is removed. Healing will then happen. However, if the organ has been badly damaged or if the area of the body has been very scarred, it may never function properly again.

General (whole body) effects of inflammation

In both acute and chronic inflammation, *certain toxins and other chemicals are put into the blood.* Some of these chemicals are made by the body to help the defensive inflammatory reaction. Some of these chemicals cause more white blood cells to be made, fever, fast pulse rate, etc. Some of these chemicals may be from the cause of the inflammation, especially if it is an organism. Some of these chemicals may be toxins which cause high fever, damage to blood vessels with bleeding, wasting of the body (muscles get thin and weak), damage to the bone marrow and blood cells with anaemia etc.

In acute inflammation, more acute changes are caused – high fever, shivering (rigors), fast pulse, bleeding, etc.

In chronic inflammation less acute changes are caused – low fever, wasting, anaemia etc.

Neoplasm (also called newgrowth or tumour or cancer)

Normal body cells grow only where and when they are needed, e.g. during growth of a child, or to repair a wound, or to make new parts for the body to replace worn out parts. These normal cells stop growing after they have done their work.

A neoplasm is the growth of *abnormal body cells* which *keep on growing either where or when they are not needed.* The body cannot stop them growing.

The cause of some neoplasms is not known. Known causes of neoplasm include:

1. Chemicals, e.g. tobacco smoke causes lung cancer; betel nut and lime causes mouth cancer.
2. Some drugs, but not those used by most health workers.
3. Some viruses, e.g. hepatitis B virus causes hepatoma.
4. Too much sunlight in people with light coloured skins (or albinos) causes skin cancer.
5. Radiation from atomic bombs, etc. causes blood cancers.
6. Hereditary factors

There are two types of neoplasm:

1. Benign (or simple) neoplasms. The cells of benign neoplasms stay in the place where they started to grow and do not spread to other organs.
2. Malignant neoplasms. The cells of malignant neoplasms do not only grow at the place where they started to grow. These cells also spread directly or in the blood or in the lymph to other parts of the body where they also start to grow. Malignant neoplasms can therefore be of two types:
   (a) Primary – the neoplasm at the place where it started,
   (b) Secondary – the neoplasm at the place it has spread to from the primary neoplasm.

Neoplasms damage the body in many ways:

1. Destruction of the tissue in which it is growing, e.g. neoplasm in the liver causes liver failure with jaundice.
2. Obstruction of the organ in which it is growing, e.g. neoplasm in the intestine causes intestinal obstruction with abdominal pain, constipation and vomiting.
3. Pressure on other important structures, e.g. Burkitt's tumour in the face pushes an eye out so that the lids cannot close.
4. Ulceration of the surface with bleeding or infection, e.g. stomach cancer causes vomiting of blood and anaemia.
5. Wasting and malaise (not feeling well).

4

A Classification of Disease – the causes of diseases

Diseases can be grouped or classified in many different ways. One good way to classify diseases in a health centre is by a *combination* of cause and pathology and clinical findings. Like this:

Congenital

These are diseases or abnormalities that were present when the patient was born. There are three subgroups:

1. inherited or hereditary, i.e. passed on from the mother or the father – these diseases are in the family (e.g. thalassaemia);
2. damage done to the baby while it was in the mother's womb (e.g. blindness or congenital heart disease from an attack of rubella (German measles) in the mother);
3. unknown (e.g. talipes or club foot).

Traumatic

These are injuries. *Causes* include:

1. mechanical injuries (e.g. cuts, bruises, fractures),
2. heat (e.g. burns).

Inflammatory

Inflammation is a reaction of part of the body to things which can injure it but do not completely destroy it. The most important part of the inflammatory reaction is that the blood vessels become wider and bring much more blood to the area. The blood vessels then allow fluid, proteins and cells to go into the area to fight the thing that is attacking the body (see Inflammation, Chapter 3).

Causes include:

1. Infection with organisms including:
   viruses, bacteria, protozoa, rickettsiae, fungi, worms and insects (called 'infestations').
2. Trauma:
   mechanical, heat.
3. Chemicals, especially:
   toxins, bites, stings and venoms (e.g. insect stings, stonefish sting).
4. Allergic reactions.
   Allergy is an inflammatory reaction of part of the body caused by some foreign substance on or in the body. This substance does not cause inflammation in the body of normal people. But if a person develops allergy to this substance, he may develop abnormal antibodies to this substance. When this substance comes in contact with the body again there is a reaction between the substance and the abnormal antibodies which causes an inflammatory reaction. (See Chapter 10 page 39.)
   (a) Allergy can be caused by substances touching the skin, e.g. skin rash due to streptomycin powder in some nurses.
   (b) Allergy can be caused by substances being inhaled (i.e. breathed in), e.g. asthma and hayfever from house dust in some people.
   (c) Allergy can be caused by substances being injected, e.g. skin rash, asthma or shock in some people after penicillin injection or certain insect bites.
   (d) Allergy can be caused by substances being swallowed, e.g. skin rash in some people after swallowing aspirin tablets or cows' milk.

Neoplastic (also called tumours, cancers, newgrowths, or growths)

Neoplasms are made of abnormal body cells. These cells grow both when and where they are not needed. They cause damage to the normal parts of the body where they are growing.

They may be:

1. simple or benign,
2. malignant, either
   (a) primary where the neoplasm started, or
   (b) secondary where the neoplasm has spread to.

(See Neoplasm, Chapter 3.)

Causes include:

1. viruses, e.g. EB virus together with malaria infection causes Burkitt's tumours;
2. chemicals, e.g. tobacco smoking causes lung cancer, lime and betel nut chewing causes mouth cancer;
3. some drugs, e.g. immunosuppressive drugs can cause lymphomas;
4. excess radiation, e.g. sun on skin of albino causes skin cancer;
5. hereditary factors;
6. other and as yet unknown causes.

Degenerative

These diseases are a wearing out of part of the body.

Causes include:

1. Old age, e.g. cataracts cause blindness in old people.
2. Habits or events during life can cause parts of the body to wear out more quickly than others, e.g. osteoarthritis when men play football and damage their knee joints many times.
3. Amyloid disease. This is an unusual condition in which an abnormal protein is put into the tissues and stops organs working properly. It happens in old age and sometimes in chronic inflammatory diseases (e.g. leprosy) and sometimes for no known cause.

Chemicals – drugs, poisons, toxins, venoms

These may have been given purposely or accidentally. They may have been given for good or bad reasons. They may have been given by the health worker, the employer, a traditional healer, an enemy or the patient himself.

1. Drugs should be given only by those who know the risks of their unwanted bad effects as well as their wanted good effects. These persons include health workers and patients who are instructed in the use of certain drugs, e.g. antimalarials. Drugs given by health workers and drugs patients themselves have taken to treat one disease, can be the cause of another disease.
   The patient may also give himself other drugs – alcohol, tobacco and lime with betel nut. These are very common causes of disease – accidents, chronic bronchitis and cancer of the mouth (respectively).
2. Poisons may be added to a person's food or drink by an enemy; but this in fact is very rare. Poisons may be taken by the patient himself to attempt suicide or attempt to treat a condition (e.g. unwanted pregnancy); but most commonly by accident (e.g. kerosene left in a soft-drink bottle).
3. Toxins may be formed by bacteria in food. When eaten, the toxins cause 'food poisoning'.
4. Venoms may be injected by insect stings, fish stings or snake bites. They may cause various changes including pain, paralysis of muscles and abnormal bleeding.

Malnutrition

Not enough food, or not enough of some foods, or too much of some foods can cause disease, e.g.:

- marasmus from not enough food,
- kwashiorkor from not enough protein,
- anaemia from not enough iron or folic acid,
- obesity from too much food.

Psychological

Situations causing worry, stress and anxiety often cause disease, e.g. tension headaches, anxiety states and 'hysterical' paralysis.

Failure of an organ or system of the body

(especially blood vessels)

Some conditions or diseases of parts of the body are caused by the failure of other parts of the body.

The most common of these conditions are those caused by the failure of the blood vessels. If an artery becomes narrowed or blocked, then little or no food and oxygen can go to the part of the body supplied by the artery. That part is then damaged and cannot function properly and may die. If veins become blocked then blood pumped into part of the body cannot go out of that part. That part then swells up, is damaged and cannot function properly. Such conditions have *vascular* causes.

Failure of one body system may cause other conditions:

1. *Blood failure* may cause shock (not enough blood volume); shortness of breath, fainting, dizziness (anaemia); bleeding (platelets or clotting protein abnormal), etc.
2. *Heart failure* may cause oedema, enlarged liver, etc.
3. *Respiratory (lung) failure* may cause wasting, cyanosis, abnormal behaviour, heart failure, etc.
4. *Liver failure* may cause wasting, oedema, bleeding, abnormal behaviour, jaundice, etc.

5. *Endocrine gland failure* (e.g. pancreatic failure may cause wasting, passing a lot of urine, unconsciousness, etc., i.e. diabetes mellitus).

All body systems must be considered; but especially important are vascular, blood, heart, respiratory, kidney, liver and endocrine.

Others

Other groups do exist but are not as common as the nine groups discussed above. Some have known causes. Some have causes not yet discovered.

Summary

When a disease or disability is discovered in a patient and the diagnosis is not obvious, answer the following questions:

Is this condition:

1. Congenital?
2. Traumatic?
3. Inflammatory, caused by:
   (a) trauma?
   (b) infection?
   (c) toxins or bites or venoms?
   (d) allergy?
4. Neoplastic?
5. Degenerative?
6. Caused by chemicals – drugs, poisons, toxins, venoms?
7. Caused by malnutrition?
8. Caused by psychological causes?
9. Caused by the failure of an organ of the body – especially blood vessels?
10. Caused by other causes known or unknown?

5

Epidemiology

It is not enough to know only the causes of illnesses.

The presence of the cause of a disease (usually called the 'specific agent') does not mean that the disease will always develop. All people have the organisms that cause pneumonia (the specific agent of pneumonia) in their respiratory tracts sometimes. But few get pneumonia. Some, however, do. Why? Smoking tobacco causes lung cancer. But many people smoke all of their lives and do not get lung cancer. Some, however, do. Why? There are certain things about the specific agent, or about the person who has the specific agent acting on him, or in the environment, that determine if disease will or will not happen.

The study of the distribution of disease in the community (i.e. when it occurs, where it occurs and who gets it) and all the things that determine if disease will or will not happen, is called epidemiology.

> Epidemiology is the study of *who* gets a particular disease, *where* and *when* these persons get the disease, and *how* and *why* they get the disease. (See Figures 5.1 and 5.2).

Epidemiology gives the known answers to these questions about a disease.

1. *Who* (including how many)
2. *When*
3. *Where*

} are the people affected?

4. *How* does the whole process including the means of transfer of the specific agent (or 'cause') happen?
5. *Why* – or what are the factors (reasons) in:
   (a) the specific agent (i.e. the 'cause'); or
   (b) the means of transfer of the specific agent; or
   (c) man; or
   (d) the environment
   which determine if the disease happens or not.

Accurate terms to describe how often a disease occurs (or the *frequency* of a disease) include:

- *Prevalence* of a disease is the *total* number of persons with the disease at a certain time in a certain population.
- *Incidence* of a disease is the number of *new* persons getting the disease during a certain time in a certain population.

See Chapter 9 for other definitions and explanations.

Epidemiology has many uses. Many of these uses are not useful in your day-to-day work. Some, however, are.

If you know the epidemiology of a disease, it will help you in the differential diagnosis (see Chapter 6) of a patient who is sick. Some diseases do not affect some groups of people but may be common in other groups of people. By knowing which group of persons your patient is in and what diseases are common in his group, it is much easier to decide which disease your patient has.

If you know the epidemiology of a disease it will help you to understand that there is often more than one 'cause' of a person getting sick. There may be more than one thing which you need to do, therefore, to make the patient well again.

If you know the epidemiology of types of disease, this may help you to find the reason for an outbreak of a disease in your community.

If you know the epidemiology of a disease it will help you control and prevent a disease. You may have to try to kill or remove the specific agent which can cause the disease. You may have to change the environment to stop its means of spread. You may have to increase the resistance of the person who is susceptible to the specific agent. It is only if you know the epidemiology of the disease, that you can decide which of these things is the best to do.

If you really want to improve the health of the people in your community, you need to use the methods of epidemiology to make a 'community diagnosis' of

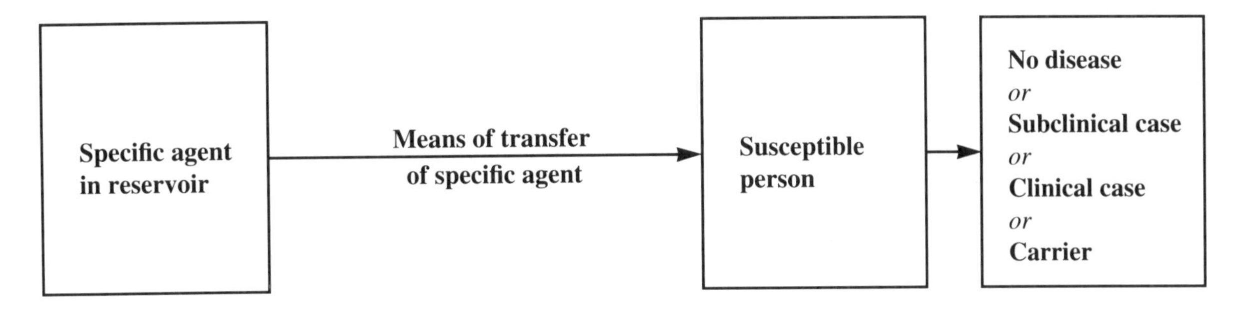

or, in more detail:

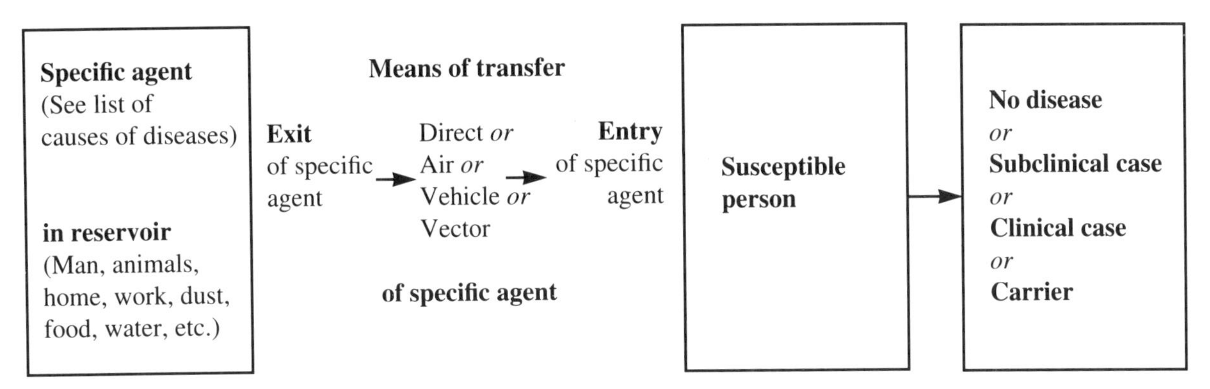

Figure 5.1 Diagrams showing how disease may be caused.

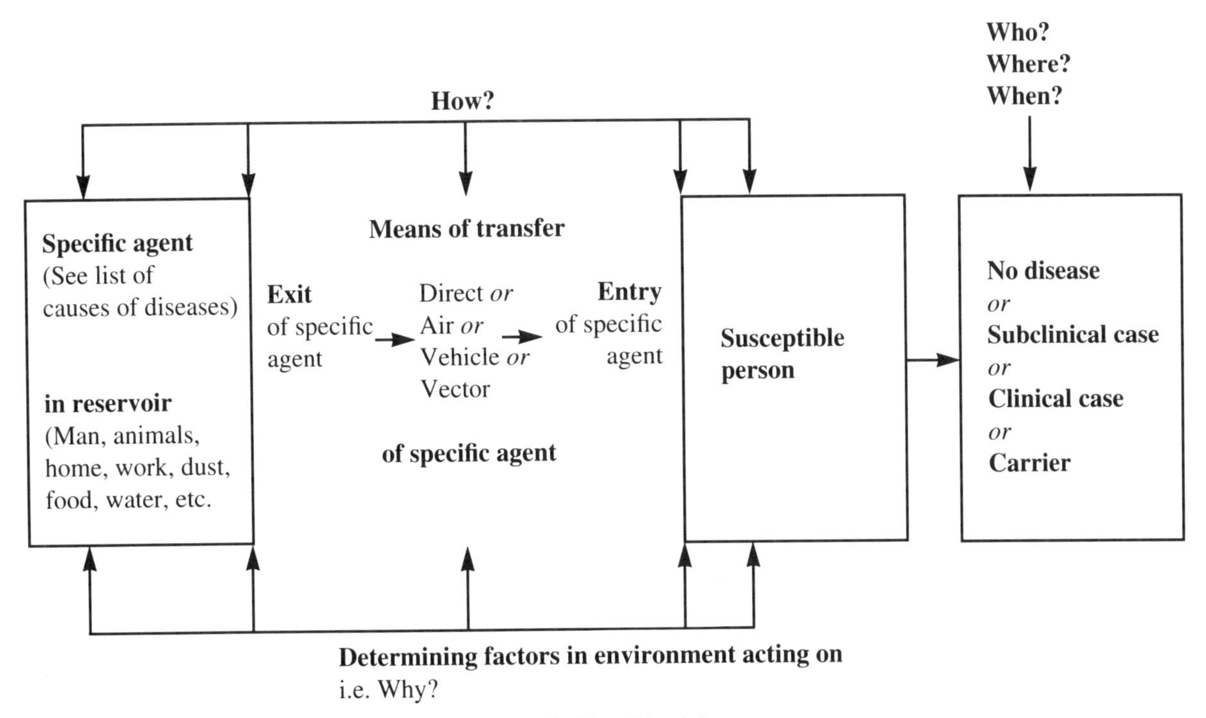

Figure 5.2 A diagram showing the things that are studied in epidemiology.

your own community. You need to find out who makes up your community and how many men, women and children there are. You need to know what illnesses really do affect these people. You need to know which members of the community have these illnesses. You need to know when and where and how and why these people get these illnesses. It is only when you have used epidemiological methods to make your own community diagnosis that you will be able:

1. to make the best use of epidemiological methods in diagnosing and treating individual patients, and
2. to give the best advice for disease prevention and health promotion to all the people of the community.

6

Diagnosis of Disease

To make the correct diagnosis you must do all of the following six things:

1. Take a medical history.
2. Do a medical or physical examination.
3. Make a differential diagnosis (or make a list of the diseases that *could* be causing the patient's main symptoms and signs).
4. Do or order any tests that are needed:
   (a) to find out which of the diseases in the differential diagnosis the patient really has; *or*
   (b) to confirm a diagnosis; *or*
   (c) to give a 'baseline' to see if the patient gets better or worse.
5. Make a provisional diagnosis and decide:
   (a) which disease (or diseases) is most likely to be causing the patient's symptoms and signs;
   (b) how severe this disease is;
   (c) how quickly this disease is getting better or worse.
6. Decide on the prognosis of the patient.

Remember: you must diagnose before you can treat.

You must first diagnose what condition or disease a patient has before you can choose the proper treatment to help the patient. The only treatment which will help the patient is the proper treatment for the condition or disease which the patient really has. Treatment (even good treatment) for a condition which the patient does not have will not help the patient.

Taking a medical history

If you know what questions to ask you can take a full history in about 2–5 minutes in most ordinary cases.

If you make the patient give you a good history, you will often hear the patient tell you a story which you recognise. The story may be one you have heard before or it may be a story that you have read about in your medical books. In either case, you will recognise the patient's story as the story of a disease about which you know. Even if you do not recognise the story of a disease, you will hear about important symptoms which you can use in making the differential diagnosis.

Also the history will often tell you how you need to examine the patient.

The medical history is in nine parts (the medical examination is in nine parts too):

1. general information and admission notes;
2. complaints and their duration;
3. history of the present illness;
4. specific questioning (or specific interrogation);
5. past history;
6. family and contact history;
7. if the patient may have a mental condition, take the history again from a relative or another witness;
8. check the patient's outpatient card and inpatient notes for any history in them;
9. tell the patient a summary of the history – ask him to correct anything wrong.

1. General information and admission notes

Write down:

Date.
Patient's name and address, etc.[1]
With whom patient lives and the address.[1]
Reason for admission.
Who referred patient.

1 The patient's exact present address and also a friend's or relative's name and address are most important. If you do not write this down it will not be possible to find the patient later if it is necessary. You may need to find the patient if he has an infectious disease (e.g. tuberculosis) and does not come for treatment.

2. *Complaints and their duration* (or how long they have lasted).[2]

Write down:

Only the main problems.[3]
Only short descriptions.
Only the patient's own way of describing them.

3. *History of present illness (HPI)*

Ask questions like these and write down the answers:

How long ago was it that something first went wrong with you?
What was this first thing that went wrong?
What was the next thing that happened?
When did this happen?
What happened next?... When?...

You should also:

- Ask for a full description of pain or any other symptom.
- Ask about *all* the symptoms of *all* the body systems in which the patient has symptoms.
- Ask about the presence or absence of all the symptoms of any possible disease.
- Ask what treatment has already been given.

4. *Specific interrogation (SI) or specific questioning*

Ask the patient about (unless already talked about in the HPI):[4]

Fever.
Cough. Sputum. Haemoptysis.
Chronic cough.
Pain in the chest.
Shortness of breath.
Eating well. Vomiting. Diarrhoea.
Pain in the abdomen.
Urinary pain, urinary frequency, abnormal colour of urine. Blood in the urine.
Date of last menstrual period.
Getting fatter or thinner or staying the same weight.
What the patient thinks is wrong.
What the patient thinks is the cause.

If the patient is *pregnant* also ask about:

Oedema? Treatment?
High blood pressure? Treatment?
Vaginal bleeding? Treatment?
Anaemia? Treatment?
Labour pains started? When?
Vaginal show or bleeding? When?
Membranes ruptured? When?

5. *Past history (PH)*

Ask about:

Drugs:

- given today,
- given for the treatment of this illness before today,
- given regularly,
- alcohol and tobacco – how much, how often.

Treatment given by traditional healers? What?
Previous attacks of this illness? When? What treatment?
Previous other serious illnesses or operations or accidents? What? When?

If the patient is *pregnant*, also ask about:

How many births? Dates?
How many miscarriages? Dates?
Any abortions? Dates?
How many stillbirths or neonatal deaths? When? Why?
Any difficult deliveries (Caesarian section, symphysiotomy, vacuum extraction, very long labour (> 24 hours)? Which births?
Any post-partum haemorrhage or retained placenta? Which births?

6. *Family history and contact history (FH, CH)*

This is especially important for those who live in the same house. Ask if there is:

anyone with this illness,
anyone with other serious illness,
anyone with tuberculosis (or cough for more than 4 weeks),
anyone with leprosy.

---

2 When you have ordered treatment, look back at this list to make sure you have done something for the patient's complaints.

3 Make sure the patient tells you all of his complaints. He may leave the most important one till last.

4 You must always get answers to all of these questions. If you already know the answers from the HPI, do not ask the questions again. You cannot think that the patient does not have these symptoms only because the patient has not told you about them. He may not think they are important. He may not want to talk about them. These questions are about the main symptoms caused by the main pathological processes in each of the major body systems. You must find out about each one of them. In some places where there are special diseases, other questions may have to be added to this list.

7. If the patient may have a mental problem or condition, take all history again from a relative or other witness

8. Look at the patient's outpatient card (also any inpatient notes) for any HPI, SI, PH, FH etc. in it. (Return the card to the patient.)

9. Tell the patient a summary of the history obtained. Then ask him to correct anything wrong

If pain (or another symptom) is present it will often help the health worker to ask about:

1. The site (or where it is).
2. The radiation (or if it spreads to any other place and where).
3. The character or type (e.g. constant [stays the same all time] or colic [comes and goes again and again in minutes]).
4. The severity (or how bad it is).
5. The frequency (or how often it comes).
6. The duration (or how long it lasts).
7. Things that start it, make it worse or make it better.

Performing a medical or physical examination

The medical examination is in three parts. The *first part or basic observations* should *always* be done on *all* patients for at least two reasons.

1. It will show you if the patient is 'sick' or not. This is not done by intuition (a feeling or an idea). This is done by observation during examination.
2. It is a simple test for the common and fatal diseases. You may need to add some other observations to this list in places where there are special diseases. The following diseases are suggested by the 'basic observations':
   - Meningitis is suggested by the change in the level of consciousness and the stiff neck.
   - Malaria is suggested by a high temperature.
   - Penumonia is suggested by a fast and abnormal type of respiration.
   - Gastroenteritis is suggested by the weight loss and signs of dehydration.
   - Malnutrition or wasting is suggested by the signs of malnutrition and wasting.
   - Anaemia is suggested by the colour.

Therefore, even if a patient has only a simple laceration, you should still do the 'basic observations' so that you can do any necessary preventive medicine. Diseases may be found while they are still mild. Treatment will stop these diseases becoming severe or causing death.

The *second part* is the examination of the part of the body which the symptoms suggests is diseased.

The *third part* of the examination is the examination of the whole body. You must examine the whole of the body if:

1. The patient is 'sick'.
2. The disease you think the patient may have could affect more than one part of the body.
3. You are not certain of the diagnosis.

In each part of a clinical examination you usually do these five things:

1. Inspection – look and see.
2. Palpation – feel and touch with hands.
3. Percussion – tap and listen (and feel).
4. Auscultation – listen (usually with stethoscope).
5. Measurement – not often done in a health centre.

It is not always possible to do all these things. But you should do them all, in this order, if possible.

The medical examination is in nine parts.

1. Basic observations.
2. Head and neck including the ears, nose and throat, thyroid and lymph glands.
3. Chest and spine.
4. Abdomen.
5. Skin and hair.
6. Muscles, bones, joints.
7. Head and neck etc. (if not done before).
8. Any special examinations suggested by previous history and examination.
9. Mental state.

1. Basic observations

Signs of meningeal irritation (drowsiness, or irritability or fitting, stiff neck, stiff back, Kernig's sign positive).

Does the patient have signs of meningitis or cerebral malaria?

Temperature (T°)
Pulse rate (PR)
Blood pressure (BP) (if needed)
Respiration rate (RR) and type of respiration
Weight

} 5 vital signs

Does the patient have signs of malaria or pneumonia or shock or weight change?

Dehydration – eyes sunken, mouth dry, inelastic skin, pulse fast, weight loss
Oedema (limbs, back, face)
Malnutrition
Wasting
Colour – anaemia, jaundice, cyanosis
} 5 general conditions

Does the patient have any of these five signs?

Is the patient 'sick'?

2. *Head and neck including ears, nose and throat, thyroid and lymph glands in the neck and axilla*

See also Chapter 20 page 198), Chapter 30 page 403, Chapter 22 page 256)
These may be left until 7.

3. *Chest*

(See also Chapter 20 page 205).
Look for:
- rate of respiration,
- type of respiration,
- deformity of spine or chest.

Feel for decreased movement of:
- all of the chest,
- part or parts of the chest.

Percuss for:
- dullness or
- increased resonance

} in { all of the chest, or, part or parts of the chest.

Listen for:
- amount of breath sounds
- breath sounds normal or bronchial
- crackles or crepitations
- wheezes or rhonchi

} in { all of the chest, or part or parts of the chest.

Ask the patient to cough – listen to the cough.
Look at sputum (is there any pus or blood?).
Does the patient have pneumonia or tuberculosis or obstruction of bronchi?

4. *Abdomen*

(See Chapter 36 page 489–502, Chapter 22 page 266, Chapter 23 page 272, Chapter 24 page 306.)
Look at:
- size (distension),
- shape (herniae, masses,)
- surface (scars),
- movement when breathing.

Feel for:
- tenderness, rebound tenderness, guarding, rigidity,
- liver, spleen, uterus and bladder,
- lumps, including herniae and lymph glands.

Percuss, if needed, for:
- organs or masses,
- fluid (e.g. ascites).

Listen, if needed, for bowel sounds.

Pelvic examination through the rectum (PR), if needed, for:
- tenderness,
- enlarged organs,
- masses,
- faeces, blood or pus in rectum.

Pelvic examination through the vagina (PV), if needed, for:
- tenderness,
- enlarged organs,
- masses,
- blood or pus in vagina.

Does the patient have signs of 'peritonitis' or an enlarged organ, or an inflamed organ or an abnormal mass?

If the patient is *pregnant*, also:
Palpate for:
- size of uterus (height of fundus),
- lie of fetus, what is presenting part.

Auscultate for fetal heart rate.

If the patient is in *labour*, also:
Palpate for:
- size of uterus (height of fundus),
- lie of fetus, what is presenting part, engagement of head,
- frequency, duration and strength of contractions.

Auscultate for fetal heart rate.
Do pelvic examination PV for:
- state of cervix and start cervicograph,
- membranes ruptured or intact,
- level of head (above or below spines),
- caput.

5. *Skin and hair*

(See also Chapter 32.)

Look for:
- scabies,
- infections,
- other rashes,
- scars.

Does the patient have scabies or impetigo or leprosy?

6. Muscles, bones and joints
(See also Chapter 28.)
Look and feel for:
- deformity,
- tenderness,
- swelling.

Does the patient have fracture, osteomyelitis, arthritis or absess?

7. Head and neck, ENT, thyroid, lymph glands (if not done)

8. Any special examination indicated by previous history and examination
Five important examinations which you may need to do:

- If gynaecological disease is possible, do pelvic examination PV (see Chapter 26 page 353).
- If leprosy is suspected, do examinations for nerve enlargement and tenderness and for loss of sensation and for paralysis (see Chapter 18 page 95).
- If there is pain in the eye or loss of sight, examine for iritis and corneal ulcer and corneal foreign body (see Chapter 31 page 411).
- If there is a wound, check that nerves, tendons and blood vessels are all working.
- If there is oedema or if heart failure is suspected, examine for raised jugular venous pressure (see Chapter 27 page 371).

9. Mental state
(See also Chapter 35 page 470.)

- Ability to communicate (hear, see, move, talk, etc).
- Level of consciousness.
- Memory – recent past – distant past.
- Orientation: person, time, place.
- Intelligence.
- Thoughts by:

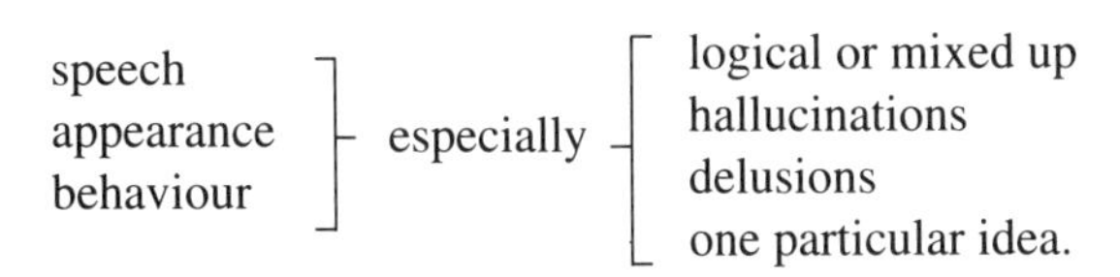

- Mood by:

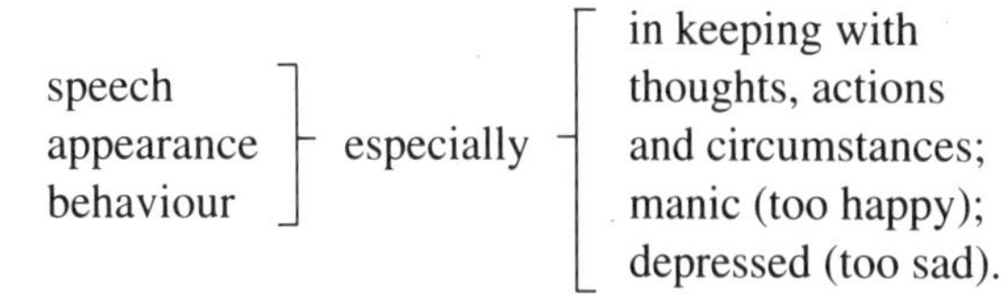

- Insight.

If you carry out a good examination you will often see in the patient a 'picture' or 'pattern' which you recognise. The 'picture' or 'pattern' may be one you have seen before in another patient or it may be one you recognise from reading about it from your medical books. In either case, you will have recognised the 'picture' or 'pattern' as a disease which you know about. Even if you do not recognise a 'picture' or 'pattern' of a disease, you will have found important signs to use in making the differential diagnosis.

Making a differential diagnosis (DD)

The patient's symptoms and signs are caused by, (1) an abnormality of the structure and/or function of a part of his or her body and (2) the cause of this abnormality.

A number of different conditions can cause the same symptom or sign. These different conditions, however, usually have other symptoms or signs or tests as well, which are not all the same. The different conditions which cause the same symptom or sign can be separated by using these other symptoms and signs and tests.

The differential diagnosis is a list of the conditions any one of which could be causing the patient's main symptoms and signs.

Write down the patient's main symptoms and signs in a row across the top of a page of paper. Then under each of these symptoms and signs, write down the list of conditions which could cause these symptoms and signs. The differential diagnosis is all the conditions in all the lists.

Next, look for a disease (or diseases) which is in each list (as a cause of each symptom and sign). This is the condition which is most likely to be the cause of the patient's condition. If there is more than one condition in all of the lists, then tests will probably be needed to find out which of the conditions is the real cause of the patient's problems.

Doing or ordering tests (or investigations)

You may need a test:

1. to decide between the possible diagnoses in the DD;
2. to confirm a diagnosis;
3. to give a base line to be able to judge if a patient is getting better or worse.

See Appendix 1 (this page) for how to take and send blood for tests in the hospital laboratory.

Making a provisional diagnosis (PD)

The provisional diagnosis (PD) is the condition you think the patient really has.

You decide the PD after considering all the conditions in the differential diagnosis that could cause the patient's main symptoms and signs. Reject the other conditions in the list if:

1. these conditions do not cause all of the patient's symptoms and signs; and
2. these conditions have other symptoms or signs or tests which do not fit the patient.

Choose the condition as the PD which:

1. is a cause of all the patient's symptoms and signs; and
2. has other symptoms and signs and tests all of which do fit the patient.

In this book, the PD of most of the common symptoms and signs is set out.

The prognosis

The prognosis is what you think will happen to the patient because of the condition you have diagnosed, e.g.

- die or live,
- improve quickly or slowly,
- not improve at all.

The prognoses of the common diseases are set out in this book.

The signature of health worker and date should always be written after any of the above are written into the patient's notes.

Summary

Diagnosis of disease includes:

1. Taking a medical history (nine parts).
2. Doing a clinical examination (nine parts).
3. Making a differential diagnosis.
4. Doing or ordering any tests needed.
5. Making a provisional diagnosis.
6. Deciding the prognosis.

You must practise doing medical histories and examinations again and again until all of the things in this chapter can be done in 5–10 minutes.

Appendix 1: Method of taking blood for tests, making blood smears and sending pathology specimens to the hospital laboratory

1. Always use gloves when taking blood or handling blood. This is to protect you from HIV and hepatitis virus and other infections which may be in the blood.
2. Always put lancets, disposable needles and other sharp pieces of equipment which may have blood on them, into the special 'sharps' disposal container. This container should be itself disposable, strong enough that none of the 'sharps' can stick through the side of it and should never be overfilled. The filled container should be got rid of as has been decided by your health department, such as by burning it and then burying it or otherwise as you have been instructed.
3. All re-useable equipment should first be washed well to remove all blood, etc. and then sterilised and not used again unless the sterilising is known to have been good enough to kill all the organisms which could be on the instrument.

Collection of blood

Skin puncture (capillary blood)

1. In adults use the patient's finger or the lobe of the ear, choosing a site free from disease.

2. In infants use the heel.
3. Squeeze or flick the ear, finger or heel a few times. Clean it with spirit or antiseptic and allow to dry.
4. Make a good prick with a quick motion, using a sterile, dry, sharp lancet.
5. Try not to squeeze the finger or ear after you have pricked it because this spoils the specimen for some methods.
6. Make a blood film straight from the drop of blood or fill a blood pipette with it.
7. Label the specimen clearly.

Venepuncture (venous blood)

1. The syringe and needle *must* be clean, dry and *sterile*. Check that the syringe will suck. Fit a sharp sterile needle.
2. Place the tourniquet around the arm above the elbow; ask the patient to open and close his hand several times.
3. Clean the skin over the veins at the fold of the elbow with iodine or spirit.
4. Pull the skin tight over the vein with the thumb of the left hand. With a quick push, puncture the skin and vein with the needle which has the bevel upwards.
5. Do not move needle or syringe after the needle is in the vein.
6. Withdraw blood by pulling on the plunger of the syringe.
7. When ready to remove syringe, put a small piece of sterile, dry cotton-wool over the needle. Remove tourniquet and withdraw needle from vein. Ask the patient to hold the cotton-wool on the needle puncture for 2–3 minutes.
8. Remove needle from syringe and gently empty blood into a sterile test tube to clot; or into a bottle containing an anticoagulant, mixing gently to prevent clotting.
9. Keep stopper in bottle to prevent evaporation.
10. Wash syringe and needle at once with cold water to remove blood before it clots.
11. The bottle containing the EDTA blood must be mixed for 3 minutes immediately before using the blood for a test.
12. Label the specimen clearly.

Anticoagulant used in haematology

1. It is necessary to have the correct proportion of blood to anticoagulant to prevent shrinkage of the cells which would give incorrect results.
2. *8% EDTA Solution*
   (a) Pipette 0.1 ml of EDTA solution into small screwtop bottles. Allow the water to evaporate completely at room temperature. Fix the screw-caps and label them.
   (b) This amount of EDTA prevents 4 ml of blood from clotting. It is important to try to add just 4 ml of blood to the bottle.

Preparation of thin blood films

To make a good thin blood film the slides must be perfectly clean; so first wash the slides in detergent and then clean water and store them in methylated spirit or 70% alcohol. Before use, wipe the slide dry with a clean cloth or paper (toilet paper will do). *Always hold the cleaned slide by the edges.*

Preparation of spreader (Figure 6.1)

Break off the corners of a glass slide, making sure that the edge of the slide is smooth. *It must not be chipped or rough* because this will spoil the blood film.

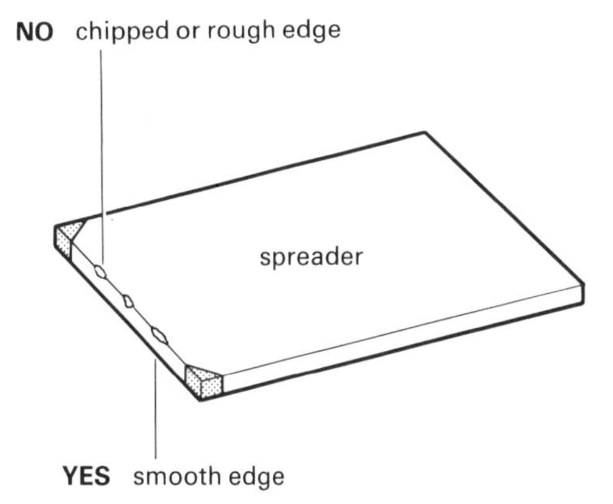

Figure 6.1

Making the film (Figures 6.2 and 6.3)

1. Place a small drop of fresh blood, about 1 cm ($\frac{1}{2}$ inch) from the end of the clean slide.
2. Hold the spreader so that it slopes backwards.
3. Place the spreader just in front of the drop of blood, then move it back till it touches the blood. The blood will then spread along the edge of the spreader.
4. Push the spreader forward smoothly and quickly.
5. Immediately, hold the slide by the edges and wave it in the air quickly until the blood film dries.

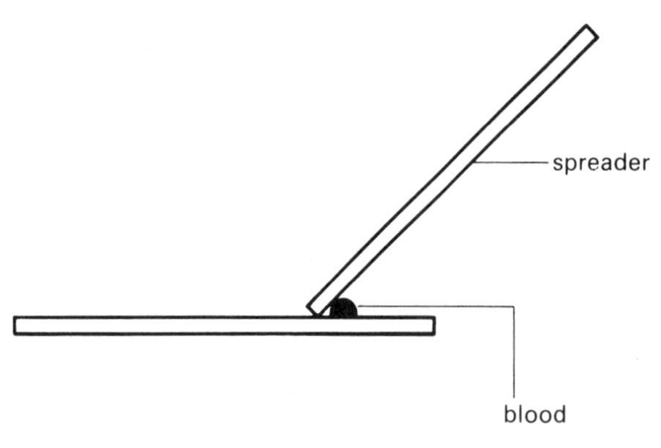

Figure 6.2

6. Write the patient's name on the end of the slide with a marking pencil, or write the patient's name in pencil on the blood film.
7. Always wash the spreader with water after use, then dry it with soft paper.

Preparation of thick blood film (Figure 6.4)

1. Place a drop or three small drops of fresh blood in the centre of a clean slide.
2. Spread the blood with the corner of a slide, making sure that it is spread evenly, until you can just see the print of a newspaper or book through it.
3. Leave the slide flat and allow to dry, protecting it from flies and insects.

Fixation of blood film

If the blood film is to be sent to another laboratory, it must be fixed immediately to preserve the blood cells.

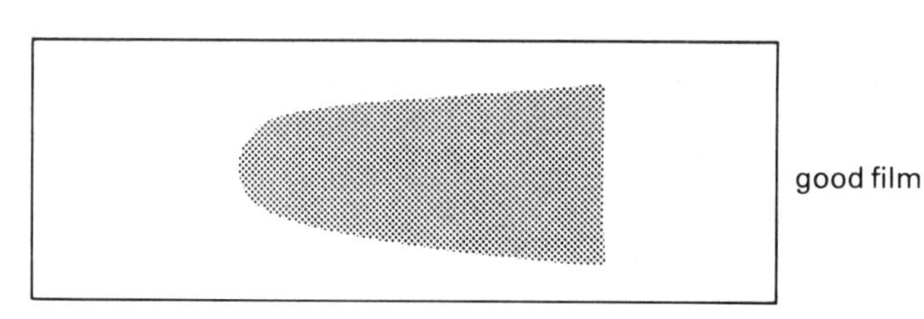

Faults

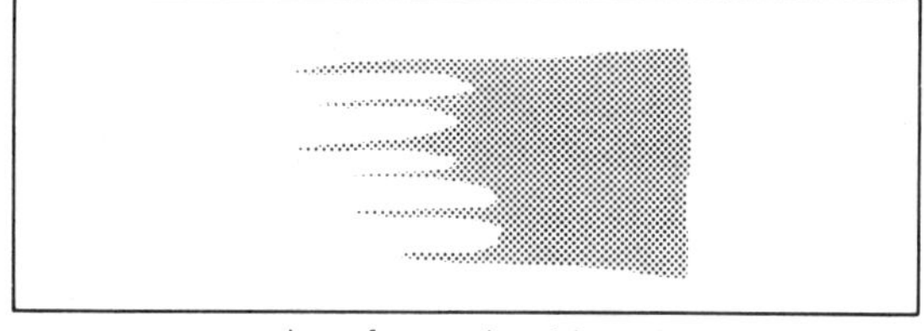

edge of spreader chipped

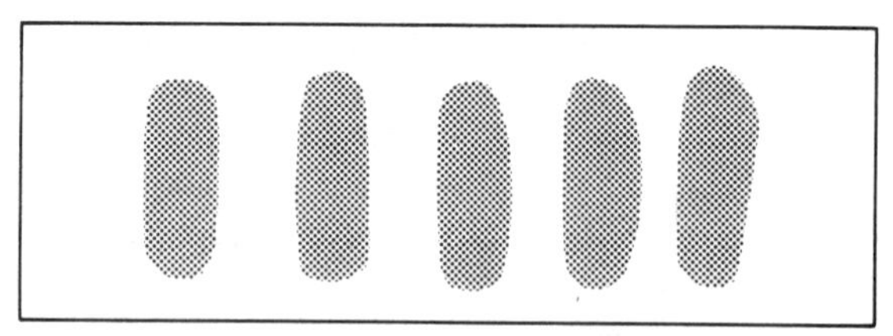

too much blood and film goes off the end

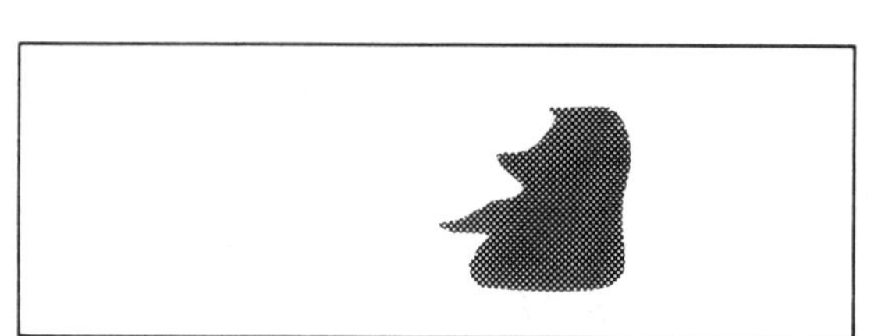

too short and thick

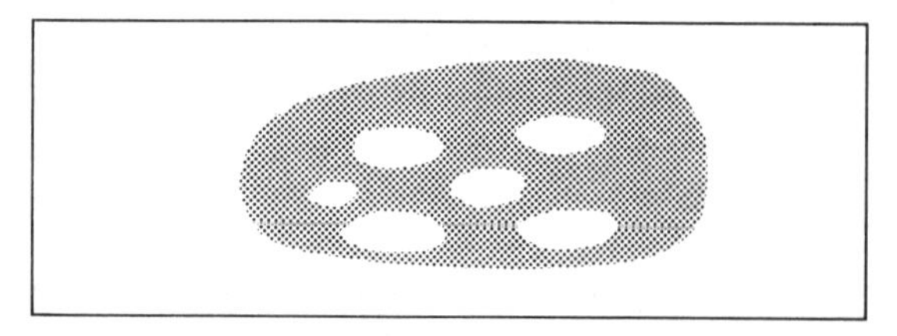

spreader not pushed smoothly

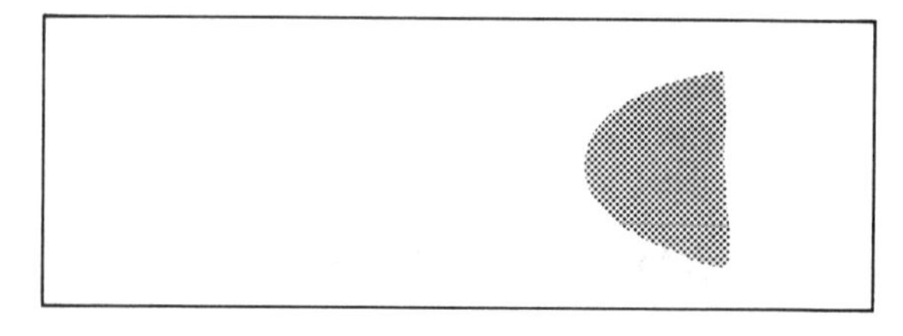

greasy slide making holes in the blood film

not enough blood film too small and thin

Figure 6.3

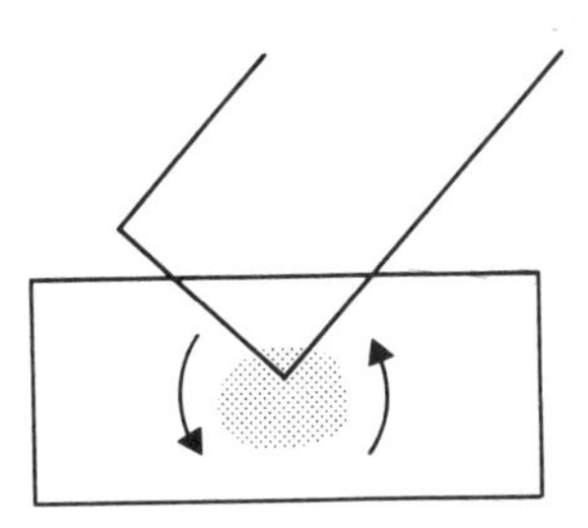

IF YOU CAN READ THE TYPE.
THEN THE BLOOD FILM IS
TOO THIN

IF YOU CA HE TYPE.
THE BLO O THICK

IF YOU C THE TYPE.
THE BLO ORRECT

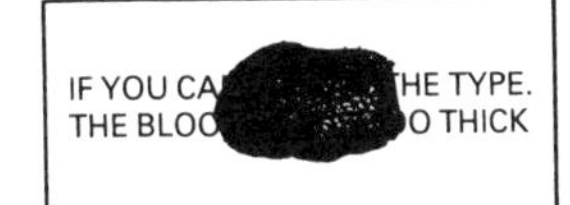

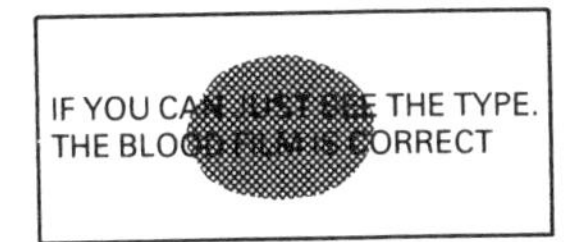

Figure 6.4

Place the prepared film in a jar filled with *pure methyl alcohol* and leave it there for *10 minutes.* Then take it out and dry it in the air. Another method is to pour a few drops of methyl alcohol over the film and allow 10 minutes for fixing before drying the film. Then wrap the fixed films in soft paper (e.g. toilet paper) and pack.

Make two films in case one is broken or damaged.

Details of how to take other tests are found in the appropriate chapters

Urethral smears for gonococci Chapter 19 page 168.
Smears for Donovan bodies Chapter 19 page 174.
Skin smears for AFB (leprosy) Chapter 15 page 107.
Skin biopsies Chapter 15 page 107.
Sputum smears for AFB (tuberculosis) Chapter 14 page 81.
Etc.

Sending specimens to laboratory

1. Some specimens must be sent from a health centre to a laboratory. It is very important that specimens are packed and sent properly so that they do not spoil before they arrive.

2. *Histology specimens* are pieces of patient's tissues which are taken in the operating theatre. The specimens are fixed in 10% formalin saline and sent to the laboratory. *Make sure that 10% formalin is used and that there is at least five times as much formalin as tissue.* The specimen must be kept in formalin for 24 hours to make sure that fixation is complete.
   Packing
   (a) Check that all specimens are labelled and see that the patient's name, age, sex, home village and census division etc. are on the laboratory request forms, as well as details of his illness. Write these details into the record book and the date the specimens were sent to the laboratory.
   (b) Small specimens such as liver biopsy, uterine scrapings and skin biopsy (in McCartney bottles) can be wrapped with cotton wool and packed with the request form in a small cardboard box.
   (c) Big specimens can be sent in a polypot. Fix them first and pack them in a polypot with some cotton wool made wet with 10% formalin saline. Wrap them several times round in a polythene bag. Then seal this bag with sticking plaster. Pack the tissue wrapped in the polythene bag and laboratory request forms in a cardboard box.

3. *Bacteriology specimens.* Send specimen in a universal container packed in a cardboard box (see above). Swabs for culture should be sent in 'Stuart's transport medium' available from the hospital laboratory.

4. *Haematology, biochemistry and serology specimens*
   (a) Blood specimens such as serum, EDTA blood and thin blood films may need to be sent. Fix the films by pouring a few drops of methyl alcohol over the films, allow 10 minutes for fixing, then dry them. Write on the laboratory request form that they are fixed with methyl alcohol. Wrap the slides separately with toilet paper and pack with the request forms in a small cardboard box.
   (b) Wrap the serum and EDTA specimens carefully in cotton wool and put them inside a plastic bag. Seal the plastic bag with sticking plaster and

pack with laboratory request forms in a cardboard box. Write '*BLOOD SAMPLES*' and '*Notify the department on arrival*' on top of the parcel.

(c) It is very important that all blood specimens should be sent by air freight or other quick delivery and *not* by ordinary post.

(d) *Specimens for biochemistry and serology.* Always send *serum*, never *whole blood*. The only time you send whole blood is for blood sugar which is collected into the special fluoride oxalate bottle. (These special bottles can be obtained from the hospital.)

7

Treatment, Drugs and Pain Relief

Treatment of the patient

Only when you have made a provisional diagnosis of the patient's problem can you decide how to treat the patient and manage the problem caused by the disease. Treatment of the patient only is not enough. You must do four things when you diagnose a disease:

1. Treat the patient (see this chapter).
2. Notify the necessary authorities and relatives (see Chapter 8).
3. Control the spread of the disease if necessary (see Chapter 9).
4. Prevent the disease occurring again in the patient and in the community if possible (see Chapter 9).

There are nine things you must do to treat a patient properly:

1. Decide on outpatient treatment or admit for inpatient treatment.
2. Order the proper nursing care.
3. Give specific treatment to cure the disease.
4. Give symptomatic treatment to relieve the symptoms.
5. Give explanation and comfort to the patient and to the relatives.
6. Give health education to the patient and to the relatives about control and prevention of the disease.
7. Consult with the Medical Officer *or* transfer the patient to Medical Officer care *or* refer the patient to the next visiting Medical Officer if necessary.
8. Discharge the patient and give final health education.
9. Follow-up the patient if necessary. *Treatment* of a patient may include any or all of these things.

1. Treat as outpatient or admit for inpatient care

2. Order proper nursing care (if necessary)

- Rest – in bed; in special position, etc.
- Special care of respiratory tract, mouth, eyes, ears, bowels, bladder, limbs, pressure areas, etc.
- Special fluids – orally or intravenously.
- Special diet.
- Special observations.
- Isolation.
- Collection of specimens for tests.

3. Give specific treatment (to cure)

- Drugs. Which drugs; by what route; how much; how often; for how long?
- Surgery. What surgery; who will do it; when?
- Dressings, plasters, etc.
- Physiotherapy.
- Fluids – orally or intravenously. Food or diet.
- Psychiatric counselling.

4. Give symptomatic treatment (to relieve symptoms)

- To make the patient *feel* better (i.e. to relieve his symptoms, especially pain).
- 'Rule' treatment, e.g. 'Give anti-malarials to every patient with a fever'. (There are different 'rule' treatments for different places and different countries).

Symptomatic treatment may include any of the things in 2 and 3 above, especially:

- drugs,
- surgery,
- dressings,
- diet,
- psychiatric counselling,
- nursing in special positions,
- special nursing care of parts of the body.

5. Give explanation and comfort

Give explanation and comfort to the patient and to his relatives.

6. Give health education

Give health education about control and prevention of the disease to the patient and relatives.

7. Consult – Transfer – Refer (if necessary)

Consult with the Medical Officer (by phone or radio if necessary) if you are not sure of the diagnosis or what the management should be.

Transfer of patient to Medical Officer care in a hospital if necessary. Transfers are of two types: urgent (emergency); or non-urgent (routine).

Arranging transfer includes the following:

- Get permission from Medical Officer if, when where, how to transfer.
- Get written permission of patient or relative for any necessary treatment.
- Tell the hospital when the patient should arrive.
- Arrange for drugs, dressings, fluids, oxygen, splints, stretcher, pillow, blanket, etc.
- Arrange for a suitable person to accompany the patient.
- Arrange transport.
- Provide a letter.

Refer problem cases who are non-urgent to next visiting Medical Officer.

8. Discharge the patient

Arrange for patient to return for review on completion of treatment if necessary.

Write up patient's outpatient health record and give it to him.

Give final health education.

9. Follow-up the patient (if necessary)

> Management of the problem caused by the diagnosing of a case of a disease includes:
> 1. Treat the patient (nine things may be necessary) (see above).
> 2. Notify the necessary authorities and relatives.
> 3. Control the spread of the disease if necessary.
> 4. Prevent the disease occurring again in this patient and in the community if possible.

Drug treatment

A *drug* is any substance that can change the body or pathological states of the body.

Drugs act by changing the function or structure of parts of the body, or by changing the structure or function of organisms or substances which have entered the body.

Always use the '*approved*' generic or '*official*' *name* for a drug. Do not use the trade names given by companies to their brands of the drug, as the health department changes the brands of the drug supplied from time to time. Also, brand name drugs are usually more expensive than generic drugs.

Drugs may be given by a number of different ways (or routes) and are absorbed by the blood vessels there:

1. GI tract by mouth (orally).
   Drugs are usually given by mouth. Drugs are not given by mouth if they would not be absorbed, because of any of the following reasons:
   (a) Their structure is such that they are not able to be absorbed from the gastrointestinal tract.
   (b) Vomiting and/or diarrhoea.
   (c) Shock (with little blood going to the gastrointestinal tract).
   (d) Swallowing not possible (e.g. unconscious).
   (e) The patient is not willing, or is not reliable enough, to swallow the drug.
2. By injection.
   Injections may be of different types:
   (a) intravenous injection (IVI),
   (b) intramuscular injection (IMI),
   (c) subcutaneous injection (SCI),
   (d) intradermal injection (IDI),
   (e) injection into special structures (e.g. intrapleural injection).
   Drugs are given by injection for any of the following reasons:
   (a) They may not be absorbed from the gastrointestinal tract (see above).
   (b) Oral administration is not possible – patient is not reliable enough, or is not conscious, etc.
   (c) Treatment needs to be effective quickly.
   (d) A high concentration in special structures in the body is needed.
3. GI tract, rectally, by suppository.
4. Lung (inhalation), skin (transdermal), under tongue (sublingual), nose (intranasal) or vaginally by pessary occasionally.

Drugs do not all go to all parts of the body. A drug has to be chosen which will go to the parts of the body where it is needed, but not go to parts of the body where it could cause damage.

Most drugs are destroyed ('inactivated' or 'metabolised') and removed from the body ('excreted') by either the liver or the kidneys. In liver or kidney diseases therefore, drug doses may have to be lower than normal.

All drugs have unwanted side effects. These may include the following:

1. Effects that are normal actions of the drug other than the one action wanted for this patient.
2. Allergy (see Chapter 10 page 39) and other effects that do not normally occur, but do occur in a few special persons.
3. Damage to an unborn child in the uterus.

Give a drug only if its possible bad effects are less than the risk of the untreated disease.

Chemotherapy

Chemotherapy is the name given to the use of chemical substances as drugs for therapy or treatment.

The term chemotherapy is usually used only when the drug is used to treat either infections in the body or cancers in the body.

You will be using chemotherapy any time you treat any infection with a drug even though you do not often use the name chemotherapy when you do this; although you may, for such things as 'short term chemotherapy' for tuberculosis. You, yourself, will not be using chemotherapy for cancer but you may send patients (with e.g. Burkitt's lymphoma) for chemotherapy for their cancer with drugs such as cyclophosphamide.

Drug treatment of pain – analgesia

The best treatment for pain is to remove the cause of the pain. While this is being done or if this is not possible, use one of the following groups of pain relieving drugs called analgesics.

1. General anaesthetics, e.g. ketamine.
2. Narcotic or opiate drugs, e.g. morphine, pethidine, codeine phosphate.
3. Paracetamol, aspirin (acetylsalicylic acid), and non-steroidal anti-inflammatory drugs (NSAIDs).
4. Other systemic drugs with various actions, e.g. chlorpromazine.
5. Local anaesthetics, e.g. lignocaine, procaine, amethocaine, local cooling agents.

Choice of analgesic

For mild pain, give aspirin or paracetamol tablets.

If aspirin or paracetamol is not enough, use compound analgesic tablets also called codeine compound tablets ('codeine co') which are a combination of aspirin and a small dose of codeine phosphate. Paracetamol and codeine tablets are also available.

For bowel colic, use codeine phosphate.

For severe pain use pethidine tablets or injection. If pethidine is not enough, use morphine injection. Do *not* use these drugs for chronic pain unless the patient is expected to die soon.

Use chlorpromazine in small doses together with the usual dose of pethidine or morphine to make these drugs more effective and last longer; but only in special cases.

For very severe pain, give a general anaesthetic, usually a ketamine injection.

For some pains in only one part of the body (e.g. a sting from a 'stonefish') you can use an injection of a local anaesthetic around the painful area.

Morphine, pethidine and codeine

These are dangerous drugs. They are also called narcotic or opiate drugs. There are special rules for storing and using them. Effects and precautions include:

1. Pain is relieved. *Never use them in abdominal pain until the cause is definitely diagnosed and proper treatment started. Otherwise, when pain and tenderness are gone, diagnosis may not be possible.*
2. Breathing and coughing is less. *Never use in chronic obstructive lung disease or asthma or if the patient might have any difficulty in breathing. Otherwise the patient might completely stop breathing.*
3. Diarrhoea is stopped and constipation can be caused. They are a very effective treatment for severe diarrhoea.
4. Vomiting is caused sometimes.
5. Itch occurs sometimes.
6. Sleepiness and change in consciousness is caused. *Never use if the patient has a head injury as level of consciousness is then difficult to interpret.*

7. Happiness is often caused. Addiction occurs quickly. *Never use for chronic pain or for more than a few days unless the patient is soon to die.* However, they are good treatment for pain in the dying patient.

Overdose is treated with artificial ventilation and naloxone or nalorphine.

Aspirin (acetylsalicylic acid)

Effects include the following:

1. Pain is relieved (mild pain only).
2. Temperature is lowered. However, treatment of the cause of the raised temperature is much more important.
3. Anti-inflammatory effects occur if large doses are given regularly. This is done for arthritis and leprosy reactions.
4. Indigestion, peptic ulcer and gastrointestinal bleeding can occur. Do not give aspirin if the patient possibly has a peptic ulcer or any bleeding.
5. Allergic reactions can occur.

Give aspirin when required for pain.

Give aspirin regularly for its anti-inflammatory effect.

If the dose of aspirin is too high, the patient may get:

1. 'ringing' or other noises in the ears; or deafness,
2. headache,
3. nausea, vomiting.

If these occur:

- stop the aspirin for 1 day,
- then give it in a lower dose.

A large overdose of aspirin is very dangerous. Immediately make the patient vomit if he is conscious. Treat immediately as described in Chapter 34.

Paracetamol

Paracetamol relieves pain and often reduces a fever. However, it is not usually as effective a drug as aspirin. It does not have the anti-inflammatory effects of aspirin. However, it does not cause gastrointestinal irritation and bleeding as aspirin does.

An overdose of paracetamol is very dangerous. Treat immediately as described in Chapter 34 and transfer the patient urgently to a Medical Officer for special treatment to try to stop severe liver damage.

Doses of analgesic drugs

Aspirin (300 mg tablets, but also others from 100 to 500 mg)

- 300–1200 mg (1–4 tabs) each 4–6 hours if required for pain.
- Use a small dose (1–2 tabs) for a small adult or for mild pain in large adult. Use a large dose (3–4 tabs) for a more severe pain in a large adult.
- No more than 4 grams in 24 hours.

Codeine compound tablets (aspirin 300 mg and codeine 8 mg in each tablet).

- 1–4 tablets each 4–6 hours if required for pain.
- Use a small dose (1–2 tabs) for a small adult or less severe pain in a large adult. Use a large dose (2–3 tabs) for a severe pain in a large adult.
- Give no more than 12 tablets in 24 hours.

Paracetamol (500 mg tablets, but also others, e.g. 100 mg)

- 500–1000 mg (1–2 tabs) each 4–6 hours if needed for pain in adults.
- No more than 4 g in any 24-hour period.

Paracetamol (500 mg) and codeine (8 mg) (co-codamol) tablets

- 1–2 tabs each 4–6 hours if needed for pain not relieved by paracetamol alone.
- No more than 8 tablets in any 24-hour period.

Codeine phosphate (30 mg tablets)

- 1 tablet each 4–6 hours if needed for pain (or diarrhoea) not controlled by the above drugs.
- Give also either aspirin or paracetamol as well as codeine.
- This will cause constipation if more than 1 dose; give also a laxative.

Pethidine (50 mg/ml – 2 ml amps of 100 mg and 1 ml amps of 50 mg by IMI or SCI)

- 1–1.5 mg/kg each 4–6 hours if required for pain
- Small adult, pain not very severe, 50 mg (1 ml).
- Small adult, severe pain, 75 mg (1.5 ml) ($1\frac{1}{2}$ ml).
- Large adult, pain not very severe, 75 mg (1.5 ml) ($1\frac{1}{2}$ ml).
- Large adult, severe pain 100 mg (2 ml).

Morphine (10 mg/ml – 1 ml amps of 10 mg by SCI or IMI).

- 0.2 mg ($\frac{1}{5}$ mg)/kg each 4–6 hours if required.
- Small adult 7.5 mg ($7\frac{1}{2}$ mg) 0.75 ml ($\frac{3}{4}$ ml).
- Large adult 10 mg (1 ml).

Lignocaine (or lidocaine) plain 1% solution (50 ml vial) and

Procaine plain 1% solution (2 ml amp).

- Inject the smallest volume needed into or around the affected area to cause analgesia of the part of the body affected.
- Never inject more than 20 ml (or 40 ml of a 0.5% solution or 10 ml of a 2% solution) at any one time into a patient.

IVI ketamine, IMI ketamine for general anaesthetic.

IVI lytic cocktail for general analgesic effect.

IVI lignocaine (or lidocaine) for regional anaesthesia.
Do *not* use these three drugs *unless*:

1. you have been trained in their use; *and*
2. you have all the necessary equipment for resuscitation and artificial ventilation available and ready.

8

Notification of Disease and Death

There are three types of notification:

1. Notification of the Provincial or District or Regional Health or Medical Officer of:
   (a) the number of cases each month of the diseases which are being monitored;
   (b) events of public health concern.
2. Notification of the coroner and the police of all cases of 'sudden and unnatural' death and cases where you do not know the cause of death – including persons who are 'dead on arrival'. Notify the police of all fights, accidents, alleged poisonings, etc. if the patient is ill.
3. Notification of the relatives and friends of the nature, treatment and prognosis of the patient's illness.

Notification of the Health Officer

If certain diseases or conditions occur you must notify these to the Health Officer.

The Health Officer can then help you in your disease control and prevention work and can send you special advice or special help.

The Health Officer may report these things to Health Department Headquarters. Headquarters need to know what diseases occur so that they can send the proper staff, drugs and equipment to help. Headquarters may also have to report certain communicable diseases (the Quarantinable Diseases) to the World Health Organization (WHO).

There are two types of condition which are notified to the Health Officer:

1. Diseases which are monitored and reported regularly at the end of each month.
   (a) Count and record every single case of these diseases (no matter whether an inpatient or an outpatient).
   (b) Send the number of cases of each disease to the Health Officer at the end of each month.

> Keep a copy of the list of diseases you must monitor and report in a safe handy place.

2. 'Events of Public Health Concern'. If any of these things happened, notify the Health Officer immediately, by the fastest possible method:
   (a) outbreaks or epidemics of known diseases;
   (b) outbreaks or epidemics of unknown diseases;
   (c) single cases of dangerous diseases not usual in the area, e.g. cholera, plague, yellow fever;
   (d) natural disasters (floods, earthquakes, etc.) which may affect people's health;
   (e) unusual events such as diseases or deaths of animals (e.g. fish or rats) which may affect people's health.

9

Control and Prevention of Disease – summary of patient management

Control and prevention of disease

To control and prevent disease, you need a knowledge of both:

1. the cause of the disease, and
2. the epidemiology of the disease.

You can then choose the most effective means (one or more) to control and/or prevent the disease. The four means for control and prevention of infectious diseases are:

1. Kill the specific agent (an infecting organism) in the body of the original host (clinical case, subclinical case or carrier) or reservoir (man, animal, dust, etc.).
2. Block the means of spread from the reservoir to susceptible persons.
3. Increase the resistance of susceptible persons.
4. Prophylactic treatment. Give a drug to stop the infection in probably infected persons before the infection produces clinical disease.

Always give *health education to the patient and to his relatives* about those things which they can do to control and prevent the disease the patient has.

Always use a case of a disease as an opportunity to give *health education to all the community.*

Never forget to use each case of a disease to give *health education to your own health workers* about that disease including its prevention.

Figures 9.1 and 9.2 illustrate important points in control and prevention of infectious disease. *Use these five methods for the prevention and control of all (non-infective as well as infectious) diseases.*

See Chapter 11 for details of control and prevention of infectious diseases.

The summary of the management of a person with a medical problem

When a patient comes to a health worker with a symptom, the management of this problem may well include some or all of these things:

1. taking a medical history;
2. doing a clinical examination;
3. making a differential diagnosis;
4. doing or ordering tests;
5. making a provisional diagnosis;
6. deciding on the prognosis;
7. deciding on inpatient or outpatient treatment*;
8. ordering proper nursing care*;
9. giving specific treatment to cure the disease*;

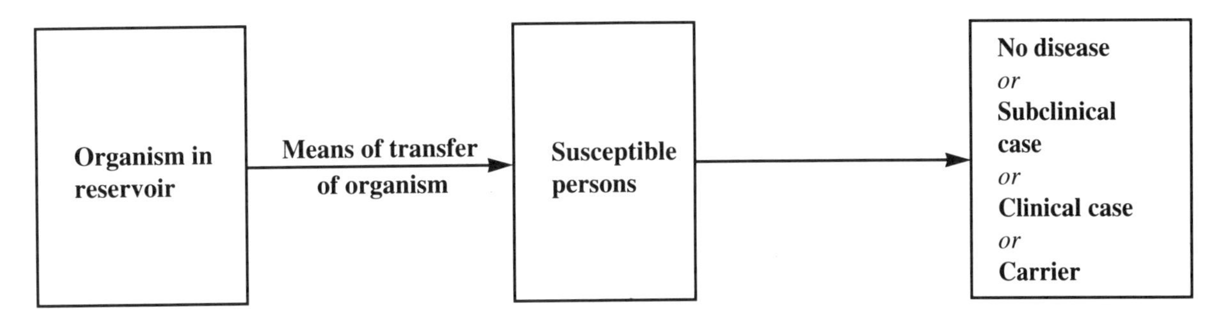

Figure 9.1 Aetiology and epidemiology of disease.

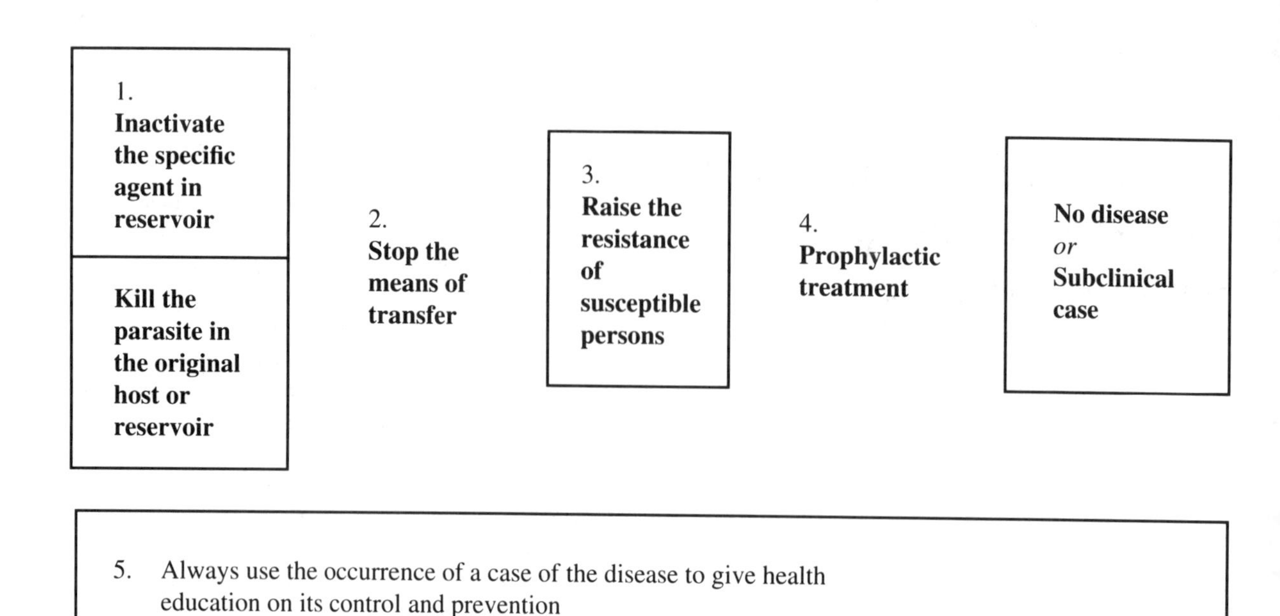

Figure 9.2 Means of control and prevention of disease.

10. giving symptomatic treatment to relieve symptoms*;
11. giving proper explanations and comfort to the patient and to his relatives*;
12. giving health education about the control and prevention of the disease to the patient and to his relatives*;
13. consulting with a Medical Officer (MO), transferring the patient to MO care or referring the patient to next visiting MO*;
14. notifying the Health Officer, the Coroner, the patrol officer, the police, the relatives, etc.;
15. controlling the spread of the disease;
16. preventing the disease occurring in the patient again and also in the community;
17. discharging the patient and giving final health education*;
18. following up the patient*.

(* These nine things were previously listed as 'treatment' of a patient.)

10

Infection, Immunity, Immunisation and Allergy

Infection

The specific agents (organisms) which cause infectious diseases are around people all the time. Why do these specific agents not cause disease in all people all the time?

There are many epidemiological answers. Here are some:

1. The specific agents – only some organisms cause disease.
2. The body – man's body has defences against the organisms that cause disease.
3. Transfer – the organism has ways of transferring to another person; sometimes it cannot use these ways of transferring.
4. The environment – changes in the environment can change the organism, man's body and the transfer of the organism.

This chapter considers:

1. the organisms which can cause disease, and
2. the body's defences against these organisms.

The specific agents which cause infections

The specific agents which cause infections are organisms such as:

- viruses,
- rickettsiae,
- bacteria,
- protozoa,
- fungi,
- worms,
- insects (called 'infestations').

Viruses

Viruses are the smallest organisms. You cannot see them with an ordinary microscope. (You can see them only with a special 'electron microscope'.) They need to be inside body cells to multiply; but they can stay alive outside body cells and pass from one person to another. Most chemotherapeutic drugs and antibiotics at present available in health centres cannot kill them.

Examples of virus infections are the common cold in the respiratory system and the polio virus in the nervous system, and the HIV virus in the immune system.

Rickettsiae

Rickettsiae are organisms that are bigger than viruses, but smaller than bacteria. You can see them, but not easily, with an ordinary microscope. Like viruses, they need to be inside body cells to multiply. Some antibiotics (tetracycline and chloramphenicol) can kill them. An example of rickettsiae is the typhus organism.

Bacteria

Bacteria are small organisms. You can see them only with a microscope. They can live in many places, inside and outside the body. Most bacteria are harmless – some are helpful to us. However, some bacteria can cause disease such as pneumonia in the lungs and leprosy in the skin and nerves. Chemotherapeutic drugs and antibiotics can kill most bacteria.

Protozoa

Protozoa are organisms of only one cell. They are much bigger than bacteria but usually you can only see them with a microscope. Some protozoa cause diseases such as malaria in the blood and amoebic dysentery in the intestine. There are chemotherapeutic drugs that will kill most protozoa.

Fungi

Fungi are simple organisms usually with more than one cell, and are something like plants. Some cause disease such as tinea on the skin and thrush in the mouth. There are chemotherapeutic and antibiotic drugs that can kill most fungi.

Worms

Worms are organisms with many cells. You can usually see them easily without a microscope. Worms are common parasites of man and animals. Many worms have complicated life cycles with different stages in man and other animals. Examples of worm infestations include filariasis in the lymph vessels and roundworm in the intestine. There are chemotherapeutic drugs that can kill most worms.

Insects

Insects are small animals that have three pairs of legs and a head, chest and abdomen. Many insects have wings. An example is the body louse, which can attach itself to hair or clothing and live by sucking blood. The bites often become infected with bacteria.

What determines if these organisms will cause infection and disease or not?

Pathogenicity

Some kinds of organisms *can cause disease* in *most* people they attack. These are called *highly pathogenic.*

Some organisms *can cause disease* in *only a few* of the people they attack. These are called *mildly pathogenic.*

Some organisms *cannot cause disease* in *any* of the people they attack. These are called *non-pathogenic.*

Virulence

The disease caused by organisms can be *mild* (e.g. common cold caused by the cold virus) or *severe* (e.g. meningitis caused by bacteria) or somewhere in between (e.g. influenza caused by influenza virus). Organisms that cause *severe disease* are called *virulent.* Organisms that cause *mild disease* are called *non-virulent*

The number of organisms

The number of organisms that enter the body can determine if they will cause disease or not. A certain number of organisms must stay alive after entry to cause disease. This number is different for each specific agent. This fact is very important.

The body defences against infection

The body surfaces

The skin and the mucous membranes (or mucosa) act as a wall which can stop many organisms entering the body.

Secretions (or fluids made by the glands) on the body surfaces can contain antibodies which kill the organisms. Secretions can also wash away organisms. Damaged or diseased skin or mucosa makes it easier for many organisms to enter the body.

The body defence cells

Some cells in the blood and in the tissues can surround and kill and digest many (but not all) organisms.

The body immune system

When organisms enter the body, some lymphocytes in the blood and in the lymph glands start to grow and change. These lymphocytes can recognise protein parts of the attacking organism as not belonging to the body and being 'foreign' and therefore try to destroy them. Proteins which are recognised as not part of the body and are 'foreign' are called 'antigens'.

1. B lymphocytes change to plasma cells and then make proteins called antibodies. These antibodies go into the blood and then spread into the tissues. These antibodies then join to the antigens on the organisms. These antibodies may damage the organism or stop it growing or spreading. These antibodies may also help other body defence cells to digest the organisms or destroy them in a number of other ways. This immune response by B lymphocytes making antibodies, is sometimes called 'humoral immunity' ('humoral' means 'travelling in the blood').
2. T lymphocytes can cause 'cell mediated immunity'. T lymphocytes can change into at least four different kinds of cells. Cytotoxic T lymphocytes destroy body cells which have organisms in them before the organisms inside them have time to grow and reproduce. (Natural killer cells, which are not T lymphocytes and do not need to be activated by antigen, can also recognise and kill such infected cells.) Helper T lymphocytes help B lymphocytes to make enough antibody. Suppressor T lymphocytes stop B cells making too much antibody and also stop the body becoming immune to itself. Other T lymphocytes are responsible for the delayed hypersensitivity reaction. All of these are part of the 'cell mediated immunity' system.

Antibodies protect the body against bacteria, bacterial toxins and viruses that are floating free in the body fluids. Cellular immunity protects the body against bacteria and viruses and protozoa that are growing inside cells and therefore cannot be reached by antibodies. Cellular immunity also protects against other protozoa, fungi and some worms.

If organisms have entered the body and caused an infection before, antibodies and the cells of cellular immunity can still be in the body. These antibodies and immune cells can then immediately attack any organisms of the same type that enter the body. If organisms have not entered the body and caused an infection before, there will be no antibodies and immune cells ready to attack them. It will take a week or more for the needed antibodies and immune cells to be made and start to attack the organisms.

Examples of infections

Acute infection with bacteria and the inflammatory reaction

This is what *can* happen:

1. The pathogenic organisms must first get onto the surface of the body (skin or mucous membrane).
2. The organisms must overcome the body surface defences. Usually the organisms must find a break in the skin or mucous membrane. However, some organisms can break through unbroken skin or mucous membranes.
3. The organisms must then grow and multiply in the tissues more quickly than the body defence cells, antibodies and cellular immunity can kill them.
4. If the organisms are not immediately killed, the body usually establishes an inflammatory reaction. The blood vessels in the area dilate (open up more widely) and bring more blood to the area. Defence cells and antibodies then go through the dilated blood vessel walls into the affected area and attack the organisms.
5. A protein from the blood called fibrin sometimes makes a wall around the area so that the organisms cannot spread to other tissues.
6. The whole body prepares to fight the infection. The body cells in the area release chemicals. These chemicals cause more white blood cells to be made, raise the temperature and make many other changes.
7. If the body defences do not kill the organisms quickly, the organisms can release poisons called toxins. The blood then carries the toxins around the body and they can poison the body in a number of ways. This is called 'toxaemia'. These toxins can cause malaise (feeling sick), raised temperature, fast pulse rate, nausea, vomiting and diarrhoea. Certain toxins can cause clinical disease, e.g. tetanus (see Chapter 25 page 330).
8. If the body defences do not kill the organisms quickly, the organisms can also destroy tissues in the area of the infection. The dead tissues and blood cells and organisms are called pus.
9. The organisms can spread through the lymph vessels to the lymph nodes and cause inflammation in these places too – lymphangitis in the lymph vessels and lymphadenitis in the lymph nodes.
10. The organisms can be carried around in the blood stream. This is called bacteraemia. The infection can spread to other organs.
11. The organisms can grow and multiply in the blood. This is a very serious and often fatal disease. It is called septicaemia.

Acute infection with viruses and the inflammatory reaction

1. There can be all the symptoms and signs of acute inflammation.
2. There is no pus (e.g. there is only a watery nasal discharge in a viral common cold).
3. There can be a loss of function of the organ that is infected (e.g. viral hepatitis).
4. There can be the general symptoms and signs of toxaemia (e.g. influenza).

Chronic infection and inflammation produced by tuberculosis

1. There are the usual symptoms and signs of chronic inflammation.
2. There is slow destruction of the body tissues.
3. Thick pus (like cheese) is formed.
4. Fibrous tissue tries to make a wall around that area of the body so that the infection cannot spread.
5. Healing is by the contraction and shrinking of the fibrous tissue. This causes scarring.

There are many other types of reaction to infection.

Immunity and immunisation

Immunity is when a person has a resistance to a disease. Sometimes immunity is complete – the immune person can never get the disease again.

More often, the immunity is relative – the body has defences against infection; but, if the body is

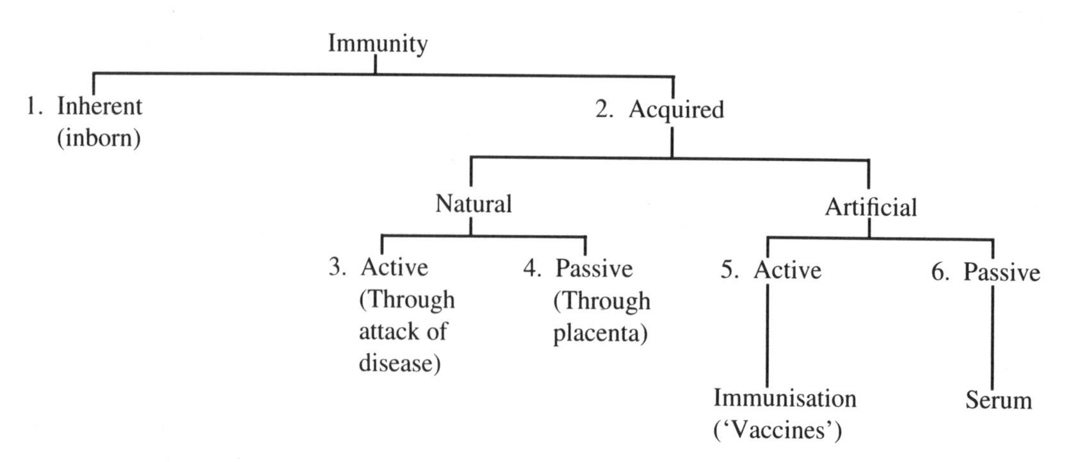

Figure 10.1 Diagram to illustrate the classification of the different types of immunity.

weakened or if the infecting agent is very strong or present in large numbers, the immunity can fail and disease can happen.

There are different types of immunity as shown in Figure 10.1.

1. *Inherent (inborn) immunity* is the immunity a person has without being infected or immunised etc. It varies with race, sex, family, etc.
2. *Acquired immunity* is due to specific antibodies or immune cells which develop in the body after an infection or immunisation. These antibodies or immune cells join onto the attacking organism or toxin and destroy it.
3. *Natural active immunity* follows a natural infection. After the infection some antibodies or immune cells can stay in the blood (or another part of the body) all the time. Also, the body 'remembers' how to make the antibodies immediately the organism tries to attack again.
4. *Natural passive immunity* is only in infants for the first few months of life. The infant gets the antibodies through the placenta or in its mother's milk if the mother has these antibodies. The antibodies do not last in the infant after 3–9 months.
5. *Artificial active immunity* is produced by immunisation (or 'vaccination') with any of the following three things:

   (a) Dead infectious organisms.

   (b) Living infectious organisms that are exactly like the organisms which cause disease, but cannot cause disease themselves (because they are avirulent or non-virulent organisms).

   (c) A substance like the poison or toxin of an organism but not poisonous itself (called 'toxoid')

   The body makes antibodies or immune cells against all of these three things. These antibodies or immune cells are also effective against the real live organisms or toxins that cause disease. Some of these antibodies and immune cells stay in the blood or other parts of the body after the immunisation. The body also 'remembers' how to make them immediately the disease-producing organism or toxin attacks.
6. *Artificial passive immunity* is produced by giving serum from another person or animal who has antibodies against the disease. This kind of immunity lasts for weeks or months, but after this time there are no antibodies left and there is no immunity.

   However, if the antibodies come from a horse or other animal, the human body can have a severe or even fatal reaction to the other proteins in the serum when it is injected. This is even more likely if the serum is used more than once.

Active immunity is always better than passive immunity.

The WHO Expanded Programme on Immunization (EPI)

Immunisation should be given to produce artificial active immunity against all infectious diseases important to a population. This should be done for all infectious diseases that are common and for all infectious diseases that may not be common but which are usually serious. This will save those in the population who would otherwise have been infected, from suffering the disease; from having permanent damage to their bodies caused by the infection; or sometimes from death. It may also allow some diseases to be totally destroyed if there is no reservoir for the infection (as everyone is immunised and immune). This is becoming more important as some diseases such as tuberculosis and malaria are becoming resistant to drugs which used to kill the organisms causing them; and some diseases, such as poliomyelitis and HIV infection cannot be cured by any drugs that exist at present. Immunisation should be given to produce artificial passive immunity for patients with infections to which they do not already have immunity, where the infection could have serious or fatal results.

The WHO has therefore recommended the programme given in Table 10.1. Your national government may have changed this programme a little or added other things to it to make it more effective for the diseases and the people affected by these diseases in your community. You must find out what your national programme is and do all you can to make sure that all people in your community get all immunisations possible. As new immunisations become available, add these to your list.

Allergy or hypersensitivity

Allergy or hypersensitivity is an inflammatory reaction of part of the body caused by some foreign substance in or on the body. This substance does not normally cause inflammation in normal people. However, some people (who are called 'allergic' or 'hypersensitive') develop an abnormal immune reaction to these substances. If these people contact the substance again there is an immune reaction between the abnormal antibodies or immune cells and the substance. In this reaction, histamine and other substances may be released. These substances cause an 'immediate' allergic reaction. Cellular immune reaction causes a 'delayed' hypersensitivity reaction.

Immunity is a helpful reaction of the immune system of the body to a foreign substance. Allergy or hypersensitivity is a harmful reaction of the immune system of the body to a foreign substance.

There are many types of allergy including:

- asthma,
- hayfever,
- urticaria ('hives')
- oedema (angio-oedema), and
- shock.

Allergic reactions can be caused by things which:

- touch the skin,
- are inhaled (breathed in),
- are swallowed, or
- are injected.

Table 10.1 The present WHO Expanded Programme on Immunization. Change this programme as your national government tells you. Add new immunisations as soon as they become available. Make sure everyone in your population gets all these immunisations.

Age	*Vaccine*	*Hepatitis B vaccine* (two alternative schemes)*	
		Alternative A	*Alternative B*
Birth	BCG, OPV-0	HB-1	
6 weeks	DPT-1, OPV-1	HB-2	HB-1
10 weeks	DPT-2, OPV-2		HB-2
14 weeks	DPT-3, OPV-3	HB-3	HB-3
9 months	Measles, Yellow fever†		

BCG, used to prevent tuberculosis
OPV, oral polio vaccine
DPT, diphtheria–pertussis–tetanus vaccine
HB, hepatitis B vaccine
* In countries with carriage rates of HBsAg of 2% or more; scheme A is recommended in countries where perinatal transmission of HBV is important (e.g. SE Asia), and scheme B in countries where perinatal transmission is less important (e.g. sub-Saharan Africa).
† In countries where yellow fever poses a risk.

Treatment includes:

1. Adrenaline (epinephrine) 1 mg/ml (1:1000 solution) injection for acute severe reactions; 0.5 ml ($\frac{1}{2}$ ml) SCI or IMI; or if near death, 0.1 ml/minute IVI (dilute 0.5 ml with 4.5 ml 0.9% saline or dextrose saline and give 1 ml/minute) (see Chapter 27 page 379).
2. Anthistamine drugs IV or IMI if life-threatening; or orally if not severe reaction; and repeat the dose if needed, e.g.
   - promethazine is long acting (e.g. 24 hours) (10 and 25 mg tablets; 1 mg/ml elixir; and 25 mg/ml injection) give 25 mg stat; and repeat once if needed; but maximum dose in 24 hours is 50 mg; *or*
   - chlorpheniramine (also called chlorphenamine) is short acting (e.g. 4 hours) (4 mg tablets and 10 mg/ml injection for IVI diluted with saline to 5 ml slowly over 1 minutes), give 4–10 mg stat and repeat soon and each 4 hours if needed but maximum dose in 24 hours is 24 mg by mouth and 40 mg by injection; *or*
   - dexchlorpheniramine is similar to chlorpheniramine but is twice as active and the dose is half that of chlorpheniramine.
3. Other special drugs sometimes used by Medical Officers, including adrenocorticosteroids, e.g. hydrocortisone, prednisolone, cortisone, dexamethasone, etc. For an acute allergic reaction threatening life 100–300 mg of hydrocortisone or dexamethasone 4–10 mg IVI would be given immediately and 100 mg hydrocortisone or 4 mg of dexamethasone each 4–8 hours until the patient could swallow prednisolone 1 mg/kg (e.g. 50–60 mg daily). However this takes some hours to work and is not the most important treatment – adrenaline (followed by antihistamine) is the important treatment.
4. The usual treatment of any complication.
5. Avoiding any further contact with the cause.

Autoimmune diseases

Very occasionally the body's immune system attacks part of the normal body and can damage this part or destroy it.

It is thought that some types of diabetes mellitus (Type I), some types of over-active thyroid glands (thyrotoxicosis) and under-active thyroid glands (myxoedema), perhaps rheumatoid arthritis and other conditions are brought about in this way.

Immunodeficiency disorders

Immunodeficiency occurs when either the antibody response or cellular immune response, or both, do not work properly to produce the immunity that would be expected in healthy people.

Causes of this include:

- congenital or inherited abnormalities;
- malnutrition (where not enough protein etc. is available for the cells and antibodies to work properly);
- old age (where immune system starts to wear out);
- use of drugs which suppress immunity especially adrenocorticosteroids (cortisone, prednisone, etc.) and some anti-cancer drugs;
- certain diseases especially diabetes and kidney (renal) failure;
- the human immunodeficiency virus (HIV) which slowly destroys some of the T lymphocytes and therefore the cellular immunity.

Sera and vaccines for prevention and treatment of infectious diseases

Table 10.2 is reproduced with thanks from the book by Drs Fr. von Massow, J.K. Ndele and R. Korte *Guidelines to rational drug use* (1997, London, Macmillan) to try to help you remember when to give immunisations. The scheme for hepatitis B prevention has been added.

This section is intended to be a reminder of the importance of the WHO Expanded Programme on Immunization (EPI). EPI activities should be included in your daily routine.

Table 10.2 Sera and vaccines for prevention and treatment of infectious diseases.

Sera and vaccines	*Indication*	*Use*			*Notes*
		In children	*In pregnant women*	*In non-immunised people*	
BCG vaccine (dried) injection	To build up immunity against: tuberculosis	*Age*: after birth	Avoid	Do not use in immuno-compromized (HIV^+)	Tuberculin test may not be used for 3 months after injection
diphtheria–pertussis–tetanus vaccine (DPT) injection	To build up immunity against: diphtheria, pertussis, tetanus	*Age*: 6 weeks 10 weeks 14 weeks		Full course of 3 doses: • 1st at the day of visit, • 2nd 4 weeks later; • 3rd another 4 weeks later	*In children* give polio **vaccine** at the same time (days) Give booster dose after 10 years
diphtheria–tetanus vaccine (DT) injection (different strengths for adults and children)	To build up immunity against: diphtheria, tetanus	*Age*: 6 weeks 10 weeks 14 weeks		**DPT** is contraindicated in patients with progressive neurological disorders or cramps; use **DT** instead	May be used instead of DPT Give booster at 7 years of age; then every 10 years
poliomyelitis vaccine (live attenuated) oral solution	To build up immunity against: poliomyelitis	*Age*: after birth 6 weeks 10 weeks 14 weeks	Avoid unless significant risk of exposure		*In children* give **DPT** at the same time (days) Give first booster dose after 5 years; then every 10 years
hepatitis B vaccine	To build up immunity against: hepatitis B	*Age*: 6 weeks 10 weeks 14 weeks *or* *Age*: after birth 6 weeks 14 weeks			Start at 6 weeks if not much infection near birth (e.g. Africa) Start at birth if a lot of infection then (e.g. Asia)

Table 10.2 (continued)

Sera and vaccines	*Indication*	*Use*			*Notes*
		In children	*In pregnant women*	*In non-immunised people*	
measles vaccine injection	To build up immunity against: measles	*Age*: > 9 months (Never before 6 months)	Avoid during first month of pregnancy		If child is vaccinated before 9 months of age give a 2nd dose after age of 9 months
tetanus vaccine injection	To build up immunity against: tetanus		Give refresher at first visit	Give in case of accidents	Give booster dose every 10 years
		Application			
	Prophylactic treatment after accident	If person is not immunized or not fully immunized give a full course of 3 doses: • 1st at the day of visit; • 2nd 4 weeks later; • 3rd another 4 weeks later.			If a booster is needed use **DT** when available Give in case of accidents or large burns; also give **antitetanus serum** or **antitetanus immunoglobulin**
antitetanus serum injection - - - - - **antitetanus immuno-globulin (human)** injection	Prophylactic treatment after accident	Apply if person is not immunized or not fully immunized			Give in case of accidents or large burns; also give **tetanus vaccine**

Table 10.2 (continued)

Sera and vaccines	*Indication*	*Application*	*Notes*
rabies vaccine injection	To build up immunity against: rabies	*Pre-exposure* give a full course of 4 doses: • at day 0, 7 + 28, and 1 year later Read manufacturer's leaflet as schedule may differ *Post-exposure* give following course *intradermally*: (a) 0.1 ml at day 0, 3, 7, 14 (b) 0.1 ml into 8 (!) different sites in 1 session; booster of 0.1 ml once at day 7 + 28	Very expensive. Use only in groups at high risk exposure: wildlife services; veterinary services, animal handlers Post-exposure prophylaxis is less expensive than pre-exposure vaccination; (a) may be the best choice for developing countries, as the antibody levels are good Give booster dose after 3 years
rabies immunoglobulin injection	Prophylactic treatment after bites		Extremely expensive
diphtheria antitoxin injection	Prophylactic treatment	Suspected cases only; sensitivity reactions are common	Also give prophylactic antibiotic treatment
meningococcal vaccine injection	Prophylaxis if significant risk of exposure	Give as *mass treatment* only after decision of national (or other relevant) health authority	
cholera vaccine injection		Has become *obsolete*	Concentrate on environmental hygiene and effective treatment

11

Infectious Diseases and Chemotherapy

Infectious diseases

Definitions

Infectious disease

Infectious diseases are also called contagious or communicable diseases, and are diseases caused by harmful organisms which can spread from one person to another.

These harmful organisms can:

1. exit from (or leave) some reservoir of infection (a person, animal or place);
2. transfer to (or spread to) susceptible persons (persons who can get the disease);
3. penetrate (or enter) susceptible persons;
4. have pathogenicity (cause disease by either multiplying or making toxic products in the body).

Endemic disease

A disease is *endemic* in an area if it happens continuously (or all the time) in the area.

Sporadic disease

A disease has a *sporadic incidence* when it does not happen continuously in the area.

Epidemic

An *epidemic* of a disease is when large numbers of people are affected in a short period of time and this causes a temporary increase in the frequency of the disease.

How diseases can be caused

(see Figure 11.1)

Organisms

The specific agent or cause of a disease is a living organism (which is a parasite). These include:

- viruses,
- rickettsiae,
- bacteria,
- fungi.
- protozoa,
- worms, and
- insects.

See Chapter 10 page 35 details of these organisms.

The reservoir of the infection

People who may spread the disease include the following:

1. people who have symptoms and signs of the disease ('cases');
2. people who are incubating the disease;
3. people who have an infection which cannot be seen (no symptoms and signs) (also called 'sub-clinical cases');
4. people who have the disease and are getting better ('convalescent carriers');
5. people who have the disease chronically ('chronic carriers').

Animals, dirt, dust, etc. can also be reservoirs.

The exit of organisms from the reservoir

If the reservoir is a person, the organisms can go out (exit) through:

1. the respiratory tract through the mouth or nose;
2. the gastrointestinal tract in faeces or vomitus;
3. the urogenital tract by semen, vaginal or urethral discharges or in urine;
4. the skin and other mucous membranes (e.g. eyes) by discharges or bleeding.

The communicable or infectious period

This is the time during which the organism can be transferred directly or indirectly from an infected person to another person (or from an infected animal to a person).

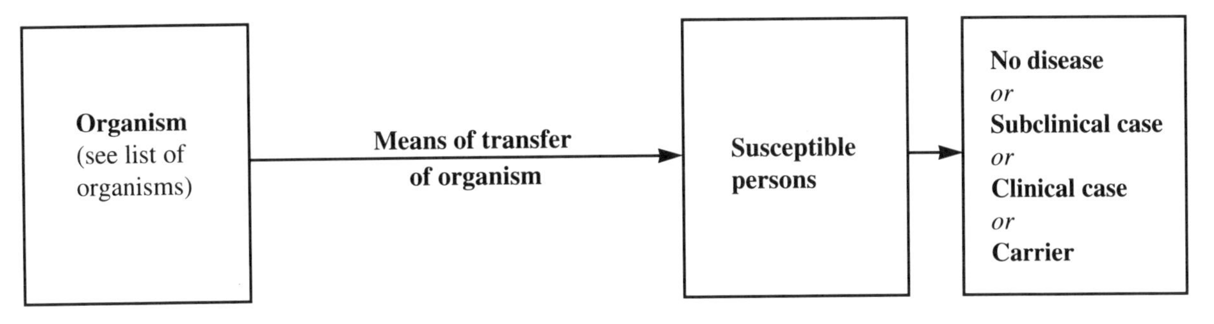

or, in more detail

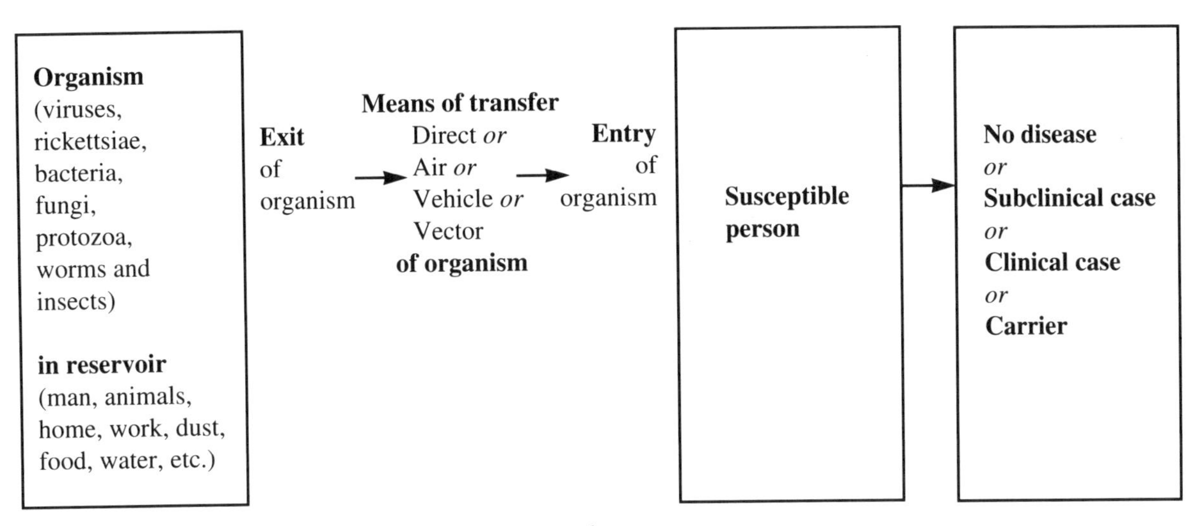

Figure 11.1 Diagrams showing how disease may be caused.

The means of transfer of organisms

Infection can be spread by:

1. direct contact (including droplets);
2. droplets, droplet nuclei and dust in the air which can be inhaled;
3. 'vehicles', such as:
   - fingers,
   - food and drink
   - water,
   - instruments, and
   - blood contaminated injections;
4. 'vectors' – usually insects

The entry of the organism (into a susceptible person)

Organisms can enter a person by:

1. inhalation (breathed into the respiratory tract),
2. ingestion (swallowed into the gastrointestinal tract),
3. inoculation (injected through the mucous membranes or the skin).

The susceptible person

A person has defences against infection (see Chapter 10 page 35):

1. skin and mucous membranes covering the body surfaces,
2. the body defence cells,
3. the body immune systems.

If an organism enters the body, the defences usually cause an inflammatory reaction.

The time that passes after a person gets an inflection and before the signs and symptoms of the disease start is known as the 'incubation period'.

Means of control and prevention of infectious disease (see Figure 11.2)

1. Kill the organism in the original reservoir (man, animal, dust, etc.).

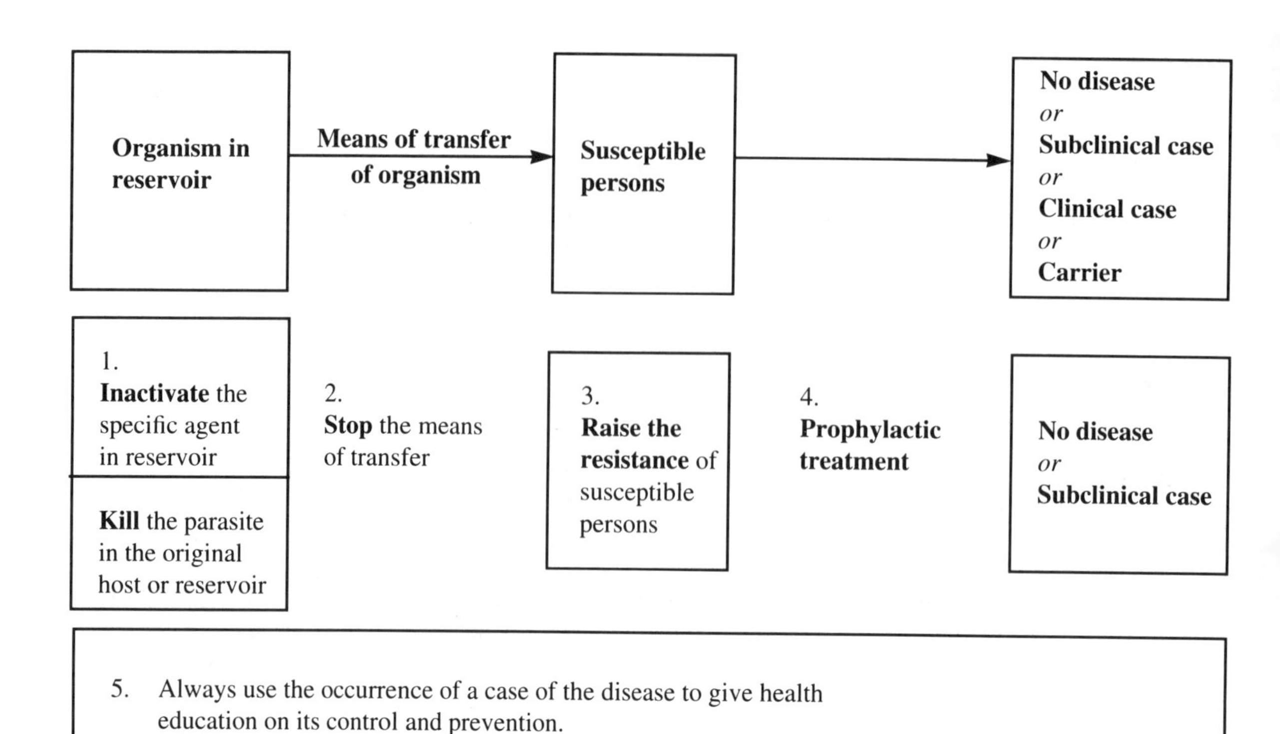

Figure 11.2 Diagrams to show the means of spread of infectious disease (upper diagram) and the means of control and prevention of infectious disease.

2. Stop the means of transfer.

   If the infection is spread by *direct contact*, then:
   - avoid exposure to carriers and persons with the disease,
   - disinfect discharges,
   - improve personal hygiene,
   - give barrier nursing to the patient.

   If the infection is spread by *droplets* etc. in the air, then:
   - cover mouth during coughing and sneezing.
   - avoid overcrowded rooms and crowds,
   - have good ventilation in all rooms.

   If the infection is spread by *vehicles*, then:
   - if instruments – improve personal hygiene, sterilisation of instruments, give barrier nursing to the patient;
   - if other people (fingers) – improve personal hygiene, give barrier nursing to the patient;
   - if food – supervise preparation, handling and hygiene of food;
   - if water – purify the water;
   - if needles or syringes – sterilise syringes and needles properly.

   If the infection is spread by *vectors* then:
   - control or eradicate the insects,
   - personal protection from insects (insect repellants, use of protective clothing, use of mosquito nets at night).
3. Raise the resistance of susceptible persons.
   - immunise these people – use active immunisation if possible, and passive if no active immunisation is available,
   - improve general health.
4. Prophylactic treatment (or 'chemoprophylaxis'). Give drugs to persons who are probably infected before the organisms cause disease. This is not often possible.
5. Use the occurrence of a case of the disease to give health education on the means of control and prevention of the disease.

Chemotherapy

Chemotherapy is giving a person a chemical that attacks the organisms that cause disease. The chemical is absorbed into the body and kills or stops the growth and multiplication of the organisms which are infecting that person. If possible the chemical will not harm the body of that person.

Chemotherapeutic drugs can sometimes cure an infection alone; but usually other treatment is needed too.

Chemotherapeutic drugs are of three kinds:

1. natural plant products (e.g. quinine, etc.);
2. antibiotics made by bacteria or fungi to kill other bacteria or fungi (e.g. penicillin, tetracycline, chloramphenicol, etc.) (now made in the laboratory);
3. chemicals first made in the laboratory (e.g. sulphadimidine, isoniazid, dapsone, chloroquine, metronidazole, diethylcarbamazine, etc.).

A chemotherapeutic drug is usually effective against only one of the groups of pathogenic organisms as shown in Table 11.1.

A chemotherapeutic drug is also usually effective against only some of the members of that group. Table 11.2 shows some examples for antibacterial drugs.

Infecting organisms that are killed or cannot grow or multiply in the presence of a chemotherapeutic drug are *'sensitive'* to that drug. Organisms that are not killed and can grow and multiply in the presence of a chemotherapeutic drug are *'resistant'* to that drug.

Some organisms have always been resistant to certain drugs. Some organisms which were sensitive to a chemotherapeutic drug can *develop resistance* to that drug. Development of resistance depends on the organism and the drug. Development of resistance can often be stopped by:

1. using the drug in the proper dose for long enough, *and,*
2. using at least two drugs to which the organism is sensitive at the same time.

Table 11.1 Examples of different types of drug.

Antiviral drugs	*Antibacterial drugs*	*Antifungal drugs*	*Antiprotozoal drugs*	*Antihelminthic drugs*
Aciclovir Zidovudine (AZT) No antiviral drugs available in most countries	Penicillin Streptomycin Tetracycline Chloramphenicol Sulphadimidine Isoniazid Thioacetazone Dapsone	Griseofulvin Nystatin Amphotericin B	Quinine Chloroquine Amodiaquine Pyrimethamine Metronidazole Mefloquine Artesunate Doxycycline	Diethyl-carbamazine Ivermectin Thiabendazole Albendazole Praziquantel

Table 11.2 Effectiveness of some antibacterial drugs.

	Penicillin	*Chloramphenicol*	*Isoniazid*	*Dapsone*
Pneumococcus (Pneumonia)	Effective	Effective	Not effective	Not effective
Salmonella typhi (Typhoid fever)	Not effective	Effective	Not effective	Not effective
Mycobacterium tuberculosis (Tuberculosis)	Not effective	Not effective	Very effective	Not effective
M. leprae (Leprosy)	Not effective	Not effective	Slightly effective	Very effective

Rules for using antibacterial chemotherapeutic drugs

1. Do not give a patient with a fever for which no cause can be found antibacterial chemotherapeutic drugs, unless he becomes very 'sick' (see Chapter 36 page 483).
2. Always use the proper dose of chemotherapeutic drugs – never use less.
3. Always give chemotherapeutic drugs for the full course. For chemotherapeutic drugs used for bacterial infections, this is:
   - mild infections – at least 5 days or for 2–3 days after clinically cured (whichever is longer);
   - severe infections – at least 10 days or 2–3 days after clinically cured (whichever is longer);
   - tuberculosis – at least 12 months unless rifampicin is used, when it will be at least 9 months, unless both rifampicin and pyrizinamide are used and rifampicin continued for the whole course, when it will be at least 6 months;
   - leprosy – at least 2 years for multibacillary (lepromatous) disease and at least 6 months for paucibacillary (tuberculoid) disease.
4. Do not stop antibacterial chemotherapeutic drugs in less than 48 hours because they do not seem to be effective. If the patient is getting worse *add* another drug before the 48 hours are finished. If the drug has no effect after 48 hours, then try another drug. However if the patient gets very sick and looks as if he will die, change to chloramphenicol (see Chapter 12 page 53).

Notes on some antibacterial chemotherapeutic drugs

Sulphonamides and trimethoprim and co-trimoxazole

Sulphonamides, (e.g. sulphadimidine) were effective against many bacteria in all parts of the body. Now some bacteria have become resistant to them. Sulphonamides alone are not used much now (except for urinary tract infection) as other drugs are more effective. The dose of sulphadimidine is 1 g (2 tabs) four times a day for 10 days.

Possible side effects include the following:

1. Formation of crystals in the urine if the patient does not drink enough when the drug is taken. Always make sure the patient drinks enough to pass a lot of urine when he takes a sulphonamide.
2. Allergic reactions, such as fever, skin rashes and jaundice.

Sulphonamides are also effective for trachoma (see Chapter 31 page 417).

Sulphonamides (and trimethoprim) also have an antimalarial effect. This is a weak effect, but if it is combined with another drug such as pyrimethamine, the effect of both drugs together is powerful. For malaria sulphadimidine is not used but a similar sulpha-drug (such as sulphadoxine) is used (see Chapter 13 page 71).

Trimethoprim acts in a similar way to sulphonamides to kill many bacteria but fewer organisms have become resistant to it and its side effects are less. It is also mildly effective against malaria. It can be used to treat respiratory infections and urinary infections. The dose is 150–200 mg twice daily or 300 mg once daily best taken with meals.

Co-trimoxazole is a combination of a sulphonamide and trimethoprim. The sulphonamide used is sulfamethoxazole 200 mg in 5 ml of mixture, 400 mg in a single strength tablet and 800 mg in a double strength tablet; the dose of trimethoprim being 40 mg in 5 ml of mixture; 80 mg in a single strength tablet and 160 mg in a double strength tablet. The drug is given twice daily. It was thought that this combination was more effective than either drug alone. Its side effects are mainly due to the sulphonamide. However the more it is used the more organisms become resistant to it. It is best not to give it to pregnant women. However, because it has become very cheap and because it has actions against many bacteria and also malaria, it is used in some places as the first treatment for many infections including upper and lower respiratory infections, urinary tract infections, gastrointestinal tract infections, skin infections and even septicaemia. Problems with cotrimoxazole used like this are:

1. It depends on the patient understanding and remembering to continue to take it after the first dose even if he feels cured (which he is not) until the whole course in finished.
2. Side effects can occur.
3. Organisms quickly start to get resistant to the drugs.

The dose is one 800 mg/160 mg tablet or two 400 mg/80 mg tablets twice daily for 5 days (or shorter or longer depending on the condition treated).

Penicillin

Penicillin is effective against most organisms that cause infections in all parts of the body, except those that cause bowel or urinary tract infections. Organisms that cause bowel or urinary tract infections are usually resistant to penicillin.

A few of the organisms that cause severe infections (including meningitis, septicaemia and pneumonia) are also resistant to penicillin. Some organisms which were sensitive have now developed resistance to penicillin.

Penicillin is given for most infections except bowel and urinary tract infections. If the infection does not improve, co-trimoxazole or tetracycline can be used instead. If the infection is a serious one which threatens life (e.g. meningitis, peritonitis, severe pneumonia, etc.), or an essential body part (e.g. eye, bone or joint, etc.), chloramphenicol is used instead.

Treatment is given for at least 5 days for mild infections and at least 10 days for moderate or severe infections.

The main side effects are allergic reactions including skin rashes, asthma, shock and fever with arthritis. If allergy happens the patient should not be given penicillin again. You must tell him he is allergic to penicillin and that he must never have penicillin again. You must tell him to tell this to any health worker who ever treats him. You must also write it on the outside of both his outpatient and inpatient notes. Penicillin is safe during pregnancy.

Benzyl (crystalline) penicillin, 1200 mg or 2,000,000 units IVI or IMI each 3 hours is given for infections which threaten life and 600 mg or 1,000,000 units each 6 hours is given for moderate infections.

Procaine benzylpenicillin, 1 g or 1,000,000 units daily is given for mild infections or severe or moderate infections which have improved after benzyl (crystalline) penicillin has been given for some days. Give procaine benzylpenicillin only by IMI.

Phenoxymethyl penicillin 250 mg and 500 mg tablets and 125 mg each 5 ml mixture is absorbed after being taken by mouth. It must be taken every 4–6 hours. It is not used much because you cannot know if the patient will remember to take it regularly. It is never used for moderate or severe infections. Normally use 250–500 mg four times daily.

Benzylpenicillin is a long acting penicillin which produces low levels of penicillin in the blood for a long time (a little up to 3–4 weeks). It is used for a 'one dose treatment' for syphilis and once each month for preventing rheumatic fever. The dose is usually 1.44 g or 2,400,000 units.

Ampicillin and amoxycillin are newer penicillins. These are often not available as they are more expensive. They can be given by IVI, IMI or by mouth. They kill many pathogenic organisms in most parts of the body including the urinary and gastrointestinal tracts. They can be used instead of penicillin and also for urinary tract infections. They have the same side effects as penicillin. In places where these drugs are scarce they are used only:

1. instead of tetracycline when a patient is pregnant (the dose is 250–500 mg (1–2 caps) orally three to four times a day – larger doses are given by injection for severe infections);
2. for gonorrhoea instead of the one large dose of procaine penicillin (see Chapter 19 page 169).

Cloxacillin (and flucloxacillin, dicloxacillin, etc.) are penicillins which kill an organism called *Staphylococcus aureus* which can become resistant to other penicillins and cause serious skin and bone (osteomyelitis) infections and at times other infections. These drugs are used only for these infections where staphylococci are known, or are very likely, to be present as they are not as effective as other penicillins against other organisms and are more expensive and have more side effects (including hepatitis).

Cephalosporins

Cephalosporins are a group of antibiotics, some of them being like benzyl penicillin (though one, cephalothin, being very effective against staphylococci), some of them being like amoxycillin and others, such as ceftriaxone being more like chloramphenicol. Some can be given orally but others including ceftriaxone only by IM injection or by IV injection. However, they are usually expensive and not available in health centres.

Chloramphenicol

Chloramphenicol is a very powerful antibiotic effective against most infecting bacteria in all parts of the body. Chloramphenicol enters all parts of the body. However, chloramphenicol can cause death in a few patients by stopping the body making blood; and is used therefore only for serious infections. It can cause shock in newborn infants and is therefore not given to them or to women just before delivery or when breastfeeding infants. Other side effects are minor, e.g. nausea, diarrhoea, headache.

It is therefore used only for:

1. severe infection which immediately threatens life (e.g. septicaemia, meningitis, peritonitis, severe pneumonia, etc.);
2. severe infection which threatens an essential body part (e.g. eye, bone or joint, etc.);
3. infection which does not respond to other antibiotics (e.g. pneumonia, urinary tract infections, etc. which has not improved on penicillin, co-trimoxazole or tetracycline);
4. Infection for which no other treatment is available (e.g. typhoid fever).

Penicillin or co-trimoxazole, or if one of these is not effective, tetracycline, are almost always effective for the treatment of infections. However, if chloramphenicol is needed for an acute severe infection which is threatening life or a vital body part (and the risk of disease is more than the risk of the drug) then the proper large dose of chloramphenicol should be used, i.e. 100 mg/kg daily or 25 mg/kg every 6 hours. When the patient is apparently cured then the dose of chloramphenicol is reduced to half ($\frac{1}{2}$) of the above, i.e. 50 mg/kg daily or 12.5 mg/kg every 6 hours to complete the treatment course. *For adults of ordinary size 1 g (1 bottle of 1 g injection or 4 caps) every 6 hours is the usual dose.* When the patient is apparently cured (or when a patient who needs long treatment improves), then, the dose is reduced to 750 mg (3 caps) for large adults (> 50 kg) and 500 mg (2 caps) for small adults (< 50 kg) each 6 hours.

Chloramphenicol is well absorbed from the intestine after it is given by mouth. Chloramphenicol is therefore always given by mouth unless:

1. The patient cannot swallow it because:
   (a) he is unconscious and there is no intragastric tube;
   (b) he is unco-operative.
2. The patient can not absorb it from the bowel, because of:
   (a) shock (little blood will be going to the bowel);
   (b) vomiting;
   (c) severe diarrhoea.
3. The patient is very sick and you cannot be sure that the drugs will be given by mouth because:
   (a) the staff are not dependable enough (staff are usually more dependable with injections than with oral drugs);
   (b) the patient is not dependable (he may refuse it or spit it out or vomit without telling the staff this);
   (c) of the other usual reasons that *very* sick patients are given injections.

Chloramphenicol acts quickly after IV injection. It acts only after some delay if given by IM injection. If it is given regularly every 6 hours this delay is not a problem after the first injection, because the effects of the previous dose will still be present. IM chloramphenicol is given if chloramphenicol by mouth is not possible (see above) and IV chloramphenicol is not needed or not possible. If IM chloramphenicol is given, it is best to give an extra injection IV with the first IM dose, if possible. If the IV injection is not possible, give the extra dose by IMI also.

Tetracycline group

Tetracycline, oxytetracycline and doxycycline are effective against most infecting bacteria in all parts of the body; but some bacteria are or have become resistant to them. Therefore they are not used for very severe infections which are threatening life or involving an essential body part. Tetracyclines are used for:

1. most infections if penicillin and/or co-trimoxazole do not cure the patient or if it is best not to give (penicillin) injections or it is not possible to give penicillin or co-trimoxazole (e.g. allergy);
2. gastrointestional or urinary tract infection if other treatment (sometimes including co-trimoxazole or just sulphonamides) does not cure them.

The dose of tetracycline or oxytetracycline is 20–40 mg/kg daily. For severe infections give 500 mg (2 caps) four times a day and for less severe infections or after severe infections improve, give 250 mg (1 cap) four times a day by mouth. Give this between meals and not with food or milk.

Doxycycline (50 or 100 mg tabs or caps) is a newer and cheaper and better form of tetracycline to use, if it is available. The dose is 2.5 mg/kg once daily, usually 200 mg for the first dose and then 100 mg daily. It should be taken just before a meal, as if it sticks in the oesophagus, it can cause severe ulceration and pain in the oesophagus. Patients should not lie down after taking doxycycline in case it comes back into the oesophagus.

Do not use a tetracycline and penicillin together as they do not kill organisms as well together.

Tetracyclines also have good activity against malaria organisms.

Side effects include vomiting and diarrhoea; discoloration of children's teeth if they are given before the teeth come through the gums, i.e. if given during pregnancy or before age of 12 years; and doxycycline can cause oesophageal ulcers.

Do not give tetracycline to:

1. pregnant women,
2. children,
3. people with kidney (renal) failure which may be made worse.

If penicillin is not effective for these patients, you can give amoxycillin or ampicillin or erythromycin or ask a Medical Officer to supply a special drug.

Macrolide or erythromycin group

These drugs act like something between penicillin and tetracycline but have some special actions against some special bacteria that cause pneumonia. They are very safe. Erythromycin itself can be used in pregnancy. Erythromycin, however, does cause nausea or diarrhoea in quite a few patients; it occasionally causes hepatitis; and it has to be taken 3–4 times daily and patients often forget to do this. As well as this, it is still expensive. Roxithromycin causes little nausea or vomiting and has to be taken only once daily but it is still expensive. However, erythromycin may be supplied for you to use in people who are allergic to penicillin (and therefore amoxycillin) but cannot take co-trimoxazole or tetracycline as they are pregnant. The dose of erythromycin is 250–500 mg 4 times daily between meals and roxithromycin 300 mg once daily.

Quinolones

This group of drugs is very effective against a large number of bacteria and protozoa. They can be given by injection or orally; can often be given once daily; do not have a lot of side effects; but as yet are very expensive. They are very unlikely to be available for some years in health centres except perhaps ciprofloxacin, which may be used for urethral discharges and perhaps later ofloxacin which may prove to be a good treatment for leprosy.

Streptomycin

Streptomycin is effective against a number of bacteria including tuberculosis organisms. However, organisms soon develop resistance to streptomycin. Therefore, you must:

1. Use streptomycin only with other drugs. Do not use streptomycin alone. National guidelines for streptomycin use must be followed.
2. Use streptomycin only for tuberculosis in adults and children (and then only with isoniazid), or for neonatal infections before tuberculosis infection is possible (and then only with penicillin).

Do not use streptomycin for any other infections.

See Chapter 14 page 189 for dose of streptomycin.

Summary of choice of antibacterial drug

For mild or moderate infection

1. In all places except the gastrointestinal or urinary tracts use penicillin[1] (co-trimoxazole[2] second choice or tetracycline[3]).
2. In the urinary tract, except sexually transmitted urethritis (gonorrhoea, etc.) use sulphadimidine[2] or co-trimoxazole[2] (tetracycline[3] second choice).
3. In the gastrointestinal tract – antibacterial drug usually not needed.

For severe bacterial infection which threatens life or a vital body part

1. In all places in adults (but not for newborn babies) use chloramphenicol in the correct *large* dose.
2. For neonatal septicaemia (before tuberculosis infection is possible) use penicillin in large doses and streptomycin (chloramphenicol is second choice; but make sure only the correct *small* dose is given).

For mild or moderate infections which do not respond to penicillin or co-trimoxazole

In all places use tetracycline.[3]

If the infection is likely to come back many times and the *patient is likely to need long or repeated courses* of antibacterial drugs, then it is very important to *USE tetracycline*; *DO NOT USE chloramphenicol* (unless the infection threatens life or a vital body part).

In some places amoxycillin may be available to use at this stage.

---

1 Penicillin. Do not give if the patient is allergic to penicillin.
2 Co-trimoxazole. Do not give if allergic to sulphonamides or if pregnant.
3 Tetracycline. Do not give if the patient is pregnant or a child or has kidney failure.

For moderate infections which do not respond to either penicillin (co-trimoxazole) or tetracycline

First look for causes of failure to respond to treatment. There is probably a cause which needs other treatment rather than changing antibiotics.

If you can find no cause then: in all places – chloramphenicol.

> Use streptomycin in adults for only TUBERCULOSIS and ONLY TOGETHER WITH isoniazid. Do not use streptomycin in any other way.

Continue the antibacterial drug for:

1. two to three days after the patient seems cured *or*;
2. mild infections – 5 days,
   moderate infections – 7 days,
   severe infections – 10 days,

whichever is longer.

For special infections

None of the above is correct for these special infections:

- urethritis – see Chapter 19 page 169,
- tuberculosis – see Chapter 14 page 84,
- leprosy – see Chapter 15 page 108.

12

Septicaemia

Septicaemia is present when organisms get into the bloodstream and multiply in it.

Septicaemia occurs only in special circumstances:

1. Organisms are put straight into the bloodstream e.g.:
   - injection of contaminated drugs or blood transfusion (with organisms in them);
   - an operation where an infected area is cut;
   - passage of a urethral catheter especially when there is infection in the urethra;
   - changing or leaving in too long an infected intravenous cannula;
   - doing a burns dressing.
2. The body is in a state of weakened immunity or resistance e.g.:
   - HIV infection;
   - malnutrition;
   - anaemia;
   - certain chronic illnesses, e.g. diabetes mellitus and kidney (renal) failure;
   - after operation or childbirth;
   - if another infection is present in the body;
   - if the patient has cancer or leukaemia, etc;
   - if the patient is taking adrenocorticosteroid drug (e.g. prednisolone) or anti-cancer drugs.
3. There is a particularly severe or widespread infection in the body, e.g. certain types of pneumonia.
4. The attacking organism is particularly virulent, e.g. certain types of organism which can cause meningitis and septicaemia.

If a patient in any of these situations suddenly gets worse, always think of septicaemia.

The first group of conditions is of particular importance in the health centre. Septicaemia can follow simple procedures. A very common cause of septicaemia is the passage of a urethral catheter. In all these procedures in Group 1, virulent organisms may be put straight into the bloodstream where they start to grow and produce septicaemia.

If septicaemia develops, the patient may have any of the following:

1. Rigor(s) (high temperature with shivering or shaking).
2. General symptoms and signs of infection which could include:
   - severe malaise and weakness;
   - nausea, vomiting, diarrhoea;
   - being not fully conscious or being psychotic or even fitting;
   - dyspnoea and fast respiration;
   - raised temperature.
3. Fast pulse, low blood pressure but skin warm (due to dilation of blood vessels in the skin) ('warm shock').
4. Fast pulse, low blood pressure, cold, cyanosed, low urine output ('cold shock').
5. Haemorrhages into the skin – petechiae (pin-point haemorrhages) or larger areas of bleeding or bruises.

> However, any patient who has an infection and gets worse or any patient who has had any type of procedure carried out on him and then gets very sick should be thought of as having septicaemia.

Management of septicaemia

1. Chloramphenicol (25 mg/kg each 6 hours). For an adult of average weight give 2 g immediately then 1 g every 6 hours.

   Give by IVI if:
   - shock (essential), or
   - IV drip needed for another reason and is running.

If a patient has a condition which makes it likely for him or her to develop septicaemia, and he or she then develops symptoms and signs suggesting septicaemia, immediately manage as follows:

1. chloramphenicol in large doses (usually 1 g each 6 hours);
2. antimalarial drug as indicated usually quinine;
3. IV drip – but only if needed for shock or dehydration, etc.;
4. treatment of any heart failure;
5. treatment of any infected body part in the usual way;
6. consult a Medical Officer if necessary;
7. do not reduce the chloramphenicol dose unless the patient seems to be cured very quickly;
8. continue chloramphenicol for *at least* 10 days.

Give by IMI *if*

- IV drip not needed, or
- IV drip not possible.

and if

- oral drugs are not reliable enough (as very sick), or
- oral drugs are not effective (as shock or not able to swallow or vomiting or severe diarrhoea).

Give orally (4 caps) *only if*

- is not very sick; or after improves (when oral drugs are reliable enough), and
- can swallow, and
- has no vomiting or severe diarrhoea, and
- is not shocked.

2. Antimalarial drug for all patients.
   Quinine 10 mg/kg (450 mg for a small adult or 600 mg for a large adult) by IMI or by a SLOW (over 4 hours) IV drip if patient:
   - is shocked or
   - is unconscious, or
   - is very sick

   and if patient:
   - is in or has been in an area where chloroquine resistant malaria occurs, or
   - has been given chloroquine and is still sick. See Malaria Chapter 13 for further treatment.
3. Set up an IV drip; but only if needed, i.e. if shock, severe dehydration, unconscious, very sick, not able to take oral fluids and drugs.
   Do not give more fluid than is really necessary (or this may cause cerebral oedema, convulsions and death).
   - When shock – see Chapter 27 page 378.
   - When dehydration – see Chapter 23 page 285.
   - When maintenance fluids only needed – give 0.18% sodium chloride in 4.3% dextrose 1 litre each 8 hours.
   - When drip for IV injections only needed – give 0.18% sodium chloride in 4.3% dextrose, 1 litre each 12 hours.
4. Look for heart failure. Treat if present. Give intranasal oxygen 2–4 litres/minute.
   Give frusemide 20 mg IVI or 40 mg orally or if not available, any other diuretic.
   Give digoxin 0.5 mg ($\frac{1}{2}$ mg) or 500 μg IVI slowly immediately or, if injection not available, 0.5 mg ($\frac{1}{2}$ mg) orally immediately.
   Give only maintenance fluids (see 3 above) (do not give 0.9% sodium chloride). Then see Heart Failure (Chapter 27 page 371).
5. Treat any infected part or any other complication in the usual way.
6. Consult a Medical Officer urgently about further management if you are not sure of the diagnosis or treatment or if transfer for surgery is likely.
7. Do not quickly reduce the chloramphenicol dose.
   If the patient is apparently cured very quickly, 12.5 mg/kg ($12\frac{1}{2}$ mg/kg) each 6 hours could be given, i.e.
   - 750 mg (3 caps) each 6 hours for a large adult (> 50 kg) and
   - 500 mg (2 caps) each 6 hours for a small adult (< 50 kg)

   However, *most patients* should continue 1 g (4 caps) each 6 hours.
8. Continue the chloramphenicol for at least 10 days. many infections will need longer treatment; however use the reduced dose (see 7) *after* clinical improvement and 10 days high dose treatment.

13

Malaria

Definition

Malaria is a disease caused by infection of the red blood cells by a protozoal organism called *Plasmodium* of which there are four types. Infection causes acute and chronic types of fever, anaemia and enlargement of the spleen. Infection sometimes causes severe disorders of the brain, kidneys, liver and other parts of the body.

Frequency

Malaria is the most common important infectious disease in the world. Malaria affects many of the people living between the latitudes of approximately 60°N and 40°S (see Figure 13.1). Malaria affects between 300 to 500 million people and each year causes over 2 million deaths.

Cause

Malaria is caused by infection with one or more of four protozoal (one-celled microscopic organism) parasites:

1. *Plasmodium falciparum* is the most common in hot, wet climates.
2. *Plasmodium vivax* is the most widespread of the parasites in the world and is more common than *P. falciparum* in places which have cool or dry seasons.
3. *Plasmodium malariae* is not common.
4. *Plasmodium ovale* is very uncommon.

Epidemiology

Man is the only host of the above malaria parasites.

Transmission of these parasites is usually from the blood of an infected person to a female *Anopheles* mosquito and then to susceptible new persons.

Occasionally transmission is through the placenta to a baby or by transfusion of blood which has malaria parasites in it.

See Figure 13.2 for details of the life cycle of the malaria parasite.

The time from when the mosquito ingests the gametocytes until it has infective sporozoites is at least 10 days. The gametocytes can develop into sporozoites only if the temperature is above 15°C (60°F).

The incubation period in man (from the bite of an infected mosquito until the start of symptoms and signs of malaria) is usually about 2 weeks. However it is often much longer. It cannot be shorter than 8 days.

Transmission of malaria can occur only if the following four conditions are present:

1. There are human gametocyte carriers present in the area.
2. *Anopheles* mosquitoes are present in the area.
3. The temperature and humidity is right for the parasite development in the mosquito.
4. There are susceptible human hosts (usually babies and children in endemic areas).

Partial or incomplete immunity to malaria (mostly due to antibodies) can develop after 4–10 years of continuous exposure to malaria (if the person does not die from chronic malaria or one of the acute attacks of malaria during this time). This means that older children or adults, who have lived continuously for years in places where malaria is present all the time, develop partial immunity. They are often called 'semi-immune'. However, to develop and keep this semi-immunity, a person has to be repeatedly sick with malaria, as well as being likely to die from malaria for 4–10 years (unless treatment for acute attacks is always immediately available).

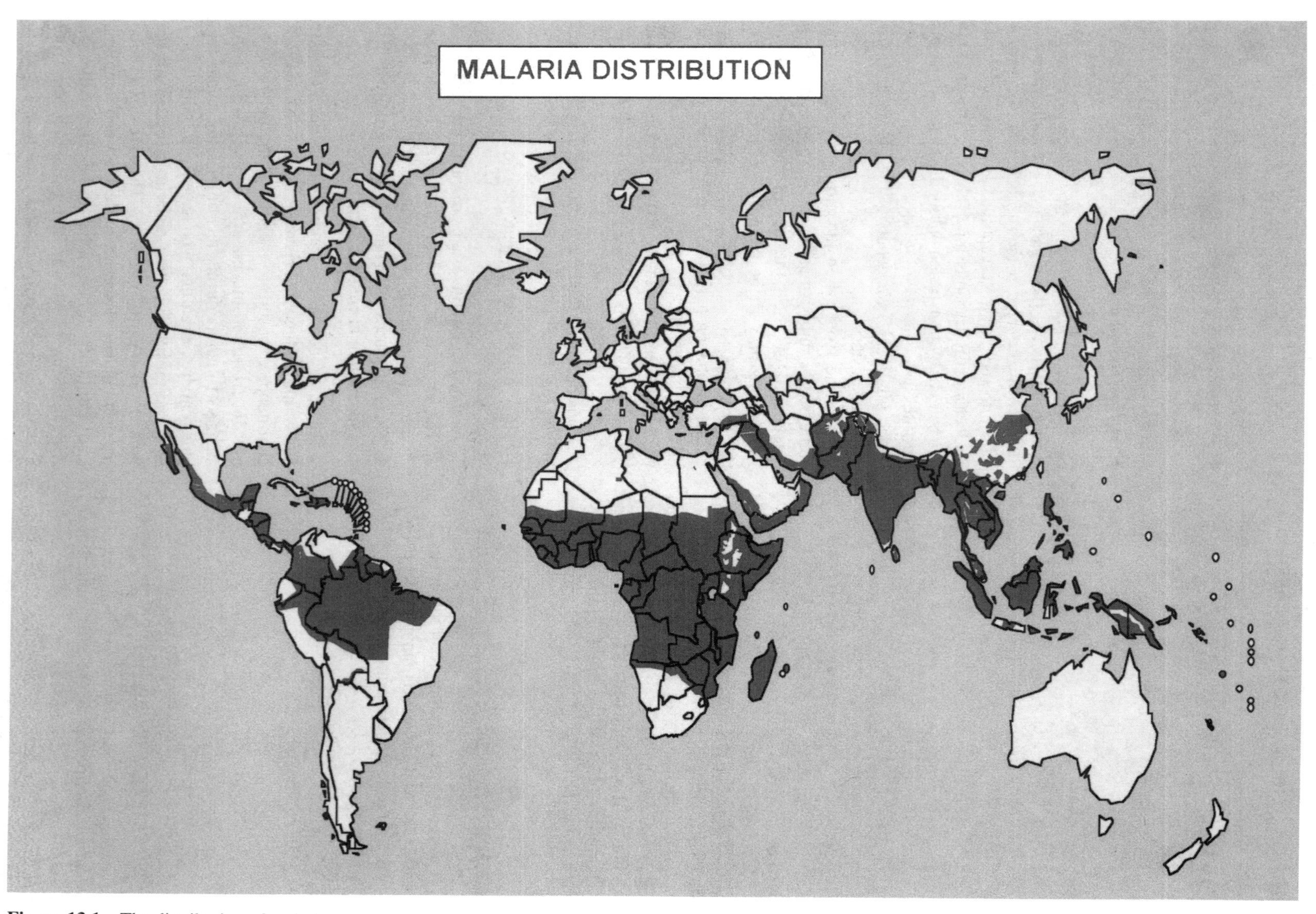

Figure 13.1 The distribution of malaria.
(Source: World Health Organization, WHO/CTD, 1998)

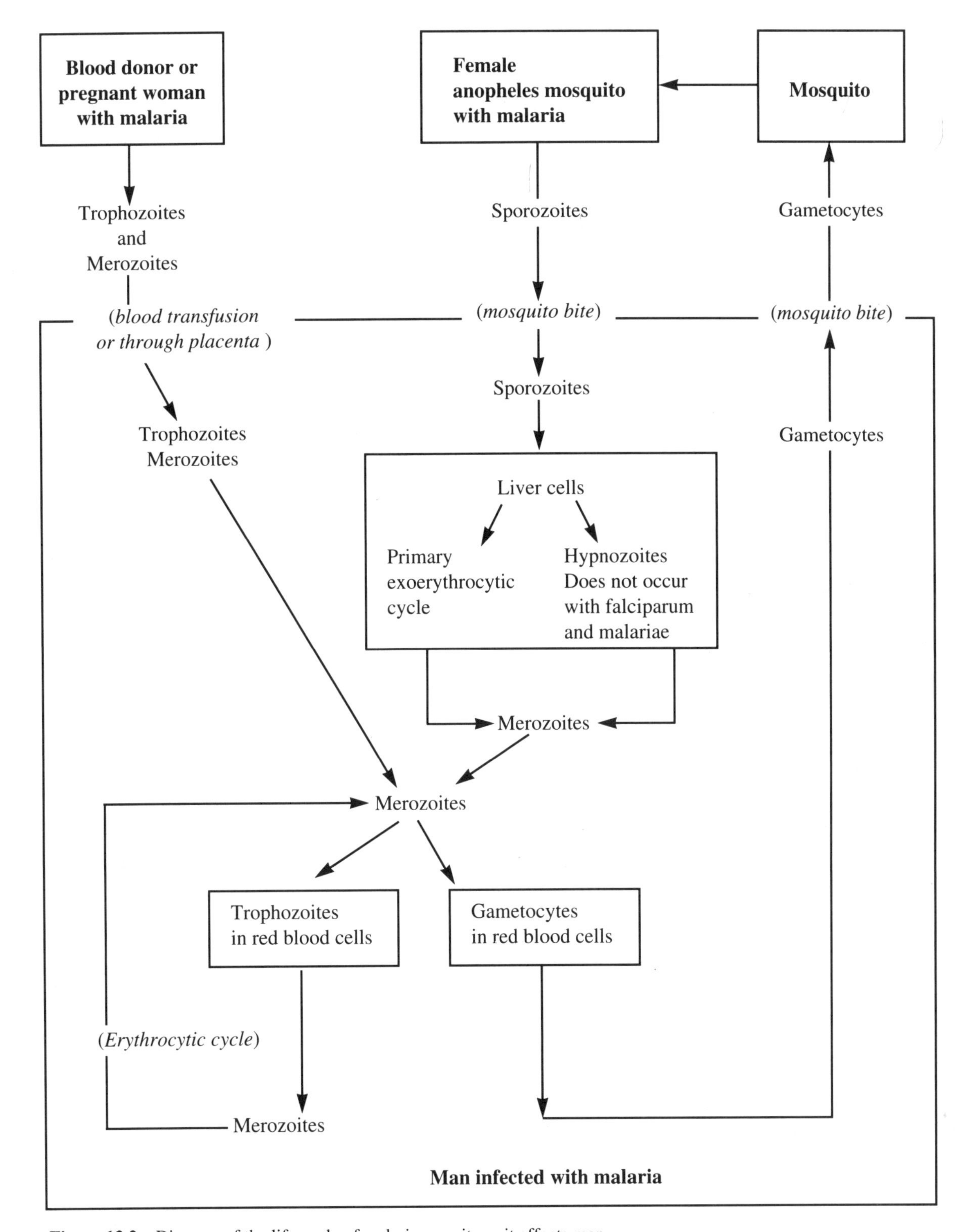

Figure 13.2 Diagram of the life cycle of malaria parasite as it affects man.

Other than these persons who have developed semi-immunity to malaria, all persons of all ages and both sexes are susceptible to malaria.

The persons most commonly affected by malaria are:

1. babies and children in areas where malaria is present all the time;
2. persons of all ages who come to malarial areas;
3. persons of all ages in areas where malaria can occur but where malaria is not present all the time if conditions suitable for transmission of malaria occur (temperature and rainfall change).

Immunity to malaria may be overcome by malaria parasites in the following situations:

1. during pregnancy (especially the last 3 months of pregnancy and especially in the first pregnancy);
2. during another illness;
3. if a person goes for a while with no malaria parasites present in his blood (e.g. the person has been taking antimalarials and stopped them; the person has been living in a screened house or dormitory; the person has been away from a malarial area, etc.);
4. if a person shifts to a place where there is more malaria or a different type of malaria;
5. if a person is given drugs such as cortisone or prednisolone which stop immunity working properly;
6. if the patient has his spleen removed.

Symptoms and signs, course and complications

Infection with malaria parasites can cause many different symptoms and signs and clinical states. Common clinical states include:

1. An acute attack of vivax (or malariae or ovale) malaria in a non-immune person.
2. An acute attack of falciparum malaria in a non-immune person. One of the nine common complications of acute malaria is likely to develop in non-immune patients with falciparum malaria.
3. Chronic malaria (in the years from the first infection until good semi-immunity has developed).
4. Malaria in semi-immunes.
5. Late complications of malaria.

Acute attack of vivax, malariae or ovale malaria in non-immune people

There may be a few hours to a few days of vague ill health (e.g. feeling cold, aches and pains, nausea, etc.) before any fever and severe disease. Attacks of fever then occur.

At first the patient is cold for $\frac{1}{4}$–1 hour and the temperature is not raised. The patient then starts to shiver and has a rigor and the temperature rises quickly up to about 40°C. The skin is cold and pale, the pulse fast and the BP often higher than normal. Vomiting, diarrhoea and urinary frequency are common.

Next, a hot stage comes for about an hour. The rigor stops, the patient feels hot, the skin feels hot and dry, the pulse is fast and the BP is often low. Headache, delirium, thirst and vomiting are common.

After this a sweating stage comes. The patient sweats a lot, the temperature falls, the pulse and BP become normal and after an hour or two the patient often goes to sleep. After waking the patient may feel reasonably well.

About a week later attacks of fever may come each third or fourth day. Until then they occur irregularly.

Jaundice may be seen after attacks of fever.

Anaemia, which causes pallor, gets worse after attacks of fever.

The spleen becomes enlarged and eventually becomes very big.

The liver enlarges but does not become very big.

If treatment is given, there is a good response to treatment within a few hours. Even without treatment the attacks of fever get less frequent. However, relapses occur (when a liver hypnozoite makes merozoites) after treatment of an acute attack.

Severe and fatal complications (see page 59) do not usually occur.

Chronic malaria (see page 60) then develops.

Acute attacks of falciparum malaria in non-immune people

The incubation period is usually 2 weeks. It can be longer; but it can also be as short as 8 days.

There may be some hours to a few days of vague ill-health (e.g. feeling cold; headache, backache and pains all over; nausea, vomiting and diarrhoea).

The attack then occurs. The attack may be like other forms of malaria. However, more often the attack does not have the three definite stages.

- In an attack the patient may appear to be very sick (as in any febrile illness).

- Pains in the head, bones and muscles are severe.
- Vomiting and diarrhoea are common.
- Mental confusion and delirium are common.
- The temperature is usually raised but rigors may not occur. Sometimes the temperature is normal. Most commonly the temperature is raised but it does not go away after an attack and may be continuous.
- Sweating is often severe.
- Pulse is usually fast.
- Blood pressure is often low.
- Respiration rate is usually fast.
- Anaemia develops quickly.
- Jaundice is sometimes present.
- The spleen is usually enlarged and tender.
- The liver is often enlarged.

If treatment is given there is usually a good response to it after a few hours.

If treatment is not given or if the treatment given is not correct or if the treatment is not given quickly enough, complications can occur and these include the following:

1. febrile fits (only in children), hyperpyrexia, (complications of fever, see this page);
2. convulsions, unconsciousness, paralysis, psychotic behaviour, etc. (cerebral malaria, see this page);
3. hypoglycaemia (low sugar (glucose) in blood);
4. acute anaemia and hypoxaemia ('anoxia'), (see page 60);
5. severe vomiting, diarrhoea and sometimes even dysentery, (gastrointestinal malaria, see page 60);
6. shock (see page 378);
7. malarial haemoglobinuria ('blackwater fever', see page 60);
8. respiratory symptoms and signs (pulmonary malaria, see page 60);
9. complicating bacterial infection (especially pneumonia, urinary tract infection and septicaemia).

Chronic malaria (see page 60) then develops if the patient does not die from an acute attack or from a complication.

Complications of falciparum malaria

Complications of fever. Febrile fit. Hyperpyrexia

Fever occurs in almost all cases of malaria.

In children, if the temperature rises very quickly, a febrile fit may occur. If the child is given an injection of an antimalarial drug and anticonvulsants and is cooled, the fitting will stop and the child will become fully conscious again. (Occasionally another fit can occur and the child not be fully conscious for an hour or so.) This is different from cerebral malaria (see below).

> Remember that all children who fit must have a lumbar puncture in case they have meningitis (as well as a blood slide taken for malaria parasites and an injection of an antimalarial drug).

Fever alone does not cause fitting in adults. *Adults do not have febrile fits.* All adults who fit must have a lumbar puncture in case they have meningitis (as well as a blood slide taken for malaria parasites, and an injection of an antimalarial drug).

Occasionally, in children and adults, the temperature rises above 40°C and stays there. This is called 'hyperpyrexia'. This is particularly dangerous if the patient stops sweating and the skin become dry. Cyanosis and mental disturbance may occur. The patient needs urgent cooling or he will become shocked and die.

Cerebral malaria

The malaria parasites may partly block the blood vessels going to the brain and may poison the brain with their toxins and cause an encephalitis (see Chapter 25 page 327). This condition is called cerebral malaria.

Cerebral malaria may cause all sorts of brain and mental symptoms and signs. These include those of depression of the brain functions such as severe headache, drowsiness, paralysis and unconsciousness. They also can include those of irritation of the brain functions such as restlessness, irritability, confusion, abnormal (psychotic) behaviour, twitching and fitting, etc. On examination, the patient is usually febrile, the neck is often stiff, the mental state is often abnormal and any of the above signs may be found.

> All patients in a malarious area
> - with a severe febrile illness for which no cause can be found, or
> - who are unconscious, or
> - who have had a fit, or
> - with a stiff neck, or
> - with an acute psychosis when not known to be previously psychotic,
>
> must have:
> 1. a lumbar puncture done,
> 2. a blood smear for malaria parasites made, and
> 3. full doses of injected antimalarials, preferably quinine.

The loss of consciousness from cerebral malaria may last for some days. Even after this, the patient may still make a full recovery.

Hypoglycaemia (low glucose in blood)
The blood sugar or glucose may become low in acute malaria. This happens especially if the malaria is severe or if the patient is pregnant or a child or if treatment is given with quinine. The low blood glucose can cause loss of consciousness or fitting.

Acute anaemia and hypoxia
Acute severe anaemia with hypoxia (symptoms and signs of a low oxygen level in the brain and the rest of the body) can occur in those who have a low haemoglobin level (usually below 5 g/dl) and who then develop an acute attack of malaria. More red blood cells are destroyed and the anaemia rapidly becomes worse. Poisons from the malaria parasites stop the body cells using what little oxygen is brought by the anaemic blood ('hypoxia' – little oxygen in the tissues). Death can occur quickly from lack of oxygen in the brain and other tissues of the body.

> Any patient in a malarious areas who is very pale and develops acute malaria needs urgent treatment for the malaria and an urgent blood transfusion.

Gastrointestinal malaria
The patient with malaria may develop repeated vomiting, diarrhoea with large volumes of watery stools, or even rarely dysentery. This loss of fluid may lead to dehydration and death.

> Any patient in a malarious area who develops gastroenteritis or dysentery needs a smear for malaria parasites taken, an injection of an antimalarial drug as well as fluids orally or IV.

Shock ('algid malaria')
The patient with malaria may become shocked with a fast pulse and a low blood pressure. The skin may feel cold but the body temperature, if taken with the thermometer in the rectum, is high. This may occur with or without vomiting and diarrhoea.

Malarial haemoglobinuria ('blackwater fever')
Malarial haemoglobinuria is very rare. It can occur in persons who have recently moved into the malarious area or have come back to the area or persons who have had irregular antimalarial drugs especially quinine. It can, however, occur in persons without either of these. Due to an abnormal immune reaction, many red blood cells are haemolysed (i.e. broken open and destroyed). Haemoglobin from inside the broken red cells is then free in the blood. This haemoglobin is also passed in the urine which becomes red or brown or black (see Chapter 26 page 355).

The patient may become very anaemic because the red cells are destroyed. Also haemoglobin free in the blood (and not in the red blood cells) is very poisonous to the body and especially the kidney. The patient may become shocked and develop kidney failure (when he will pass only a very little urine which is red or brown and has a lot of protein in it). Unless he is given urgent treatment, he will die of the anaemia, the shock or later the kidney failure.

Pulmonary malaria (pulmonary oedema)
The respiration rate is usually raised in malaria. In severe cases there may be some respiratory distress. Occasionally, a cough may occur and some crackles may be found in the chest.

> *Never* assume that chest symptoms or signs are due to malaria alone. They always must be treated as due to bacterial infections and the patient given antibiotics as well as antimalarials.

Chronic malaria (before immunity is fully developed)

Chronic malaria occurs in persons from the time they are infected with malaria until the time they become semi-immune, i.e. until they develop enough immunity against malaria to overcome most of the malaria parasites and most of the effects of the malaria parasites, most of the time.

This may take 4–10 years. Some people never develop enough immunity and continue to have chronic malaria all their lives.

Symptoms and signs of chronic malaria include:

1. recurrent attacks of acute malaria,
2. anaemia,

3. enlarged spleen,
4. enlarged liver,
5. poor appetite and other gastrointestinal symptoms and signs,
6. wasting of muscles (abdomen often very enlarged in comparison),
7. reduced resistance to other diseases especially recurrent attacks of bacterial infections and gastroenteritis.

The above are especially severe in children and often lead to death.

Malaria in persons with immunity ('semi-immunes')

1. Irregular short attacks of malaise, headaches, backaches, loss of appetite, fever and sweating occur.
2. Mild anaemia may be present all the time.

Late complications of malaria

After many years a few patients may develop the following:

1. hyperreactive malarious splenomegaly or tropical splenomegaly syndrome (see Chapter 21 page 243), or
2. nephrotic syndrome (see Chapter 26 page 356).

Tests

1. Make a blood smear for malaria parasites from all patients with fever or suspected malaria (see Appendix 1, page 68).
2. Do a haemoglobin estimation on anyone who is pale (see Chapter 21 page 248).

Diagnostic features

1. Fever (*all* patients with fever must be treated with antimalarials unless it can be proved that they do not have malaria).
2. Anaemia (*all* patients with anaemia must be treated with antimalarials unless it can be proved that they do not have malaria).
3. Splenomegaly (in non-immunes).

Management

Management may include five things:

1. Give antimalarial drugs (see page below).
   Chloroquine for 3 days – if usual case.
   Quinine for 3 days *then also* pyrimethamine and sulphadoxine once or doxycycline for one week or continue quinine for one more week
   - *if* chloroquine resistant malaria proven or possible or
   - *if* a complication especially cerebral malaria or shock.

   Use oral tablets usually.
   Use injection if:
   - unconscious or fitting, or
   - vomiting or severe diarrhoea, or
   - shock.

   See page 62 for which drugs to give by what route.
2. Treat symptoms (see page 65).
3. Treat complications (see page 65).
4. Do not give primaquine also unless in special areas and also the Medical Officer tells you to.
5. Give drugs for prophylaxis only if needed (see page 66).

Note on antimalarial drugs and[1] chloroquine resistant malaria organisms

Drugs for malaria include those listed below. Some are very expensive or not available. The most suitable drugs and doses for your area will have been worked out by your Health Department and you must follow your Health Department's recommendations.

Those drugs marked with an asterisk (*) are the ones often used in health centres.

1. Quinolone related drugs
   - chloroquine* tablets or injection
   - amodiaquine tablets
   - quinine* tablets or injection
   - quinidine tablets or injection
   - mefloquine tablets (e.g. Lariam, Mephaquin)
   - halofantrine tablets (e.g. Halfan)

1 For chloroquine resistance, see Appendix 3, page 72.

- primaquine tablets
- atovaquone (with proguanil, e.g. Malarone) tablets

2. Antifolate drugs
   - pyrimethamine* tablets (combined with another drug, e.g. Fansidar if combined with sulfadoxine and Maloprim if combined with dapsone)
   - proguanil tablets
   - chlorproguanil tablets
   - trimethoprim* tablets or injection (also combined with another drug usually sulphamethoxazole as co-trimoxazole (in e.g. Septrin or Bactrim) and this then combined with another drug)
3. Artemisinin/qinghaosu
   - artemisine* tablets and suppositories
   - artemether IM injection
   - artesunate tablets and IV injection
4. Antibacterial drug with antimalarial actions
   - sulphonamides* (e.g. sulfadoxine or sulphamethoxazole) tablets or injection and sulphones (e.g. dapsone)
   - tetracyclines* (e.g. tetracycline, doxycycline) tablets or caps
   - macrolides (e.g. erythromycin, roxithromycin) tablets or injection
   - quinolones

Chloroquine at present is still the best drug to use for malaria.

In many parts of the world however many strains of *P. falciparum* have become resistant to chloroquine. Also, in some parts of the Pacific and Asia, some strains of *P. vivax* have become resistant to chloroquine. These strains of *P. falciparum* and *P. vivax*, however, are usually sensitive to quinine. However, quinine would need to be given for 7(–14) days to kill all the parasites. To make the treatment shorter, 3–5 day courses of quinine are followed by 1 dose of pyrimethamine and sulphadoxine. If there is resistance of the malarial organisms to pyrimethamine and sulphadoxine the quinine is followed by a course of tetracycline or doxycycline.

Quinine is a quick acting drug as well as very effective against chloroquine-resistant malaria. Quinine is therefore always used in cases such as cerebral malaria where you have to be sure:

1. the drug will be effective, and
2. action will be quick.

Artemisinin is a drug which probably soon will become more and more available. Suppositories are quick acting and effective. Especially where injection of quinine is not immediately possible, artemisinin suppositories may be the best immediate treatment; being followed, of course, by further artemisinin suppositories or tablets and then, as with quinine, by pyrimethamine and sulphadoxine or doxycycline. Artemether IM injection or artesunate IV injection or tablets may at some time replace quinine.

For details about chloroquine resistant malaria and for further details about some of the presently available antimalarial drugs, see Appendices 2 and 3 pages 70 and 72.

Note

- Tetracycline and doxycycline should not be used at any time during pregnancy or in childhood.
- Sulphadoxine and sulfamethoxazole should not be used just before delivery.
- Halofantrine should not be used at any time in pregnancy.
- Mefloquine and artemisinin/artemether/artesunate should not be given in the first 3–4 months of pregnancy.

Note on management of malaria

All patients with a fever who are in or who are from areas where malaria occurs are assumed to have malaria unless it can be proved otherwise. *But always look for other causes*, especially severe infections. Always do a full history and examination and test the urine.

Even if there appears to be another cause of fever, *treat all such patients with a fever with a full treatment course of antimalarials unless it can be proved that they do not have malaria.* Treat any other cause as well.

Admit for inpatient treatment if there is a severe attack or a complication.

Treat as an outpatient in a mild attack.

Give antimalarial drugs

Choose drugs according to severity of attack.

- Usual attack. See next page about oral chloroquine.
- Usual attack with vomiting or diarrhoea.

See page next page about IMI chloroquine.

- Usual attack but not cured by chloroquine. See next page about oral pyrimethamine and sulfadoxine or quinine and doxycycline.

- Severe attack if patient in or from an area where chloroquine-resistant malaria common. See page 64 about oral or IMI quinine and oral pyrimethamine and sulfadoxine or doxycycline.
- Patient unconscious or fitting or shocked or very 'sick'. See page 64 about IMI or IVI quinine or rectal or IMI artemisinin and treatment of complications.

Usual attack. No vomiting. No diarrhoea.

Give oral chloroquine

- Give 10 **mg/kg** of the base immediately;
  if cannot weigh patient
  small adult (< 50 kg) – 400 mg
  large adult (> 50 kg) – 600 mg.
- Give 5 mg/kg of the base 6 hours later;
  if cannot weigh patient
  small adult (< 50 kg) – 200 mg
  large adult (> 50 kg) – 300 mg.
- Give 5 mg/kg the following day – see above.
- Give 5 mg/kg the following day – see above.
- Give therefore 25 mg/kg over 3 days.

If the patient immediately vomits the tablets, give the same dose again; but do not repeat the dose if the patient vomits more than $\frac{1}{4}$ of an hour later; but if nausea still present when the next dose is due, start with the first dose of IM chloroquine.

In many health centre areas the dose of chloroquine as above may be too complicated for your staff and your patients to remember. A very simple dose (Table 13.1) was used for many years in Papua New Guinea and has been effective and safe and easy for staff and patients.

Table 13.1 Chloroquine dosage.

	Using 150 mg base/tablet		
Size of adult	Dose on Day 1	Dose on Day 2	Dose on Day 3
Small (less than 50 kg)	3 tablets	3 tablets	3 tablets
Large (more than 50 kg)	4 tablets	4 tablets	4 tablets

You, however, will have to follow the rules laid down by the Health Department where you work.

Usual attack but vomiting or diarrhoea

Give IM chloroquine.

When possible use oral instead of IM chloroquine.
Do not give both oral and IM chloroquine at the same time to a patient.

Give 3.5 mg chloroquine base/kg patient's body weight (maximum dose 200 mg) each dose.

The dose if you cannot weigh the patient is:

- small adult (< 50 kg) – 150 mg
- large adult (> 50 kg) – 200 mg

After 6 hours if the patient cannot take oral chloroquine, repeat the *same* dose of IM chloroquine. However, if patient can take oral drugs, give the first dose of the three daily doses of chloroquine tablets instead (see above).

If the patient still cannot take oral chloroquine, then, instead of the once daily dose of tablets, give IM chloroquine each 6 hours. Use the *same* IM dose (see above). As soon as possible change to oral chloroquine.

Stop chloroquine after a total of 25 mg/kg of treatment, i.e. after 7th dose or after 36 hours.

Usual attack not cured by chloroquine

1. Check that the correct dose of chloroquine was ordered.
2. Check that the chloroquine was ordered for the correct length of time – 7 doses for IMI *or* 3 days if orally.
3. Check that *every* dose of the chloroquine was really given.
4. Check that the chloroquine was absorbed (i.e. was not vomited and that the patient did not have diarrhoea if oral treatment was given).
5. Look carefully for other causes of fever and treat any found.

If the correct dose of chloroquine was not properly given for the correct time, *then* give the correct dose properly for the correct time.

If the correct dose of chloroquine was properly given, *then* make another smear for malaria and treat as chloroquine-resistant malaria with pyrimethamine 25 mg and sulfadoxine 500 mg tablets (e.g. Fansidar).

- Small adult (< 50 kg) $2\frac{1}{2}$ tabs
- Large adult (> 50 kg) 3 tabs
- Give one dose only.
- Do not give if pregnant.
- Do not give if resistance to these drugs known in the area but instead treat as follows:

If the patient is not cured by chloroquine then pyrimethamine and sulfadoxine or

If it is known that *P. falciparum* malaria is resistant to pyrimethamine and sulfadoxine or it is known that the organism is *P. vivax* resistant to chloroquine, then treat with both:

1. quinine (see below) and
2. doxycycline for one week in all patients but not if pregnant (see below).

Some health centres may be instructed to try mefloquine before quinine and doxycycline.

Severe attack if patient in or from an area where chloroquine-resistant malaria common

1. Make a (or another) blood smear for malaria parasites.
2. Look carefully for other causes of fever and treat any you find.
3. *If* the blood smear shows trophozoites ('troph' or 'T') or *if* the blood smear result is not immediately available *then* give quinine 10 mg/kg patient's body weight twice or three times daily for 3 days.

Give quinine orally if possible (quinine sulphate 300 mg).

Give quinine by IMI if vomiting or diarrhoea or very sick (quinine dihydrochloride 300 mg/ml (600 mg in 2 ml amps)). Change back to oral quinine as soon as the patient can take oral drugs.

The dose of quinine is:

- small adult (< 50 kg) – 450 mg each 8–12 hours
- large adult (> 50 kg) – 600 mg each 8–12 hours

Quinine is given twice daily in areas where the malaria organisms are known to be very sensitive to quinine but otherwise three times a day.

The dose of quinine will be reduced to half of the above if the patient is very sick or jaundiced or has kidney (renal) failure or develops side effects of quinine. If the patient is semi-immune, 3 days of treatment with quinine may be enough, otherwise 7 days or other drugs are needed.

If the patient is not immune or is pregnant and is unable to take any other drugs, it would be safer to give quinine for 10 (or even 14) days.

Then, after the 3 days of quinine, give *also* one of the following:

1. One dose only of pyrimethamine 25 mg and sulfadoxine 500 mg tablets (e.g. Fansidar tablets):
   - small adult (< 50 kg) – $2\frac{1}{2}$ tabs
   - large adult (> 50 kg) – 3 tabs

   but not if pregnant or if malaria in the area is resistant to these drugs.
2. If there is *P. falciparum* resistance to pyrimethamine and sulfadoxine as well as chloroquine, or it is known that the organism is *P. vivax* resistant to chloroquine, give instead:
   - doxycycline 2.5 mg/kg daily (200 mg daily) *or*
   - tetracycline 4 mg/kg 4 times a day (250 mg 4 times a day) and continue for 7 days but not if pregnant.
3. Continue quinine tablets for a total of 10–14 days (usual treatment if pregnant).

> A 3-day course of quinine must ALWAYS be followed by one of the above even if the patient seems to be cured by 3 days of quinine.

Patient unconscious or fitting or shocked or very 'sick'

Give quinine dihydrochloride (300 mg/ml) (600 mg in 2 ml amp) by IMI or by SLOW IV drip (see page 73), 10 mg/kg each 8 hours. The dose, if the patient cannot be weighed, is:

- small adult (< 50 kg) – 450 mg
- large adult (> 50 kg) – 600 mg

The drip should run for over 4 hours. Use 5% dextrose in the drip.

> IMI is usually the easiest method for giving quinine in a health centre. IV drip is however needed for giving quinine if the patient is shocked. (See Appendix 4 page 73 for method).

If chloroquine has already been given, give no more chloroquine and immediately start the quinine. Do not continue to give chloroquine as well as quinine to a patient.

See previous section for details about continuation of quinine in the drip or IMI injections; change to oral quinine; and then addition of other drugs. These things are essential.

If quinine injection is not available:

1. give artemisinin injections;
   or if not available:
   give artemisinin suppositories;
   or if not available:
2. give chloroquine injections and
   give pyrimethamine and sulfadoxine
   injection *or* if not available
   put down an intra-gastric tube and:
   (a) give pyrimethamine and sulfadoxine, and
   (b) start doxycycline or tetracycline, and
   (c) change IM chloroquine to quinine through the tube but only if or when not shocked and no vomiting and no diarrhoea;
   (d) transfer urgently (emergency).

If no injections possible:

1. give artemisinin suppositories;
   or if not possible:
2. put down an intra-gastric tube and through this tube:
   (a) give pyrimethamine and sulfadoxine tablets crushed one dose,
   (b) start quinine tablets crushed 8th hourly,
   (c) start doxycycline tablets twice daily or tetracycline tablets crushed four times daily,
   (d) transfer urgently (emergency).

Treat the symptoms

- Rest
- Pain – aspirin 600–1200 mg (2–4 tabs) 4th hourly if needed. Give no more than 4 g in 24 hours.
- Fever – aspirin and sponge or wrap in wet sheet and fan.
- Vomiting many times – chlorpromazine 0.5 mg ($\frac{1}{2}$ mg)/kg IMI once (dose in ml is patient's weight in kg divided by 2 with maximum dose 25 mg (1 ml)). Do not give if systolic blood pressure < 80.

Treat any complications

Cerebral malaria

Give quinine by IMI or by *slow* IV drip (see above and Appendix 4 page 73) immediately.

Do lumbar puncture *always*.

Treat for meningitis also if CSF is not clear or is bloody or is not obtained (failed LP) (see Chapter 25 page 323).

Paraldehyde 5–10 ml deep IMI; or diazepam 5–10 mg over 2–4 minutes if convulsions. (Then see Chapter 25 page 325.)

Give glucose 1 ml/kg if blood glucose test shows glucose less than 2.2 mmol/ml or 40 mg/dl or if test not available. Repeat each 4 hours.

Care of unconscious patient (see Chapter 25 page 332).

If not improved in 24 hours do a repeat lumbar puncture. If CSF still clear continue treatment. If CSF not clear or is bloody or is not obtained (failed LP) treat for meningitis also.

When unconsciousness lasts more than 24 hours transfer to Medical Officer care.

Acute severe anaemia

If Hb less than 5 g/dl and malaria (fever), transfer urgently (emergency) for blood transfusion.

Give IM antimalarials first if vomiting of oral antimalarial drugs is likely during transfer.

Gastroenteritis or dysentery

IV fluids as for dehydration (see Chapter 23 page 285).

Give IM chloroquine or IM quinine.

Shock

Give quinine by slow IV drip (see Appendix 4 page 73).

IV fluids in another drip as for shock (see Chapter 27 page 378).

Blackwater fever

Do *not* give quinine. Give instead IM or rectal artemisinin or if not available IM chloroquine.

Immediate treatment for shock or acute kidney failue if present. Transfer urgently (emergency) to Medical Officer care.

Very high fever

Up to 40°C:

- Aspirin 600–1200 mg (2–4 tablets) 4th hourly if needed. No more than 4 grams in 24 hours.
- Sponge or wrap in wet sheet. Fan.

Above 40°C:

- Emergency – as above and wrap in a wet sheet, repeatedly wet the sheet and fan vigorously.

- IMI chlorpromazine 0.5 mg ($\frac{1}{2}$ mg)/kg (maximum 25 mg or 1 ml).
- Watch carefully for shock and treat if it occurs (see Chapter 27 page 378).
- When improved and treatment stopped, watch carefully for rise in temperature again which needs treatment again.

Give IMI, not oral, antimalarials.

Hyperreactive malarious splenomegaly or tropical splenomegaly syndrome

See Chapter 21 page 243.

> *If* the patient is very sick or unconscious *then* treat this patient with quinine (not chloroquine) by IMI or by slow IV drip.
> This is especially important:
> *If* the patient is in or is from an area where chloroquine-resistant malaria occurs, *or*
> *If* the patient has not responded to chloroquine already given.

> *If* the patient is very ill or shocked and has some history or some signs that suggest he may have an acute severe bacterial infection: *then* treat for septicaemia too (see Chapter 12).

Transfer to Medical Officer care

This is required only *if* complications occur *and* if is not possible to treat the complications properly in the health centre, e.g.:

1. cerebral malaria with unconsciousness which has lasted more than 1 day;
2. acute anaemia (Hb less than 5 g/dl and fever);
3. shock which cannot be corrected;
4. blackwater fever.

Prevention and control

Eradication is not possible in most areas.

The best methods of control for your area will have been worked out by your Health Department. You need to follow their policy. It may include the following.

Eliminate reservoir. Stop transmission.

Killing all the malarial parasites in the bodies of all the original hosts (by giving antimalarial drugs, including primaquine to kill gametocytes, to all of the population until all mosquitoes carrying malaria have died) is not possible in most areas.

A previous eradication programme depended on spraying all indoor surfaces of all dwellings regularly with DDT or another residual insecticide. Anopheles mosquitoes bite at night when most people are indoors or near a house. After feeding, the mosquito likes to rest on a wall, which should have been covered with insecticide. Before there was time for the malaria to develop in the mosquito, the insecticide was to have killed the mosquito. The aim of spraying was to kill all anopheles mosquitoes that had bitten human beings in their houses (the aim of spraying was not to kill all mosquitoes). Unfortunately for many reasons this method has failed in most areas.

However bites from anopheles mosquitoes which are usually at night, can be reduced greatly by the following:

1. Cover the body with clothing, e.g. long-sleeved shirts and long trousers to be put on as daylight goes.
2. Use insect repellents (DEET) on uncovered areas, e.g. face and hands
3. Use insect screens on windows and doors.
4. Use insecticides in the house or at least burn 'mosquito coils'.
5. Use insecticide-treated (e.g. permethrin) nets to cover people at night when sleeping. (See Appendix 5 page 74 for ways to prepare these nets.)

In some areas methods may be able to be used to decrease the number of mosquitoes, e.g. drain breeding sites, introduce fish which eat mosquito larvae, put things on the surface of the water to kill larvae, etc.

Raise the resistance of susceptible persons

This is not possible; but immunisation with a malaria vaccine is the main hope for control of this disease for the future. At present a number of vaccines are under trial.

Prophylactic treatment

Regular prophylactic antimalarial drugs will stop the development of malaria parasites in the blood (trophozoites). They will therefore prevent clinical malaria. But they will also prevent the development of semi-immunity to malaria. And after a variable period of time (often about a year) they will cause the loss of any existing semi-immunity to malaria.

Prophylactic antimalarial drugs are therefore given only to certain groups of people.

1. People who
   - have no immunity to malaria, *and*
   - have come to a malarious area, *and* who
   - do not need to develop semi-immunity to malaria (e.g. they will not live in the malarious area for the rest of their lives or for many years), *or*
   - do not wish to suffer the ill-health needed to develop semi-immunity to malaria, i.e. chronic malaria with repeated acute attacks of malaria for 4–10 years (see page 55); although the danger and severity of this ill-health can be greatly reduced by quick correct treatment of any acute attack which occurs.

   This group will include:
   (a) adults from areas where malaria does not occur,
   (b) adults from areas where the same kind of malaria is not present all the time,
   (c) children under 6 years; but only in *some* countries (after the age of 6 the children can clearly complain of the symptoms of malaria and be given quick drug treatment of the acute attack and are then allowed to develop chronic malaria and semi-immunity).

2. People who do have some immunity to malaria but this immunity is reduced for a while due to another condition.
   This group will include:
   (a) women when they are pregnant;
   (b) people sick from another illness, e.g. pneumonia (stop antimalarials as soon as the pneumonia is cured) or anaemia (stop antimalarials as soon as haemoglobin is 10 g/dl).

3. People who cannot develop normal immunity to malaria. This group will include:
   (a) patients with hyper-reactive malarious splenomegaly or tropical splenomegaly syndrome;
   (b) possibly people who have had their spleens removed.

Chloroquine (300 mg) (2 tablets) each week is used for adults in most areas.

In some countries in areas where 10–20% of falciparum parasites are resistant to chloroquine, it has been made a policy to give pyrimethamine 12.5 mg and dapsone 100 mg combined in one table (e.g. Maloprim) one tablet each week. However, before you give this drug, check that it is policy to do so in your area. Also check whether it is safe for you to give it to women who are, or may be, pregnant. This drug also may not always prevent attacks of vivax malaria and chloroquine may have to be taken as well. Doxycycline is an alternative to pyrimethamine and dapsone and may be more effective and safer but should not be given to pregnant women or children as severe teeth discoloration and deformities may occur. The dose is 100 mg daily.

For most people who live all their lives in areas where malaria is endemic, they are best to develop semi-immunity by not taking prophylaxis all the time. Any acute attack of malaria should be treated fully and immediately before it becomes severe or complicated. By doing this, they can slowly build up their immunity and not risk dying from an acute attack in the meantime. If people live far from health care, they will need to be supplied with drugs and taught how to use them. These drugs may be chloroquine or other drugs for chloroquine resistant malaria. They also may include artemisinin suppositories for treatment of those who cannot swallow. Your Health Department will give you instructions about this.

Appendix 1 Malaria blood smear

You should take a blood smear for examination for malaria parasites ('MPs') from all patients who have a fever. Even though you usually cannot examine the slide in the health centre you should still take one. At the end of the month you should send all the slides to the Malaria Control Office. This will help them tell how much malaria and what kind of malaria is occurring in the area.

Method of making malaria blood films

Both thick and thin blood films are used to detect and identify malaria parasites. These are usually made on the same frosted ended slide. See Chapter 6 page 23 for details.

1. For best results make a spreader. Break off the corners of a glass slide making sure that the edge of the slide is smooth. It must not be chipped or rough because this will spoil the thin blood film.

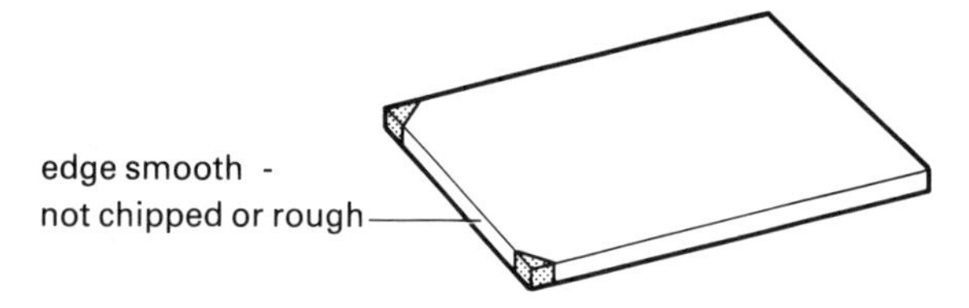

2. Imagine that the non-frosted area of a standard clean slide is composed of three equal parts.

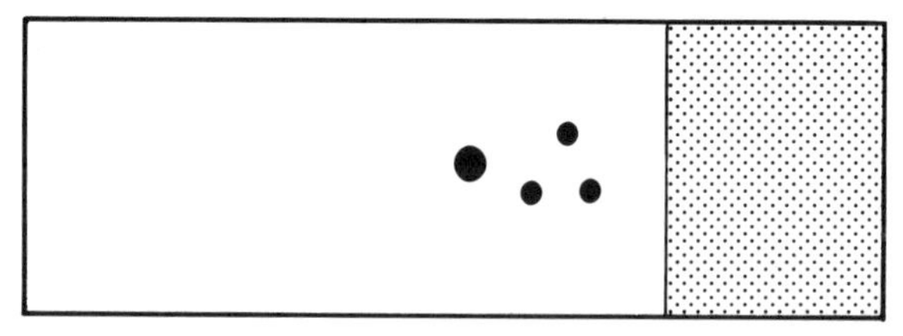

3a. Put one large or preferably three small drops of blood in the middle of the part nearest the frosted end.

3b. Put one small drop of blood at the beginning of the next part.

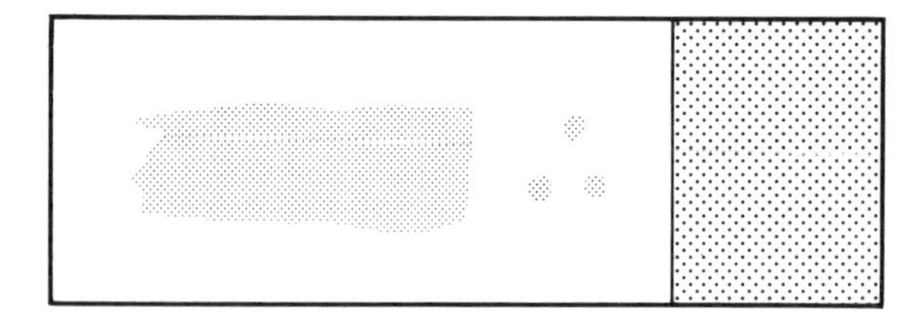

4. Bring the edge of a second slide to contact the surface of the blood slide just in front of the one drop of blood – push this spreader slide backwards until it just touches the drop of blood, which will then spread along its edge.

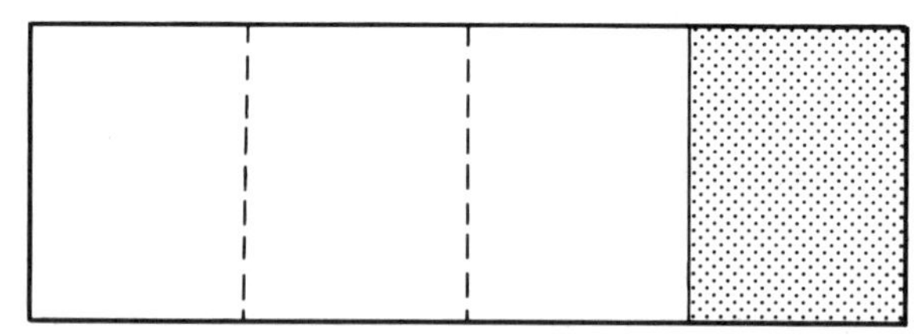

5. Hold at an angle of 45° and spread the drop of blood by pushing the spreader forward. (See Chapter 6 page 23 for details.)

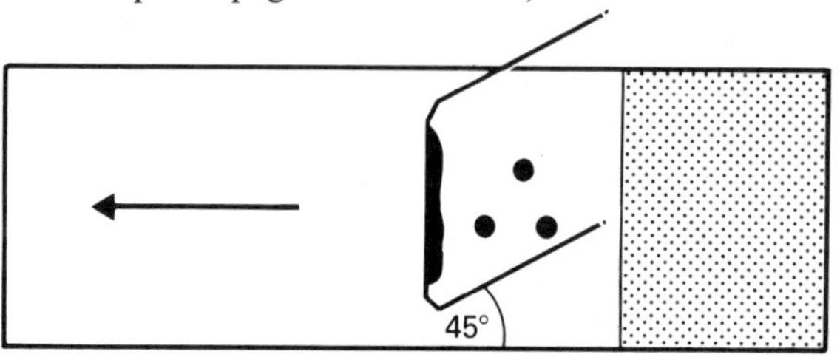

6. With the corner of the spreader slide, spread the 3 drops to form a circular thick film about 1 cm in diameter. Spread the blood evenly. If you can just see the print of a newspaper through it, the smear is the right thickness.

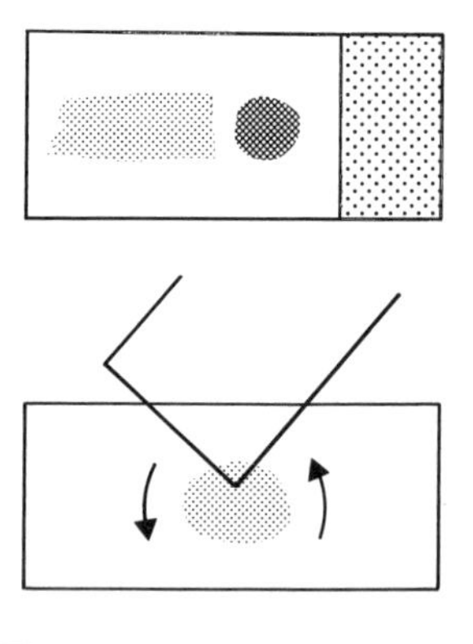

IF YOU CAN READ THE TYPE. THEN THE BLOOD FILM IS TOO THIN

IF YOU C
THE TYPE.
THE BL
OO THICK

IF YOU CAN JUST SEE THE TYPE.
THE BLOOD FILM IS CORRECT

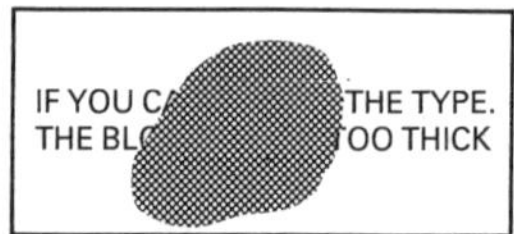

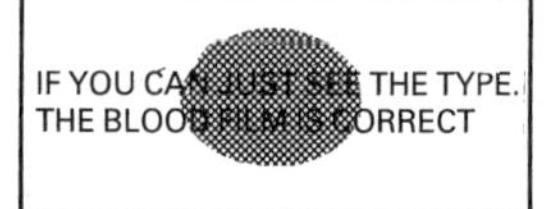

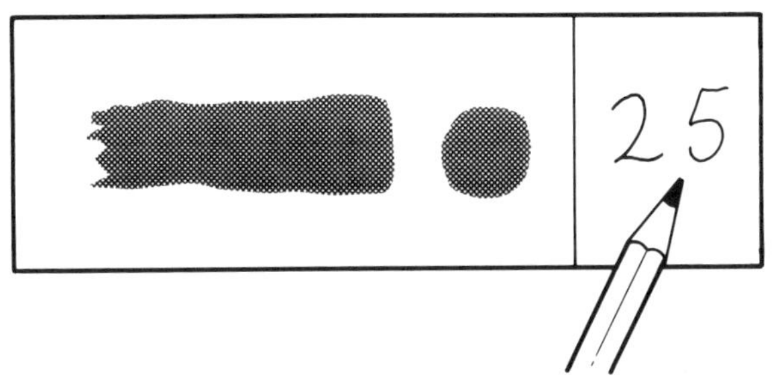

7. Leave the slide flat so that the thick film will dry evenly. Use a pencil to write the slide number on the frosted end of the slide.

Interpretation of reports of malaria smears

A report of 'negative' means that after the examination of 100 high power fields under the microscope, no malaria parasites were seen. Therefore it is very unlikely that the patient's illness is caused by malaria.

If malaria parasites are found, the number of parasites per field is counted and recorded like this:

1. If the number of parasites in an average field is higher than 20 (e.g. 43) only one field is counted and the total number of parasites reported (e.g. 43/1).
2. If the number of parasites present in an average field is between 3 and 19, (e.g. 14) then ten fields are counted, and the total number of parasites reported (e.g. 140/10).
3. If the number of parasites present in an average field is less than 3 (e.g. 1 or 2) in most fields, then 100 fields are counted and the total number reported (e.g. 120/100).

If mixed infections are found, then each species is reported separately.

Trophozoites and *P. falciparum* gametocytes are reported separately.

The presence of trophozoites or gametocytes shows infection with malaria parasites. But only trophozoites harm humans. Trophozoites indicate the patient's illness may be caused by malaria. Gametocytes do not harm humans. The presence of gametocytes in the blood does *not* suggest that the patient's illness may be caused by malaria. Chloroquine treatment may cure a patient of falciparum malaria and trophozoites will disappear from his blood within one week. However, as chloroquine does not kill *P. falciparum* gametocytes, the smear may show gametocytes for another 3–4 months although the patient is cured. The gametocytes are however infectious for mosquitoes.

Trophozoites ('Troph' or 'T') present in a slide mean the patient may be sick with malaria.

Gametocytes ('G') do not mean the patient may be sick with malaria (but the patient can pass on the disease to mosquitoes).

A more accurate method of estimating parasite density is to estimate the number of parasites present in 1 cubic mm of blood (1 microlitre of blood). When examining the film, the laboratory worker counts 200 white cells and all the parasites present in the fields which contained the 200 white cells. He then multiplies the number of parasites by 40 (as there are about 8000 white cells per cubic mm) to give the number of parasites per cubic mm. Again mixed infections are reported separately, and trophozoites and *P. falciparum* gametocytes are reported separately.

Another method of recording parasite density is as follows:

- Fewer than 10 parasites in 100 fields. +
- More than 10 parasites but fewer than 100 parasites in 100 fields. + +
- More than 100 parasites in 100 fields but fewer than 10 parasites in 1 field. + + +
- More than 10 parasites in one field. + + + +

Again, mixed infections are reported separately and trophozoites and *P. falciparum* gametocytes are reported separately.

Appendix 2 Drugs used for treatment of malaria

Quinolone related drugs

Chloroquine tablets, syrup and injection

Dose is ordered in mg of chloroquine base (not in mg of sulphate or phosphate salt).

Many different strengths and sizes of tablets or injections are available.

As chloroquine overdose is likely to be fatal, ensure the correct dose is ordered and the correct strength of tablets or strength of injection is used.

- Tablet – 75 mg, 100 mg, 150 mg, 200 mg of chloroquine base and 300 mg of hydroxychloroquine as sulphate or (di)phosphate.
- Syrup – 10 mg base/ml as sulphate.
- Injection – 40 mg base/ml as sulphate; 50 mg base/ml as diphosphate.
- Chloroquine by IMI or IV drip
  100 mg base/ml as diphosphate.

IMI chloroquine base dose is 3.5 mg/kg body weight (maximum dose 200 mg) give immediately and give every 6 hours until a total dose of 25 mg is given, i.e. 7 doses over 32 hours.

If the chloroquine has to be given intravenously (e.g. shock) then:
10 mg/kg (maximum 600 mg) in normal saline slowly over no less than 8–16 hours then:
5 mg/kg (maximum 300 mg) over 8 hours starting on the 16th hour until total dose of 25 mg/kg given, i.e. 32 hours.

However most cases who are this sick should be given quinine instead.

As soon as the patient can swallow and has no diarrhoea or vomiting and is not shocked, change to oral chloroquine. Oral chloroquine is just as effective and is safer and easier.

If the patient cannot be weighed:

- Small adult (< 50 kg) – 200 mg each 8 hours.
- Large adult (> 50 kg) – 300 mg each 8 hours.

Chloroquine by mouth – see Chapter 13 page 63.

Side effects of chloroquine include nausea, vomiting, visual disturbances, itch not helped by antihistamines, fall in blood pressure and rarely other conditions. Regular use over years can cause eye problems.

Amodiaquine tablets and syrup

Amodiaquine is similar in action and dose to chloroquine. It may be more effective than chloroquine against resistant organisms. However if used for a long time it can occasionally cause fatal blood disorders. It is therefore not much used now.

Quinine tablets and injection

Dose is usually ordered in mg of the salt but can be ordered in the mg of base (Table 13.2).

The tablets come in two sizes and the injections in two or three strengths.

- Tablets
  300 mg sulphate or bisulphate,
  200 mg sulphate or bisulphate.
- Injections
  300 mg/ml dihydrochloride,
  150 mg/ml dihydrochloride,
  60 mg/ml dihydrochloride.

As an overdose is likely to cause death, make sure you know what dose of salt or base is ordered and what strengths of tablets and injections are available to be given.

Dose 10 mg/kg patient's body weight
each dose each 8–12 hours for 3–7 days.

- Small adult (< 50 kg) – 450 mg
  ($1\frac{1}{2}$ of 300 mg tabs or 1.5 ml of 300 mg/ml injection).
- Large adult (> 50 kg) – 600 mg
  (2 of 300 mg tabs or 2 ml of 300 mg/ml injection).

Quinine is given twice daily in areas where the malaria organisms are known to be very sensitive to quinine but otherwise three times a day.

The dose of quinine will be reduced to half of the above if the patient is very sick or jaundiced or has kidney failure or develops side effects of quinine.

If the patient is semi-immune, 3 days of treatment with quinine may be enough, otherwise 7 days is given.

Table 13.2 Quinine: salt–base equivalents.

	Salt (mg)	*Base (mg)*
Quinine sulphate	363	300
Quinine bisulphate	508	300
Quinine hydrochloride	360	300
Quinine dihydrochloride	366	300
Quinine hydrobromide	408	300
Quinine ethylcarbonate	366	300

If the patient is not immune or is pregnant and is unable to take any other drugs, it would be safer to give quinine for 10 or better 14 days.

Mefloquine tablets (Lariam, Mephaquin)

- Tablet 250 mg base

Mefloquine is used for treatment and prevention of chloroquine resistant *P. falciparum* although some of these are now becoming resistant to mefloquine.

It is very expensive.

The dose is 15–25 mg for treatment and if the total dose is more than 1000 mg, give only 1000 mg immediately and give the rest of the dose 12 hours later.

Do not give until 12 hours have passed since the last dose of quinine.

Nausea and dizziness or mental upsets are side effects.

Do not give within 4 weeks of halofantrine as this may cause death.

Prevention is 5 mg/kg (usually 1 tablet) weekly.

Halofantrine (Halfan)

- Tablet 250 mg
- Syrup 100 mg/5 ml

Halofantrine is used for treatment of chloroquine resistant *P. falciparum* although some of these organisms are now becoming resistant to halofantrine.

It is very expensive.

The dose is 8 mg/kg usually 2 tablets of 250 mg every 6 hours on an empty stomach for 3 doses. Repeat these 3 doses after 1 week.

Do not give within a month of mefloquine or death from heart problems may occur.

Atovaquone and proguanil (see page 74)

Primaquine tablets

Used to treat hypnozoites of *P. vivax* and *P. ovale* and gametocytes of all types.

Give only at the direction of a Medical Officer or for special malaria control programmes.

Antifolate drugs

Pyrimethamine is almost always combined with another drug.

Pyrimethamine 25 mg and sulfadoxine 500 mg (Fansidar) is used for treatment of chloroquine resistant malaria.

Pyrimethamine 12.5 mg and dapsone 100 mg (Maloprim) is used for prophylaxis against chloroquine resistant malaria.

Side effects from the pyrimethamine are occasional anaemia or blood disorders. Sulphadoxine and dapsone however can have significant side effects including severe skin rashes which can include the mucous membranes, loss of appetite, vomiting, diarrhoea, headache, hepatitis, anaemia, other blood disorders, etc.

Proguanil tablets.

Chlorproguanil tablets.

Trimethoprim tablets or injection (also combined with other drug, e.g. Septrin or Bactrim if combined with sulphamethoxazole)

See Chapter 11 page 48.

Artemisinin/Qinghaosu

Give another long acting drug, usually mefloquine (usually 25 mg/kg), or a single dose of pyrimethamine and sulfadoxine or doxycycline for 1 week together with these drugs to prevent early relapse.

Artemisinin tablets and suppositories

- By suppository – 10 mg/kg immediately and 4 hours later, followed by 7 mg/kg at 24, 36, 48 and 60 hours if needed.
- By mouth – 25 mg/kg on the first day followed by 12.5 mg/kg on the 2nd and 3rd days.

Artemether IM injection only: 3.2 mg/kg initially followed by 1.6 mg/kg at 24-hour intervals for a total of 5–7 days.

Artesunate IV injection: 2 mg/kg immediately followed by 1 mg/kg 4–12 hours later and 1 mg/kg once daily for 5 days.

Artesunate tablets: 5 mg/kg on the first day; 2.5 mg/kg on 2nd and 3rd days.

Side effects of all of these drugs so far have been minimal. These drugs, however, should, as yet, not be given in the first part of pregnancy.

These drugs should not be used for prophylaxis. Suppositories are good treatment if vomiting; or injection not possible.

Antibacterial

- Sulphonamides (e.g. sulfadoxine and sulphamethoxazole) and sulphones (e.g. dapsone) tablets or injection.
- Tetracyclines (e.g. tetracycline, doxycycline) tablets or caps.
- Macrolides (e.g. erythromycin, roxithromycin) tablets or injection.
- Quinolones.

See Chapter 11 pages 48–51.

Appendix 3 Chloroquine resistant malaria

In some parts of the world, especially in South-East Asia, the Pacific, South America and now also in parts of India and Africa (See Figure 13.1 page 56), some malaria parasites have become resistant to treatment with chloroquine and the related drug, amodiaquine. This has happened with only some *P. falciparum* parasites. A full treatment course of chloroquine does not 'cure' the patient as it previously did, i.e. make the patient clinically well *and* clear the blood of all the asexual parasites (trophozoites in the red blood cells (RBCs)).

Resistance against chloroquine is divided into three types depending on the results of blood slides taken after a proper 3-day treatment course of chloroquine. The first day of treatment is called day 0. For exact details of the tests see the WHO publications. A simplified explanation is as follows.

S Sensitivity *P. falciparum* trophozoites are cleared from the blood within 7 days and do not later appear (unless reinfection). (In fully sensitive parasites the trophozoites have usually all gone within 2 days.)

R_1 Resistance *P. falciparum* trophozoites disappear from the blood slides within 7 days as in S; (however they are *not* all killed); trophozoites reappear in the blood slides before 4 weeks have gone.

R_2 Resistance The number of *P. falciparum* trophozoites in the blood slides is reduced but the blood is not cleared of trophozoites within 7 days; also the number of trophozoites rises again before 4 weeks have gone.

R_3 Resistance The number of *P. falciparum* trophozoites in the blood smears is not significantly reduced by treatment. (It may even rise.) Trophozoites therefore are still present after 7 days.

The definitions are further explained in the following graphs.

These tests are difficult to do in areas where malaria is common as most patients will be infected with malaria again before 4 weeks have gone. However, the time from the bite of an infected mosquito until an attack of that malaria infection (with a significant number of malaria parasites (trophozoites) in the blood slide) is usually (10–) 14 days. Therefore, any trophozoites in the blood after 7 days and before 14 days

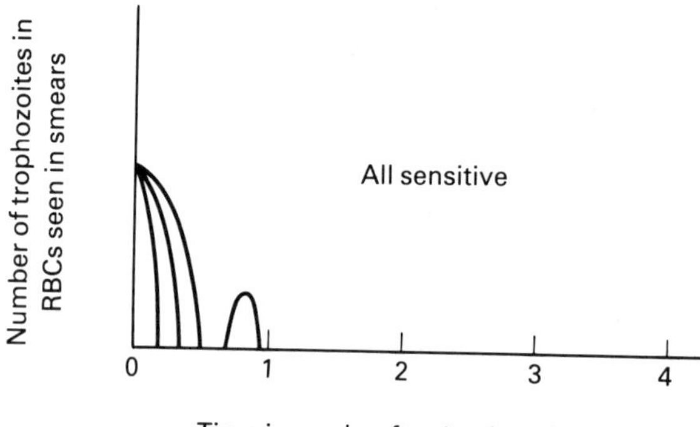

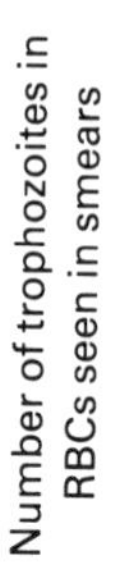

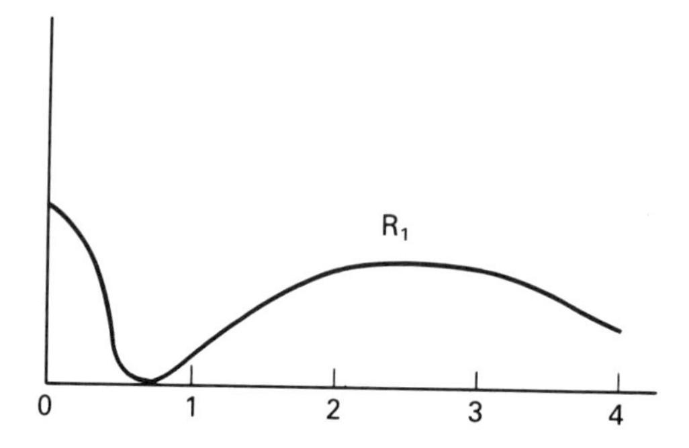

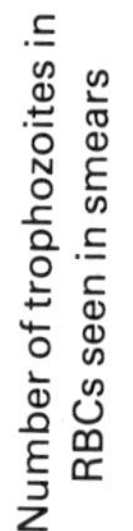

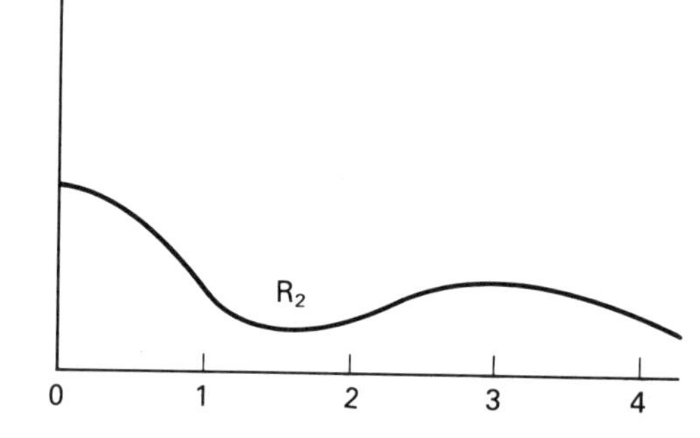

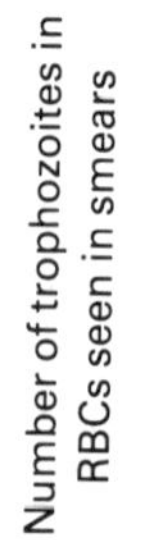

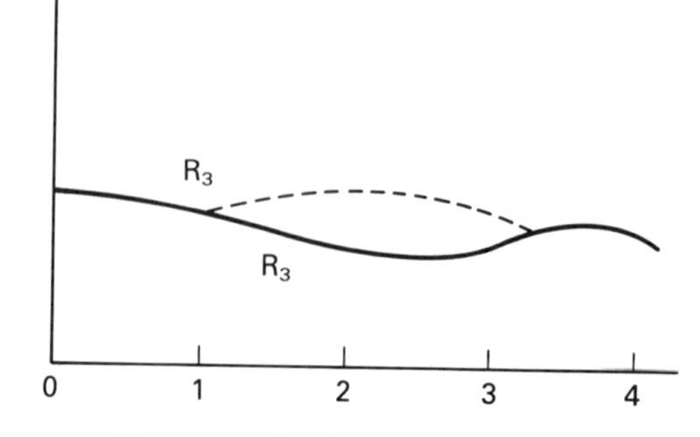

(from the first day of the chloroquine treatment course) are almost certainly because of chloroquine resistance malaria in the body.

Before deciding that a patient has chloroquine resistant malaria:

1. Make sure it is falciparum and not one of the other types of malaria which have a delayed liver cycle and are not 'cured' by chloroquine.
2. Make sure that the patient did swallow and did absorb the chloroquine (i.e. did not have vomiting and/or diarrhoea).

Appendix 4 Method of giving quinine by slow IV drip

Give quinine by a slow IV drip *only if*:

1. It has been possible to get a drip running immediately (before 15 minutes have passed). (An immediate IMI is better than a late IV drip.)
2. The staff are able to keep the drip running.
3. The staff will not let the drip run in quickly. (A rapid IVI of quinine will cause sudden death.)

If not, it is better to give the quinine by IMI.

Give quinine by IMI *when*:

1. IV drip was not started immediately (before 15 minutes have passed).
2. The staff are not capable of keeping the drip running.
3. You are not certain that the staff will not let the drip run quickly.

IM quinine is not as effective as IV quinine especially if the patient is shocked. Also it may cause an injection abscess.

Method of giving quinine by slow IV drip

Use 10 ml/kg patient's body weight of 5% dextrose or 4.3% dextrose in 0.18% sodium chloride solution to dilute the quinine. Glucose is needed as both quinine and malaria can cause hypoglycaemia (low blood glucose). Let the fluid run out of a flask of dextrose saline until the required amount is left (e.g. 500 ml for an adult).

Add the dose of quinine to the solution by injecting the quinine into the flask.

Mix well.

Run the drip *slowly over four (4) hours.*

- Order the number of drops per minute.
- Mark on the IV flask the level for each hour.
- Then, every hour check that the fluid has fallen to the level of this mark, but *no more.*

Appendix 5 Method of making insecticide treated bed nets

Permethrin can be purchased as a 5% emulsifiable concentrate Ambush (ICI) and Perigen (Wellcome) or a wettable powder Coopex WP (Wellcome).

Each square metre of net (m^2) will need 0.5 g of permethrin. A 6 m^2 net will therefore need 3 g permethrin or 6 ml of 50% emulsifiable concentrate or 12 g of wettable powder. Mix this with 150 ml water.

Place the net in a large plastic bag.

Pour the diluted permethrin on top of the net in the bag, making sure none spills.

Screw up the top of the plastic bag in your hand so that no liquid can come out of the bag.

Squash the net and the fluid in the bag until all the fluid is absorbed into all parts of the net.

Then take the net out and hang it up to dry.

Store the dry net in a plastic bag when it is not being used so that the permethrin stays in it.

A net treated like this will give a lot of protection for 3 months from mosquitoes which bite at night.

If curtains over windows and doorways are treated, this will give a lot more protection to those in the house.

Appendix 6 New antimalarial drugs

Add new drugs here as they become available.

Atovaquone 250 mg and proguanil 100 mg tablets (e.g. Malarone)

This drug combination is effective against chloroquine resistant malaria.

The adult treatment dose is 4 tablets in a single dose with a meal once daily for 3 days and all doses *must* be taken.

It is very expensive.

Side effects include nausea, vomiting, abdominal pain, diarrhoea, headache, cough and possibly anaphylaxis.

14

Tuberculosis

Definition, cause, pathology and epidemiology

Tuberculosis is a disease that mainly affects the lungs but also other parts of the body. Man, and sometimes other animals, are affected. It is usually a chronic disease but sometimes it can be acute.

Tuberculosis is caused by an infection by a bacterial bacillus called *Mycobacterium tuberculosis* and occasionally *M. bovis* and other mycobacteria. When the *M. tuberculosis* bacillus is stained in the laboratory and then covered with acid, it keeps the colour of the stain. (Most other organisms lose their colour.) *M. tuberculosis* is therefore called an acid-fast bacillus. This is shortened to AFB. (*M. leprae* is also an AFB. See Chapter 15 page 93).

Tuberculosis is very common in developing and tropical countries especially in urban areas and especially where there is poor general health, malnutrition, overcrowding in housing and not enough public health services to quickly diagnose and treat infectious cases of tuberculosis.

Tuberculosis has recently become more common where many people's resistance to tuberculosis has been damaged by HIV infection. Tuberculosis now causes about 3 million deaths each year. There are about 9 million new infections with tuberculosis each year, about 90% of these being in the developing world. About 30% of the world's population has been infected with tuberculosis. About 10% of people infected with *M. tuberculosis* organisms will develop disease from these tuberculosis organisms during *their whole lifetime*. However in people who have HIV infection *as well as* the tuberculosis infection, about 10% will develop disease from the tuberculosis organisms *each year they live*. In some areas of the developing world, up to half of all new cases of tuberculosis are found to have HIV infection also.

Tuberculosis is nearly always spread by persons with tuberculosis of the lungs who are not being treated. These people cough out tuberculosis organisms in droplets and droplet nuclei into the air. These droplets or droplet nuclei are then inhaled into the respiratory tract of another person. The *M. tuberculosis* organisms then start to grow, if the person does not have some immunity to the organism.

Some immunity against infection with tuberculosis organisms can be given by previous infection with *M. tuberculosis* from which the person has recovered or by deliberate immunisation using mycobacterial organisms that are able to cause no more disease than a skin sore for a couple of weeks (e.g. BCG).

If the organisms grow, they cause a small area of bronchopneumonia. The organisms then spread to the lymph nodes in the chest. They are then carried by the lymph into the blood. Then the blood spreads the organisms to the whole body. In the 1–2 months while it is happening, the body is slowly developing cellular immunity to the organisms (see Chapter 10 page 36). When this immunity has properly developed, the body usually then kills the organisms and the infection heals. This is called '*primary tuberculosis*'. A few organisms may remain alive (in the lungs or any other part of the body to which they spread) for many years or the rest of the person's life and are called 'persistors'. But these organisms are usually surrounded by scar tissue and are not able to cause disease.

'*Post-primary tuberculosis*' happens if the organisms start to grow again and escape from their surrounding scar tissue. This can happen at any of the places they spread to in primary tuberculosis. It happens most commonly in the lungs; but it can also happen in lymph glands, meninges, bones and joints, kidneys, etc.

Sometimes in primary or post-primary tuberculosis, when the organisms are in the blood and spread to many or all organs of the body, they continue to grow and multiply in all these places and cause '*miliary tuberculosis*'. Figure 14.1 shows the stages of infection with tuberculosis organisms.

During primary tuberculosis or post-primary tuberculosis, the *M. tuberculosis* organisms can grow

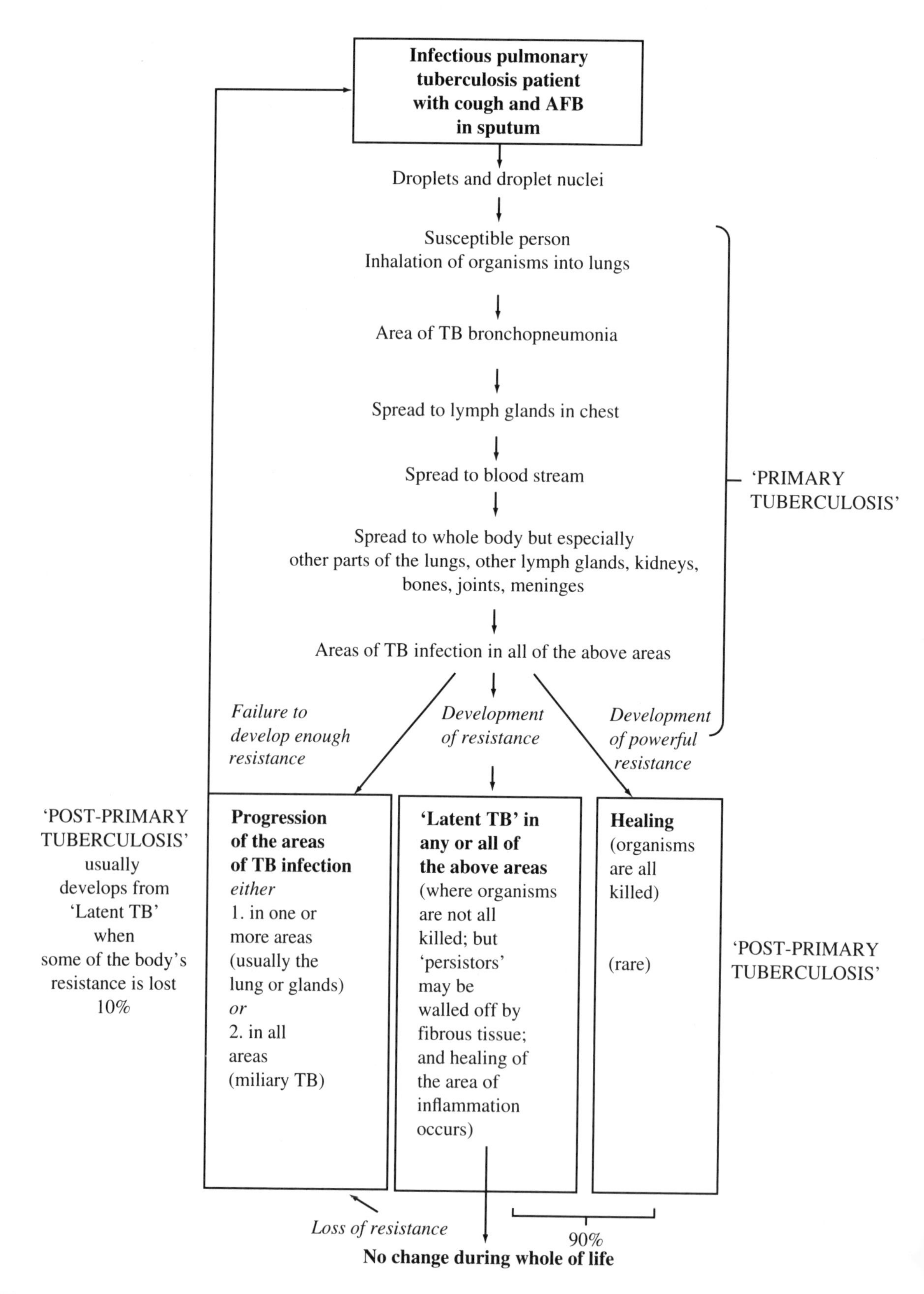

Figure 14.1 Diagram showing the stages of infection with tuberculosis organisms.

without being stopped by the body's defences if the cellular immunity is decreased by malnutrition, another disease such as measles, certain drugs especially adrenocorticosteroids (e.g. cortisone and prednisolone) and anti-cancer drugs, but most especially if cellular immunity is damaged by HIV infection.

Symptoms and signs

Symptoms and signs of tuberculosis are caused by:

1. disease of the organ infected by the *M. tuberculosis* organisms – destruction of the organ and the formation of pus in it; and
2. toxins made by the *M. tuberculosis* organisms – causing general symptoms and signs of infection.

The symptoms and signs of primary tuberculosis, post-primary tuberculosis and miliary tuberculosis are outlined in this section.

Primary tuberculosis

The body's defence system usually wins the fight before any organ is badly damaged. Usually there is only a mild febrile illness, the cause of which is not found out by the health worker.

Post-primary tuberculosis

Pulmonary tuberculosis

Symptoms include the following:

1. Chronic cough, almost always. The cough stays and does not go away even after treatment with antibiotics. *Anyone who has a cough for more than 3 weeks must be examined for tuberculosis.* Often a cough is the only symptom or sign of tuberculosis.
2. Sputum, usually – usually made of pus.
3. Haemoptysis, sometimes – it can be large or small.
4. Pain in the chest, usually of pleuritic type; but this is not common.
5. Shortness of breath, sometimes. This comes early in the disease if the disease is severe (e.g. miliary tuberculosis) or there is a large pleural effusion; otherwise it only comes after years when most of the lungs are destroyed.
6. Fever, sweating etc. especially at night. (i.e. general symptoms of infection) – not very common.
7. Loss of weight – only if acute severe disease or late disease.

Signs include the following:

1. Sometimes mild fever; usually only in severe or late disease.
2. Sometimes wasting and weight loss; usually only in acute severe or late disease.
3. Sometimes anaemia; usually only in acute severe or late disease.
4. Sometimes abnormalities on chest examination; but often not. If abnormalities in the lung are present, they are most likely to be those of upper lobe disease or of pleural effusion. However, patients who also have HIV infection may have pneumonia from tuberculosis in the lower lobes of the lung.

Patients with tuberculosis can also get ordinary pneumonia or acute bronchitis. When you ask how long they have had a cough, they often say for only as long as their acute chest infection. They think the previous chronic cough was normal. Therefore always ask all patients with acute chest infections if they *also* had a chronic cough before the start of this present infection. Send sputum from such patients for AFB tests.

Pneumonia or other chest infection which is unusual or not 'typical' in anyway, may be caused by tuberculosis. Suspect pneumonia of being caused by tuberculosis if *any* of the following are true:

1. it is in an upper lobe of the lung;
2. the signs in the chest are much worse than you expect because the patient does not seem very 'sick';
3. the pneumonia does not get better as quickly as it should with proper treatment; or
4. the patient had a chronic cough before the start of the pneumonia.

Send sputum from such patients for AFB tests. If the patient is still not cured after 2 weeks of proper treatment send three more sputum slides for AFB tests.

> *Everyone* who has had a cough for more than 3 weeks *must* have three samples of sputum sent for AFB (TB) tests even if the person has no other symptoms or signs (see exception later).

Lymph node (gland) tuberculosis

Usually children or young adults are affected; but anyone can be affected.

Usually neck nodes are affected; but nodes in other areas can be affected (see Figure 14.2).

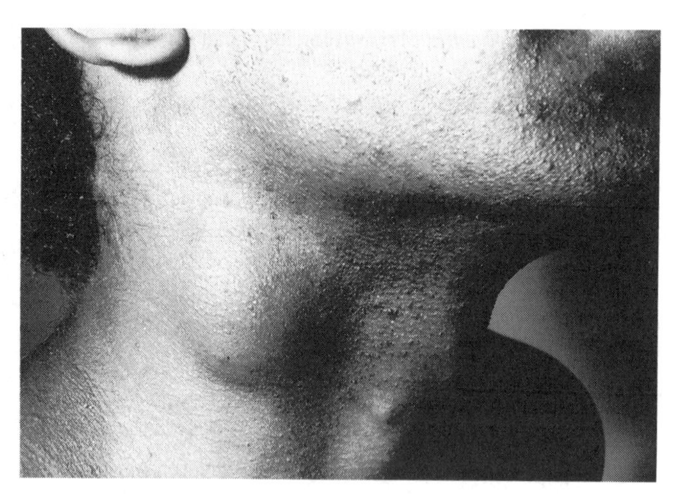

Figure 14.2 Tuberculous cervical lymphadenitis. An aspiration or biopsy must be done.

Usually the only symptom is a lump which does not go away, but gets bigger.

Usually the only sign is enlarged firm lymph nodes which are matted (or joined) together and which are not tender or red or hot. Sometimes there may be a sinus (hole) discharging pus over the nodes.

> Any chronic enlargement of cervical lymph nodes with no obvious cause (e.g. infection in the ENT or head) which does not improve after antibiotics for 3 weeks, must be aspirated or biopsied to look for tuberculosis (especially if the tuberculin test is positive).

Kidney tuberculosis

Symptoms are those of an urinary tract infection or blood in the urine.

Signs are often not present; but there may be kidney tenderness or epididymitis (inflammation of the tubules at the back of the testis).

Tests usually show pus or blood or protein in the urinc.

Treatment with sulphadimidine and then tetracycline or chloramphenicol does not cure the patient. Refer or non-urgently transfer such patients to a Medical Officer for definite diagnosis and treatment.

> Any patient with a urinary tract infection which does not improve after proper treatment, must be transferred to a Medical Officer for diagnosis and treatment.

Vertebral tuberculosis (see also Chapter 29 page 397)

Symptoms and signs include the following.

The patient has back pain and stiffness which lasts for months, which never improves but instead becomes steadily worse.

When you examine the back it is stiff (i.e. it will not bend normally). When you feel (or gently hit with the side of your hand) all along the spine, you find a tender part.

If no treatment is given the infected bones of the spine collapse and a lump or deformity occurs in the line of the spinal bones (see Figure 14.3).

If treatment is not quickly given, weakness or paralysis or loss of sensation in the legs may occur and the patient may not be able to pass urine (because of pressure on the spinal cord).

Suspect vertebral tuberculosis if there is chronic increasing backache with tenderness and stiffness.

Transfer such patients for X-ray and definite diagnosis.

> Any patient who has chronic backache which is becoming worse and who has a stiff spine with a tender part, must be transferred for examination for spinal tuberculosis.

Tuberculous arthritis (see also Chapter 29 page 396)

The hip or knee joints are most often affected, but any joint can be affected.

Children or young adults are most often affected, but anyone can be affected.

Symptoms are usually chronic continuous pain and stiffness of the joint or a limp which slowly becomes worse.

Signs include:

1. *chronic arthritis which slowly becomes worse* (swelling, tenderness, warmth, pain on moving joint, limited movement of joint, not able to use joint properly, etc.);
2. *wasting of muscles, usually severe*, which move the joint is typical;
3. nearby lymph nodes are usually enlarged;

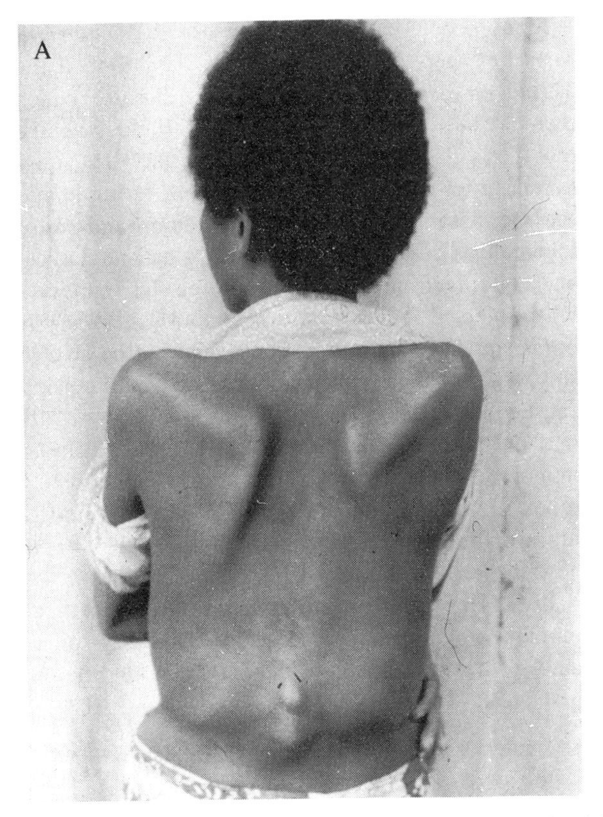

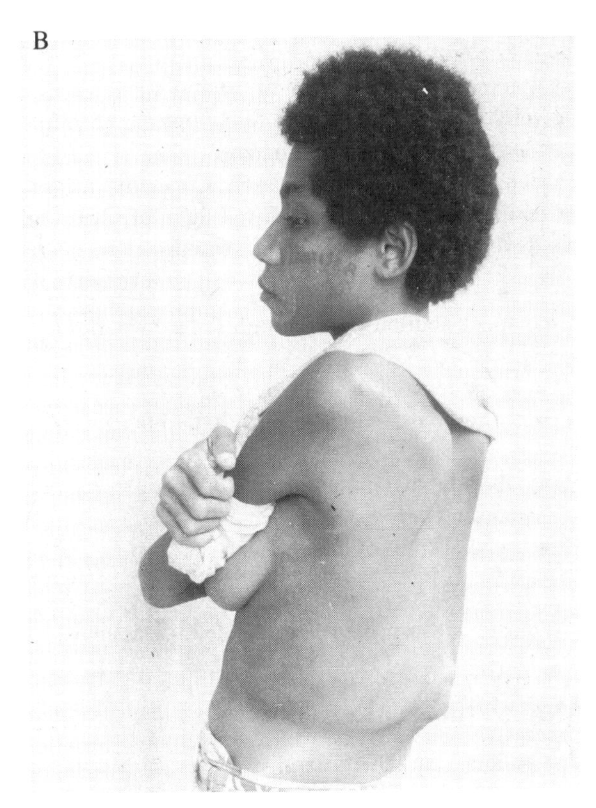

Figure 14.3A and B Tuberculosis of the spine. Note the deformity of the spine (often called a 'gibbus'). Tuberculosis of the spine is often called 'Pott's disease'. This patient needs urgent transfer for treatment before she becomes paraplegic

4. a sinus discharging pus may be present over the joint late in the disease.

Any chronic arthritis which becomes progressively worse over months should be suspected of being tuberculous arthritis.

Transfer all such patients for definite diagnosis.

> Any chronic arthritis (i.e. with inflammation of the joint) which becomes progressively worse over months, should be suspected of being tuberculous arthritis. Tuberculosis is even more likely if only one joint is involved, and especially if the tuberculin test is positive. Such cases should be referred or transferred for tests.

Meningeal tuberculosis (see also Chapter 25 page 326)

Most often the patient is a child, but the patient can be any age.

Symptoms and signs are the same as for acute bacterial meningitis (see Chapter 25 page 322) but the disease is less acute.

The history is usually much longer (i.e. more than a few days). A contact may have tuberculosis or a chronic cough not yet diagnosed as tuberculosis – check the family.

At first the patient is usually not as sick and febrile as you would expect for bacterial meningitis. Also, the patient may be wasted and have signs and symptoms of tuberculosis elsewhere. The patient does not improve as he should on proper meningitis treatment. (See Chapter 25 page 323.)

The CSF is sometimes yellow or forms a web after standing; but it can appear normal to naked eye examination.

> Transfer urgently:
> 1. all cases with the above history, examination and tests,
> 2. all cases of meningitis or encephalitis or cerebral malaria which do not improve after 2 days of proper treatment,
>
> for definite diagnosis and special drug treatment as meningeal tuberculosis is likely.

Abdominal (peritoneal, intestinal or lymph node) tuberculosis

Symptoms include: swelling of the abdomen, usually; bowel colic, sometimes; general symptoms of infection, e.g. weight loss, fever, malaise, often.

Signs include: abdominal ascites, usually; masses or tenderness sometimes; general signs of infection, e.g. fever, weight loss, anaemia, sometimes.

> Suspect abdominal tuberculosis in a patient with ascites if:
> - no oedema of the back or legs, *or*
> - no response to treatment with diuretics, *or*
> - abdominal masses or tenderness are also present, *or*
> - general signs of infection are present.

Transfer all suspected cases for definite diagnosis.

Miliary tuberculosis

The patient may have a family or contact history of tuberculosis or a past history of a chronic cough or another condition which suggests tuberculosis.

Symptoms are usually not specific but are severe – malaise, fever, sweating, weakness, nausea, vomiting, diarrhoea, cough, shortness of breath, headache, etc.

Signs are usually not specific but are severe – not fully conscious, fever, fast pulse, dyspnoea, weight loss, anaemia, etc.

Antibiotics and antimalarials do not help the patient who quickly becomes worse.

Transfer such cases urgently if they do not improve with proper treatment for septicaemia (see Chapter 12) and chloroquine-resistant malaria (see Chapter 13 page 64) within 48 hours.

Natural history of untreated tuberculosis

If patients with pulmonary tuberculosis are not treated, within 5 years 50% will be dead, 25% will be alive and well having overcome the disease themselves by their cellular immunity, and 25% will be alive but sick from the disease and be spreading tuberculosis.

HIV infection and tuberculosis

Tuberculosis may occur at any stage of an HIV infection (see Chapter 19 page 183).

Many people have been infected with *M. tuberculosis* but their cellular immunity has stopped the *M. tuberculosis* growing and causing disease, though there are still 'persistors' in the body. If a person like this then gets an HIV infection, once the HIV infection destroys enough of the body's cellular immunity, the 'persistors' can start to grow again and cause tuberculosis disease. At other times, a patient may get an HIV infection and have poor cellular immunity when infected for the first time with *M. tuberculosis* organisms. This sort of person would not be able to stop these organisms growing and they would quickly cause tuberculosis disease.

If the HIV infected person still has some cellular immunity, the tuberculosis infection may be just like tuberculosis infection in non-HIV patients and is most often in the upper part of the lungs or as described above.

If the HIV infected patient has very poor cellular immunity, then the tuberculosis infection may spread quickly into many parts of the body and be different in the following ways:

1. Lung disease may be unusual. It may be more in the lower rather than the upper lung.
2. Lung disease may be little or none and most of the tuberculosis infection may be in other parts of the body. Sputum for AFB may be negative.
3. Lymph node, bowel, meningeal and miliary tuberculosis are most likely.
4. The tuberculin test (Mantoux) is often negative.
5. Unusual mycobacterial organisms, which usually do not cause infection and could be resistant to the usual anti-tuberculosis drugs can infect these patients.
6. Reactions to anti-tuberculosis drugs, especially thiacetazone, are much more common and severe.

If a patient with HIV infection develops a new cough and sputum, which becomes chronic, and it is not due to pneumonia or empyema, these symptoms are often due to tuberculosis. If these symptoms do not respond to treatment for pneumonia (see Chapter 19 page 220) and the sputum examination is negative for AFB, find out from your Medical Officer if you should start such patients on antituberculosis treatment or whether you should send them to the hospital for further investigation. If antituberculosis drugs are started, unless another diagnosis for the cough and sputum is proven, the whole treatment for tuberculosis *must* be given until it is all finished.

Tests

Sputum tests for AFB

This is how to do the sputum test for AFB:

1. *Saliva* from the mouth is *no use* for this test. *Sputum* coughed up *from inside the chest* and spat out is *essential.*
2. Give the patient a container (such as a bottle or plastic bag), or if one of these is not available, something such as a banana leaf. Ask the patient to stand either outside in the open air or facing an open window. Ask the patient to breathe deeply three times, then to cover his mouth and then to cough deeply when he feels ready to cough. When he coughs deeply to produce sputum, tell him to spit the sputum into the container holding it close to his mouth.
3. Now look to see if the specimen is suitable for examination. A proper specimen is thick with solid pieces of pus or yellowish material and 2–5 ml in volume.
4. If the sputum is not suitable ask the patient to repeat the process until a good specimen is obtained. At times it is necessary to give physiotherapy (hit the patient on the back when he coughs or make him bend or lie down with the head lower than the chest and hit his back while he coughs) to get a proper specimen.
5. This first specimen, which you collect when you first see the patient at the health centre, is called specimen 'A'.
6. Tell the patient to collect another specimen of sputum in the same way at home immediately when he wakes the next morning and then return with it. This is called specimen 'B'.
7. When the patient comes back the next day with the specimen 'B', collect the third specimen at the health centre. This is called specimen 'C'.
8. To make a smear from the sputum specimen, take a clean slide and mark it on the rough end with the patient's name, address, etc. With an applicator stick (or any kind of stick), lift out one or two thick yellow solid pieces of sputum. Then spread this sputum around the other two-thirds of the slide thickly and evenly.
   Allow the slide to dry in the air (for about 15 minutes). Make sure it is protected from flies and insects. After it is dry, 'fix' it by passing it 3 times through the flame of a spirit lamp (or over any non-smoky flame, e.g. over a hurricane lamp if a spirit lamp is not available), until it is just hot enough to be uncomfortable if held on the back of the other hand. Make sure the patient's sputum and name are facing upwards. Place the slide into a slide box, or protect it with another slide tied to it but separated from it by broken applicator or matchsticks. It must be kept away from cockroaches or other insects. Burn the specimen containers and applicator sticks.
   Stain the slide for acid-fast bacilli (AFB) by the Ziehl–Neelsen method or other method as taught. Examine under the microscope with oil immersion lens for AFB. Otherwise send the prepared slide for examination.

The sputum smear will show AFB in almost all cases if the patient has pulmonary tuberculosis causing symptoms. In some early cases, before a bronchus is broken open by the disease, the sputum will be negative. The most common causes of slides being negative, when, in fact the patient does have pulmonary tuberculosis, are:

1. saliva and not sputum was put on the slide,
2. errors were made in the laboratory.

In places where tuberculosis is common any patient who has a cough which has lasted for more than 3 weeks or who has any other symptoms or signs suggesting pulmonary tuberculosis, should have his sputum tested for AFB three times.

Take one specimen of sputum *immediately* (specimen A). Ask the patient to cough up a second specimen early the next morning (specimen B). Collect a third specimen the day the patient brings back specimen B (specimen C).

From each sample, make a smear of the sputum, fix it by heating it, and send it to the laboratory with a request for tests for AFB.

If a patient has negative slides for AFB and you still strongly suspect pulmonary tuberculosis, repeat the slides ('A', 'B' and 'C').

If the patient has these repeated slides negative for AFB and you still strongly suspect tuberculosis, discuss the case with the Health or Medical Officer to see if non-urgent transfer for chest X-ray is needed.

In places where tuberculosis is not common and HIV infection is not common and chronic bronchitis (COLD) is very common,[1] if a patient has a true chronic

1 These rules will probably not apply in your area, unless there are particular environmental conditions. Unless your Health Department tells you that these rules can apply in your place, cross them out of this book.

cough treat with procaine pencillin or co-trimoxazole for 1 week. If the patient is then cured, discharge him.

If he is not cured treat with tetracycline for 1 week, and if he is then cured, discharge him.

If he is still not cured *and* he is over 40 years old *and* has never been where tuberculosis is common *and*:

- has never lived in the same house as a person from an area where tuberculosis is common, *and*
- has never had contact with a tuberculosis patient, *and*
- has no other symptoms or signs of tuberculosis, *and*
- has no history or signs to suggest he could have HIV infection,

then discharge with PD of chronic bronchitis (COLD).

All other cases: continue the tetracycline for 2–4 weeks and send sputum smears for AFB.

Gastric aspirate examination for AFB

This is done for children or adults who are not able to produce sputum.

Three (3) fasting morning specimens are collected.

This test is not as accurate as sputum (false negative and false positive results can occur).

Tuberculin test (also called 'Mantoux' test)

Part of dead *M. tuberculosis* organisms called purified protein derivative or 'PPD' can be injected intradermally (into the skin). If the body's defence cells have learned to fight tuberculosis organisms, there will be an acute inflammatory reaction in the skin at the site of the injection within a couple of days.

Give PPD by *intradermal* injection only.

At 72 (or up to 96) hours, measure and write down on the patient's chart the diameter in mm of the swelling (not the redness).

- 0–9 mm negative in everyone
- 10+ mm positive if patient has not had BCG
- 15+ mm positive if patient has had BCG

If the reaction is negative there is no immunity to tuberculosis organisms and, as long as the PPD was active and the test was done properly, infection with tuberculosis organisms is unlikely (but still possible).

A positive reaction means that there is some 'immunity' against tuberculosis organisms: tuberculosis organisms have been in the body in the past or are there at present.

But, remember that:

1. The tuberculin test may be negative when the patient does have active tuberculosis disease. Times when this occurs include:
   (a) when the tuberculosis infection is very severe, e.g. miliary tuberculosis or tuberculous meningitis;
   (b) when another illness is present (such as measles or chickenpox);
   (c) when the patient has malnutrition;
   (d) when the patient has HIV infection;
   (e) when the patient is taking certain drugs (especially prednisolone or cortisone-like drugs);
   (f) when the patient has some cancers;
   (g) when the PPD was not reliable, or the test was not done properly.
2. The positive tuberculin test does *not* mean that the patient is sick with tuberculosis disease. It means only that tuberculosis organisms are or were alive in his body. Do *not* diagnose tuberculosis disease just because the tuberculin test is positive.

BCG immunisation which causes an ulcer in a few days (instead of the usual few weeks) has the same meaning as a positive tuberculin test, and is called an accelerated BCG reaction.

Lymph node aspiration

This is nearly as accurate as a biopsy in diagnosing tuberculosis in a lymph node.

Inject local anaesthetic, e.g. 1% lignocaine (lidocaine) into the skin over the node and on top of the node.

Put 2–3 ml of 0.9% saline into a 10 ml syringe. Put a large, e.g. 18 gauge needle on the syringe. Hold the node between the finger and thumb, or better get an assistant to hold it. Make sure if the needle goes too far, it cannot go into any important structure such as an artery, trachea or especially lung. Push the needle through the skin until it is in the middle of the node held between the finger and thumb. Suck out any material possible into the syringe. If it is not possible to suck out any material, inject the 2–3 ml of saline into the node and then suck this, with any other material it has mixed with, back into the syringe. Use the material in the syringe to make a slide just as you would make a slide from sputum, for examination for AFB; and send this to the laboratory.

Lymph node biopsy

Lymph nodes near the body surface, i.e. just under the skin and can be easily held between the finger and thumb – the biopsy can be done at the health centre. However, do not try to do this unless you have been taught to do it and have done it under supervision (it is harder to do than it looks).

Deep lymph nodes – refer or transfer to a Medical Officer for biopsy.

Chest X-ray

A chest X-ray is not possible at a health centre and is almost never necessary for diagnosis.

A normal chest X-ray makes pulmonary tuberculosis unlikely.

An abnormal chest X-ray means further tests (mainly sputum for AFB) are needed to see if the abnormality on the X-ray is caused by tuberculosis or another disease.

Diagnostic features

1. A cough that has lasted for more than 3 weeks.
2. A chronic cough is especially suspicious when there is also – sputum, or haemoptysis, or chest pain, or fever or weight loss.
3. Swollen lymph glands in the neck with no obvious cause (especially no ENT or scalp infection) which do not go away after treatment with antibiotics.
4. Tuberculin test usually (but not always) positive. The positive tuberculin test diagnoses only infection (past or present), *not* disease.

Possibility that patient with tuberculosis also has HIV infection

Whenever a patient has tuberculosis diagnosed, ask yourself if the patient could also have HIV infection. This is likely especially if he has a history of, or present evidence of, any of the following:

1. a sexually transmitted disease of any (other) type and/or unsafe sexual practices (see Chapter 19 page 155);
2. non-sterile skin piercing (tattooing etc.);
3. previous blood transfusion;
4. intravenous drug abuse;
5. persistent generalised lymphadenopathy;
6. itchy macular skin rash of unusual type;
7. minor injuries in the skin causing large infections;
8. herpes zoster especially if it is in a young person or if it is affecting more than 1 nerve or if it comes back again soon after it goes;
9. pneumonia that is severe;
10. high fever for which no obvious cause can be found;
11. chronic diarrhoea which does not respond to the usual treatment; and/or
12. progressive weight loss of more than 10 kg or 20% of original weight;
13. candida infection in the mouth or unexplained pain on swallowing which suggests candida of the oesophagus in anyone; and severe and recurrent candida of the vagina in a woman who is not a diabetic;
14. oral hairy leukoplakia;
15. herpes simplex which spreads further than usual, lasts longer than usual or comes back again after it settles;
16. kala azar in someone not expected to get it;
17. Kaposi's sarcoma;
18. burning sensation in the feet from peripheral neuropathy;
19. unexplained change in behaviour or organic psychosis or unexplained nervous system changes especially without a stiff neck.

If any history or symptoms or signs suggest that the patient has HIV infection, see Chapter 19 page 188 about doing a blood test for HIV antibodies.

If a patient who has tuberculosis also has HIV infection, his tuberculosis treatment is not changed and is exactly as if he did not have the HIV infection apart from one thing. He is not given thiaocetazone as this drug often causes severe skin rashes in patients who have HIV infection.

If the patient is given DOTS treatment, it would be expected that his chance of cure from the tuberculosis is good. He is of course more likely to die than other tuberculosis patients. In fact, about 20% will die before the tuberculosis is cured. Many of these deaths are from other complications of the HIV infection and not due to the tuberculosis or its treatment. If a patient with HIV infection is cured of his tuberculosis by DOTS treatment it is claimed that he is no more likely to get a relapse of the infection (the infection coming back) than other tuberculosis patients without HIV who are treated.

Treatment

The two most important things in the treatment of the patient are:

1. Give only the recommended drugs in the recommended combinations. Three or four drugs will be given at the beginning of treatment. Never fewer than two drugs are used even for the continuation of treatment.
   Never give one anti-tuberculosis drug by itself – at least two are always given together.
   Never change the drug combinations yourself and never add only one new drug if the patient is not being cured by his drugs.
2. Give these drugs *regularly* for *at least* the shortest amount of time that is needed for them to cure the disease. If rifampicin is not available, this means at least 12 months. If rifampicin is available, this means 9 months. If rifampicin and pyrazinamide are both available, this means 6 months.
3. Make sure that every dose of every drug is taken – watch the patient swallow every dose of every drug for the whole course.

Treatment is divided into two parts:

1. Short-term intensive chemotheraphy daily for 8 weeks (2 months) with four (or at least three) drugs to try to kill most of the *M. tuberculosis* organisms during this time.
2. Maintenance treatment for 4 or 6 or 10 or more months (depending on what drugs are available for short-term intensive chemotherapy and for maintenance therapy) to kill the rest of the organisms especially the 'persistors'.

This treatment should be:

1. fully supervised treatment every day *or*, in some cases in maintenance treatment, three times weekly: where a health worker watches the patient swallow each drug;
2. only very occasionally, for some very special reason, unsupervised home treatment daily where the patient gives the drugs to himself.

WHO and other trials have shown that if a health worker watches to make sure that all patients swallow all doses of the drugs for the whole length of the treatment (directly observed treatment or 'DOT'), then almost every patient is cured by the recommended drugs. These trials have also shown that if a health worker does not watch that all doses of all drugs are swallowed by all patients for the whole course, then many patients are not cured. Some patients do forget to take some doses or some drugs or stop the drugs before all the course is taken; and are not cured.

The combination of drugs recommended by WHO is called short-course treatment ('S') because although the length of treatment is still 6(–12) months, this is much shorter than the old 'standard' treatments which were 12–18 or more months. Modern treatment is therefore called 'Directly observed treatment short course' or 'DOTS'.

Do not start treatment unless:

1. sputum is positive for AFB; *or*
2. lymph gland (or other) aspirate or biopsy is positive for tuberculosis; *or*
3. patient has suspected severe tuberculosis and would die before test results could be obtained or transfer was possible (diagnosis *must* later be confirmed in these cases or the full length of treatment completed); *or*
4. tuberculosis has been diagnosed by a Medical Officer in another way.

Always do a full medical history and physical examination and test the urine first.

Diagnose and treat any other conditions present especially anaemia and other bacterial chest infections.

Treatment of the patient only is not the proper management of the problem caused by the diagnosis of a case of tuberculosis. Remember the other things needed in the management of the patient.

- Do all the administrative duties.
- Arrange for a place and health worker, convenient for the patient, to get his DOTS treatment, unless he is to be admitted to the health centre to start treatment.
- Start patient and family education about the disease, the treatment, the possible side effects of treatment and when to return if worried about possible side effects. Explain that he will be cured if he takes his treatment and will probably die and infect his family and friends if he does not take his

treatment. Say that any of his contacts who think they may have tuberculosis, should come for examination and, if necessary, treatment.

- Arrange for contact education, examination and treatment, if needed, of the patient's family, schoolmates or workmates and especially anyone who has slept in the same room as him.
- Arrange for check sputum examinations for AFB after 2 months of treatment, 5 months of treatment and at the end of treatment.
- Check the patient's attendances for treatment each month.
- Arrange for a home visit if the patient does not attend for every treatment.

Most countries have only certain drugs available and have National Tuberculosis Programmes using these drugs. You must find out what your programme is and follow it. If there is no programme, then there are two essential parts to the only really effective tuberculosis treatment programmes which you must do. First, use one of the new 'short-course' treatments using rifampicin and pyrazinamide as well as other drugs. Second, use fully supervised or directly observed treatment. If you do these two things you will be using Directly Observed Treatment Short-Course or 'DOTS', which is the most and only really effective treatment known. If rifampicin and pyrazinamide are not available, one of the old standard courses may have to be given. Details of both of these follow.

The first 2 months of all treatments should always be fully supervised by a health worker, i.e. he should give the drugs and watch and see that they are actually swallowed. The second part, or maintenance phase of the treatment, should also be fully supervised. Only for very special reasons should unsupervised treatment be given and then only if the patient can be trusted to take the drugs and continue to take the drugs to the end of the course and return for review each month and be supplied with new drugs, and it is possible to find the patient if he does not return. However, if the *M. tuberculosis* organisms in the community have some resistance to the drugs available, and especially if the patient cannot be trusted to take all the drugs for the whole of the course, and definitely if the patient has previously been treated and not completed the treatment properly, or tuberculosis has come back again, then fully supervised or directly observed treatment must be given. Fully supervised or directly observed treatment for the first 2 months is every day. The following 4–7 months in short-term therapy or 10 months in standard therapy may be daily or may be three times a week, using larger doses of the drugs as shown in Table 14.1.

Table 14.1 The dose of the usual drugs for treatment of tuberculosis (maximum doses in brackets).

Anti-TB drug (abbreviation)	*Recommended dose (mg/kg)*		
	Daily	*Intermittent*	
		3×/week	2×/week
Isoniazid (H)	5 (300 mg)	10 (600 mg)	15 (900 mg)
Rifampicin (R)	10 (600 mg)	10 (600 mg)	10 (600 mg)
Pyrazinamide (Z)	25 (2 g)	35 (3 g)	50 (4 g)
Ethambutol (E)	15 (1.2 g)	30 (2 g)	45 (2 g)
Thioacetazone (T)	3	not applicable	

Table 14.2 The usual combination of drugs used in DOTS treatment for tuberculosis.

2 months intensive chemotherapy	*4–6 months continuation chemotherapy*
Isoniazid (H) daily *and*	Isoniazid (H) and ethambutol (E) daily for 6 months *or*
Rifampicin (R) daily *and*	Isoniazid (H) and thioacetazone (T) daily for 6 months *or*
Pyrazinamide (Z) daily *and*	Isoniazid (H) and rifampicin (R) daily for 4 months *or*
Ethambutol (E) *or* Streptomycin (S) daily	Isoniazid (H) and rifampicin (R) 3 times a week for 4 months

Note: that only if both rifampicin and pyrazinamide (as well as isoniazid) are used for the first 2 months, can the whole course be short (6–8 months)

Note: that only if rifampicin (as well as isoniazid) is used for continuation therapy (and only after the above drugs are all used for the first 2 months intensive chemotherapy), can the continuation course be as short as 4 months (and the whole course be as short as 6 months).

Treatment has a number of aims.

1. To cure the patient
   DOTS does this more quickly.
2. Kill the *M. tuberculosis* as soon as possible before they do further damage to the body.
   DOTS does this more quickly.
3. Kill the *M. tuberculosis* as quickly as possible so that there is less chance of them spreading to other people.
   DOTS does this more quickly
4. Prevent *M. tuberculosis* organisms becoming resistant to the drugs used.
   DOTS treatment does this best.

In all populations of *M. tuberculosis* organisms, there are occasional ones that will be resistant to one drug but not the others. If only one drug is used, all the sensitive ones will be killed off but later the resistant one will grow and cause the disease. If two drugs are given, it is unlikely, but possible, there will be some organisms there which are resistant to both drugs and when all other organisms are killed, these organisms may grow and cause disease. If three, and if particularly four drugs are given, this is very unlikely to happen.

If, however, not every single dose of the drugs is taken, organisms which are sick but not killed by the drugs, may recover and then be resistant to those drugs from then on; and after all the other organisms are killed, these resistant organisms can grow to cause the disease again. This patient's disease and anyone else who is infected by him, will then not be helped by the drugs to which the *M. tuberculosis* organism has become resistant.

To stop the above problems occurring, treatment must be with more than one drug (it is best to give four at the beginning of treatment); and treatment must never be stopped and started and stopped and started, etc. As well as this, various combinations of drugs have been tried out and found to work. Only these combinations should be used. It is not possible to make up a treatment of your own as there may be a reason you do not know about as to why your treatment will not work.

It is important to get the patient to understand that he does not take the drugs only until he feels well and then stop, but must continue until all the treatment is taken. Doctors Crofton, Horne and Miller have made a list of important things for you to remember when talking to the patient about these things. (See their book *Clinical Tuberculosis*, second edition.)

1. Be kind, friendly and patient.
2. Explain the disease to the patients and relatives. In doing this, remember there may be local beliefs about tuberculosis which you must explain.
3. Explain the importance of full treatment to the patient and relatives.
4. Show him and his relatives the kind of pills he will take and tell him how to take them.
5. Tell him and his relatives about possible reactions to the drugs. Tell him to come and see you if he gets a reaction.
6. Give him a leaflet about tuberculosis and its treatment.
7. Tell him and his relatives about your local arrangements for supervision of treatment, e.g. admission to ward/hostel *or* attendance at a centre near his home *or* supervision by volunteer or responsible person in his village.

   Arrange treatment as near as possible to his home or his work. If needed, time the clinics so that the patient does not have to miss work. Try not to keep a patient waiting. If he has long waits he may not come back.
8. Carefully tell him, and give him a card, the date and place of his next attendance. If there is a local calendar different from the standard international calendar, give him the date in the local calendar. He will understand that better.
9. Check on his/her personal problems, e.g. job, marriage, 'what the neighbours will say', etc. Give him/her kind and friendly advice about any problem. Because such counselling often takes time, in some clinics it is found best to get a nurse or an assistant with a good and friendly personality to do the counselling.
10. If he is not having DOTS, when he comes back for a new supply of drugs, remember to check the number of the pills left over. This will tell you whether he has taken all the doses, ask him in a sympathetic way why he has not. This will help you to give him the right advice about taking his full treatment. However it would be best to have him changed to DOTS.
11. If a patient does not get better or does not return for review, the best and quickest way to get the patient back is by a home visit to persuade him to return. This can be done by a specially trained 'home visitor' or 'defaulter tracer'. A good, sympathetic, persuasive personality is important. Alternatively, a nurse or other health workers may do it.

It is important to know the patient's correct address. For an illiterate patient, ask him to get his postman to write the address on a card. In order to find the patient easily, some clinics ask the patient to give three addresses:

- his home address,
- the address of a friend or relative who lives nearby,
- the address of a shop or restaurant or teahouse which knows the patient and knows where he lives or can be found.

For daily treatment Table 14.3 shows details about the drugs that you use.

A modification of this table will be supplied by your Health Department to tell you exactly what drugs, what doses and how often they are to be given for standard short-course chemotherapy, which is best given fully supervised (DOTS).

Intermittent treatment is given with the following drugs and doses. Note that thioacetazone cannot be used for intermittent treatment. See also Table 14.1.

1. Isoniazid 10–15 mg/kg max. 750 mg
   Pyridoxine 10 mg
2. Rifampicin 10–15 mg/kg max. 600 mg
3. Pyrazinamide 35–50 mg/kg max. 3 g
4. Ethambutol 30 mg/kg max. 2 g
   or
   Streptomycin 15 mg/kg, maximum 1 g (i.e. the same as for daily treatment).

But check the doses used by your Health Department for your population or otherwise use the lower of the doses given here.

- All given together in one dose.
- All on an empty stomach.
- All three times every week (e.g. Monday, Wednesday and Friday).
- All preferably fully supervised, i.e. given by the health worker who actually watches that they actually swallow the drugs
- All for 6 months if there is no initial intensive course *or*
  just isoniazid and pyridoxine and rifampicin if for continuation phase after 2 months of daily treatment, *but*
  if there is a lot of drug resistance, all four may be continued for 4 months after the initial 2 months of intensive treatment.

Drugs given to kill *Mycobacterium tuberculosis* are powerful drugs, which sometimes have side effects (Table 14.4). Some side effects are mild and will be ignored by the patient if they are explained to him. Other side effects are serious and can be fatal (Figure 14.4). If serious side effects occur, you must change the treatment (see Table 14.5).

Make sure you never stop a patient's antituberculosis treatment and do nothing more about it. The patient must have another drug put in the place of any drugs stopped and you should always talk to your Medical Officer about this. If all antituberculosis drugs have to be stopped, transfer the patient to the Medical Officer for further care, unless the patient is about to die and shortly does die.

Make sure each month, by reviewing your records, that all your patients are getting all the treatment. If not, arrange for a visit to fix up any problem that is stopping regular treatment.

Make sure that you send progress sputum tests from those patients who had a positive sputum at the beginning of the treatment:

1. at 2 months (at the end of the intensive phase of treatment),
2. at 3 months if the one at 2 months was not negative,
3. at 5 months,
4. at the end of the treatment.

If the sputum is not negative at the end of 5 months the treatment has failed. The most common cause is that the patient is not taking the treatment correctly. The most serious cause is that the tuberculosis organisms are resistant to the drugs. It is

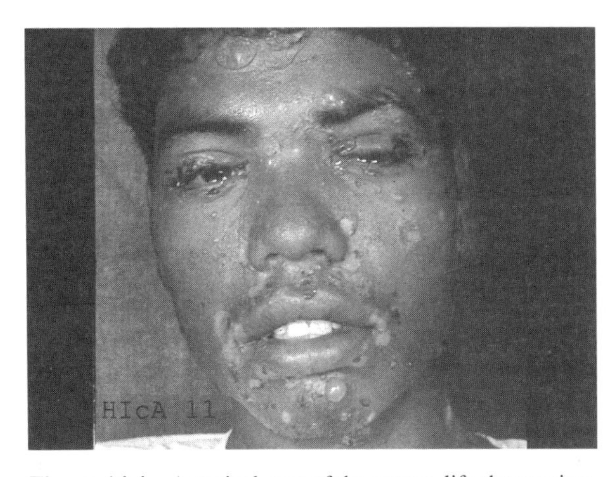

Figure 14.4 A typical case of the severe, life-threatening skin rash (Stevens–Johnson Syndrome) that can be caused by thioacetazone. It seems to be more common in some populations than others. It is much more common if the patient also has HIV infection. Do not give thioacetazone to patients who may have HIV infection. (Source: TALC)

Table 14.3 Standard short course chemotherapy.

	Initial phase: 2 months				
Body weight in kg at beginning of treatment	Isoniazid (H) and rifampicin (R) both drugs in the one tablet tabs 100 mg H and 150 mg R or tabs 150 mg H and 300 mg R	Pyrazinamide (Z) tabs 500 mg	Ethambutol (E) tabs 400 mg	or	Streptomycin (S) Powder for IM injection 1 g base in vial
< 33	2 tabs @ 100 mg H and 150 mg R daily	2 tabs daily	2 tabs daily	or	500 mg daily
33–50	3 tabs @ 100 mg H and 150 mg R daily	3 tabs daily	2 tabs daily	or	750 mg daily
> 50	2 tabs @ 150 mg H and 300 mg R daily	4 tabs daily	3 tabs daily	or	1 g daily but not if over 50 years 750 mg daily if over 50 years
All weights	Pyridoxine 10 mg daily to prevent brain and nerve problems from isoniazid				

	Continuation phase: 4 months	*or*	*Continuation phase: 6 months*		
Body weight in kg at beginning of treatment	Isoniazid (H) and rifampicin (R) both drugs in the one tablet tabs 100 mg H and 150 mg R		Isoniazid (H) and thioacetazone (T) both drugs in the one tablet tabs 100 mg H and 50 mg T or tabs 300 mg H and 150 mg T	or	Isoniazid (H) and ethambutol (E) tabs 100 mg (H) and tabs 400 mg E
< 33	2 tabs daily		2 tabs @ 100 mg and 50 mg daily	or	$1\frac{1}{2}$ tabs @ 100 mg H and 1 tab @ 400 mg E
33–50	3 tabs daily		1 tab @ 300 mg and 150 mg daily	or	$2\frac{1}{2}$ tabs @ 100 mg H and $1\frac{1}{2}$ tabs @ 400 mg E
> 50	4 tabs daily		1 tab @ 300 mg + 150 mg daily	or	3 tabs @ 100 mg H and 2 tabs @ 400 mg E
All weights	Pyridoxine 10 mg with each dose of isoniazid to prevent brain and nerve problems				

Notes:
1 There are fixed dose combinations available of isoniazid + rifampicin (H + R: 100 + 150 mg or 150 + 300 mg) and isoniazid + thioacetazone (H + T: 100 + 50 mg or 300 + 150 mg). Where available, WHO strongly recommends the use of fixed dose combination as they improve patients' compliance and cure rates. In addition, rifampicin combinations reduce the risk of drug resistant TB.
2 Ethambutol 15 mg/kg with maximum dose of 1800 mg should be used in place of thioacetazone in proven or suspected HIV-positive patients.

Table 14.4 Antituberculosis drugs and common side effects to watch for and what action to take. (Adapted from von Massow *et al.* (1997) *Guidelines to Rational Drug Use*. London, Macmillan)

Drug/Tablet size	*Do not give if*	*Side effects*	*Notes*
Isoniazid 100 mg alone 100 mg with 150 mg rifampicin 150 mg with 300 mg rifampicin	• Allergy to it • Hepatitis	• Encephalitis/fits. Loss of feeling or movement in legs and arms • Hepatitis/jaundice	• Pyridoxine prevents (stops) nervous system side effects • Stop if hepatitis and transfer to MO
Rifampicin 150 mg alone 300 mg alone 150 mg with isoniazid 100 mg 300 mg with isoniazid 150 mg	• Allergy to it • Hepatitis	• Hepatitis/jaundice • Fever/flu like • Bleeding due to platelet damage (rare) • Shock (rare) • Red urine and tears • Stops oral contraceptives working • GI symptoms	• Stop if hepatitis bleeding or shock and transfer to MO • Advise about contraceptives • Give dose at night if nausea, abdominal pain, etc.
Pyrazinamide 500 mg	• Allergy to it • Hepatitis	• Nausea/vomiting • Joint pain/gout • Hepatitis	• Anti-nauseants p.r.n. and/or give at night • Give aspirin for mild arthritis • Stop if severe gout and transfer to MO • Stop if hepatitis and transfer to MO
Streptomycin for IMI injection 1 g 500 mg	• Allergy to it • Already deaf • Pregnancy • Not able to ensure needles and syringes sterilised properly • Kidney damage/renal failure	• Dizziness and pins and needles at time of injection not important • Dizziness all the time especially if eyes closed or in dark • Deafness • Kidney damage	• Stop if getting dizzy on exertion, unsteady on feet (e.g. heel toe walking straight line) and change to ethambutol • Check with MO about reduced dose if kidney disease
Ethambutol 100 mg 400 mg	• Allergy • Poor vision not normal if wears spectacles • Kidney damage/renal failure • Young children not able to tell you if sight affected	• Rashes • Nausea/vomiting • Loss of vision	• Stop if sight getting worse – check vision with chart before starting treatment • Check with MO about reduced dose if kidney disease

continued

Table 14.4 (continued)

Drug/ Tablet size	*Do not give if*	*Side effects*	*Notes*
Thioacetazone 50 mg 150 mg 150 mg with 300 mg isoniazid	• Allergy to it • It has been proven to have a lot of side effects in your population • Patient has also HIV infection	• Nausea/vomiting • Rashes which can be severe and damage all skin and mucous membranes of mouth, etc.	• Stop if itch or rash and transfer to MO if rash gets worse • Use ethambutol instead if patient has HIV infection

Table 14.5 Symptoms which may be side effects of antituberculosis drugs and what to do about them. (Adapted from Harries, A.D. and Maher, D. (1996) *TB/HIV A Clinical Manual*. Geneva, WHO)

Side effects	*Drug(s) probably responsible*	*Management*
Minor		Continue anti-TB drugs
Loss of appetite, nausea, abdominal pain	Rifampicin	Give tablets last thing at at night but still without food
Joint pains	Pyrazinamide	Aspirin
Burning sensation in feet	Isoniazid	Pyridoxine 100 mg daily
Orange/red urine	Rifampicin	Reassurance
Itch but no rash	Thioacetazone, streptomycin, or others	Stop thioacetazone and streptomycin
Major		Stop drug(s) responsible
Skin rash	Thioacetazone, streptomycin, all others if not these	Stop all anti-TB drugs and transfer to Medical Officer
Deafness (no wax blocking canal)	Streptomycin	Stop streptomycin, use ethambutol instead
Dizziness (vertigo and nystagmus)	Streptomycin	Stop streptomycin, use ethambutol instead
Jaundice (other causes excluded)	Most anti-TB drugs	Stop all anti-TB drugs and transfer to Medical Officer
Vomiting and confusion (possible drug-induced early severe hepatitis before jaundice)	Most anti-TB drugs	Stop all anti-TB drugs transfer to Medical Officer if no other cause found due to treatment (e.g. malaria, meningitis, etc.)
Difficulty seeing or loss of colour vision	Ethambutol	Stop ethambutol
Generalised, including shock and bleeding	Rifampicin	Stop rifampicin and transfer urgently to Medical Officer

essential that you immediately report such cases to your Medical Officer.

Make sure that you do all the recording and reporting needed by your Health Department. Then they can see how your patients are doing and give you help if needed. It also shows how the tuberculosis control programme in the country is going and what changes may need to be made.

Transfer

Transfer to Medical Officer care any of the following:

1. patients who are strongly suspected of having tuberculosis; but you cannot prove the diagnosis at the health centre;
2. patients who develop serious drug reactions (urgent);
3. patients with complications, especially significant haemoptysis (urgent);
4. patients with suspected drug resistant infection, i.e. patients who continue to have positive sputum for AFB after 5 months supervised regular treatment which you know has been given and taken (non-urgent).

Note on health education and contact tracing

The patient

Teach the patient about the disease and the need for regular treatment. Get the patient to memorise the month and the year he should finish treatment (if all goes well).

Tell him if he does not take treatment the disease will destroy his lungs and infect others. Tell him if he takes regular treatment he will be cured and he will not infect others.

Tell him to come to the treatment centre immediately if he gets itch, rash, blisters, nausea, fever, jaundice, etc.

Tell him to tell the treatment centre if he intends to move to another place or go on holiday.

Ask if he has any worries or questions, and answer them.

See also p 86.

Family, other contacts and community education

All contacts (family, those who live in the same house, friends, workmates, schoolmates, etc.) should be seen.

Educate them about the symptoms of the disease and tell them that drugs cure it and tell them to come back if symptoms develop.

Question and examine them for cough, enlarged lymph glands and wasting, etc. Any who have chronic cough or other symptoms or signs should have sputum tested for AFB, and aspirate or biopsy of any enlarged lymph nodes.

If tuberculin testing or X-rays are available, do these especially in children who cannot produce sputum. Give any child under 7 years who has a positive tuberculin test but is otherwise well prophylactic isoniazid for 6 months. Give newborn (and probably all young children) who are close household contacts of infectious sputum-positive pulmonary tuberculosis patients, prophylactic isoniazid even if the tuberculin test is negative (especially if the patient is the mother). (*Make sure that the child does not have tuberculosis as then the child needs at least 2 drugs, i.e. proper treatment for tuberculosis disease.*)

Give BCG to other children and to adults who have a negative tuberculin test.

Educate everyone to come to the Health Centre if symptoms develop.

Explain to all the family and contacts how tuberculosis can be treated and how they can help the patient and *make sure* he or she gets regular treatment.

Control and prevention

Get rid of the reservoir of infection

Persons with pulmonary tuberculosis spread the disease by coughing.

Almost as soon as a patient starts on antituberculosis drugs (certainly by 2 weeks), he becomes non-infectious.

If all pulmonary cases of tuberculosis could be found and kept on treatment, the disease could no longer spread.

Therefore, every time you see any patient for any reason, ask if he has a cough. If it has been present for more than 3 weeks, send sputum for tests for AFB.

Once a case is found, it is important to examine all the patient's contacts to find who gave him the disease and to whom he has given the disease, before they spread it further (see above).

Stop the means of spread of the organisms

Measures to stop droplet spread help. Educate people to cover the mouth when coughing. Encourage housing with plenty of windows and which is not overcrowded (especially where people sleep).

Raise the resistance of susceptible persons

The resistance of the general population can be raised by general public health measures (malaria control, prevention of malnutrition, treatment of anaemia and especially prevention of HIV infection). Do all you can to stop HIV infection spreading in your community. (HIV infection is the main reason tuberculosis is becoming more and more common today. See Chapter 19 page 183.)

The resistance of individual persons can be greatly increased by BCG immunisation given before tuberculosis infection usually happens. In places where infection happens all the time and where it is not known how long the effect of BCG lasts, give BCG when your national tuberculosis programme tells you to; or, if it does not:

1. at birth or as soon as possible after;
2. at 7 years or the first year at school;
3. at 13 years or the last year at school;
4. to adults who have not had BCG before;
5. to contacts with a negative tuberculin test and no evidence of disease (if you give prophylactic isoniazid to an infant, give BCG after isoniazid completed).

Check all patients for BCG scars. If the correct number of BCG scars is not present, give BCG.

Prophylactic treatment

You should give prophylactic treatment to contacts of infectious patients who have been infected. This is to kill the few organisms in the infected contact before the organisms multiply and produce clinical *disease*. In practice this is usually done only for children under 7 years with *M. tuberculosis* infection shown by a positive tuberculin test. It is also given to newborn children (and probably best given also to all children under the age of 3) who are household contacts of sputum-positive tuberculosis patients (especially if this person is the mother), even if the tuberculin test is negative. These children are given isoniazid 10 mg/kg for 6 months. Do not give isoniazid alone if there is any evidence of tuberculosis disease (as well as tuberculosis infection); give full treatment for tuberculosis. After a course of isoniazid is finished, then give BCG.

Do not treat adults who are well and have a positive tuberculin test with isoniazid as this would mean most of the population in some places would need treatment, although only 5–10% of patients with a positive Mantoux would ever get tuberculosis during their lifetime. A more worthwhile use of the effort and money to do this would be to find infectious patients and treat them all with DOTS.

There are reasons for and against giving prophylactic isoniazid to patients with HIV who have been infected or may be infected with tuberculosis. At present the reasons for not giving it are more than the reasons for giving it in most countries. The present WHO policy is that HIV patients should not be given prophylactic isoniazid treatment except in very special circumstances (and in these, the patient will need X-rays and perhaps other tests to make sure he does not have unusual tuberculosis infection and does not need full treatment and not just isoniazid).

15

Leprosy

Definition, cause, pathology

Leprosy is a chronic bacterial infection of man. It is common in parts of the world where there is poverty, overcrowding, poor general health and infectious patients are not diagnosed and treated quickly. The infection causes chronic inflammation and destruction of the skin and the peripheral nerves. Sometimes it can also cause inflammation and destruction of the eyes, the mucous membrane of the upper respiratory tract, the muscles, the bones, the testes and other organs. Multi-drug therapy is able to cure the infection in 6–24 months. Patients need to be taught how to care for parts of their body already damaged or made anaesthetic before cure of the infection.

Leprosy is caused by an infection with *Mycobacterium leprae*, a bacterial bacillus. If you stain the *M. leprae* bacillus in the laboratory and then cover it with acid, it keeps the colour of the stain. (Most other organisms lose their colour.) *M. leprae* is therefore called an acid fast bacillus. This is shortened to AFB. (*M. tuberculosis* is also an AFB, see Chapter 14 page 75.)

M. leprae grows very slowly inside body cells. It likes to grow in skin and in nerve cells more than in other cells. It also likes to grow in cool areas of the body more than in warm areas of the body. It therefore grows best in cool areas of the skin and in nerves which are cool near the surface of the body. It also grows well in the cool nasal mucosa and testes. However, if there is not much body defence against the organism, *M. leprae* can grow in all organs of the body.

The body defends itself against *M. leprae*. It does this by its immune cells (see Chapter 10 page 36). (The body also makes antibodies against *M. leprae*; but these do not kill the organism or stop it growing.)

In most people, the body has very powerful cellular immunity. This destroys all the *M. leprae* organisms before any damage is done to the body. The infected person does not get the disease.

If the body has bad cellular immunity (or none), the *M. leprae* organisms grow and multiply and spread through all parts of the body and cause disease. This is called '*lepromatous leprosy*'.

If the body has good cellular immunity but not enough to kill all the M. leprae *organisms*, the body fights the organisms and keeps them in 1–3 places in the skin and/or in 1–3 of the nerves. But, the skin and nerves can be severely damaged in the fight. This is called '*tuberculoid leprosy*'.

There are also *people with intermediate cellular immunity, which is neither good nor bad.* They can get disease with features of both lepromatous and tuberculoid leprosy. The organisms grow and multiply, but the intermediate strength cellular immunity stops them spreading to all of the body. Disease occurs in many parts of the skin and many nerves. This is called '*borderline leprosy*'.

Table 15.1 shows the relationship between cellular immunity and the outcome of *M. leprae* infection.

Epidemiology

Organisms can only spread from patients with lepromatous and borderline leprosy. The organisms spread only from their upper respiratory tract secretions and lepromatous ulcers and ulcerated erythema nodosum leprosum (ENL) lesions.

Spread is by direct or indirect contact; but probably mainly droplets from the respiratory tract.

Organisms spread to the respiratory mucous membrane or the skin of another person.

The incubation period is usually 2–4 years; but it can be shorter or very much longer at times.

All persons are susceptible; but children and males more commonly get the disease. However, most people (99%) infected with *M. leprae* organisms overcome the organisms by powerful cellular immunity and get no leprosy disease.

Table 15.1(a) This table shows how the body's resistance (cellular immunity) to *M. leprae* organisms determines what happens after the body is infected with *M. leprae*.

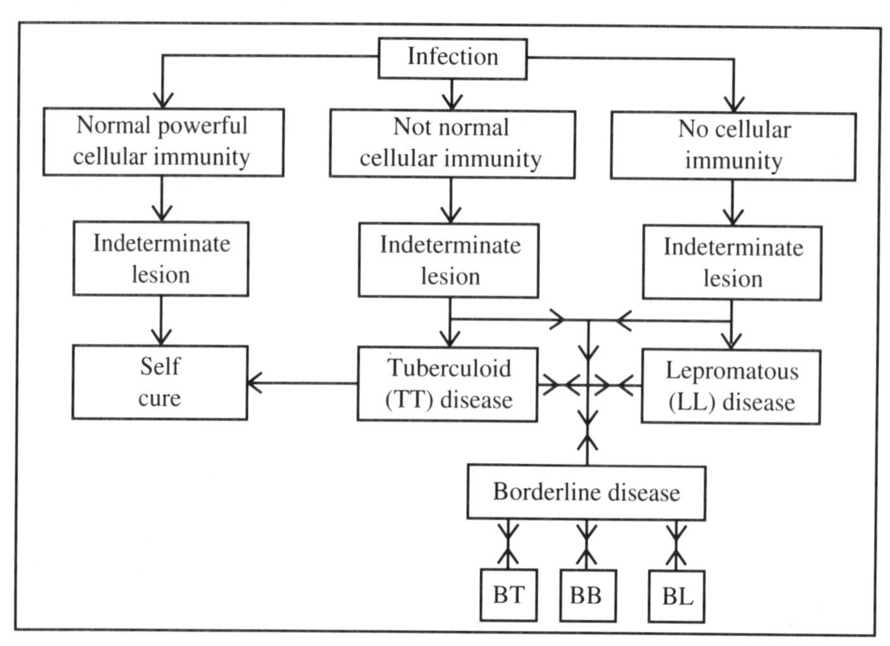

Table 15.1(b) and in more detail

Body resistance to organism	*None*	*Between none and good*	*Good but not quite normal*	*Normal powerful*
Number of M. leprae *which grow in skin*	Many	Many; but not as many as lepromatous; but more than tuberculoid	Some but not many	None
Where M. leprae *grow*	Everywhere in all organs	In skin – in many areas In nerves – in many areas	In skin – in 1–3 areas In nerves – in 1–3 areas	Nowhere
Name of disease	Lepromatous (L)	Borderline (B)	Tuberculoid (T)	No leprosy
	(LL) (BL)	(BB) (BT)	(TT)	
Number of people in the population	Very few	A few	A few	Most
	Of the few (1%) of people infected with *M. leprae* who develop leprosy only 10–20% of these few (1%) develop this lepromatous type of leprosy	Of the few (1%) of people infected with *M. leprae* who develop leprosy, most of these few (1%) develop this tuberculoid or borderline type of leprosy		Most of the people infected with *M. leprae* (99%) do not develop leprosy disease

Those people who do not overcome the infection probably have a special abnormality of just one part of their cellular immune system which does not kill the leprosy organisms. Other parts of their cellular immunity may be normal.

Leprosy occurs in areas where there is poverty, a lot of people live crowded together and there are no good health services to diagnose and cure infectious patients quickly.

The world distribution of leprosy is shown in Figure 15.1 on page 96.

There were at any time in the 1980s about 12 million cases but multi-drug therapy may have reduced these to about 1 million.

Symptoms and signs

Leprosy causes:

1. Skin patches or infiltrations (see below).
2. Nerve enlargement and/or tenderness and/or loss of function (motor and/or sensory) (see page 97).
3. Anaesthesia (loss of sensation) of areas supplied by affected nerves. Injuries, burns, ulcers and destruction occur in anaesthetic areas.
   The parts affected are especially the hands and feet and eyes (see page 98).
4. Weakness, wasting, paralysis of muscles supplied by affected nerves. Deformities of affected areas can then occur.
   The parts affected are especially the hands and feet and eyes (see page 99).
5. Changes in other organs (only in lepromatous leprosy) – the eyes, upper respiratory tract, bones, muscles, joints, testes, etc. (see page 103).
6. 'Reactions' (see page 103).

Skin patches or infiltration

Look at all the skin of the body. Remove as many clothes as possible. Ask the patient to stand in good even natural light or sloping sunlight.

Look very carefully at the face. Examine especially the ears, eyebrows, forehead, cheeks and nose for infiltration and nodules.

Firstly, look for all lesions present. Find out their type (see below), number, size, if they are all the same, and if they are symmetrical (same number on both sides) or not symmetrical.

Next look at the individual lesions and find out what type they are. Find out if they are flat or raised, if the edges are definite or not definite, the appearance of the centre, the appearance of the surface, the colour, and if the lesion is anaesthetic.

If: the lesions are 1–5 patches of any size, that are not all the same and are not symmetrical, *and*
if: the individual lesions are raised with a distinct edge, healing in the centre, dry, pale, without hair, and anaesthetic,
then: the patient has *tuberculoid type skin lesions.* (See Figures 15.2 and 15.3.)

If: the skin lesions are very many (too many to count), small, all the same and symmetrical, *and*
if: the individual lesions are flat, without a clear, edge the same all over, shiny (red, not pale) and not anaesthetic,
then: the patient has *lepromatous type skin lesions.* (See Figure 15.4.)

If: there are no individual lesions and all the skin is affected, so that the skin of the whole body is thick with deep lines, folds and nodules, which are shiny and perhaps anaesthetic at the ends of the limbs,
then: the patient has *late lepromatous type skin changes.* (See Figures 15.5, 15.6 and 15.7.)

If: the patient has many patches (but which still can be counted) and which are various sizes and which may or may not be symmetrical, *and*
if: the individual patches are different (some looking like tuberculoid patches and some looking like large lepromatous patches)
then: the patient has *borderline type skin changes.* (See Figures 15.8 and 15.9.)

Sometimes in borderline type skin changes the patches merge into normal skin and this normal skin merges into other patches. It is then difficult to see which is normal and which is abnormal skin, and the skin looks like a relief map in an atlas. These changes are characteristic of borderline leprosy.

Test any skin patches for loss of sensation (anaesthesia) with cotton wool or a pin (see Figure 15.10). First touch some normal skin with a piece of cotton wool when the patient has his eyes open. Ask the patient to put a finger on the same place as you touched. Then ask the patient to close his eyes. Touch normal skin again. Ask the patient to put a finger on the place you touched. Do this several times on normal skin with the patient's eyes closed until you

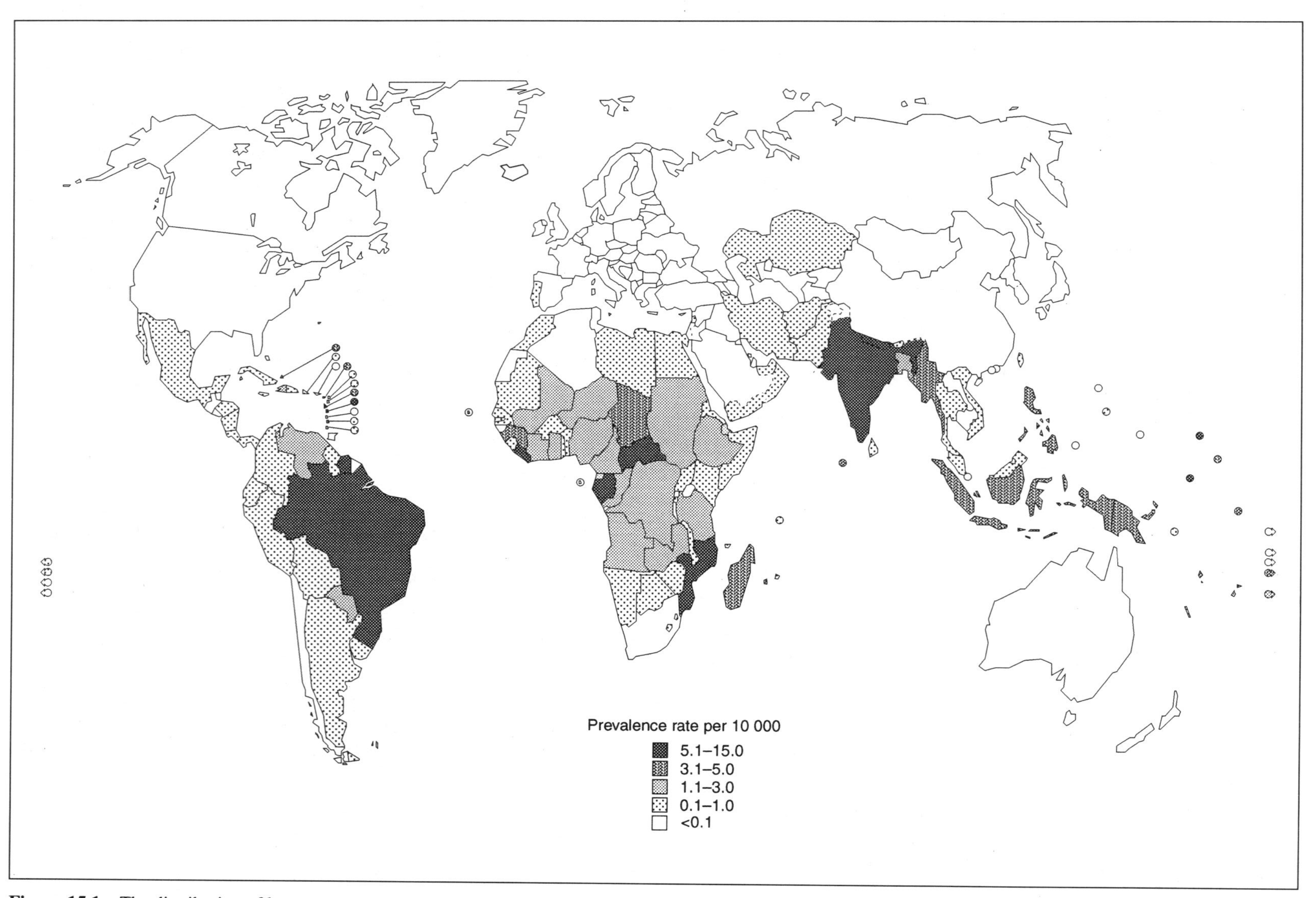

Figure 15.1 The distribution of leprosy.
(Source: *WHO Technical Report Series* No. 874, 1998)

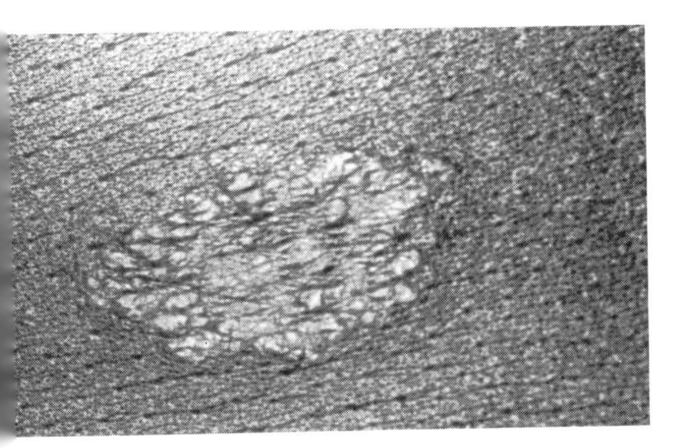

Figure 15.2 Close up view of an early tuberculoid type skin lesion.

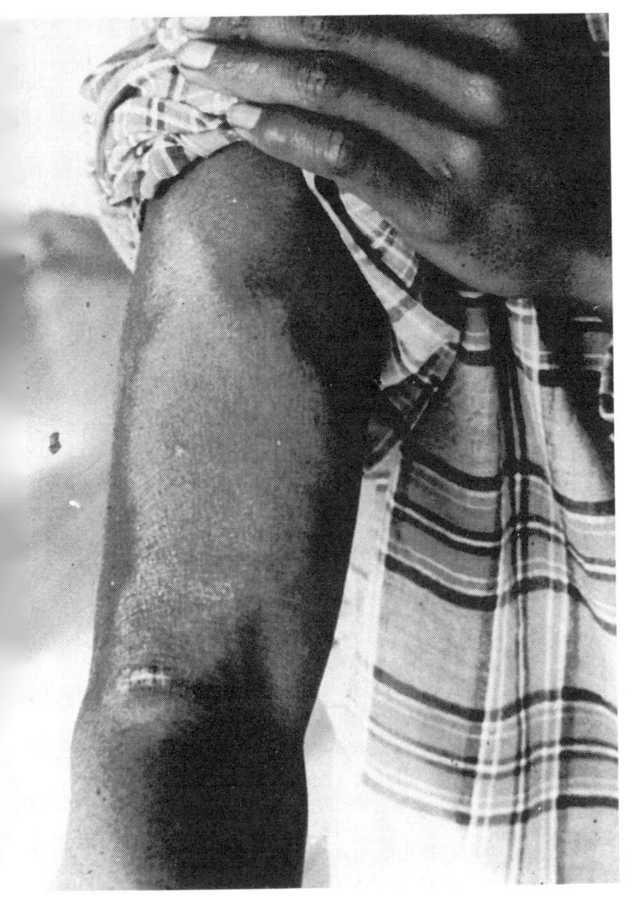

Figure 15.3 A typical large tuberculoid type skin lesion of the arm.

are sure that he understands what to do. Then touch the skin in places where there may be loss of sensation as well as places where there is normal skin. If the patient does not put his finger on places you

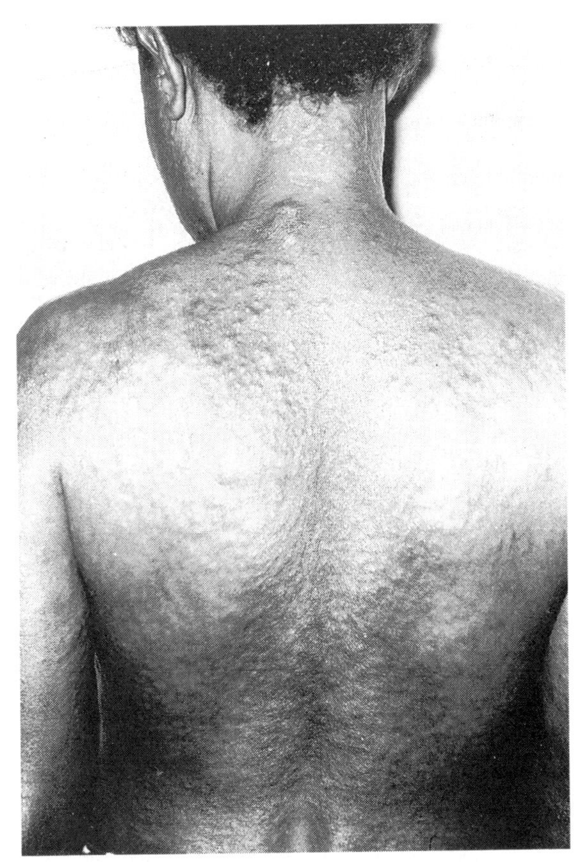

Figure 15.4 Well advanced lepromatous leprosy.

touch, then he feels nothing in these areas. He has anaesthesia in these areas. Repeat this several times on places which appear to be anaesthetic. Check the opposite side of his body in the same places.

Make sure the patient has leprosy and does not have dermal leishmaniasis (see Chapter 18 page 139) or a fungus infection of the skin (see Chapter 32 page 429).

Nerve damage – enlargement and/or tenderness and/or loss of function

The important nerves most commonly affected by leprosy which can be palpated (felt) are the ulnar, median, radial, lateral popliteal and posterior tibial (see Figure 15.11).

Feel for enlargement or tenderness of the:

- ulnar nerves at inside of elbows (Figure 15.12),
- posterior tibial nerves behind the inside of the ankle joints (Figure 15.13),
- lateral popliteal nerves at the outside of the knees (Figure 15.14).

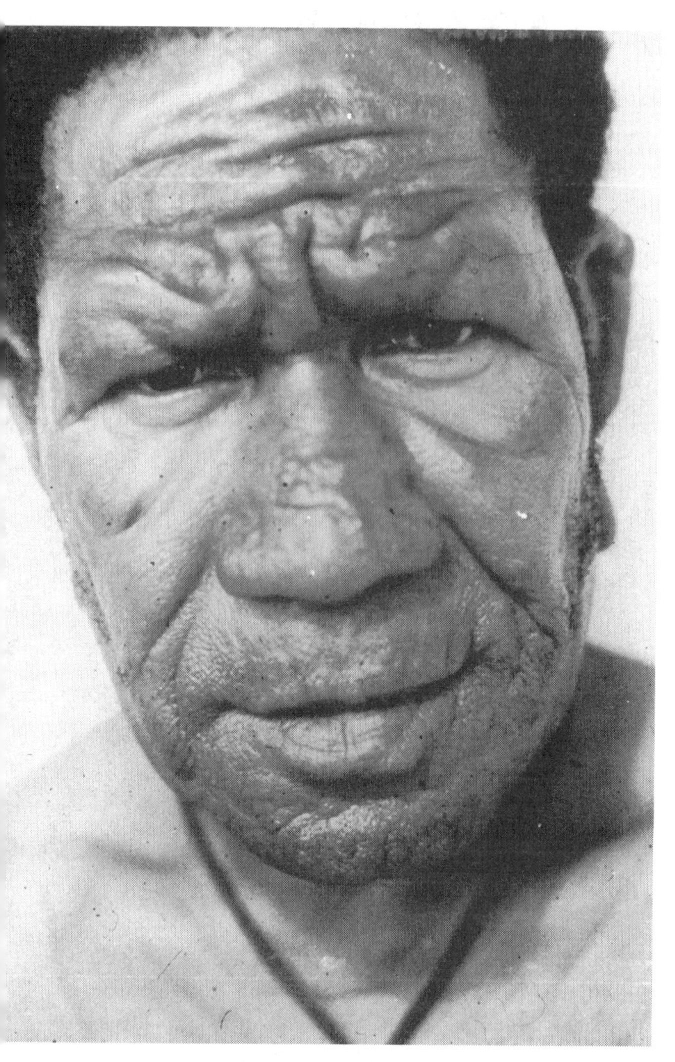

Figure 15.5 Late lepromatous leprosy.

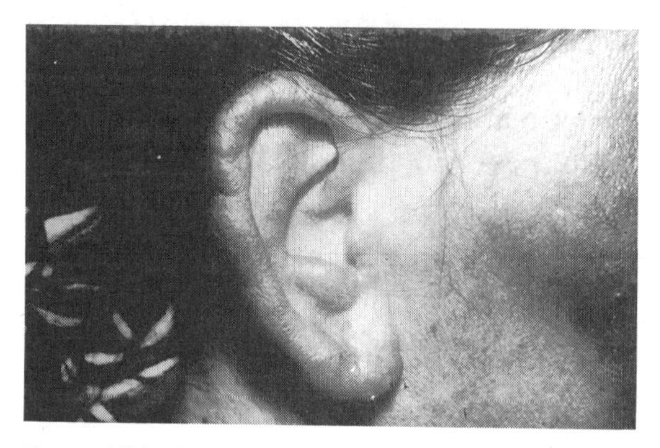

Figure 15.6 Lepromatous leprosy with nodules on the ear. Nodules are more easily seen on the ear than other places. You can see nodules on the ear even more easily if you examine the patient from behind.

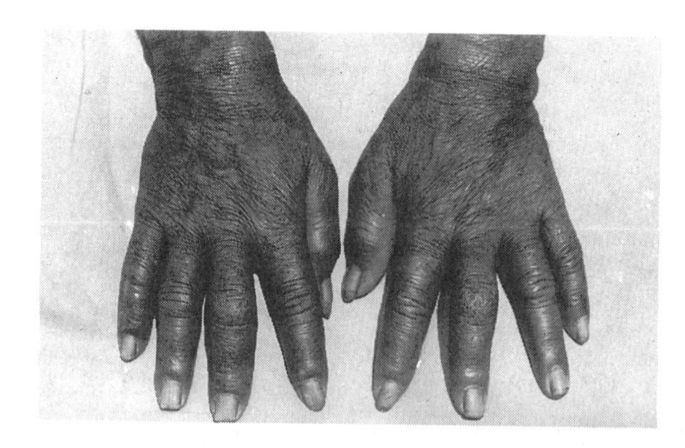

Figure 15.7 Late lepromatous leprosy. Swelling of all the skin of the body is often more easily seen in the swelling of the fingers and hands, as in this patient.

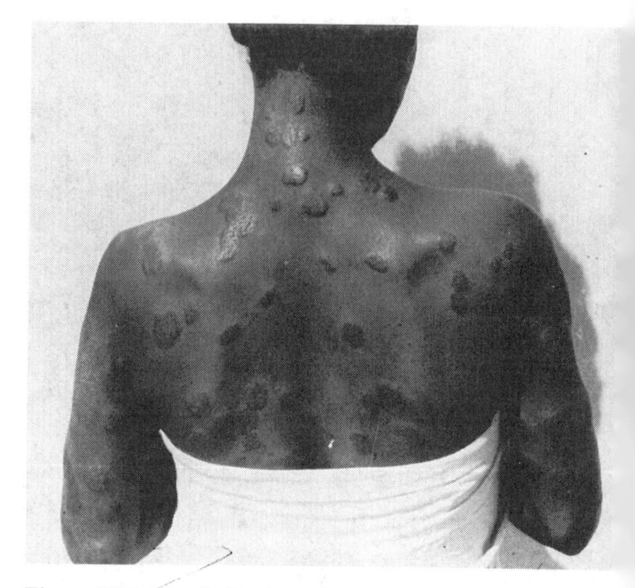

Figure 15.8 Borderline leprosy.

Nerves in the skin near a patch may be enlarged.

Nerves going to the face and the eye may be affected; but these cannot be felt easily.

Anaesthesia of areas supplied by affected nerves (hands, feet and eyes)

Ulnar nerve damage causes anaesthesia in the little finger and half of the next finger.

Median nerve damage causes anaesthesia in the rest of the hand.

Lateral popliteal nerve damage causes anaesthesia in the outside part of the leg.

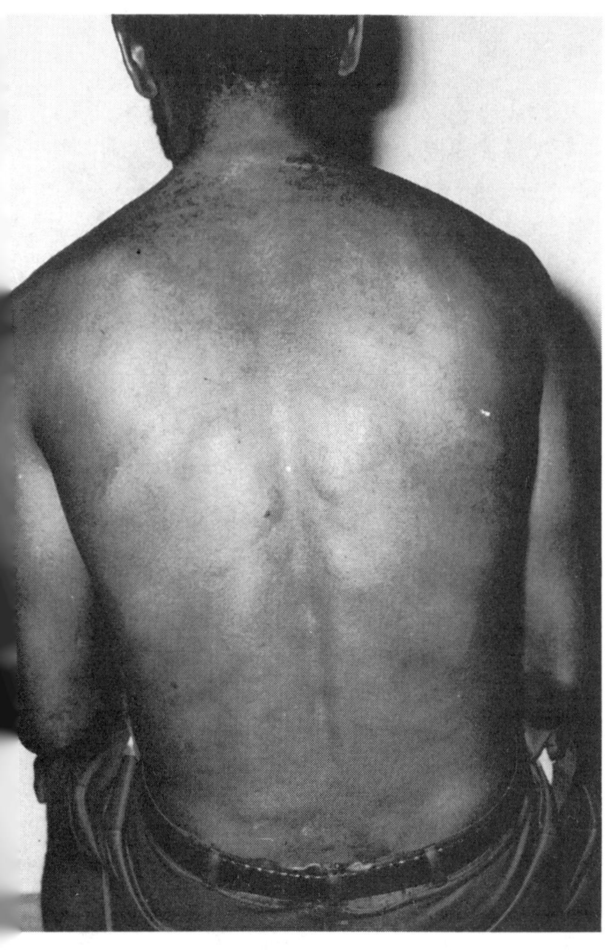

Figure 15.9 Borderline leprosy.

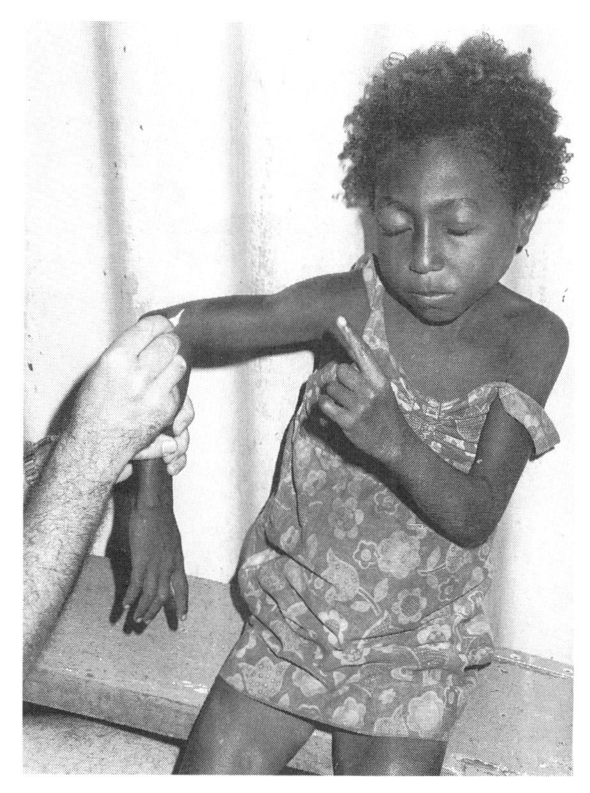

Figure 15.10 Testing for anaesthesia of a patch in the skin. (See text for description.) Compare with testing for anaesthesia in hands and feet. (See Figure 15.15.)

Posterior tibial nerve damage causes anaesthesia underneath the foot.

Damage to the nerve going to the eye causes anaesthesia of the cornea of the eye.

1. Test the hands feet and eyes for anaesthesia, (see Figure 15.15 and below).
2. Look and feel for burns, blisters, cuts, ulcers, swellings, hot areas, etc. on the hands and feet. These can be present in anaesthetic areas without patient noticing (see Figure 15.16).
3. Look for severe destruction of the hands or feet which can be caused by the anaesthesia and injuries which the patient does not notice because there is no pain (see Figures 15.17 and 15.18).

Test for anaesthesia in the eye by getting the patient to look upwards and towards his nose and then touch the cornea with a small piece of cotton wool from the side of his face. If the patient still has sensation, the eye will blink.

Weakness, wasting or paralysis of muscles supplied by affected nerves (hands, feet and eyes)

Ulnar damage causes a claw hand, affecting mostly ring and little fingers. The patient cannot straighten or bend these fingers properly (see Figure 15.19).

Median damage causes claw hand of the other fingers which the patient cannot bend or straighten properly, and paralysis of thumb so that the patient cannot pinch or lift it away from the palm of the hand (see Figure 15.20).

Radial damage causes wrist drop or the wrist cannot bend backwards (see Figure 15.21).

Lateral popliteal damage causes foot drop or the foot cannot bend up at the ankle (see Figure 15.22).

Posterior tibial damage causes paralysis of small muscles of the foot, and claw toes.

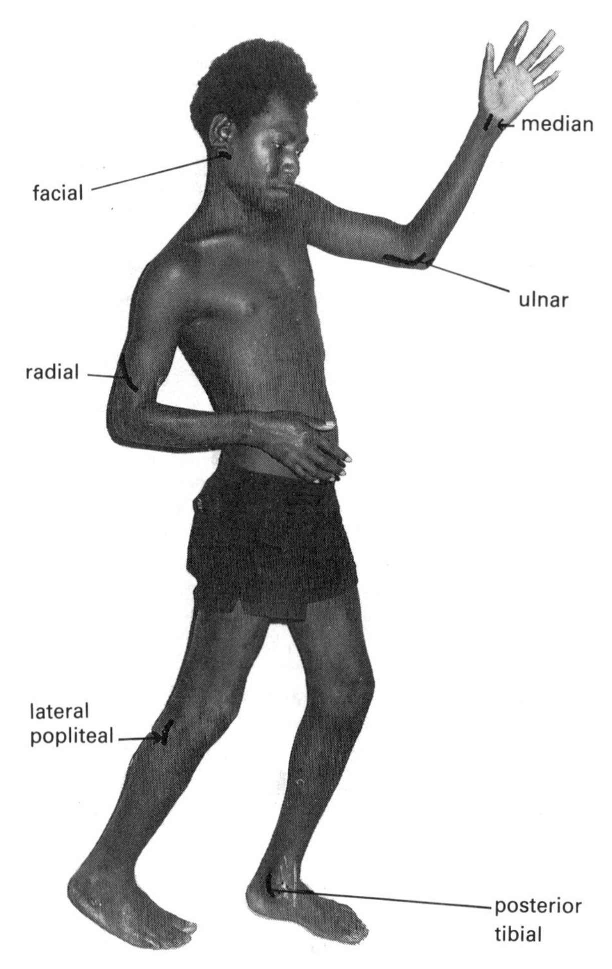

Figure 15.11 The position of nerves commonly affected in leprosy and which can be felt to be abnormal – enlarged or tender. The method of examining the three most important areas are shown in Figures 15.12, 15.13 and 15.14.

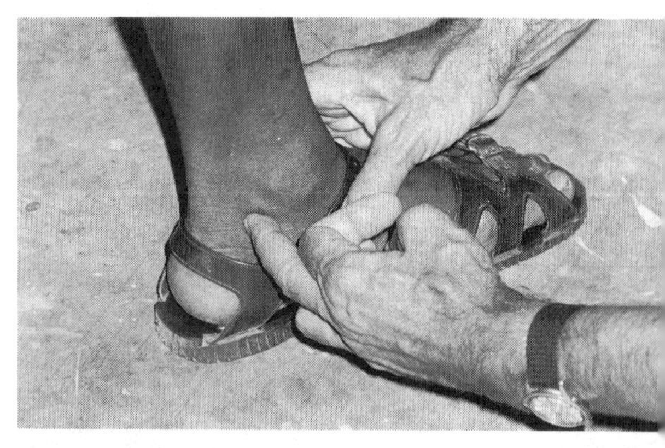

Figure 15.13 Method of palpating for tenderness and/or enlargement of the posterior tibial nerve.

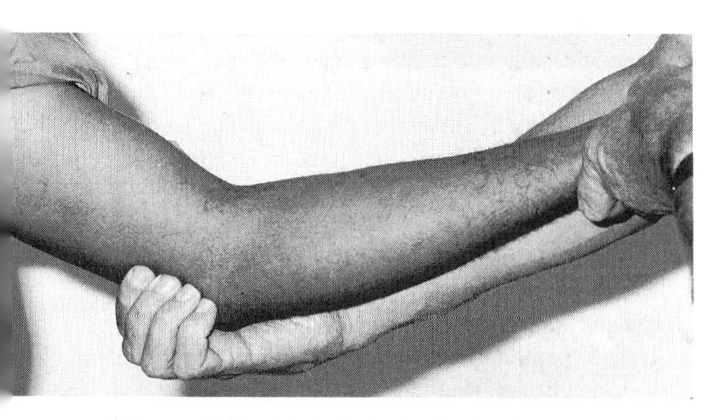

Figure 15.12 Method of palpating for enlargement and/or tenderness of the ulnar nerve.

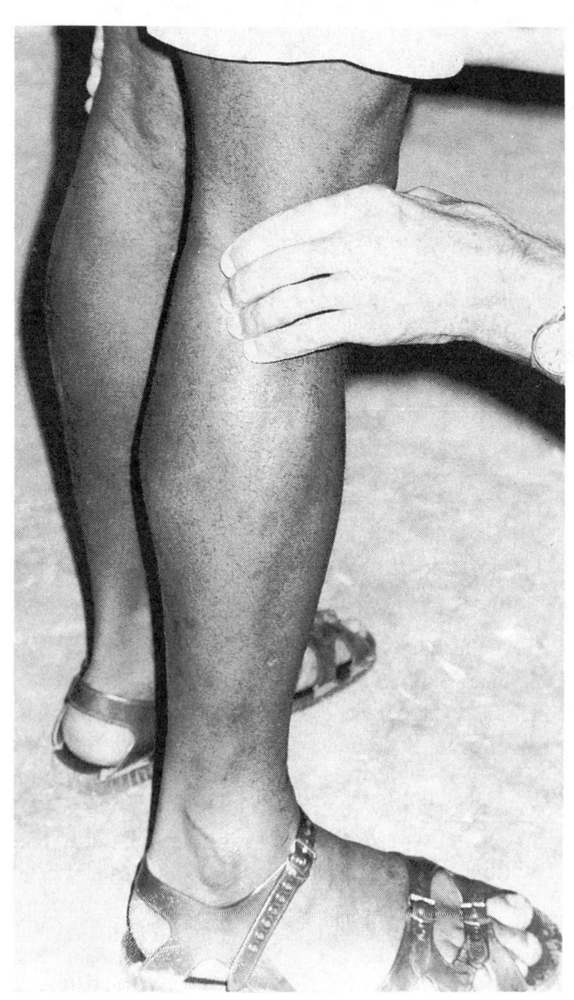

Figure 15.14 Method of palpation for tenderness and/or enlargement of the lateral popliteal nerves.

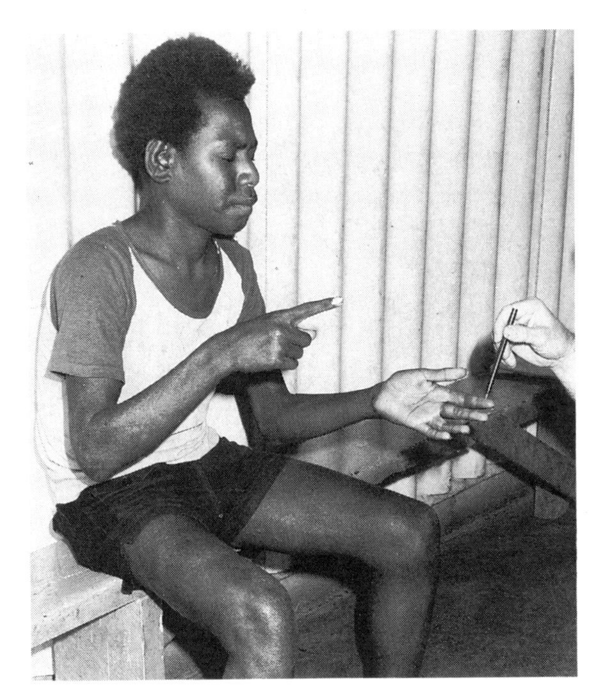

Figure 15.15 Testing for anaesthesia in the hands and feet. Note the difference from testing for anaesthesia in a skin patch (see Figure 15.10). Gently but firmly touch the palms of the hands and soles of the feet with the tip of a pencil or a piece of wire. With his eyes closed, the patient must put a finger close to the place you have touched. If he puts his finger more than 2 cm away from the place you touched, he has lost enough sensation for him to severely damage this part of his body without knowing it.

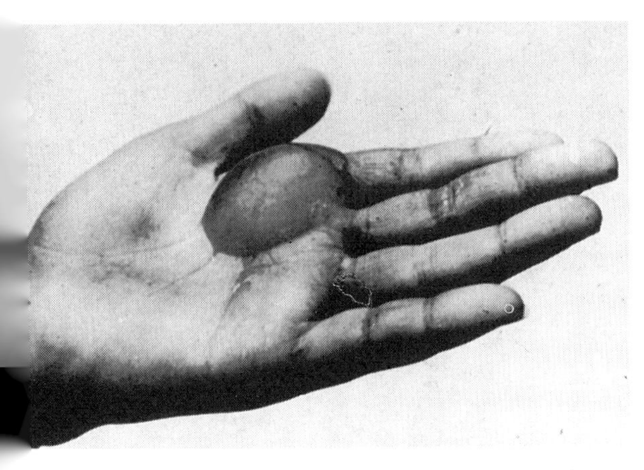

Figure 15.16 Blister from burn due to loss of sensation.

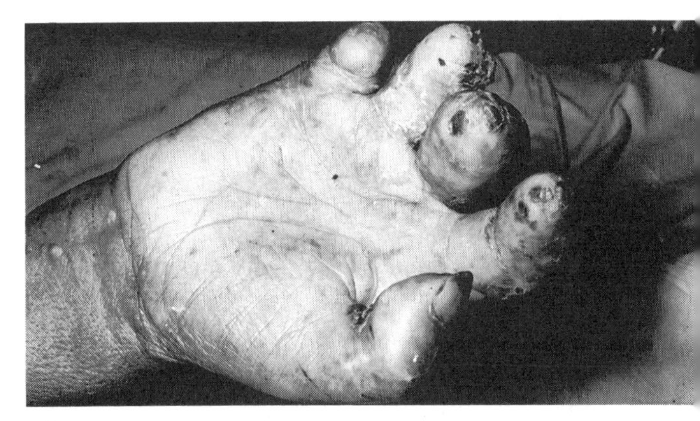

Figure 15.17 Hand destroyed because of loss of sensation and lack of special care of the anaesthetic hand. The patient has trauma including burns, cuts, blisters, etc., as the patient has in Figure 15.16, but they did not hurt and as he did not know how to look after his hand, this is what happened.

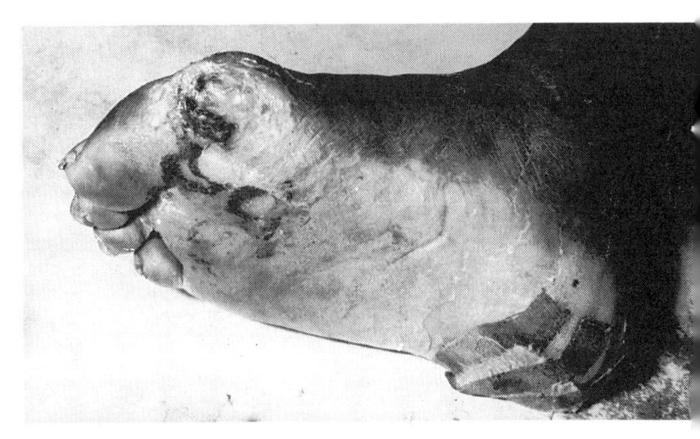

Figure 15.18 Photograph of plantar ulcers (i.e. ulcers on the sole of the foot). These ulcers were caused by injuries (such as cuts and bruises) which the patient did not worry about or care for because there was no pain. If the patient had cared for his feet properly (see page 111), he need not have got these ulcers. If the ulcers had been treated properly they would have healed. The dressings used by the health worker for this patient were useless. For proper treatment of plantar ulcers see page 112. Note that these ulcers are NOT caused by the leprosy organisms in the ulcer. These ulcers are caused by nerve damage with loss of sensation under the foot.

Facial damage causes paralysis of eyelid – the patient cannot close his eye properly (lagophthalmos) (see Figure 15.23).

A quick test for paralysis of hand muscles is as follows (see also Figure 15.24):

1. Ask the patient to hold his hand like the hand on the left of Figure 15.24 (wrist up, fingers straight but bent to 90° where they join the palm, and thumb across the palm).
2. Look for clawing of little and ring fingers (both of patient's hands) from ulnar weakness.
3. Look for clawing of other fingers (patient's left hand) for median weakness.

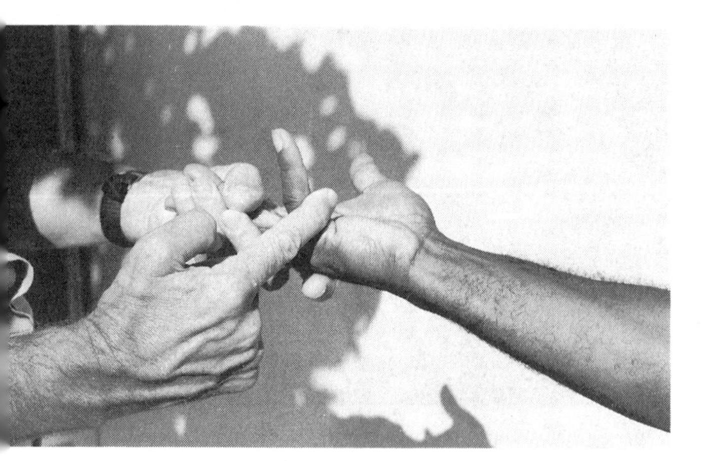

Figure 15.19 Testing for weakness of one of the muscles supplied by the ulnar nerve.

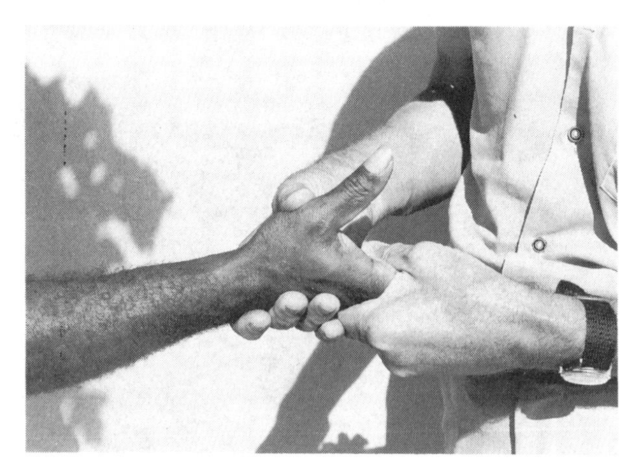

Figure 15.20 Testing for weakness of one of the muscles supplied by the median nerve.

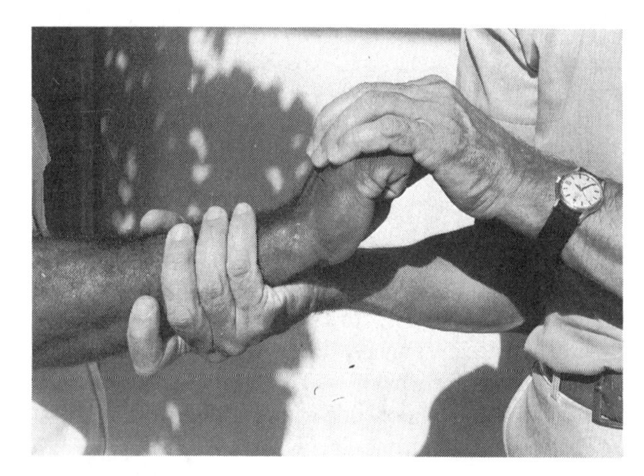

Figure 15.21 Testing for weakness of muscles supplied by radial nerve.

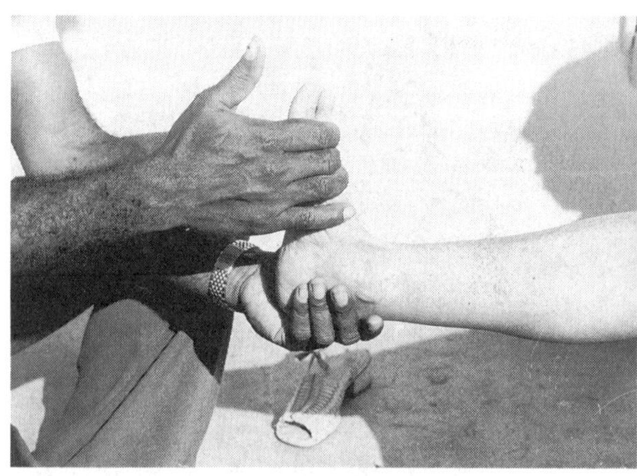

Figure 15.22 Testing for weakness of muscles supplied by the lateral popliteal nerve.

4. Look for wrist drop (not present) from radial weakness.
5. Check if the thumb cannot go across the palm (not present) from median weakness.

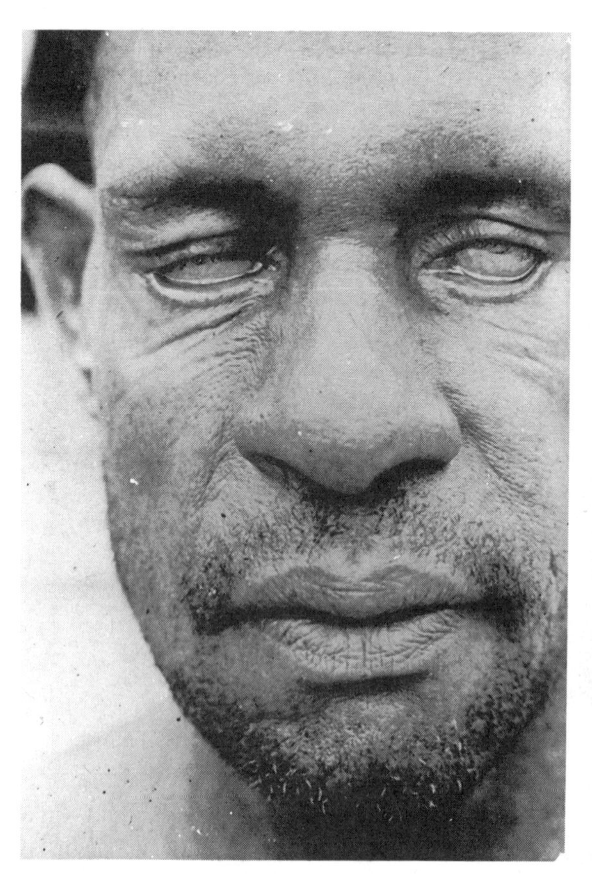

Figure 15.23 Bilateral lagophthalmos. The patient is trying to close both eyes. The eyes turn upwards, but the eyelids will not close.

Later effects

Fixed deformities occur later in the disease if treatment is not successful. The joints become stiff in the position in which they are paralysed and cannot be straightened even with another hand helping.

Damage of other organs – only in lepromatous leprosy

Nose – swollen mucous membrane causes blocked up nose which can bleed. Later, the bone collapses and the nose becomes flat.

Bones of hands and feet – these become weak and easily crushed, and the fingers and toes, etc. become shorter.

Testes – these become smaller, and sterility and gynaecomastia (swollen breasts) develop.

Eyes – iritis with loss of vision can occur (see Chapter 31 page 420).

'Reactions'

There are two types of reaction. It is more important to recognise that a reaction is occurring than to remember which type it is.

Type I reaction occurs in borderline leprosy and affects the nerves and the parts of the skin that are already affected by leprosy. The edges of the skin patches may become swollen, painful and tender. More seriously, the affected nerves may become swollen, painful and tender. There may be a sudden loss of sensation. There may be sudden paralysis.

Type II reactions occur in lepromatous leprosy. Small, painful lumps called erythema nodosum leprosum (ENL), may develop in the skin so this reaction is often called an ENL reaction (Figure 15.25). There may be also acute inflammation of any of the organs involved in lepromatous leprosy. Especially important are acute iritis (painful red eye with some loss of sight), acute orchitis (painful swelling of a testis or both testes) or painful swelling of nerves with sudden loss of sensation or paralysis.

If a reaction occurs there may also be general symptoms and signs of inflammation – fever, fast pulse etc.

Classification of types of leprosy

Lepromatous, tuberculoid and borderline leprosy are the three main types of leprosy.

But leprosy can be divided clinically into six types:

1. indeterminate,
2. tuberculoid,

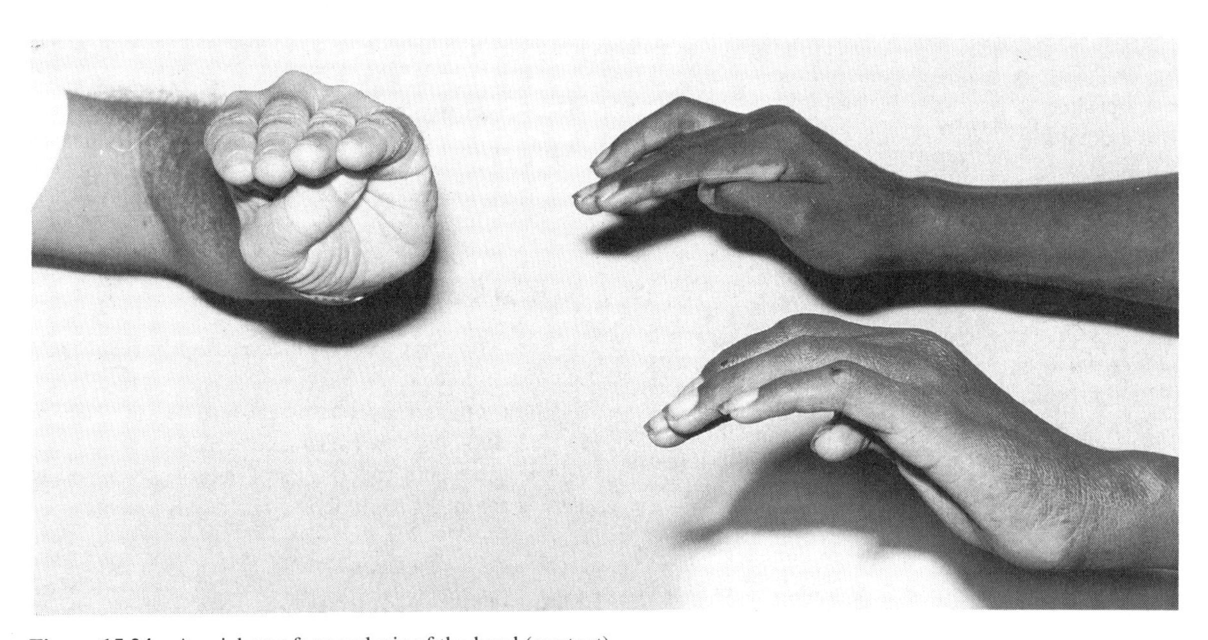

Figure 15.24 A quick test for paralysis of the hand (see text).

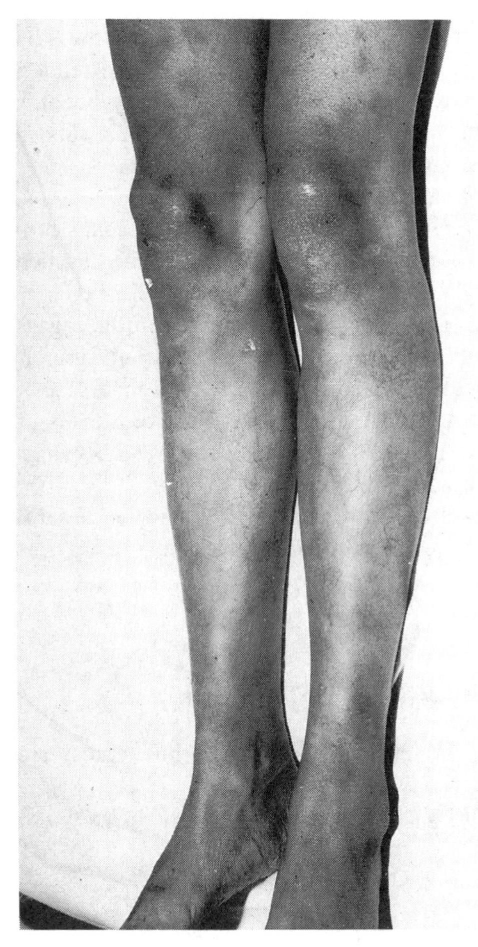

Figure 15.25 Leprosy reaction with ENL. ENL are inflamed tender nodules, most common on the front of the legs and the backs of the arms and on the face.

3. borderline,
4. lepromatous,
5. neural, and
6. clinically drug resistant leprosy.

Leprosy can also be divided into two types by the results of skin smears for bacillary index (BI) or biopsy.

1. *Multibacillary.* These patients have many AFBs in skin smears. They will usually be LL, BL, BB or at times BT cases. They are called 'multibacillary' as multi means many and bacilli refer to AFBs.
2. *Paucibacillary.* These patients have few AFBs in skin smears or biopsy. They are clinically usually TT and indeterminate cases although some may be BT. They are called 'paucibacillary' as pauci means few.

Leprosy may soon also be divided into three clinical types according to the skin lesions. This may be particularly useful where there are no laboratories to do examinations for AFB. This classification would then help in deciding what type of treatment to give (see page 109).

1. Single (1) skin lesion – single lesion leprosy
2. Two to five (2–5) skin lesions – Paucibacillary (PB) leprosy
3. More than five skin lesions – Multibacillary (MB) leprosy

Indeterminate leprosy

Indeterminate leprosy may occur soon after the leprosy organisms have entered the body and started to grow, but before it has been decided if the body's defences or the organisms will win the fight.

One (or a few) flat (or slightly raised), indistinct, slightly pale, sometimes slightly anaesthetic patch in the skin may be found. Skin smears (see page 108) may show a few AFB, but may be negative.

Unless the smear is positive for AFB, do not diagnose indeterminate leprosy. Either biopsy the lesion (see page 107) (*but* do *not* biopsy a lesion on the face), or see the patient each 6–12 weeks until either the lesion goes away, or the lesion is obviously leprosy, or the lesion is examined by a Medical Officer. Many people with a diagnosis of 'indeterminate leprosy' do not have leprosy at all.

Tuberculoid, borderline and lepromatous leprosy

See Table 15.2.

Neural leprosy

Some cases only involve nerves and have no skin lesions.

Some cases may have had skin lesions which healed, and only nerve changes remain.

These are both called 'neural' leprosy, or, if many nerves are involved, 'polyneuritic' leprosy.

Drug resistant leprosy

See page 113.

Table 15.2 Main features of the main three types of leprosy.

	Type of leprosy			
	Tuberculoid (TT) Type (Paucibacillary)	*Borderline (BB) Group* (Multibacillary)	*Lepromatous – early (LL) Type* (Multibacillary)	*Lepromatous – late (LL) Type* (Multibacillary)
1. Skin				
(a) Lesions				
• type	Patches	Patches	Patches	The patches join; all the skin is affected
• number	1 – 5	Many – but can be counted	Many – cannot be counted	
• size	Small or large	Vary	Small	
• all the same	No	No	Yes	
• symmetrical (i.e. same both sides)	No	Sometimes	Yes	
(b) Individual lesions				
• flat or raised	Raised at edge	Some flat; some raised	Flat	The skin is all thickened with folds and nodules
• edge distinct or indistinct	Distinct	Some distinct; some indistinct	Indistinct	
• appearance of centre	Healing and scarring	Some healing; some not	All the same	
• appearance of surface	No sweating; no hair	Some normal; some not sweating; no hair	Sweating; hair	
• colour	Pale at edge	Some pale; some shiny	Shiny (red) not pale	Shiny (red) not pale
• anaesthesia	Anaesthetic	Some anaesthetic but not complete	No anaesthesia	Anaesthesia
2. Nerves				
Cutaneous (skin) (sensory)	Only nerves going to a patch	Nerves going to patches	Hands and feet both sides	Much of arms and legs both sides
Peripheral and cranial number	1–3	Many	None or all	All
Symmetrical (i.e. same both sides)	No	Sometimes	Yes	Yes
• swollen	Yes (very)	yes	Only a little	Yes
• tender	No	No; yes if in reaction	No; yes if in reaction	No; yes if in reaction

Table 15.2 (continued)

	Type of leprosy			
	Tuberculoid (TT) Type (Paucibacillary)	*Borderline (BB) Group* (Multibacillary)	*Lepromatous – early (LL) Type* (Multibacillary)	*Lepromatous – late (LL) Type* (Multibacillary)
3. **Anaesthesia** of area supplied by affected nerves	Yes (usually)	Yes	No	Yes
4. **Paralysis** and wasting of muscles supplied by affected nerves	Yes (usually)	Yes	No	Yes
5. **Other organs affected**				
(a) mucous membranes of URT	No	Not marked	Yes	Yes
(b) bones	No	Not marked	Yes	Yes
(c) muscles	No	Not marked	Yes	Yes
(d) testes	No	Not marked	Yes	Yes
(e) general symptoms and signs	No	Not marked	Yes, especially if reaction	Yes, especially if reaction
6. **Reactions**	No	Yes (Type 1)	Yes (Type 2)	Yes (Type 2)

URT, upper respiratory tract

Tests

Skin smear for BI and MI

Do a skin smear in all cases of suspected leprosy – especially lepromatous or borderline leprosy.

How to make a skin smear

Take smears from the ear lobes, the eyebrows and any suspicious skin lesions. Pinch the skin firmly between your thumb and forefinger so that it cannot bleed. With a sharp scalpel, make a slit in the skin 2–3 mm deep and 5 mm long. Then scrape the tissues from the bottom of the wound with the point of the scalpel blade. Use the material on the scalpel blade to make the slide. Warm the slide over a flame until it is just too hot to hold on the back of the hand.

Pack the slide where no insects can reach it, and send it to the laboratory with a request form asking for examination for AFB, including both BI and MI (see Figure 15.26).

Bacillary index (BI) tells how many *M. leprae* organisms there are in the slide. The bacillary index is high (e.g. BI 6 +) in lepromatous cases. Some bacilli may be seen in borderline cases (e.g. BI 1–4 +). No bacilli are seen in tuberculoid cases (BI negative or 0). If originally high, the BI takes years to become negative, even during successful treatment.

Morphological index (MI) tells the percentage of the *M. leprae* organisms that are seen which are morphologically normal (or solid staining or in one piece). The morphological index therefore shows what percentage of organisms are alive. Before treatment MI may be up to 60%. (It is never much more than 60% and never 100%.) MI should fall to 0% after 6 months of successful treatment. The MI should stay at 0% if treatment is effective.

Repeat the smear (for MI and BI) each 3 months (e.g. 1st week of each January, April, July and October), if the original smear was positive.

Skin biopsy

Do a skin biopsy if the diagnosis of tuberculoid or borderline leprosy is not certain.

Take a skin biopsy from the edge of the patch. The bigger the biopsy the better the report can be; but an oval piece of skin about 1 cm in length is enough. Infiltrate the area with local anaesthetic. Mark a narrow oval of skin 1 cm in length to be cut out. With a sharp scalpel cut along the mark you have made,

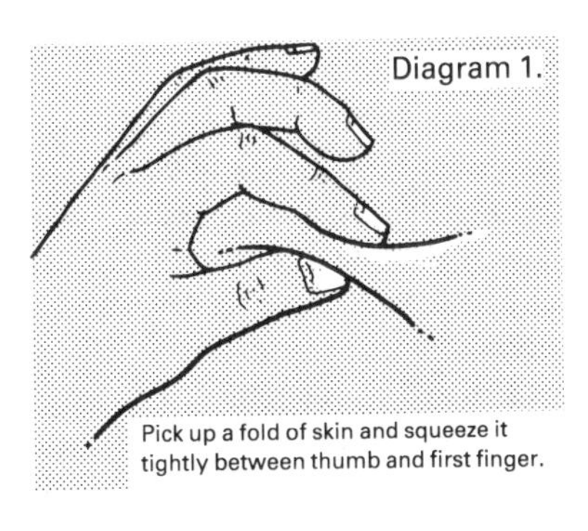

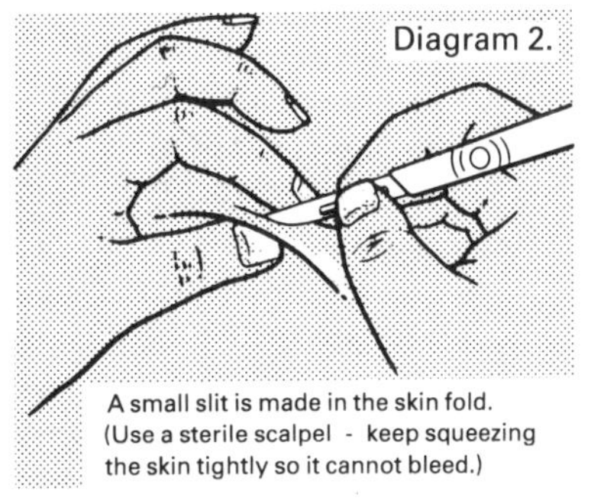

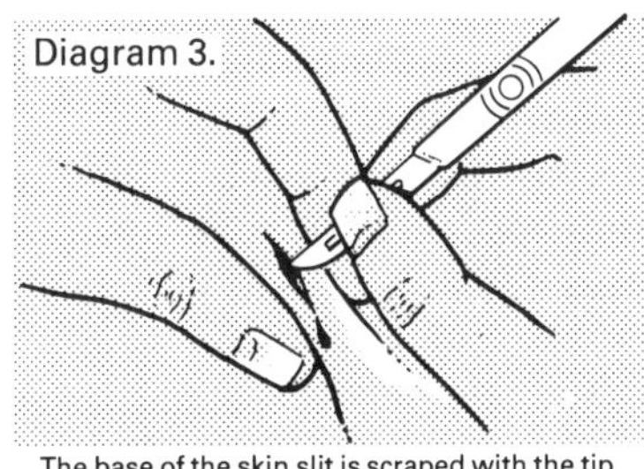

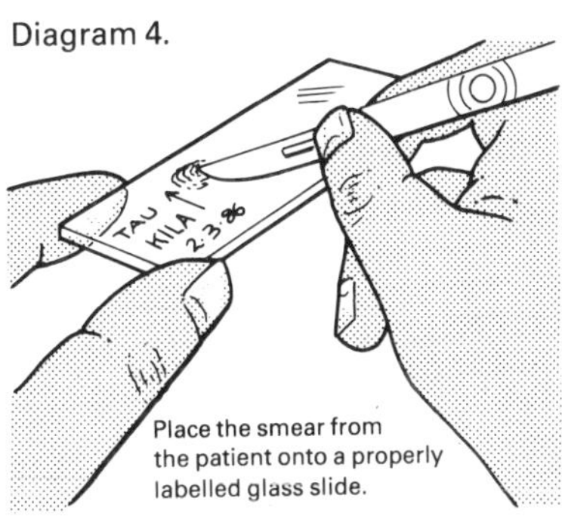

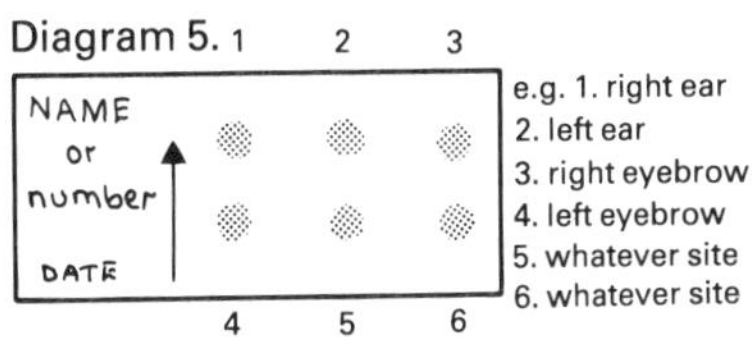

This is how to label and place the patient's smears on the slide. Use a diamond pencil or sticking plaster to label. Do NOT use pencils or paper labels which can rub off. The arrow is to show where you start numbering the smears. Place the smears ON THE SAME SIDE of the glass as the LABELLING. On the requisition slip - use the same numbering as shown in the diagram. Give the actual site from which each smear came.

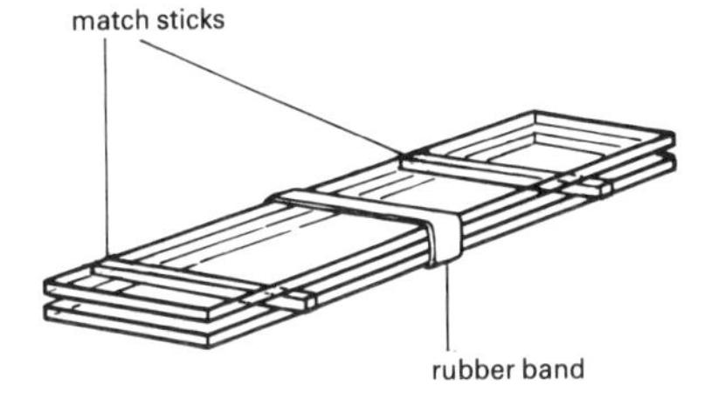

Slides can be packed in pairs like this. The smears must face inwards.

Figure 15.26 Diagrams 1–6 show how to make skin smears for AFB (see text). Wear gloves to do this test.

down to the *fat* under the skin. Lift the biopsy up by the fat underneath the skin *very carefully* (with the smallest forceps you have), and cut through the fat to remove the skin biopsy. Do not squeeze the skin with the forceps because this will make it difficult to examine under the microscope. Drop the biopsy into 20–30 ml fixative solution or formal-saline. Stitch up the skin. For best results, ask your laboratory to send you Ridley's FMA for fixative solution. Leave the biopsy in this solution for 2 hours; then rinse it with water and put it in 70% alcohol. If you do not have this special fixative, use formalin and leave the specimen in the formalin.

Course and complications

Indeterminate leprosy cures itself without treatment in three out of four cases. Treatment will cure the other types.

Tuberculoid leprosy will often cure itself without treatment. But before this happens, severe nerve damage can occur. Treatment will kill the infection and soon stop more nerve damage occurring.

Lepromatous leprosy never cures itself but becomes worse. Reactions are common. Many organs are damaged. Treatment can cure the infection. After some time of regular correct treatment, reactions become less common and then stop.

Without treatment, borderline leprosy will later become like either tuberculoid or lepromatous leprosy. Meanwhile severe nerve damage occurs. Treatment can cure the infection and after some time the reactions will stop.

When the infection is stopped and the *M. leprae* all killed, damaged nerves and other organs cannot recover. But, further damage can be stopped by proper treatment. Proper treatment before much damage occurs is the most important thing.

Treatment

The most important things in the treatment of the patient are:

1. Give anti-leprosy multidrug therapy (MDT) according to the type of leprosy the patient has and using the drugs recommended by your Health Department for as long as they say to give them.
2. Give the patient education about:
   (a) the need for regular treatment
   (b) the care for hands/feet/eyes if these are anaesthetic, and
   (c) the need for quick and proper treatment of reactions, for when reactions occur later.

Until the early 1980s treatment was by giving dapsone alone for 5 years for tuberculoid disease and for life for lepromatous disease. Patients often did not take the drug, so they were not cured. Dapsone-resistant organisms started to occur.

Since 1982, WHO has recommended:

1. Multi-drug therapy (MDT) with dapsone and rifampicin for paucibacillary or tuberculoid patients; and dapsone, rifampicin and clofazimine for multibacillary or lepromatous patients and
2. Supervised taking of the absolutely essential parts of this drug treatment by the health worker – watching to see that the drugs are really swallowed.

This has reduced the number of registered cases from 5.4 million in 1985 to 0.9 million in 1996. Leprosy has relapsed (come back) in fewer than 1% of these properly treated cases.

Other effective and quick-acting drugs such as ofloxacin (a quinolone group drug) as well as other drugs such as clarithromycin (a macrolide group drug) and minocycline (a tetracycline group drug) and fusidic acid are being tested in regimes of treatment which last for shorter periods than the present MDT. These new regimes include MDT (as above) for 1 year only if ofloxacin also is given daily for the first 4 weeks for multibacillary disease; and rifampicin and ofloxacin and minocycline daily for only 4 weeks for paucibacillary disease; or a single dose only of rifampicin and ofloxacin and minocycline for indeterminate leprosy. We do not know yet which of these new regimes will work and which one your Health Department will decide for you to use.

You need therefore to find out what drugs and what doses and what length of treatment your health department is using and, if necessary, change the following presently recommended WHO regime.

Paucibacillary leprosy (indeterminate; TT; and some BT)

As long as the bacterial index is 1 or less (i.e. fewer than 10 AFBs seen in 100 oil-immersion fields) use the following treatment regime.

1. Rifampicin 600 mg for a normal sized adult or 450 mg for an adult < 35 kg; once a month for 6 months, supervised by the health worker.
2. Dapsone 100 mg every day for 6 months, unsupervised, i.e. taken by the patient himself at home. Supply 30 × 100 mg tablets or 60 × 50 mg tablets each month. If the patient is having treatment for reaction with corticosteroid (e.g. prednisolone or cortisone) when the 6 months course ends, continue the dapsone until the corticosteroid treatment finishes.

Multibacillary leprosy (LL, BL, BB, and some BT)

If the bacterial index is 2 + or more (10 or more AFBs in 100 oil-immersion fields) the following drugs are given regularly for 2 years then stopped.

1. Rifampicin 600 mg for a normal sized adult or 450 mg for a small adult (< 35 kg), each month, supervised by the health worker.
2. Clofazimine 300 mg each month supervised by the health worker.
3. Clofazimine 50 mg daily unsupervised, to be taken by the patient himself at home. Supply 30 capsules of 50 mg each month.
4. Dapsone 100 mg daily, unsupervised, to be taken by the patient at home. Supply 30 × 100 mg tablets or 60 × 50 mg tablets each month.

New recommendations mean that the following even simpler regimes may be effective using the simple clinical classification of leprosy (see page 104). Do not use these doses unless told to do so by your *Health Department.*

For paucibacillary and multibacillary leprosy – possible future treatment

	PB for 6 months	MB for 12 months
Dapsone	100 mg daily	100 mg daily
Rifampicin	600 mg 4-weekly supervised	600 mg 4-weekly supervised
Clofazimine		50 mg daily 300 mg 4-weekly supervised

In some areas for single lesion PB leprosy

A single dose rifampicin 600 mg and ofloxacin 500 mg and minocycline 100 mg (but not if pregnant or a child)

Notes

1. If the morphological index (MI) is not zero at the end of 6 months, it is most likely that the patient has not been taking the drugs regularly. It is possible, although unlikely, the patient's organisms are resistant to the drugs. All such cases must be seen as soon as possible by the supervising Medical Officer. (The BI may take years to become zero.)
2. If clofazimine will not be taken by people as it make their skin too red, refer the patient to your Medical Officer about the use of either prothionamide or ethionamide 250 mg for a small adult and 375 mg for a large adult once daily in a single dose after the main meal of the day. These drugs cause more gastrointestinal and liver side effects than clofazimine, which is by far the better drug for them to use.
3. If no 50 mg and only 100 mg capsules of clofazimine are available give 100 mg every two days or three times a week, e.g. Monday, Wednesday and Friday (instead of 50 mg daily).

Side effects of anti-leprosy drugs

Rifampicin

1. Red brown urine and sputum colour. If this does not occur, the patient is not taking his rifampicin. Warn the patient about the colour of his urine and explain that it is a good sign.
2. Gastrointestinal upsets. Even if these occur, rifampicin must be taken on an empty stomach, and no food must be eaten for half an hour after the rifampicin. At home, if first thing in the morning causes too many side effects, try last thing at night. In supervised treatment, tell the patient not to eat for 2 hours before he is seen, when he will be given the drug.
3. Influenza-like reaction after the dose.
4. Hepatitis is the most serious side effect. The rifampicin, but also other anti-leprosy drugs, should be stopped and the patient immediately sent to the Medical Officer's care. Do not just stop the rifampicin.
5. Oral contraceptives may not work. Tell the patient to use other forms of contraception while taking rifampicin.

Clofazimine

1. The skin becomes red and later darker but fades when the clofazimine is ceased.
2. Gastrointestinal symptoms, mainly abdominal pain – this usually occurs only if the dose is larger than 100 mg.

Ethionamide and prothionamide

1. Gastrointestinal upsets.
2. Hepatitis, especially if used in rifampicin. If this occurs, all anti-leprosy drugs must be stopped immediately and the patient sent immediately to the Medical Officer.

Fluoquinolones, e.g. ofloxacin

1. Gastrointestinal upsets.
2. Central nervous system upsets including dizziness.

Dapsone

1. Gastrointestinal upsets.
2. Blood abnormalities including anaemia.
3. Skin rashes.

Before treatment

Do not start treatment unless:

1. the diagnosis is certain because of typical symptoms and signs, or
2. the diagnosis was not certain but is now confirmed by a test (skin smear or biopsy).

If the diagnosis is not certain:

1. do a skin smear for AFB if you suspect lepromatous or borderline leprosy;
2. do a skin biopsy if you suspect tuberculoid or borderline leprosy;
3. if a biopsy is not possible, then, review the patient each 6–12 weeks instead;
4. wait for the results before starting treatment.

Always do a full medical history and physical examination and test the urine. Diagnose and treat any other conditions you find, especially anaemia or tuberculosis.

Treatment of the patient only is not the proper management of a case of leprosy. Remember the other things needed in the management of the patient. (See box.)

Management includes nine things:

1. Register patient. Fill in index and treatment cards. Arrange treatment and patient follow-up. Arrange contact tracing.
2. Give supervised multidrug therapy.
3. Treat reactions quickly and effectively.
4. Educate about the care of anaesthetic hands/feet/eyes and the use of footwear.
5. Physiotherapy for weak, paralysed or deformed hands/feet/eyes.
6. Plaster of Paris casts, footwear, etc. for plantar ulcers.
7. Arrange surgery if necessary.
8. Check that the infection is controlled by drugs.
9. Transfer to Medical Officer care if necessary.

Do all necessary administrative procedures

1. Confirm the diagnosis (if the diagnosis was made by another health worker).
2. Register the patient in the register book and give him a number from the register.
3. Fill in details on the index card. Put the card in the index card file.
4. Fill in details of the treatment plan on the treatment card. Send the card to the treatment centre with the patient.
5. Start patient education and family education.
6. Arrange contact education and examination.
7. Arrange for a skin smear for BI and MI of AFB immediately, and then (if positive) every 3 months (e.g. 1st week of January, April, July, September) until MI = 0: then every year.
8. Check smear results and attendances on the treatment charts every 3 months (e.g. 1st week of February, May, August, November). Write the results on the index cards.
9. Notify the Health Department in the monthly report. (The Leprosy Report form is filled in from the index file every month.)

Give supervised antileprosy multidrug therapy

Give education to the patient about the importance of regular treatment for 6 months for paucibacillary leprosy and 24 months for multibacillary leprosy.

Arrange for the patient to attend the most suitable treatment centre for both the patient and that health centre.

Supply dapsone and if needed clofazimine for him to take home to take daily.

Visit all the patients who do not come for treatment (see the rules for 'defaulter action'). The treatment centre worker visits if the patient misses one treatment. The Officer in Charge (OIC) of the supervising centre visits if the patient still does not attend for treatment.

Notify the OIC of the Leprosy Control Unit at the Provincial or District Health Officer if the patient does not have his treatment for 3 months.

See Chapter 14 page 86 for advice on how to organise successful treatment and follow-up of patients – what applies to tuberculosis, applies to leprosy also.

Treat any reaction

Give health education to the patient about the symptoms and signs of reaction. Tell him that he should immediately report to the health worker if he gets any of these symptoms or signs: lumps in the skin; swelling of skin patches; nerve pain; sudden paralysis; sudden loss of sensation; painful eyes; any loss of sight; painful and swollen testis.

Treat reactions as follows:

1. Treat anything which may have caused the reaction (e.g. illness, accident, anxiety, etc.).
2. Make the patient rest in bed if possible. Support any affected part in a sling or a well padded splint.
3. Continue the full dose of all antileprosy drugs.
4. Aspirin 900–1200 mg (3–4 tabs) four times a day until reaction stops, or for 3 weeks.
5. Chloroquine 300 mg base (2 tabs of 150 mg base) daily for up to 3 weeks; but stop if not being effective within 1–2 weeks.
6. If the reaction is a Type 2 reaction (that is, reaction with ENL) and if the reaction does not quickly improve with the above treatment give clofazimine:
   - 300 mg daily (1 cap three times a day) until it stops, *then*
   - 200 mg daily (1 cap twice a day) for 1 month, *then*
   - 100 mg daily (1 cap once a day) for 1 month, *then*
   - 100 mg (1 cap) three times a week for 1 month then stop treatment.

   Do not give clofazimine for a Type 1 reaction (i.e. reaction without ENL).
7. Transfer any cases as recommended on page 115 as they may need tests for other possible diagnoses and adrenocorticosteroid drugs (prednisolone or cortisone) and (if not a woman of child-bearing age), thalidomide or even surgery for decompression of a nerve.

If the patient has anaesthetic hands or feet or eyes, give education about their care and supply protective footwear

Give a copy of a suitable booklet in the patient's own language for him to read.

Special care for anaesthetic hands includes:

1. Soak in water every day.
2. Precautions to stop burns.
3. Precautions to stop injuries.
4. Every night and morning look at both sides of the hands for burns or injuries, and feel for hot areas.
5. Wash, dress and splint any burn or injury.
6. Get medical treatment if the burn or injury does not improve quickly (dressings, splint, antibiotics, etc.).

Special care for anaesthetic feet includes:

1. Soak in water every day.
2. Always wear footwear to stop injuries or burns from the outside.
3. No running, jumping, long steps, long walks, etc. to prevent injuries to the foot from the inside.
4. Every night and morning: look for lumps, wounds or ulcers; feel for hot areas; feel for deep tenderness.
5. Wash and dress any injury and do not use the foot until it is better, (i.e. go to bed or use a crutch or stick).
6. Ask for medical treatment if the injury does not improve quickly (usually a plaster of Paris (POP) cast is necessary).

Special care for anaesthetic eyes includes:

1. Look at the eye every night and morning.
2. If the eye becomes red, ask for medical help (i.e. to remove any foreign body (not felt by the patient), to treat any infection and to treat any reaction if necessary).

If the patient has weakness or paralysis or deformity of hands, feet or eyes, start physiotherapy

1. Any recent paralysis is probably caused by a reaction. Transfer the patient for special drugs, special plasters and special exercises.
2. Any foot drop, which has started in the last 6 months, is also treated as a reaction. Transfer for treatment with special plasters and special drugs.
3. In other cases, ask the patient to do the special exercises.

Treat any plantar ulcer with a plaster of Paris (POP) cast and footwear

> These ulcers are not caused by leprosy organisms in the ulcerated areas. These ulcers do not happen without a definite cause. These ulcers are always caused by an injury or pressure on part of the foot.

Because of anaesthesia, the patient does not feel the cause of injury. So he does nothing about this cause. The injury becomes worse and worse. Even when he does know of the injury he continues to walk on the foot. This makes the damage worse and stops healing. (A person with normal sensation would have too much pain to walk.)

Abnormal positions of parts of the feet due to muscle weakness or deformity cause a lot of pressure on some areas of the foot. This can damage the skin and other tissues in this area, and ulcers then form.

Secondary bacterial infection usually occurs and makes the ulcer worse.

Note that the ulcer is *not* caused by leprosy organisms or bacterial infection but *is* caused by anaesthesia and injury.

It is important that you tell the patient how to prevent ulcers. Treatment for ulcers includes the following:

If there is secondary bacterial infection

(i.e. if the foot is hot, red, swollen, etc. or pus is discharged from the ulcer).

1. Rest the foot:
   - Rest in bed with the foot higher than the rest of the bed.
   - Use crutches to walk (to toilet, etc.).
   - The foot must *not* be put on the ground.

   This is the most important part of the treatment.
2. Antibiotics – give penicillin at first; give tetracycline if penicillin is not effective.
3. Use dressings with Eusol.
4. Cut away any thick dead skin. Do not cut any living tissue (which will bleed).
   Do not cut out bone from inside the ulcer. Remove *loose* pieces of bone with forceps.

Prepare suitable footwear (before POP applied)

1. If the foot is not deformed, get a sandal or shoe of the patient's size. Get a soft rubber insole and stick it inside the sandal or shoe.
2. If the patient's foot is deformed, take a POP cast of the foot. Send the cast to the leprosy shoe workshop. They will make a suitable shoe with an insole shaped to fit the patient's foot and send it back to you.

When infection is controlled

1. Apply a below knee POP cast (see Figure 15.27).
2. When the cast is dry apply a wooden rocker or walking iron to the POP (see Figure 15.28).
3. The patient can then walk on the POP.
4. The patient may be kept in the health centre or discharged and checked every week, to make sure the POP is not damaged.
5. Remove the POP (and apply a new one) if there is pain under the POP or any other suspicion of pressure.
6. After 6 weeks remove the POP cast. In most cases the ulcer will be healed. If it is not healed remove any dead hard skin, treat any infection, and then re-apply a POP cast.

After removing the POP cast (when the ulcer is healed)

1. Immediately tell the patient to put his new shoes on.
2. The patient must *always* wear these shoes. He must never walk anywhere without these shoes.
3. Allow the patient to walk only a little the first day and then a little more every day. After 3–6 weeks he can walk normal distances.
4. Get new shoes for the patient before the old ones wear out. Do not allow anyone to repair the shoes with nails or wire. These could damage the patient's foot.

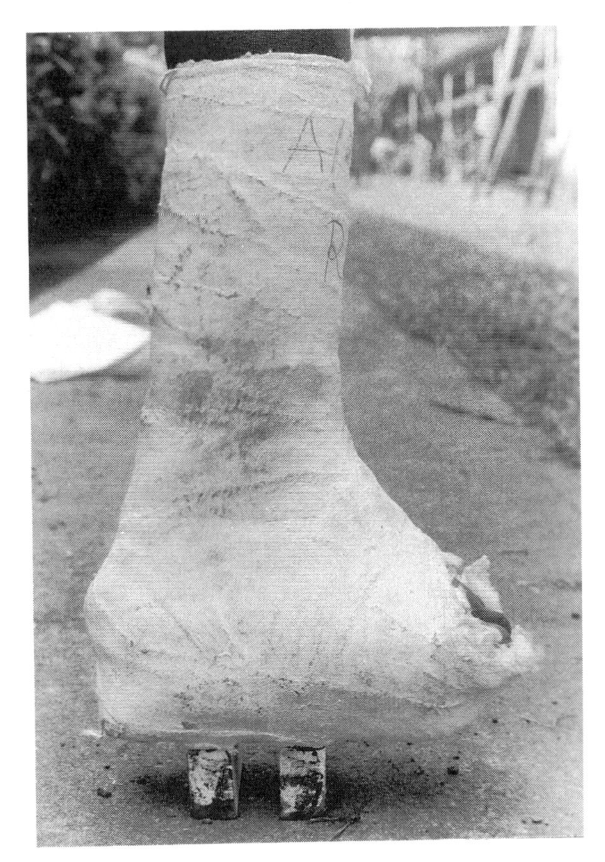

Figure 15.27 A below-knee plaster of Paris cast fitted with a 'home made' walking rocker made out of scrap wood and an old car tyre. The whole job was done by an orderly, and although it was not perfect, the ulcer was completely healed in 6 weeks.

Surgery

If physiotherapy is not successful, surgery may help. Cases which surgery may help include patients with:

1. completely wasted hand muscles;
2. foot drop for more than 6 months;
3. lagophthalmos for more than 6 months.

Check that the infection is controlled by drugs

Look for signs of drug resistance.
Do smears for BI and MI every 3 months on borderline or lepromatous patients.
Do clinical examination at least every 12 months.

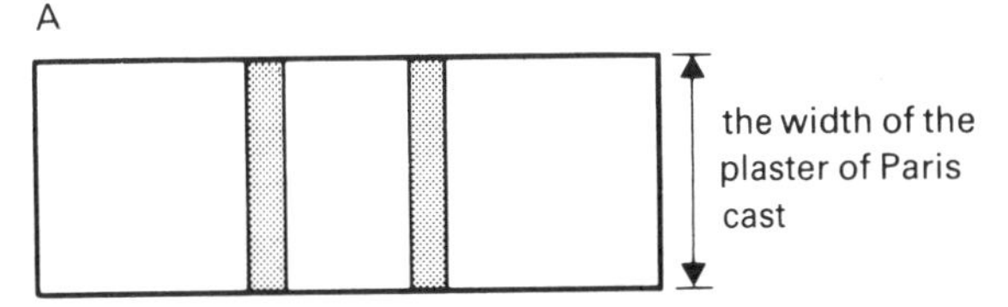

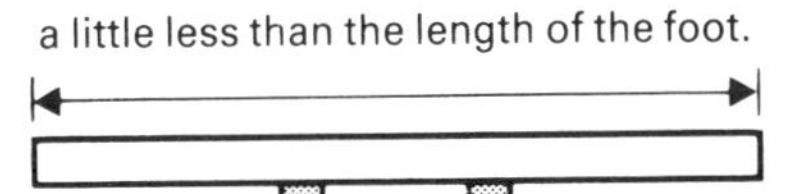

Figure 15.28 Diagram of a simple rocker: (A) from underneath; (B) from the side. The main part or platform is made from 3- or 5-ply or a piece of wood such as the top of a packing case. The rockers are made of 2 pieces of wood nailed on across the whole width of the platform. Underneath these, rubber cut from an old car tyre is nailed on. Apply the below-knee POP one day and do not let the patient walk on it. The next day make the bottom of the cast flat with POP and then plaster the rocker on with a POP bandage. Do not allow the patient to walk on it until the next day.

Patients likely to develop drug resistant leprosy include:

1. patients who have lepromatous leprosy,
2. patients who have not had regular treatment in the correct dose,
3. patients who have had only dapsone (and no other antileprosy drug),
4. patients who have had only small doses of dapsone,
5. patients who have had irregular dapsone, either because they were unreliable or because it was reduced during repeated reactions.

Signs of drug resistant leprosy (Figure 15.29) include:

1. A mixture of old and new lesions.
   - There may be the wrinkled ears and resolving nodules etc. of treated leprosy.
   - There are *also* new lesions, especially nodules.
2. Some of the new lesions may not be typical.
   - Nodules are often in unusual places, e.g. on the eyes, abdomen, front of elbows, etc.
   - Lesions may not be symmetrical.
   - Some lesions may be large and raised.
3. The new lesions will have a high BI and MI when the rest of the body and old lesions have a much lower or negative BI and MI.
4. The MI of the new lesions will not fall to 0 after 6 months of daily supervised treatment.

Make sure the nodules are not just one of the following:

1. ENL nodules. These are usually tender and come and go over a few weeks.
2. Recurrence of leprosy because the patient has stopped taking his drugs.
3. Dermal leishmaniasis (see Chapter 18 page 139).

Patients with suspected drug resistance should have supervised treatment.

If they do not greatly improve in 3–6 months and the MI does not fall to 0 (the BI will not change in 6 months) they must be transferred to Medical Officer care for special tests and treatment.

Control and prevention

Kill the organism in the body of the original host or reservoir

Discover and treat all the infectious (lepromatous and borderline) cases. When they start treatment, leprosy patients become non-infectious within a couple of weeks and cannot spread the disease.

How to find cases of leprosy:

1. Contact education and examination.
   You should see all contacts (family, those who live in the same house, friends, workmates, schoolmates, etc.) and educate them about the symptoms of leprosy and tell them it can be cured. You should then examine and test them all. You should tell them to come to the health centre if symptoms develop later. All contacts of lepromatous patients should be examined every year for 5 years.
2. You should educate and examine special groups during other health examinations – especially school children.
3. You should educate the general public.
4. You should arrange surveys in areas of known or suspected high prevalence of leprosy. (Whole population surveys are not usually as useful as using your available resources or (1) and (2).)

Follow-up of treated patients is not needed as a routine if they actually took their MDT regularly for the correct time, as relapse is so uncommon. It is better to teach the patients the signs of leprosy and tell them to come back for examination and tests at any time they have symptoms or signs which could be due to leprosy coming back.

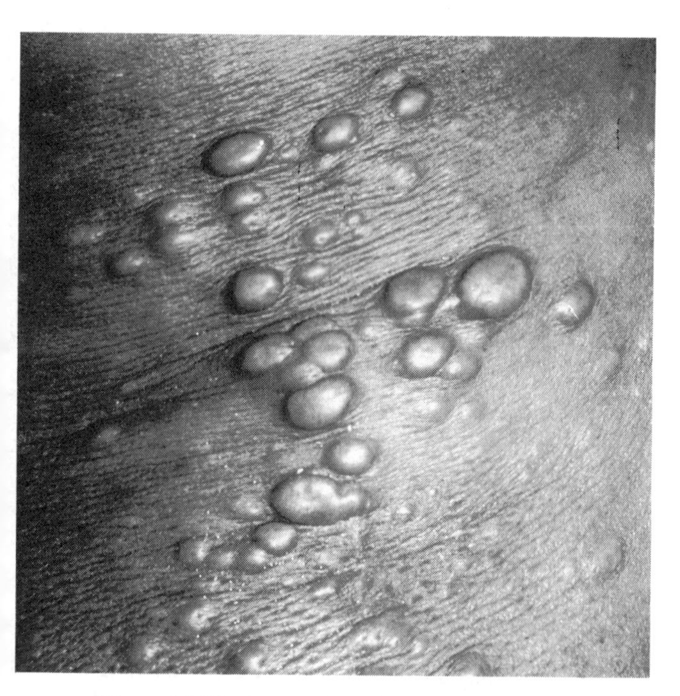

Figure 15.29 Drug resistant leprosy. A close-up photograph of new nodules in a patient, who also has signs of old treated lepromatous leprosy. The nodules are on the front of an elbow. The outer elbow was not affected. The lesions are raised and some have a sunken central part. The lesions had a B1 of 5 and an MI of 50% whereas the smear from the ears had a B1 of 1 and an MI of 0.

Stop the means of spread of the organism

This is not possible and is not worth trying.

Isolation of cases is not possible and should not be tried, especially as this stops patients coming for diagnosis and treatment and they then spread the disease to many people.

Improvement in housing, especially so that a lot of people do not live close together in a few rooms, and living standards and general public health will do far more to stop the spread of leprosy than any special rules for leprosy patients (as long as the infectious leprosy patients take their anti-leprosy drugs).

Raise the resistance of susceptible persons

1. The resistance to leprosy of the general population is raised by better housing, stopping of overcrowding, better nutrition, the treatment of other diseases and general public health methods.

2. The resistance of individual persons in some groups of people in some countries is raised by childhood BCG immunisation. This resistance may then be raised even more by further BCG vaccination after childhood and in some areas up to 80% protection is gained although this is mainly against tuberculoid type leprosy.
3. Specific immunisation against leprosy is not available at present but it is hoped that it soon will be.

Prophylactic treatment

This is not given (except in very unusual circumstances in infants).

Transfer

Transfer to Medical Officer care the following cases:

1. All *new* cases who before treatment is started, have:
   (a) reaction, and/or
   (b) tender nerves,
2. All cases with a *reaction* which
   (a) involves vital body parts (especially the nerves or eyes), or
   (b) is severe, or
   (c) does not stop with treatment.

   These include patients who have:
   - tender nerves,
   - acute paralysis or loss of sensation (and foot drop starting within last 6 months),
   - acute orchitis (painful, swollen testis),
   - iritis (eye red or painful, or sight becoming worse),
   - severe general signs and symptoms,
   - reaction which does not stop after 3 weeks of treatment, or
   - reaction which returns after reaction treatment has stopped.
3. All patients who have drug reactions especially hepatitis, which stops them taking their drugs (do not just stop treatment and do nothing else).
4. Any patient who may have drug resistant organisms.

Refer to visiting Medical Officer – any case with complications especially paralysis or deformity, for advice and assessment for possible surgery.

Elimination of leprosy as a public health problem

If the above treatment and control processes can be kept in place, and especially if better methods become available, it is hoped that by the year 2000 leprosy can be reduced to less than 1 case for each 10,000 members of the population.

16

Some Common Infectious Diseases

Figure 16.1 A close-up photograph of the measles skin rash. The rash is often very hard to see on a dark skin.

This chapter covers some acute specific infectious diseases that cause fever and occur everywhere.

Measles (morbilli)

Measles is caused by the measles virus and is a common, very infectious disease. It usually affects children but can affect adults. It is endemic, but small epidemics occur.

Spread is from the respiratory tract of an infectious patient by direct contract or by droplets.

The incubation period is of medium length (1–2 weeks).

The pattern of the disease is as follows:

1. At first the symptoms and signs of a quite severe viral-type upper respiratory tract infection (URTI) and conjunctivitis with fever develop. This lasts for about a week.
2. Then Koplik spots appear in the mouth. The Koplik spots are like white grains of salt on the red mucous membrane, usually on the inner side of the cheek. If you see Koplik spots, the disease is not a usual URTI, but measles.
3. After about 4 days, the typical measles rash comes (see Figure 16.1). There are many slightly red and raised patches of various sizes on the skin. These start on the face and shoulders and then spread to the rest of the body. The other symptoms improve as the rash appears.
4. Secondary bacterial infection of the respiratory tract often occurs, especially otitis media and pneumonia. This usually happens when the rash is improving.

Treatment of measles itself is symptomatic only – rest, aspirin, and antimalarials (if in a malarious area).

Treatment of secondary bacterial complications is with antibiotics.

If otitis media occurs see Chapter 20 page 212. If pneumonia occurs see Chapter 20 page 220. If gastroenteritis occurs see Chapter 23 page 285.

If the patient is a child see a textbook on children's diseases.

Immunise all children at the age of 9 months and certainly before the age of 1 year with an injection of live virus vaccine.

German measles (rubella)

Rubella is not a commonly diagnosed disease. It usually affects children and young adults.

It is endemic but small epidemics occur. The cause if the rubella virus.

Spread is by direct contact or by droplets from the respiratory tract of adult patients, or by any discharge from an infant with congenital infection.

The incubation period is of medium length (2–3 weeks).

The patient is infectious from 1 week before the rash appears until 4 days after it appears.

The symptoms and signs are usually mild – mild fever, etc. then a rash like mild measles and enlarged lymph nodes behind the neck.

Treatment is symptomatic only.

The disease is important only because pregnant women infected in the first 4 months of pregnancy may have deformed babies.

> Patients with rubella should not be allowed to come into any type of direct or indirect contact with pregnant women. Infectious patients include normal child or adult patients and babies born with the disease.

Young girls should try to have the disease before the age when they may become pregnant. Immunisation is possible with a live virus vaccine either before puberty or immediately after delivery.

Chickenpox (varicella)

Chickenpox is a common infectious disease. The cause is the chickenpox or varicella-zoster virus. It usually affects children, but can also affect adults.

It is endemic, but small epidemics occur. Spread is by direct contact and by droplets from the respiratory tract of infectious patients (but not from the crusts of the sores). The incubation period is of medium length (2–3 weeks). The patient is infectious from the day before the rash appears until 1 week after it appears.

The disease causes:

1. Mild general symptoms and signs of infection (fever, malaise, etc.).
2. A typical rash (see Figure 16.2):
   - macules, papules, vesicles, pustules and crusts (see Figure 32.2),
   - mostly on the trunk and face,
   - with new lesions appearing from time to time (so that at any one time in any one place there are lesions at different stages).

In adults a severe chickenpox virus pneumonia sometimes occurs.

Treatment is symptomatic only, with aspirin and calamine lotion and antimalarials (if in a malarious area). If the skin lesions become infected by bacteria,

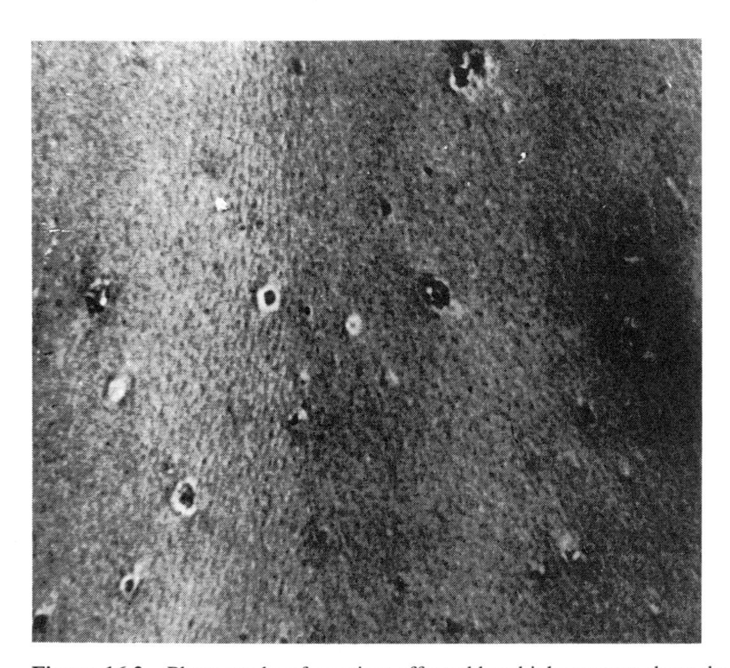

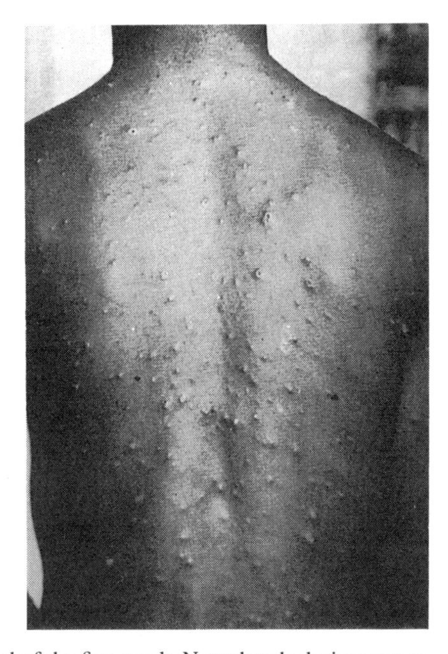

Figure 16.2 Photographs of a patient affected by chickenpox at about the end of the first week. Note that the lesions are at different stages.

give antibiotics by injection or by mouth and skin preparations (see Chapter 32 page 432).

If pneumonia occurs see Chapter 20 page 220.

> If the patient is a child, see a textbook on children's diseases

Varicella zoster or herpes zoster

Varicella zoster or herpes zoster or shingles is caused by a re-activation of the chickenpox or varicella zoster virus in someone who has had chickenpox before. This can happen for no apparent reason, but it can be because the person's immunity has decreased, e.g. old age, cancer and especially HIV infection.

A rash like the chickenpox rash appears (see Figure 16.2 and Figure 16.4) *but*

- it is in the area of skin supplied by only one nerve (see Figure 16.3),
- it is usually on only one side of the body,
- it stops exactly at the midline of the body,
- it usually appears on the trunk or the face,
- there is severe pain in the affected area often before the rash appears, as well as during the rash, and sometimes for months or years after the rash goes.

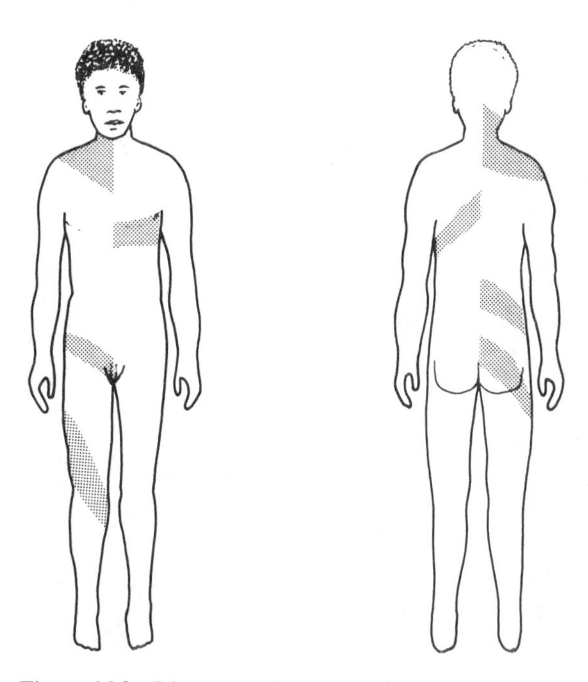

Figure 16.3 Diagram to show some of the possible distributions of the herpes zoster rash.

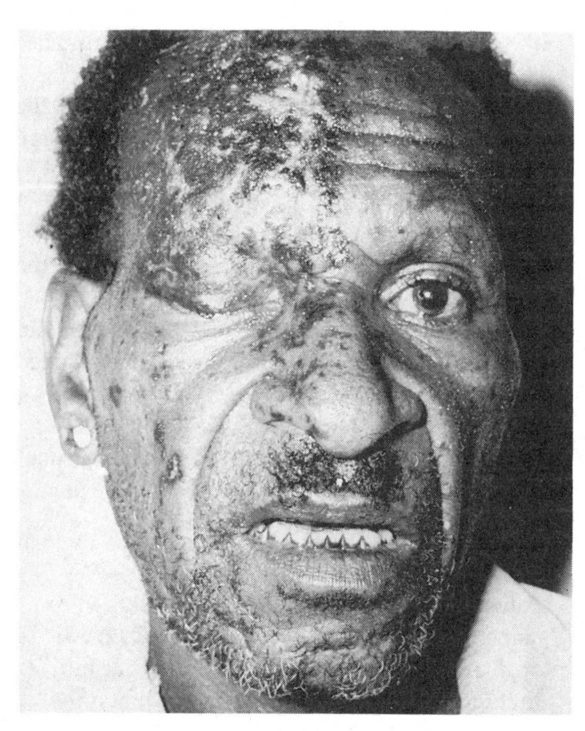

Figure 16.4 Herpes zoster of the right side of the face. Note that the lesions stop exactly at the midline. Note that the eye is affected and the patient therefore needs urgent treatment and transfer to Medical Officer care. Note that the patient is elderly (probably not HIV infection too).

Management is as for chickenpox, but powerful drugs, including codeine or even pethidine may be needed to control pain at first. If the eye is affected, put chloramphenicol ointment into the eye every 3 hours, keep the eye covered and transfer the patient urgently to Medical Officer care.

If the patient is young (less than 50 years old) or if the infection involves more than one nerve at one time or if the infection comes back again after going, always think of an underlying HIV infection allowing the herpes zoster virus to grow. See Chapter 19 page 186).

Other viral diseases with skin rash

The diseases described so far have:

1. fever and other generalised symptoms and signs of infection,
2. skin rash – which is typical of the disease, and
3. other complications.

There are many other viral diseases which are similar, except that the rash is not typical of only one disease. These viral infections cannot therefore be identified by most health workers, but this does not matter.

If the patient is not very 'sick', treat only the patient's symptoms and give antimalarials (if in a malarious area – see Chapter 36 page 482).

If the patient is very 'sick' treat him for septicaemia and malaria (see Chapter 12). If he does not improve, transfer him to Medical Officer care. If complications such as encephalitis occur, transfer the patient to Medical Officer care.

Infectious mononucleosis or glandular fever – Epstein–Barr virus infections

Epstein–Barr virus (EBV) is a virus that affects the squamous epithelium (surface cells) and the B lymphocytes (which make antibodies) of the body. Almost everyone is eventually infected. Infected patients become carriers for life. The infection usually occurs from infected material spread by close oral contact although possibly at times through sexual intercourse. In developing countries, most infections occur in infancy and cause little or no clinical illness. As health standards improve, infections occur later in life in adolescence and often cause the illness called 'infectious mononucleosis' or 'glandular fever'. The EBV however, is also associated with the development of Burkitt's lymphoma, anaplastic nasopharyngeal carcinoma (malignant tumour of the back of the nasal cavity), some lymphomas (especially in immunosuppressed people) and also a condition of the mouth called oral hairy leukoplakia.

Infectious mononucleosis causes fever, sore throat, neck swelling, pains in various parts of the body and malaise. On examination the tonsils are enlarged and often coated with a white material (which can look like bacterial tonsillitis), lymph nodes are enlarged especially in the neck, the spleen is usually slightly enlarged and there is often a maculopapular rash. The patient usually recovers without treatment in 6–8 weeks. Ampicillin or amoxycillin, if given, often cause a severe rash. Other complications include hepatitis (viral), meninginitis or encephalitis (viral) and blood disorders. Diagnostic blood tests (atypical mononuclear cells in the blood smear and a positive infectious mononucleosis test) can be done in a laboratory.

EBV infection is of importance because of the following. Infectious mononucleosis has the same symptoms and signs as the 'sero-conversion' reaction of HIV infection (though infectious mononucleosis is not related to HIV infection). EBV infection commonly causes lymphomas in patients who have HIV infection once they develop immunosuppression. EBV infection occasionally causes the development of lymphomas and other tumours in non-HIV infected patients.

No treatment except of symptoms helps; but do not give amoxycillin or ampicillin which may make a severe rash occur. Vaccines are being tested to see if they can prevent the infection.

Mumps

Mumps is a common disease which usually affects children. It is not very infectious, so not all children get it. Many adults are therefore not immune to mumps and so it can also affect adults. The cause is the mumps virus.

Spread is from an infected patient from the respiratory tract and mouth by direct contact and by droplets. The incubation period is of medium length (2–3 weeks). The patient is infectious from a week before the salivary gland swelling appears until all the swelling goes. One attack gives immunity against mumps for life.

The disease causes the following:

1. mild general symptoms and signs of infection,
2. painful, tender swelling of one parotid gland, which lasts for about a week (see Figures 16.5 and 16.6),
3. often painful, tender swelling of the other parotid gland as the first one improves.

Complications include:

1. acute orchitis (painful tender swelling of one or both of the testes) – common in adults;
2. acute pancreatitis with upper abdominal pain and vomiting;
3. viral meningitis and/or encephalitis (see Chapter 25 page 326).

Make sure the patient does not have acute bacterial parotitis. This is an acute severe inflammation of the parotid gland with severe pain, severe tenderness and a lot of swelling as well as fever. It usually occurs in someone who is already sick and not drinking much

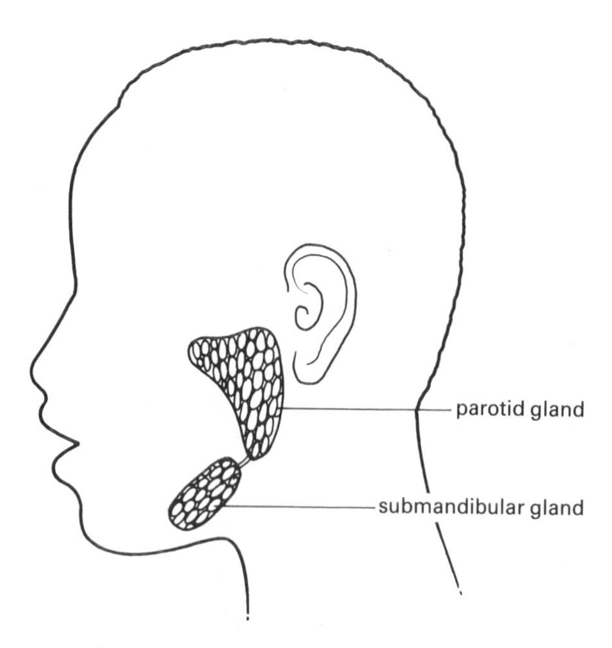

Figure 16.5 Diagram to show the anatomical position of the parotid and submandibular salivary glands.

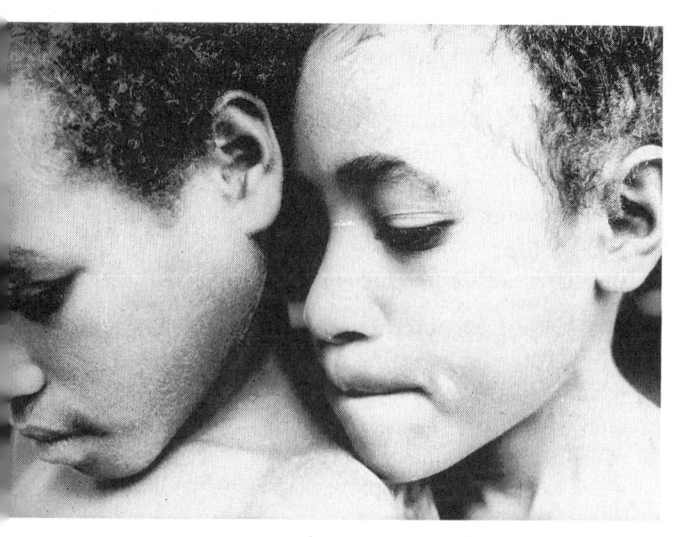

Figure 16.6 Mumps. The child on the left has parotitis with swelling in front of and below his left ear – in the position of the parotid gland (see Figure 16.5).

and not keeping his mouth clean. Acute bacterial parotitis needs urgent treatment with antibiotics.

If the patient has only mumps, treat the patient's symptoms with aspirin and antimalarials (if in a malarious area). If severe orchitis occurs, transfer the patient for Medical Officer care.

Encourage boys to get mumps before puberty as orchitis is less likely. Mumps complications are not common enough to spend money on the live mumps vaccine for developing countries.

Whooping cough (pertussis)

Whooping cough is uncommon in adults. A 'whoop' is not usual in adults who have whooping cough.

But whooping cough may be the cause of some attacks of respiratory illness with chronic cough which last for many weeks and have sputum negative for AFB (see Chapter 14 page 77).

> If the patient is a child, see a textbook on children's diseases

17

Some Serious Acute Infectious Diseases with Limited Distribution

This chapter is about some acute specific diseases which cause fever but which occur only in certain parts of the world:

1. Bacterial infections
   - Relapsing fever
   - Leptospirosis
   - Melioidosis
   - Bartonellosis
   - Plague
2. Rickettsial infections
   - Typhus fevers
3. Virus infections
   - Arborvirus infections in general
   - Dengue fever
   - Yellow fever
   - Haemorrhagic fever due to arborvirus infections
   - Japanese encephalitis
   - Haemorrhagic fever due to other viral infections

Find out which of these diseases occur in your area. If any of these diseases do not occur in your area, do not learn about those diseases.

See Chapter 36, page 482 for diagnosis and management of a patient who has a fever and you are not sure of the cause of the fever.

Relapsing fever

Relapsing fever is an acute bacterial infection which causes repeated attacks of acute severe fever and damage to the blood, blood vessels, liver, spleen, eyes, nervous system and heart.

There are two types of relapsing fever. One type is caused by a bacterium which normally lives in small animals and is spread by ticks. This is called endemic tick-borne relapsing fever (Figure 17.1). The other type is due to a bacterium which normally lives in man and is spread by lice. This is called epidemic louse-borne relapsing fever (Figure 17.2). The two diseases are clinically similar but the epidemic louse-borne type is the more severe.

Endemic tick-borne relapsing fever

There are many areas where this disease occurs (Figure 17.1). Find out if it occurs in your area.

The bacteria (*Borrelia*) which cause endemic relapsing fever normally live in small animals (such as rats and bats). Ticks bite these animals to suck their blood, and bacteria are carried from an infected animal to another animal by the ticks. These ticks like to live in the cracks of walls and floors of houses. During the night these ticks come out and bite animals and people (to suck their blood). The ticks can pass on the bacteria to any person they bite. The infected tick also passes on the bacteria to its offspring through its eggs. An infected woman can pass on the disease to her child through her placenta. Figure 17.3 shows the means of spread.

The symptoms and signs of the infection include:

1. A high fever with chills, headache and body pains; often nausea and vomiting; often liver enlargement and, in severe cases jaundice. After 4–5 days the temperature goes down and the patient stays well for 4–5 days or longer.
2. Then a relapse occurs with the same signs though usually they are less severe.
3. This cycle of a fever for 4–5 days and then being reasonably well for 4–5 days may happen up to 10 times.

Complications occur. These include:

1. meningitis with CSF that is clear to naked eye examination (see Chapter 25 page 322);
2. encephalitis (with unconsciousness or fitting) (see Chapter 25 page 327);
3. iritis (see Chapter 31 page 420) and loss of sight.

Apart from loss of sight, relapsing fever can look exactly like malaria; it is not possible to tell if the

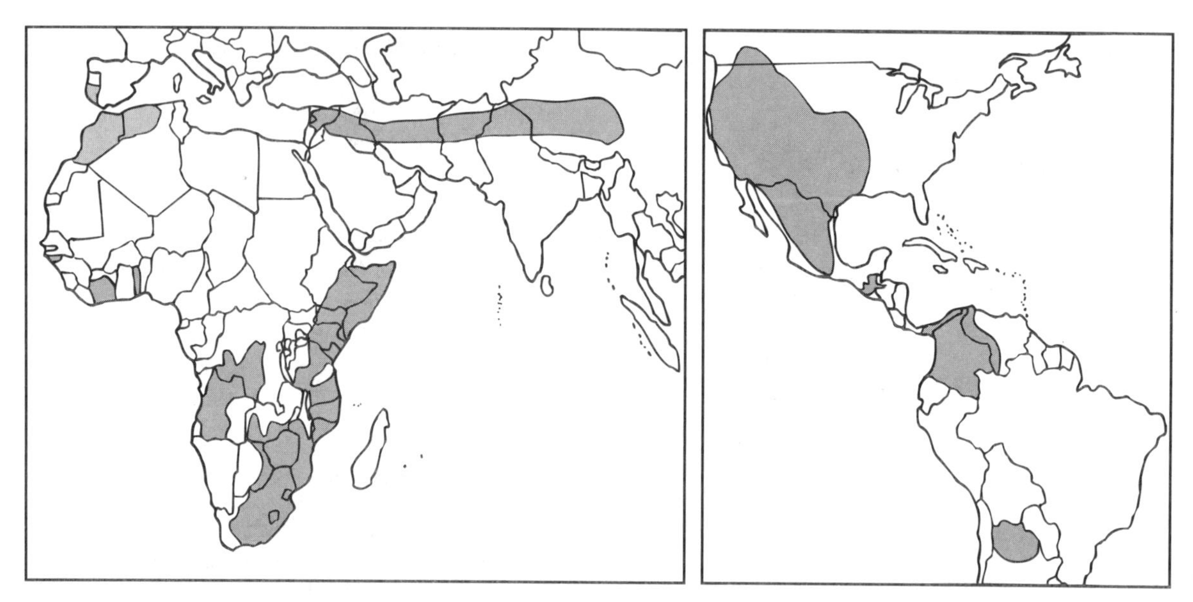

Figure 17.1 Geographical distribution of tick-borne (endemic) relapsing fever in (a) the Old and (b) New World. (Redrawn from map from Department of Entomology, London School of Hygiene and Tropical Medicine.)

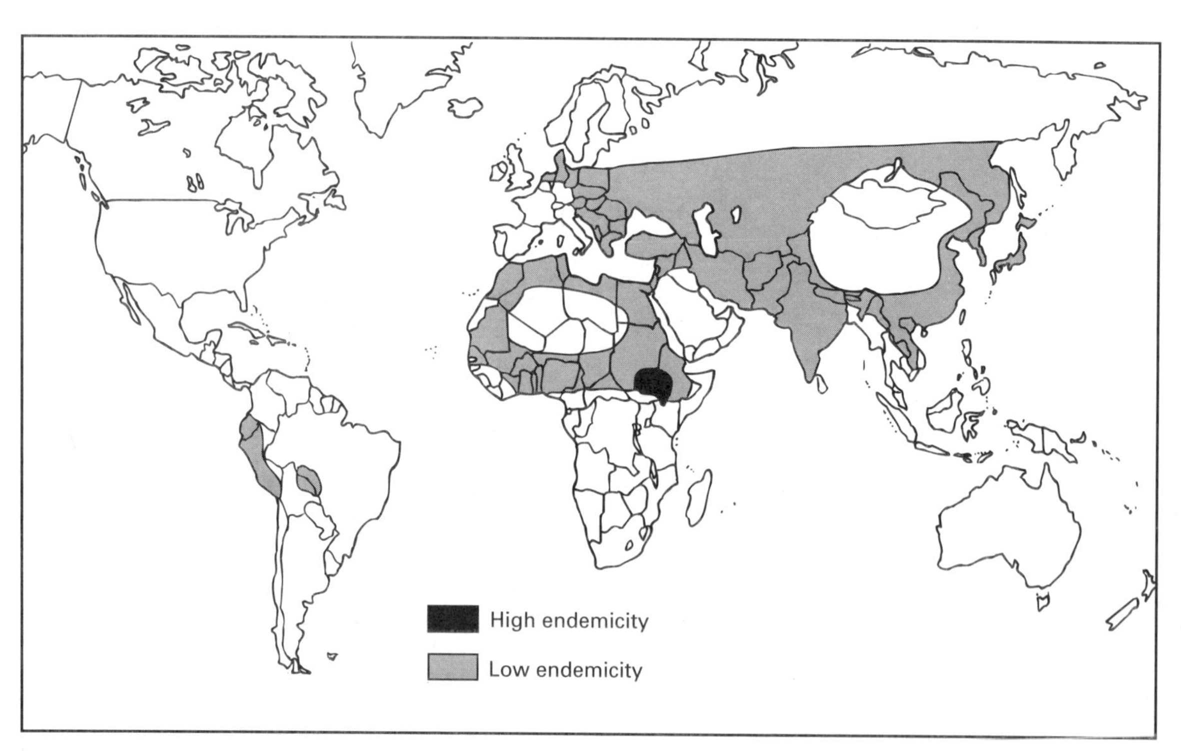

Figure 17.2 Geographical distribution of louse-borne relapsing fever (*Borrelia recurrentis*). (Redrawn from map from Department of Entomology, London School of Hygiene and Tropical Medicine.)

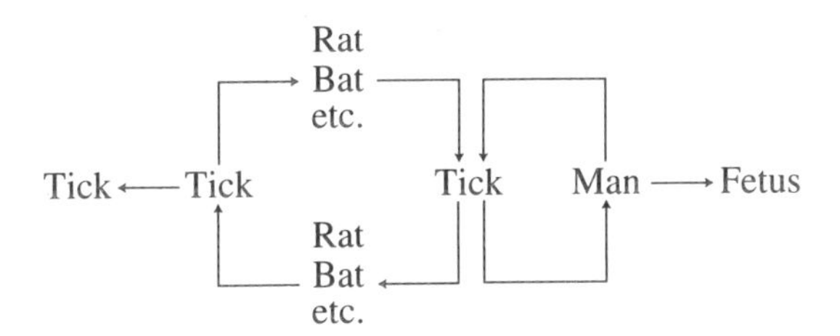

Figure 17.3 Diagram showing the means of spread of endemic tick-borne relapsing fever.

patient's condition is caused by malaria unless his blood slide is examined.

Like malaria, people who do not die from the relapsing fever, should become immune to it. The people most affected by relapsing fever are therefore (1) new-comers to the area, (2) infants and children, (3) pregnant women.

If women are infected during pregnancy they usually have a miscarriage, stillbirth or premature labour; but, if the baby is born alive, it can be born infected and will soon have the symptoms and signs of relapsing fever.

Differential diagnosis

This includes malaria and all the causes of fever (see Chapter 13 and Chapter 36 page 482).

If the patient is in or from an area where malaria occurs it is not possible to tell without tests if his fever is caused by relapsing fever or malaria. Always take a blood slide (see Figure 17.4). If possible have the slide examined immediately. If the bacteria (*Borrelia* or *Spirochaetes*) are seen and no malaria parasites are seen the patient has relapsing fever. If malaria parasites (plasmodia) are seen but no bacteria are seen the patient has malaria. If it is not possible to have the slide examined immediately you must treat the patient for both conditions.

If the patient has jaundice see Chapter 24 page 314.

Treatment

Penicillin, tetracycline and chloramphenicol all kill the bacteria of relapsing fever. However some of the bacteria are becoming resistant to penicillin.

When antibiotics kill many bacteria quickly, the toxins from the dead bacteria often cause a severe reaction. This reaction can include a high fever, fast breathing and cough, fast pulse and low blood pressure, encephalitis, shock or heart failure and death. Do three things to avoid this reaction.

1. Keep the patient in bed for the first 2 days of treatment.
2. Keep everything needed for treatment of the reaction ready (see Chapters 10 page 39, 12 and 37).
3. Give only a small dose of antibiotic at first.

Start treatment with procaine benzylpenicillin 200 mg or 200,000 units IMI. Give the same dose for the next 4 days; or on the second day change to oral tetracycline 250 mg (1 cap) four times a day for a week or doxycycline. However do not give tetracycline or doxycycline to pregnant women or to children.

Always treat with antimalarials too (see Chapter 13 page 61) unless you are certain (from good blood slide results) that the patient does not have malaria.

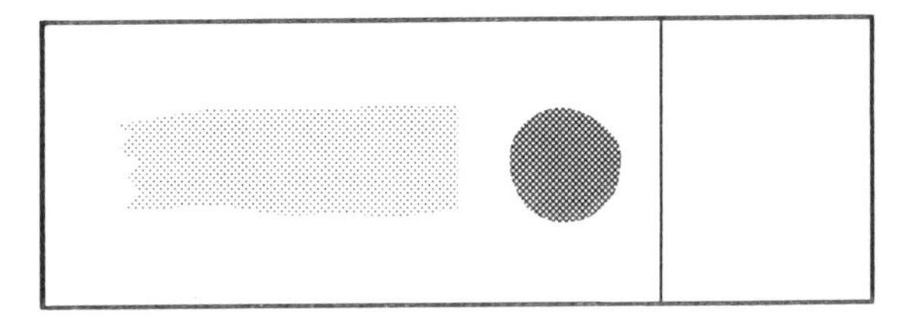

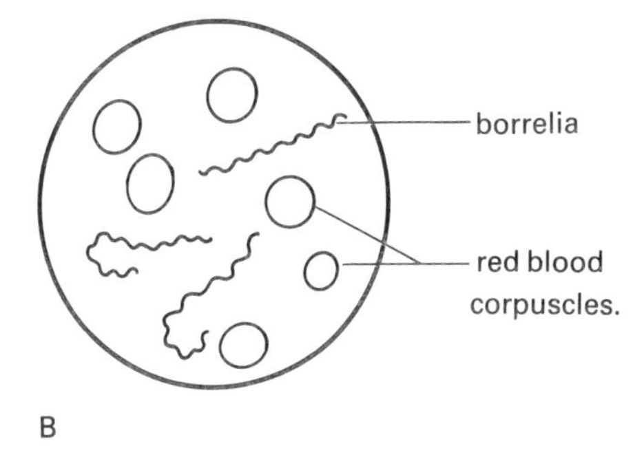

Figure 17.4 Always take a thick and thin blood slide (A) from every patient with any illness and in an area where malaria and relapsing fever occur. Ask for examinations for both malaria and relapsing fever parasites. The appearance of relapsing fever parasites (*Borrelia*) under the microscope is shown in B. They are seen between the red cells; malaria parasites are seen in the red cells.

Control and prevention

The only effective way is to stop the spread of the organism by getting rid of the ticks.

1. Treat the home with gamma BHC regularly. This is expensive.
2. Make better houses with no cracks in the walls, floors, ceilings in which the ticks can live.
3. Personal protection with repellents, use of insecticide-treated bed nets, and always sleep above the floor level, etc.

Epidemic louse-borne relapsing fever

See page 121, Relapsing Fever, first.

Cause and epidemiology

The type of bacterium (*Borrelia*) which causes epidemic louse-borne relapsing fever is a parasite of men and lice only. The lice do not pass on the disease to their offspring (see Figure 17.5). This disease starts when an infected person or an infested louse brings the disease to a group of people who are infested with lice. People have lice because they do not wash themselves or their clothes properly. Epidemic louse-borne relapsing fever is normally less common than the endemic type; but large epidemics can occur especially in times of famine or war, in refugee camps, etc.

The *symptoms and signs* are similar to the symptoms and signs of the endemic type (see page 121) though there are some differences:

1. The attacks are often more severe with fever and bleeding nose at first, hepatitis with jaundice, enlarged spleen, bleeding, meningitis and encephalitis, and then shock or heart failure as the attack ends.
2. The attacks last longer (up to 10 days) and there may be less time between attacks; but there are usually fewer attacks.
3. Half the people affected may die if they are not treated.

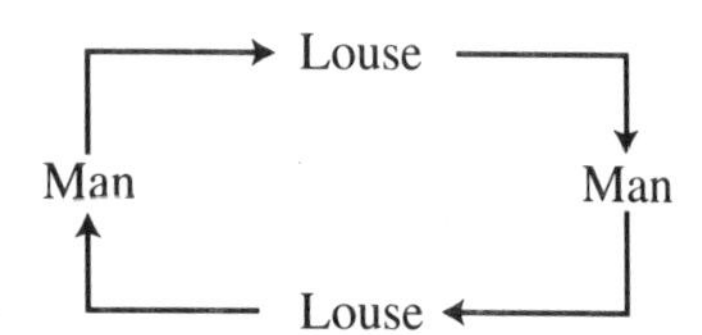

Figure 17.5 Diagram showing the means of spread of epidemic louse-borne relapsing fever.

Treatment is the same as for the endemic type (see page 123).

Control and prevention

1. All cases must be treated to reduce the reservoir; but there will still be infected lice.
2. The main means of control is therefore to stop the means of spread. All lice both on patients and other people and in clothing and bedclothes should be killed. People should try to not get lice from other people. See Chapter 17, page 128 for details of how to do this. As soon as possible, regular washing of their bodies and clothes should start.
3. Immunisation is not possible.
4. Prophylactic treatment is not needed if precautions about lice are taken.

Leptospirosis

Leptospirosis occurs in most parts of the world. It is a bacterial infection of the whole body but affects mostly the liver and kidneys.

Leptospirosis is normally an infection of rats, pigs and dogs and the organisms are excreted in the urine of these animals. Leptospirosis in man is therefore common (1) where rats are common; (2) if there is rat urine in water which people use and (3) when people live and work with animals.

Infection with the bacteria can cause the following:

1. fever of unknown cause (this may be mild or severe);
2. hepatitis with jaundice, tender liver and bile in the urine;
3. kidney damage with a lot of protein in the urine;
4. meningitis;
5. heart failure or shock.

If a white blood cell count is done, it is high. The disease can last about 3–4 weeks. For differential diagnosis see Table 17.1 page 133.

Antibiotics such as penicillin or tetracycline but not chloramphenicol improve the patient – especially if given early in the disease. Treatment of the other conditions (see above) caused by the infection is also needed.

Melioidosis

Melioidosis is an acute or chronic infection caused by a bacterial organism (*Burkholdia pseudomalleri*).

This organism usually lives in soil, ponds, rice paddies, etc. in South-East Asia but also Australia and other tropical countries and is more common in the rainy season. It gets into people by being breathed in or through cuts etc. on the skin. It does not spread person to person.

Many infections cause no symptoms or signs. There may however be acute bronchitis, pneumonia or lung abscess. At other times a chronic infection in the lung develops with symptoms and signs like tuberculosis (but of course sputum is negative for AFB). Skin infections with pus formation and lymphangitis or lymphadenitis may occur. Chronic discharging abscesses may follow. The infection can get into the blood at any time and cause septicaemia and usually death follows quickly. Any part of the body may be affected with acute or chronic infection but the lungs, liver, parotid glands and skin are those parts most often affected.

People with decreased immunity from, e.g. chronic renal failure, diabetes mellitus, chronic liver disease, alcoholism, old age and possibly HIV infection are more likely than others to develop the disease and more likely to get septicaemia.

Diagnosis is difficult and is made by seeing the organism under the microscope or by special serological blood tests.

Treatment is difficult as special antibiotics such as ceftazidime as well as co-trimoxazole or amoxycillin and clavulanic acid are needed for many weeks to many months – as well as surgery to drain any collections of pus.

In the health centre the condition may be suspected if a pneumonia does not respond to correct treatment or a liver or parotid abscess occurs; but all such cases would be transferred urgently to the hospital for Medical Officer care.

Bartonellosis

Bartonellosis is a bacterial infection (with *Bartonella*) of the red blood cells and the cells which line the inside of blood vessels. The bacterium is carried by sandflies. It occurs only in parts of South America.

The acute stage is caused by the bacteria breaking many red blood cells open (haemolysis). The symptoms and signs are: high fever, pains all over the body, vomiting and diarrhoea, enlargement of liver and spleen, anaemia and often unconsciousness and death.

If the patient does not die, he then improves for a month or so. Then many small red lumps full of blood come up on the skin. These are most common on the head and toward the ends of the arms and legs. These lumps go away after 2–3 months.

Treatment is by antibiotics. Chloramphenicol is best as secondary infections, which may be sensitive to only chloramphenicol, often occur. Other treatment and often blood transfusion are usually needed also. A severely affected patient usually needs transfer for Medical Officer care after antibiotics and treatment of the patient's other conditions are started. (See Chapter 12 page 53).

People who live in the area where bartonellosis occurs, and do not die from the infection, become immune. It is mostly new-comers to the area and children who are severely affected.

Prevention is by spraying sandfly breeding areas with insecticide and the use of repellents and protective clothing, bed nets, etc.

Plague

Plague is an acute infection with bacteria (*Yersinia pestis*) which causes:

1. inflammation of lymph nodes,
2. septicaemia, and
3. pneumonia.

Plague occurs in parts of North and South America, Africa and Asia (see Figure 17.6).

In most of these places plague is endemic and is a disease passed from one bush animal to another, often rats, by infected fleas. The infected bush animals often do not die.

If infected fleas from bush animals infect village or town rats, these newly infected rats often die and the fleas then look for a new host and may find man. Man can also be infected when hunting among infected bush animals.

After a bite from an infected flea the person develops bubonic plague – fever, severe sickness and swelling of the lymph nodes (called a bubo) near the flea bite. He then develops septicaemia. He may also develop pneumonia and cough up many of the plague bacteria. These plague bacteria can be breathed in by other people and these people then develop a severe plague pneumonia and usually die quickly. One patient with pneumonic plague can cause an epidemic. An

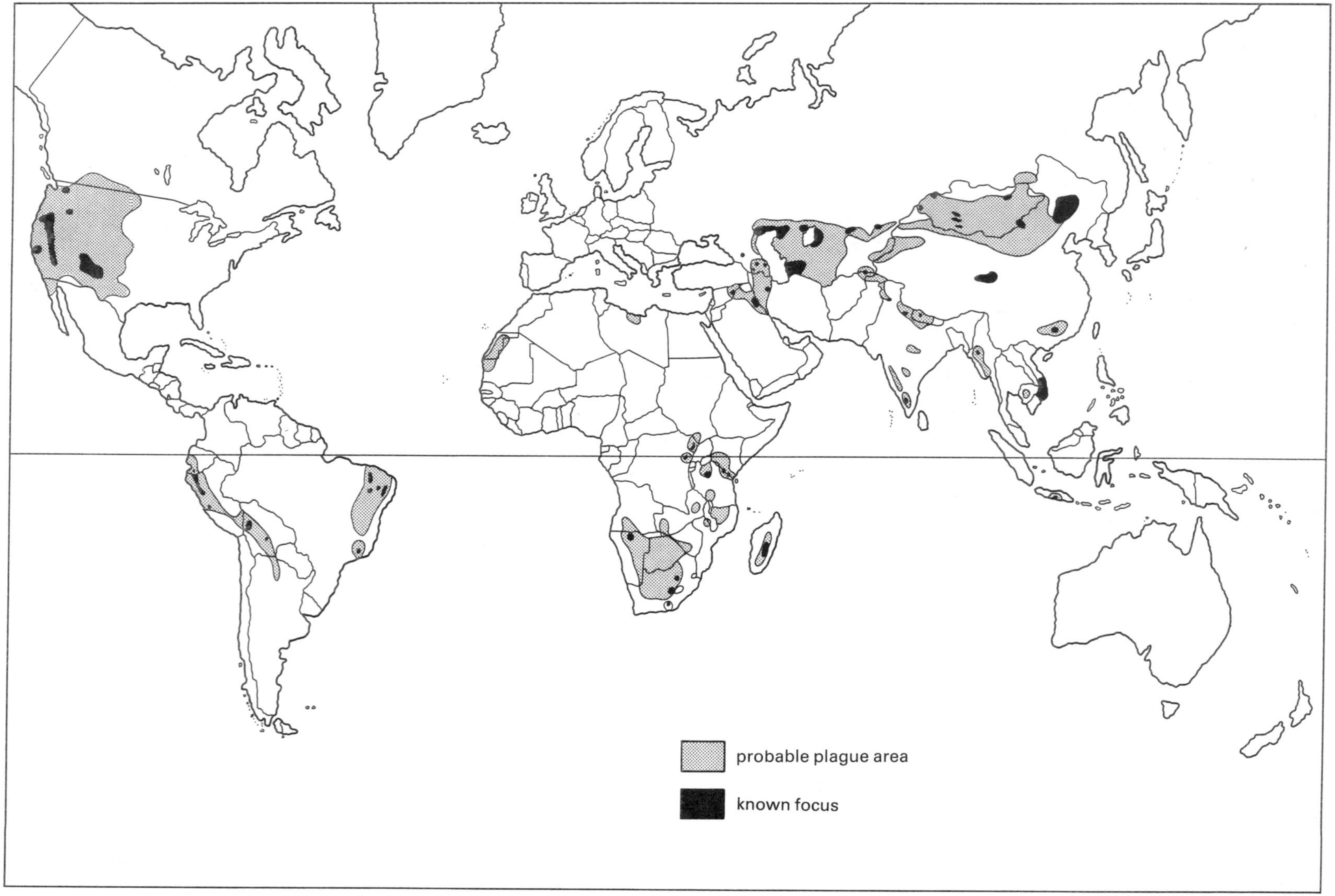

Figure 17.6 The distribution of plague.
(Source: *Weekly Epidemiological Record*, Vol. 55, p. 244 (1980))

epidemic can also be caused by infected fleas passing from one person to another.

The clinical features are therefore as follows.

Bubonic plague

Usually fever with rigors and severe generalised symptoms and signs of infection occur.

Swelling of the lymph nodes near the flea bite, called a bubo, also occurs. The bubo may become very tender. The swelling is often the size of a chicken's egg. If the patient lives, after a week or so the bubo bursts through the skin and pus comes out.

Usually the patient gets worse with severe toxaemia, bleeding into many parts of the body, septicaemia, sometimes pneumonia and death in 1–2 weeks.

Septicaemic plague

The patient becomes so ill so quickly with the septicaemia that he dies in coma and shock within 3–5 days, before the bubo can become very big.

Pneumonic plague

This may appear in a patient who has bubonic plague or in a person who has inhaled plague bacteria coughed out by a patient.

The onset is acute with fever, rigors and marked toxaemia. There is severe shortness of breath and a cough. At first the sputum is watery but it soon becomes bloodstained. Often the clinical signs in the chest are not marked.

The patient dies in 1–2 days.

Minor plague

An occasional patient (usually during an epidemic) who has bubonic plague is not very sick and the bubo bursts and discharges pus. The patient can walk around; but his pus may infect others.

Diagnosis of plague can be confirmed by the examination of:

1. fluid aspirated from a bubo,
2. 10 ml of venous blood, and
3. sputum.

Take these samples to send to the laboratory and immediately start treatment. Do not wait for any results if you strongly suspect plague. *Treatment* can be with chloramphenicol, tetracycline or streptomycin. As streptomycin should not be used in a health centre except for tuberculosis and as the patient is usually very sick, treat with chloramphenicol as in Chapter 12. It is most important to give immediate treatment to try to save the patient's life and also to try to stop spread of the disease.

As soon as the disease is suspected start *control* methods immediately.

1. Take the necessary tests from the patient.
2. Start the patient on treatment.
3. Isolate the patient (reverse barrier nursing) until 48 hours of treatment has been given and the patient is improving. Disinfect discharges of body fluids.
4. Start all contacts including yourself on prophylactic treatment (usually tetracycline 500 mg (2 caps) four times a day for a week but sulphamethoxazole/trimethoprim (co-trimoxazole) also effective).
5. Notify the Health or Medical Officer who will immediately confirm the diagnosis and take over control procedures.
6. Kill all fleas on the patient and his clothes and bedclothes and goods. Treat all the patient's contacts and their clothes, etc. similarly. Treat staff who care for the patients similarly. Use permethrin 1% as for lice (see page 128). Treat the whole health centre with insecticide (e.g. permethrin) to kill fleas.
7. Apply insecticides to places where rats run.
8. Kill rats.

If you do these things you may save many lives.

Plague is a Quarantinable Disease and the Government will notify its occurrence to the World Health Organization and neigbouring countries.

Typhus fever

Typhus fevers occur only in special areas or in special conditions. Only one type is likely to occur in your area although the epidemic type can occur anywhere if the conditions are right (see page 128). Find out if typhus occurs in your area; and if so, what type.

The typhus fevers are acute infectious diseases caused by rickettsiae (see Chapter 10 page 35). These organisms are carried to people by infected insects. These rickettsiae cause inflammation of the inside of blood vessels going to all parts of the body. The damage to blood vessels and toxins produced by the organisms cause the symptoms and signs of typhus.

The onset is usually sudden with fever and a rigor; the fever usually lasts for about 2 weeks.

Pains and weakness in the muscles are marked.

Headache is severe. Mental disturbance and deafness can occur. In severe cases encephalitis and unconsciousness follow.

The face is usually flushed and the conjunctivae are red.

A rash comes by about the fifth day. At first the rash is like measles and is of pink macules which go pale when pressed. However, unlike measles, it starts near the axillae and spreads mainly to the trunk. Later on it does not go away when it is pressed, as bleeding occurs into that part of the skin.

In the second week, especially in older people, the condition may get worse and often leads to death.

- The spleen becomes enlarged.
- The pulse becomes faster and the blood pressure lower.
- The encephalitis gets worse.
- Blood vessels can block and cause death of parts of the skin or the fingers or the toes etc.
- Bleeding can occur.
- Kidney failure can occur.
- Heart failure or shock can occur.

After the second week, those who have not died, usually improve slowly.

Treatment is usually very effective – as long as it is given soon enough.

1. Give tetracycline or chloramphenicol. Tetracycline is used if the diagnosis is certain. Chloramphenicol is used if the other differential diagnoses of relapsing fever, typhoid, meningococcal meningitis, etc. are not excluded.
   - Give the antibiotic as soon as possible before the serious effects of the disease occur, which the antibiotic cannot cure.
   - Give a large dose for the first dose, i.e. tetracycline 1 g (4 caps) or chloramphenicol 2 g (8 caps).
   - After the first dose give the normal dose for any severe infection, i.e. tetracycline 500 mg (2 caps) each 6 hours or chloramphenicol 1 g (4 caps) each 6 hours.
2. Take a blood smear and start treatment for malaria. (See Chapter 13 page 61).
3. Give good nursing care and the usual treatment of any of the complications which have already occurred.

Control and prevention depend on the type of typhus that is present (see below). There are four main groups or types of typhus.

Epidemic louse-borne typhus

Epidemic typhus is carried from person to person by the human body louse (see Figure 17.7). This disease occurs in places where a lot of people are crowded together and people do not wash themselves and their clothes properly. Suspect epidemic typhus if an illness that could be typhus occurs in a group of people, e.g. famine or war refugees in a camp.

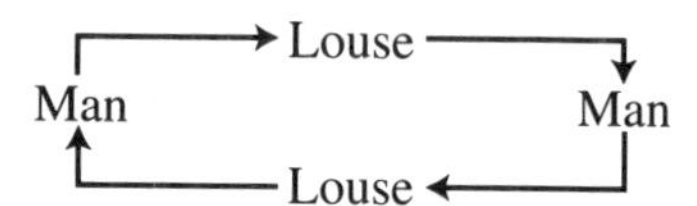

Figure 17.7 Diagram showing the spread of epidemic louse-borne typhus.

Control of the disease will include treatment of the patients to reduce the reservoir of infection. However, infected lice still remain. Control of epidemic louse-borne typhus is therefore best done by killing all lice on patients and on all other people, as well as on their clothing and bedclothes. This is done with a suitable insecticide, at present 1% permethrin or malathion, and it is also helped by better personal washing and hygiene.

1. Wash the patient. Put clean clothes on the patient. Then treat the patient, the clothes and the bedclothes with insecticide (1% permethrin or malathion powder).
2. Sterilise the patient's clothes by heat. If a steriliser is not available use a hot iron. If ironing is not possible treat the clothes with insecticide powder as above and leave them for 2 weeks before they are worn again.
3. Get staff to apply insecticide powder to their own clothes.
4. Treat the whole population with insecticide. Special blowers are available which can blow about 60 g of insecticide powder into a person's clothes without their undressing. This should be repeated 1 week later.

5. Regular washing of their bodies and their clothes should start as soon as possible.

A typhus vaccine exists to raise the resistance of people to the disease. However the vaccine is usually not available where epidemic typhus occurs. The dose for adults is 1 ml by subcutaneous injection repeated after 2–4 weeks. Booster doses are needed each year to keep up the immunity but are often given each 3 months during an epidemic.

Prophylactic treatment of close contacts and staff with tetracycline is needed only before the control measures listed above are in place.

Endemic flea-borne murine typhus

Endemic flea-borne typhus is carried to people from fleas which have fed on infected rats (see Figure 17.8).

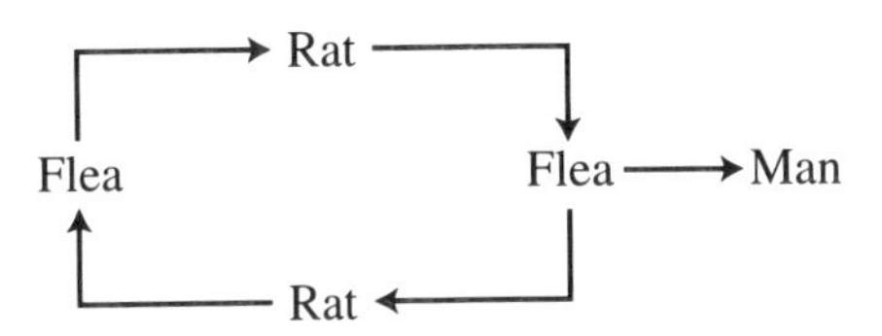

Figure 17.8 Diagram to show the spread of endemic flea-borne murine typhus.

Endemic flea-borne typhus is a much milder disease than epidemic louse-borne typhus and death rarely occurs. It is usually a short-lived 'fever of unknown cause'. Treatment is as described above.

Control is by control of rats and fleas. Insecticides are often put where rats are known to run. Typhus vaccine can be used in special circumstances.

Sporadic tick-borne typhus

Tick-borne typhus is normally a disease of small animals and ticks. Occasionally an infected tick may bite a person. Infected ticks may be brought into a house by dogs which do not themselves suffer from the disease (see Figure 17.9).

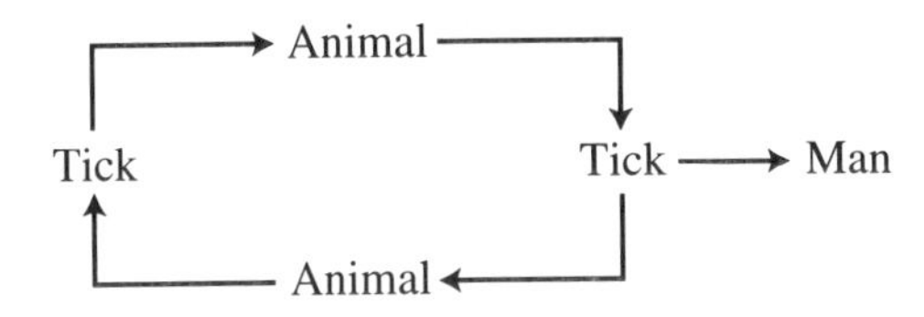

Figure 17.9 Diagram to show the spread of sporadic tick-borne typhus.

The disease is usually mild. However at the place where the tick bit the person, a black ulcer (called an eschar) usually appears and the nearby lymph nodes are usually enlarged.

However in America a severe form of typhus called Rocky Mountain spotted fever is carried by ticks.

Treatment is as described for fever typhus (see above).

Control and prevention is the avoidance of bites from ticks. Treat ticks on dogs. Do not allow dogs to sleep on beds.

Sporadic mite-borne scrub typhus

Mite-borne scrub typhus is normally a disease of small animals and mites in jungle areas of Asia and the Pacific, especially where jungles have been cleared and scrub or bush is regrowing. People are affected if they are bitten by infected mites (see Figure 17.10).

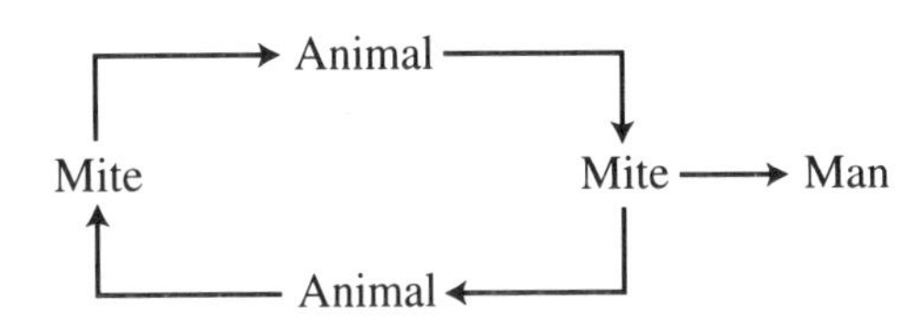

Figure 17.10 Diagram to show the spread of mite-borne scrub typhus.

The disease can be quite severe and cause death. Also a black ulcer (eschar) can form at the mite bite. Nearby lymph nodes become enlarged. Numerous eschars can be present and many lymph nodes enlarged if many infected mites bit the person.

Prevention is by keeping away from areas known to have infected mites or by people wearing protective clothing and repellents if they have to go to that area.

If an area where people must live becomes affected, then the bush has to be cleared, small animals killed and the area treated with insecticide or burned.

Arborvirus infections

Arborviruses usually live in animals (not man, except dengue) and are carried (or borne) from one animal to another by insects (mosquitoes, sandflies, ticks).

(Insects are also called arthropods and 'arborvirus' is short for '*ar*thropod-*bor*ne *virus*'.)

Man is affected by these viruses when an insect carries the virus to him instead of the normal host, although occasionally the virus can be spread another way.

Arborviruses are often localised to one area. They depend on an animal host, which may be localised to one area, and an insect vector, a particular species of which is needed for spread, possibly being localised to one area.

Most of the infections are mild and some possibly occur during infancy when the infant has partial protection from his mother's antibodies. Many local people are immune therefore to the viruses in their own area.

Human epidemics can occur:

1. at the edge of an area of endemic infection;
2. if there is a change in land use which changes the number of animal hosts or vectors (e.g. new irrigation areas allowing more mosquitoes to breed);
3. if there is a change in the human population with non-immune immigrants shifting to the area.

Symptoms and signs can include:

1. spread of the virus from the site of the bite throughout the body, with growth of the virus causing fever for some days;
2. often then an improvement for a day or more;
3. if the virus grows and damages further parts of the body, the following can occur:
   - fever again,
   - skin rash,
   - gastrointestinal symptoms with diarrhoea or vomiting,
   - hepatitis,
   - kidney damage,
   - arthritis,
   - meningitis/encephalitis,
   - immune system damage with blood platelets, blood vessel wall lining, etc. being damaged and allowing serum or even blood to leak out of the vessels and produce bleeding and shock ('haemorrhagic fever').

These symptoms and signs can look very like severe falciparum malaria or septicaemia as well as a number of other infections.

There are very many arborviruses and very many different languages and therefore very many names given to the diseases that they may cause. On most occasions they will not be able to be diagnosed at the health centre and would need special serology blood tests done in a laboratory to be able to diagnose them. This, however, does not matter as most will get better. Tests will be needed only if severe cases occur or if an epidemic occurs.

Special infections are:

- *Dengue fever* – the most common.
- *Yellow fever* – one of the severe types affecting liver and kidneys.
- *Haemorrhagic fever* – the possible result of either of the above but possible with any arborvirus infection, some other viral infections but also at times almost any type of infection.
- *Japanese encephalitis* – one of the severe arborvirus infections affecting the brain.

Dengue fever

Dengue occurs in most parts of the world. Four types of dengue virus can cause this disease. Dengue viruses are spread by mosquitoes (*Aedes aegypti*). Man is the only host in urban areas although monkeys can be affected in rural areas. Dengue usually occurs in small epidemics.

Infection with one of the dengue viruses can cause:

1. no symptoms,
2. viral type fever only,
3. typical dengue fever as below,
4. haemorrhagic fever as follows.

Typical dengue fever begins with fever and headache. After this there is often mild upper respiratory tract and conjunctival inflammation, worsening of the headache, severe pain on moving the eyes, severe backache and severe joint pains. The patient may not be able to eat or sleep and may be weak and depressed. Later abdominal pain may occur.

On examination there is fever, the pulse is not fast, conjunctival inflammation, tender eyes, various rashes on the skin (often like measles though more often red in colour and starting on the trunk and spreading to the arms and face), small vesicles on the palate and enlarged non-tender lymph glands.

In some cases after 2–3 days, the patient improves for 1–2 days but the disease returns again and lasts for about 7–10 days in all. Often at the stage of fall of fever, small spots of bleeding (petechiae) are seen in the skin especially on the lower legs and arms.

In some epidemics in some countries, especially in children, bleeding and shock can occur at this stage. Dengue therefore is one of the viral causes of 'haemorrhagic fever' (see next heading and page 134).

There is no improvement in the patient when antimalarials or antibiotics are given.

The patient may feel unwell for months.

Unless a blood slide can be examined for malaria and is negative, all cases of dengue in malarial areas must be treated with antimalarials (see Chapter 13 page 61) as well as rest and other symptomatic treatment. However do not give aspirin which could make any bleeding worse. Use paracetamol instead. If the patient is very ill, treat for septicaemia (see Chapter 12 page 53). If bleeding or shock occurs, treat as in Chapter 27 page 378.

The means of control and prevention is to kill mosquitoes, especially around houses and prevent mosquitoes breeding.

Dengue haemorrhagic fever

This complication of infection with a dengue virus is common in all areas except Africa. It almost always occurs in children under 16 years. It is thought to be due to a second infection with a different dengue virus. The antibodies from the first infection do not control the second infection but in fact help to cause even more damage than ordinary dengue infection to the blood vessels (making them leak plasma and even blood) and to the blood clotting systems (allowing bleeding to occur).

The first 2–7 days of the illness are like (and are) ordinary dengue fever with high fever. *(First point in diagnosis – fever for 2–7 days.)*

After this, there are small bleeding spots in the skin (petechiae) but these are often in the skin over all parts of the body. Bleeding from the nose, gums or gastrointestinal tract, and rarely urinary tract, can occur. If a blood pressure cuff is used on the arm after this, a number of new petechiae may be seen – especially if the cuff is left up between systolic and diastolic pressure for 2 minutes. *(Second point in diagnosis – bleeding.)*

The liver can be felt enlarged and tender but soft. *(Third point in diagnosis – tender liver.)*

Soon after, the temperature drops; the patient develops cool skin; becomes restless and over the next few hours develops definite shock with fast pulse, low blood pressure, poor peripheral circulation, low urine output, decrease in level of consciousness, etc. and often is dead within 24 hours unless treated correctly. *(Fourth point in diagnosis – shock.)*

If blood tests are available, these show a low platelet count and a high haemoglobin and haematocrit due to more plasma than red blood cells leaking from the damaged vessels. *(Fifth point in diagnosis – typical blood tests.)* Blood tests such as these and a (MAC) ELISA test to quickly diagnose the dengue virus infection are not usually available.

Treatment includes the following:

1. Give symptomatic treatment; but no aspirin which may cause more bleeding.
2. Give oral rehydration fluid if at any stage of a dengue-like illness the patient is not eating or drinking, so that they will always have adequate hydration and can withstand plasma leak better.
3. Watch carefully at the time of the temperature drop (3–7 days) for cool skin, restlessness, abdominal pain, low urine output and any bleeding into the skin or elsewhere which would mean development of leak of plasma from the vessels and shock developing. Immediately start intravenous rehydration to replace the fluid inside the vessels (see Chapter 23 page 286). Treatment is usually needed for no more than 48 hours.
4. Make sure not too much intravenous fluid is given, as this could cause heart failure. Once the pulse rate, blood pressure, urine output and skin circulation are normal, reduce the IV fluids to just maintenance fluid. If the jugular venous pressure becomes raised, stop the intravenous fluid until it becomes normal.

If cases occur, always urgently notify your Medical Officer as treatment of an epidemic of patients and control of the mosquitoes causing the epidemic, may need special organisation.

Yellow fever

Yellow fever occurs only in western and central Africa and the north part of South America. It may spread to other tropical areas (see Figure 17.11).

Yellow fever is an acute viral infection which can cause:

1. fever,
2. liver damage with jaundice (hepatitis),
3. kidney damage with protein in the urine and sometimes kidney failure, and
4. bleeding into all parts of the body.

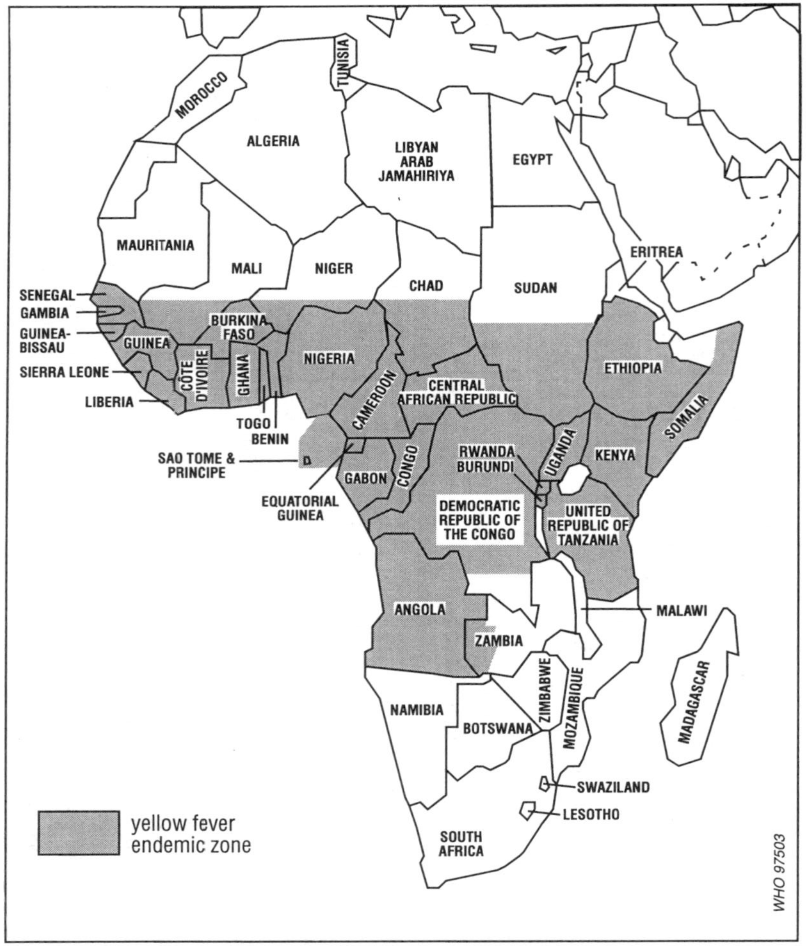

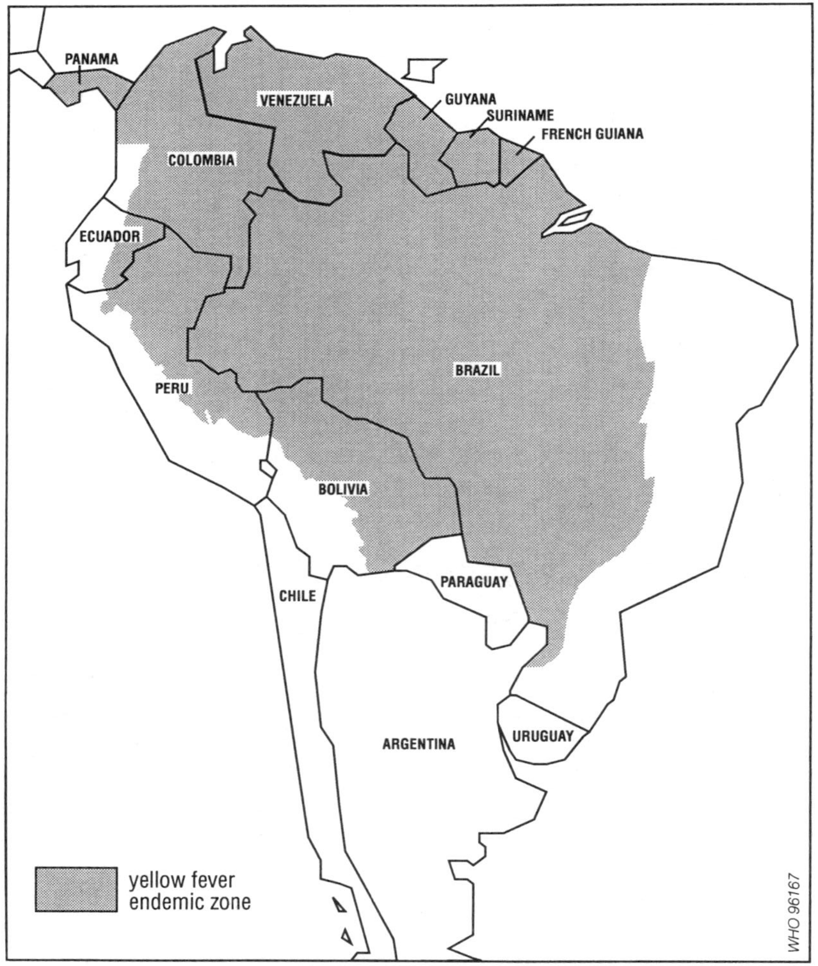

Figure 17.11 The distribution of yellow fever.
(Source: World Health Organization)

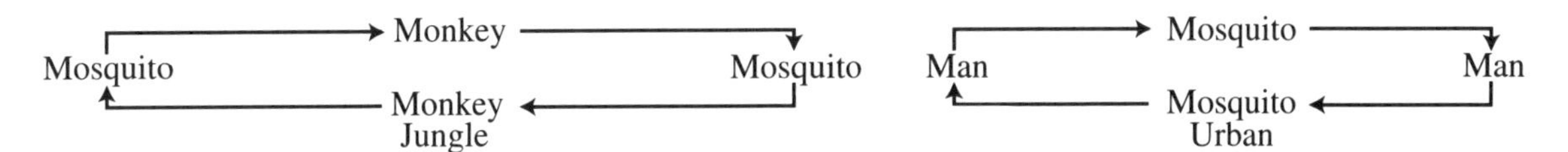

Figure 17.12 Diagram to show how yellow fever virus spreads.

The yellow fever virus is usually passed between monkeys and mosquitoes. A person can be infected if he is bitten by an infected mosquito in the jungle (jungle yellow fever). If an infected monkey, mosquito or person comes to a town, the disease can then be passed between people and mosquitoes in the town (urban yellow fever) (see Figure 17.12).

People who live in an area where yellow fever is common and do not die from an attack usually become immune or suffer only mild attacks. Severe attacks occur especially when people from other areas go to an infected area or the disease spreads to a new area.

A typical severe attack is as follows:

1. At first there are severe general symptoms and signs of a viral type infection, similar to dengue fever – fever; pains in the head, eyes, back and joints; red watery eyes; nausea, vomiting etc. The pulse is usually slow, not fast.
2. After a few days the temperature falls and the patient may improve.
3. After some hours or a day or so, however, the patient may get much worse. He or she develops a high fever (although the pulse is still slow), jaundice and a tender liver and bile in the urine (hepatitis), a lot of protein in urine and also bleeding into the skin and from the nose, mouth, lungs, intestine, etc.
4. Death occurs from liver or kidney failure or bleeding. If these can be successfully treated and the patient lives for about 12 days, the patient usually recovers.

Yellow fever is therefore one viral cause of 'haemorrhagic fever'.

The differential diagnosis includes malaria, septicaemia, relapsing fever, leptospirosis and viral hepatitis. If laboratory tests are available these would help (see Table 17.1).

For treatment of yellow fever in a health centre, see page 134.

Prevention is by immunisation with living 17D strain of yellow fever virus which does not cause disease but gives immunity for 10 years.

Japanese encephalitis

Japanese encephalitis is one of the arborviruses which causes the most severe type of encephalitis.

Most infections, however, produce only a fever, then complete recovery and immunity to reinfection. In a few, however, the virus reaches the brain and causes the neck to be arched backwards, loss of full

Table 17.1 Table to show the differential diagnosis of some causes of a fever with jaundice if you have laboratory tests to help. Remember that pneumonia is also a very common cause of fever and jaundice; but there are also signs in the chest.

Causes of jaundice and fever	*Proteinuria*	*White blood cell total*	*Blood slide*
Yellow fever	A lot	Low	Negative
Malaria	Little or none	Low or normal	Plasmodia
Relapsing fever	Some	High	Borrelia
Septicaemia	Little or none	Variable – often high	Negative
Leptospirosis	A lot	High	Negative
Viral hepatitis	Little or none	Low or normal	Negative

consciousness (the patient may be sleepy, drowsy, unconscious, etc.), signs of irritation of the brain (the patient may be restless, irritable, confused, delirious, psychotic, twitching, fitting, etc.) and then the patient within a few days, becomes unconscious and paralysed. Many die, although some slowly recover with mental abnormality, paralysis, etc. The lumbar puncture shows clear cerebrospinal fluid (CSF).

Many of the other arborviruses produce much less severe encephalitis from which there may be much better or even complete recovery.

For management, see Chapter 25 page 327.

Immunisation is possible against this particular arborvirus.

Other viral fevers similar to dengue or yellow fever causing 'haemorrhagic fevers'

There are a large number of arborviruses as already mentioned (page 130) which can cause symptoms and signs similar to dengue or yellow fever.

These diseases can cause fever, often with a slow pulse (which should make you suspect some unusual or viral disease), generalised aching and pains all over the body, rash, liver damage (hepatitis), kidney damage (proteinuria or kidney failure), bleeding, shock and other conditions.

There are other groups of virus infections, which are not arborviruses, but which can cause a similar clinical disease. The disease can be complicated by shock from blood vessels leaking fluid or bleeding through many blood vessels (haemorrhagic fever) with shock.

Lassa fever in West Africa and Junin virus in Argentina and Mochipo virus in Bolivia are one group of these other viruses. They are spread from man to man by body fluids or body secretions including urine, during close personal contact. They may also be spread to man from rats living in a person's house.

Marburg disease and Ebola fever are from another group of these other viruses which affect monkeys. Close contact with the monkey's blood or body fluids causes infection. This infection is then spread among people by contact with the infected person's blood or body fluids.

Diagnosis of any of these viral diseases is not possible (unless a known epidemic of one of them is occurring) without special laboratory tests not available at a health centre. The Medical Officer must be notified so that he can make arrangements for these tests to be done. Unless a definite diagnosis is made, the best treatment, control and prevention measures cannot be carried out.

There is no specific cure for any of these diseases. Special antiviral drugs, almost certainly not available in the country, might help. However if the patient can be kept alive until his body can make enough antibodies to kill the virus, he will probably recover. In a severe case Medical Officer care in a hospital will be needed to do this.

However, there are also a number of diseases, other than viral diseases, which also can cause similar symptoms and signs. Make sure the patient does not have one of these and die from it. Treat for all of these diseases that are treatable if they cannot be ruled out. These diseases include the following:

1. malaria,
2. septicaemia (especially meningococcal and plague),
3. relapsing fever,
4. leptospirosis,
5. typhus,
6. typhoid,
7. acute viral hepatitis.

Management

Management in a health centre of an unusual severe acute disease of unknown cause, which causes fever, abnormalities of many body systems, but especially haemorrhage in many places of the body and shock, therefore includes the following. When a diagnosis is made, those measures that are not needed can be stopped.

1. Do *not* transfer the patient unless the Health or Medical Officer tells you to do so, as epidemics can be caused by transfer.
2. Immediately notify the Medical Officer and the Health Officer and ask for advice and help.
3. Barrier nurse the patient.
   - Staff must take care not to get blood, urine, saliva, etc. onto themselves as the infection may get through normal skin.
   - Staff should wear gloves, gown, mask and goggles.
4. Staff should put insecticide (e.g. 1% permethrin powder) on their clothes if the case is possibly epidemic typhus. Treat the patient and his clothes and his bedclothes with 1% permethrin powder.

5. Treat for septicaemia (see Chapter 12 page 53).
6. Treat for falciparum malaria (see Chapter 13 page 61).
7. Treat shock if it occurs. (See Chapter 27 page 378.) Start IV fluids immediately.
8. Do not give aspirin which may make bleeding worse. Instead give paracetamol.
9. Treat bleeding if it occurs (see Chapter 27 page 378).
10. Treat for hepatitis if it occurs (see Chapter 24 page 307).
11. Treat for kidney failure if it occurs (see Chapter 25 page 347). However, unless kidney failure does occur make sure you give the patient enough fluid to give a good urine output (2 litres/day).
12. Nurse the patient under a mosquito net (and, if possible, in a room which has insect screens on the door and windows). Treat the net and screens with insecticide (permethrin) (see Chapter 13 page 74).
13. Have the patient's room and the whole health centre sprayed with a residual insecticide.
14. Destroy or treat any breeding places for mosquitoes around the health centre.
15. Treat the patient's room with gamma BHC if ticks occur in the area.
16. Try to kill any rats by poison or other means. Also put insecticide along known rat runs.
17. Take 20 ml of blood and keep it in the refrigerator at 4°C for special laboratory tests. Take and keep blood and urine for the usual laboratory tests (see Chapter 6 pages 22–26). If the patient dies, get permission to take at least a piece of liver for examination (a piece aspirated (sucked back into a syringe) through a very thick needle put into the liver through the skin, is better than none).

Make sure no blood or tissue fluid gets on you through your gown, gloves, mask and goggles.

18

Some Serious Subacute and Chronic Infectious Diseases with Limited Distribution

This chapter is about the following diseases:

1. Bacterial infections
   - Typhoid fever
   - Brucellosis
2. Protozoal infections
   - Leishmaniasis
   - Trypanosomiasis
3. Worm infections
   - Schistosomiasis

Typhoid fever (enteric fever)

Typhoid fever is an acute or subacute disease caused by the typhoid bacteria. At first it causes malaise, fever, abdominal pain and constipation. Later, it causes diarrhoea, rash, enlargement of the spleen and very severe toxaemia. This stage may be complicated by intestinal haemorrhage or perforation. Sometimes, mild cases may cause only a non-specific illness and fever.

Cause, epidemiology, pathology

Typhoid fever is caused by infection with typhoid bacteria *(Salmonella typhi).* The reservoir is persons infected by the typhoid bacteria.

The faeces or urine of infected people may contaminate food or the water supply. This may occur if they handle food, or if they do not use a toilet. It may also occur if the water supply is not safe from contamination by excreta or is not treated. Sometimes flies carry the bacteria from faeces to food.

The bacteria, when swallowed, multiply in the bowel and then spread through the whole body. They grow best in the lymph glands, spleen, gall bladder and parts of the wall of the intestines.

The faeces of the patient are often infectious for weeks or months; and the patient may become a carrier for life.

An attack of the infection usually produces considerable immunity.

A similar but less severe disease caused by *Salmonella paratyphi* types A, B or C is called 'paratyphoid fever' and is occasionally also carried by domestic animals.

Symptoms and signs, course and complications

For the first week the patient has the general symptoms and signs of infection with some special features. He has malaise, headache, pains all over and fever. He may have a cough and nose-bleeds. He usually has mild abdominal pain and constipation. On examination, the patient has fever but the pulse may be slower than expected. Nothing else special is found.

During the second week the patient becomes worse. General symptoms and signs may be severe. Abdominal pain becomes more severe and diarrhoea occurs. On examination the patient may not be fully conscious. The fever and slow pulse are still present. There may be signs of bronchitis in the chest. The abdomen is usually distended and may be tender especially in the right iliac fossa. The spleen is enlarged. A rash made up of red spots, each of which lasts for a day or so, may be seen, especially on the abdomen.

During the third week, the general and abdominal symptoms and signs become worse. The patient may become unconscious and die.

During this third week two special complications may also occur.

1. The bowel may perforate (get a hole in it through to the peritoneal cavity). The pulse gets faster, the temperature falls, the abdominal pain and tenderness get worse and signs of generalised peritonitis may develop.
2. Haemorrhage may occur from the intestinal wall into the intestine. The patient may pass blood from the rectum; or simply become pale and shocked (and later pass blood).

If the patient does not die he or she usually starts to recover quickly after the fourth week. However, in some cases, after about 2 weeks, there is a return of the symptoms and signs, though usually not as severe as before.

A much milder disease often occurs. Sometimes it may be only a fever with perhaps a mild gastrointestinal upset, or some of the other symptoms or signs of the more severe disease.

Tests
None are available at the health centre.

The white cell count is usually not raised unless a complication has developed when it may be high.

Blood and faeces cultures may grow the typhoid organism.

Diagnostic features

- Generalised symptoms and signs of infection (often pyrexia of unknown origin ('PUO'), 'sick', and no response to antimalarials, see Chapter 36 page 482).
- Slow pulse.
- Constipation at first, then diarrhoea.
- Abdominal distension and tenderness.
- Persistence of temperature, after treatment with antimalarials, without any focal signs.

Differential diagnosis
- Other causes of fever (see Chapter 36 page 482)
- Other causes of gastroenteritis have to be differentiated from typhoid (Chapter 23 page 282–283)
- Other causes of septicaemia (Chapter 12 page 53)

Treatment
Transfer the patient to Medical Officer care, if this is possible.

Dispose of faeces carefully. Disinfect the bedpan and other articles used by the patient, and carefully wash your hands after caring for the patient.

Give chloramphenicol 1 g (4 caps orally or 1 bottle by injection) each 6 hours. When the fever stops reduce the dose to 500 mg (2 caps) four times a day. However, continue the chloramphenicol for 2 weeks. In some areas sulphamethoxazole/trimethoprim (co-trimoxazole) or even amoxycillin/ampicillin may be more effective. (See Chapter 11 page 48–51.) You need to find out what antibiotic to give for your area.

Treat as for other cases of gastroenteritis. (See Chapter 23 page 285.)

Treat any complication in the usual way.

Treat schistosomiasis if present so that the worm does not become a carrier. (See Chapter 18 page 154).

Transfer
Transfer these cases:

1. All diagnosed cases (especially if laboratory tests have shown many *S. typhi* organisms in your area to be resistant to drugs available to you and therefore need ciprofloxacin or ceftriaxone etc.; or in case injected adrenocorticosteroid drugs or a blood transfusion or an operation is needed). (Start antibiotics first.)
2. The diagnosis is suspected but cannot be made and the patient is very 'sick'.
3. A complication occurs especially intestinal perforation or haemorrhage.

Control and prevention
1. Kill the organism in the body of the host (reservior) (patients and carriers).

   If typhoid fever is uncommon in the area, investigation is needed to find out where the infection came from. A carrier is usually responsible. A Medical Officer may be able to treat such a carrier. However, *if typhoid is common in an area,* a search would not be made for the source of infection.
2. Stop the means of spread of the organism.
   - Patients and carriers should not be allowed to handle food for others.
   - Proper community disposal of faeces and urine is essential.
   - Safe community water supply is essential.
   - Careful nursing of cases that are infectious is important. Staff must wash their hands carefully after caring for a patient.
3. Raise the resistance of susceptible persons.

   An oral, live typhoid vaccine (three or four doses 2 days apart) or injected Vi capsular polysaccharoid typhoid vaccine (one dose) (but not if taking antibiotics or mefloquine) is far more effective than the whole cell TAB vaccine subcutaneous injection. Immunisation will make it less likely for an immunised person to get typhoid. This is given, however, only to a person who has a particular risk of getting typhoid. These vaccines are used only for travellers or occasionally in an epidemic.

Brucellosis

Brucellosis is due to an infection with the *Brucella* bacteria. The infection is normally one of cattle, goats and pigs and it can cause abortions in these animals. The bacteria can spread to people who live with or work with infected animals or who drink raw untreated (unpasteurised) milk from infected animals.

The *Brucella* bacteria live mainly in the lymph tissues; but can affect joints and other parts of the body.

At first there can be a fever with severe pains and malaise which lasts for a few weeks. After this the patient usually slowly improves.

However, the fever may come back many times every week or every few weeks. The spleen sometimes becomes enlarged and sometimes very enlarged. Pain in a joint, especially the hip, is common. Chronic osteomyelitis of the spine or infections in almost any part of the body sometimes occur. Weight loss is common. Depression is common.

In most people this prolonged infection is usually overcome by the body itself after a year or so; but in a few, the infection continues.

Diagnosis can be made only by special blood tests (serology) not possible in a health centre.

Treatment is by tetracycline 500 mg four times a day for 4 weeks; or if this fails, other special drugs in combination.

Refer or *transfer* suspected cases to a Medical Officer for diagnosis and treatment.

Leishmaniasis

Leishmaniasis is a group of diseases caused by an infection with protozoal organisms called *Leishmania.* About 12 million people are affected and there are about 2 million new cases each year.

There are two main types of leishmaniasis.

1. Skin leishmaniasis (skin only).
   Skin and mucous membranes leishmaniasis which occurs only in South America and is called 'espundia'.
2. Skin, blood, bone-marrow, spleen, liver and lymph node leishmaniasis called visceral leishmaniasis or 'kala azar' ('visceral' means 'of the organs inside the body').

The reservoir of infection includes not only infected people but also some infected dogs, rodents and many other animals.

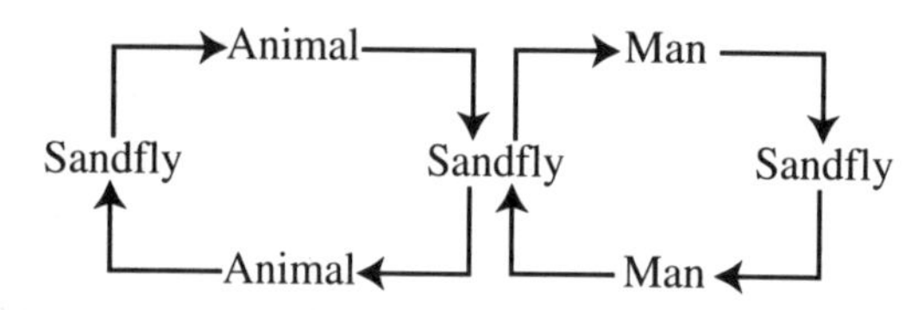

Figure 18.1 Diagram to show the means of spread of leishmaniasis.

The organisms are spread to man by the bite of a sandfly which has been infected from an infected man or infected animal (see Figure 18.1).

Control and *prevention* of leishmaniasis follow the usual rules.

1. Kill the parasite in the original host or reservoir.
   (a) Find and treat patients with the disease; but this works only if man is the only host of that *Leishmania* in that area.
   (b) Find and kill any dogs or rodents or other animals with the disease; but first special tests are needed to prove that these animals do have the same *Leishmania* organism that is causing the human disease and not another *Leishmania*, before all of these animals are killed.
2. Stop the means of spread.
   Sandflies breed in places like animal houses, rubbish dumps, anthills, crumbling stonework etc. They do not usually fly more than a few hundred metres from where they breed. The following may therefore be effective:
   (a) Move houses away from places where sandflies breed.
   (b) Kill sandflies with regular spraying of insecticide where they breed.
   (c) Protect people from sandflies by clothing, repellents and fine sleeping nets or door and window covers treated with insecticide.
3. Raise the resistance of possible new hosts.
   This can only be done for skin leishmaniasis. A sore used to be started by injecting material into an area of the skin where a scar would not matter. This sometimes did stop sores starting in other areas such as the face where a scar would matter.
   It is however dangerous, as hepatitis or HIV infection may also be passed on. Vaccines for immunisation are now available in some areas.
4. Prophylactic treatment is not yet practicable.

Skin leishmaniasis

Skin leishmaniasis occurs in many Old World countries; that is Africa, the Mediterranean, the Middle East and Asia where it is called 'oriental sore'. It also occurs in the New World, that is Central and South America, where it is often more severe or widespread and can involve also the mucous membranes (see Figure 18.2). It has been divided into five types of increasing severity. At times these differences are due to different strains of the organism, but more importantly the differences are due to different types of cellular immunity in the patient (similar to leprosy, see Chapter 15 pages 93–95)

1. *Single non-ulcerated or dry ulcerating lesions (e.g. 'oriental sore').*
   Children are most often affected as most adults have been infected and have become immune.
   The incubation period is from weeks to months.
   At first a small reddish itchy lump appears in the skin where the patient was bitten by the sandfly. A crust forms on top of the lump. The lesion gets bigger and usually becomes a rounded ulcer. The ulcer has thick raised edges and a discharge of blood and pus, which dries to form a dark crust (see Figure 18.3). Small new lumps may start around the edge of the ulcer. These lumps then get bigger and ulcerate. Eventually, as these join, a large ulcer up to 10 cm in diameter may be formed. Sometimes the lesion does not ulcerate and stays as a large lumpy mass. The ulcer is not painful. The ulcer usually lasts for months to a year and then heals leaving a thin scar.
2. *Multiple discharging lesions.*
   Sometimes there may be more than one lesion if the patient was bitten in several places. Sometimes new lesions form on the skin between the first lesion and the nearby lymph glands. Eventually all heal.
3. *Relapsing lesions.*
   These lesions heal or nearly heal only to get worse again, although eventually they do heal. If the condition goes on for a long time, severe scarring can result.
4. *Diffuse lesions.*
   If cellular immunity is poor, some organisms spread through all the skin producing nodules and loss of colour which can look like lepromatous leprosy. Ulcers do not heal.
5. *Skin and mucous membrane leishmaniasis (New World cutaneous leishmaniasis).*
   This occurs in Central and South America. The worst kind is called 'espundia' in Brazil. In espundia the first lesion (see 'Skin leishmaniasis') may be on the face, ears, elbows or knees. Either then, or months or years later, lesions appear in the mucous membrane of the nose and mouth. The nasal mucous membrane swells up and then ulcerates. The ulcer may slowly destroy all the tissues of the nose so that a terrible-looking hole is left in the centre of the face. The mouth, lips and throat may be affected.

The patient does not have a fever or feel ill because of the infection.

The diagnosis can be confirmed by aspirating some fluid through a fine needle from the edge of the ulcer and examination of this fluid under the microscope for the *Leishmania* organisms. (See Figure 18.3.)

Treatment includes the following:

1. Eusol dressings two or three times a day until the crust is gone and the ulcer is clean.
2. If there is a lot of secondary bacterial infection, give antibiotics such as penicillin or tetracycline; this is usually not needed.
3. Then keep the ulcer clean and dry under a dressing and it will probably heal in a few weeks.
4. Treat with aminosidine (paromomycin) 15% and urea 10% ointment for 4 (up to 12) weeks if available, as this usually halves the time to heal.
5. Transfer or refer to a Medical Officer for consideration for treatment with drugs as for kala azar
   - if the ulcer does not heal after the above treatment, or
   - if the ulcer is on the face, or
   - if there are a number of large ulcers (more than 4 ulcers) or very large ulcers,
   - if there are disseminated or diffuse lesions,
   - if there is mucous membrane as well as skin disease.

Epidemiology, *control* and *prevention* – see page 138.

Visceral leishmaniasis (kala azar)

Visceral leishmaniasis occurs in many countries (see Figure 18.4).

A person is infected by the bite of an infected sandfly. The *Leishmania* organisms spread to the bone marrow where they damage the cells that make new blood. The organisms spread also to the lymph nodes, liver and spleen which are damaged and

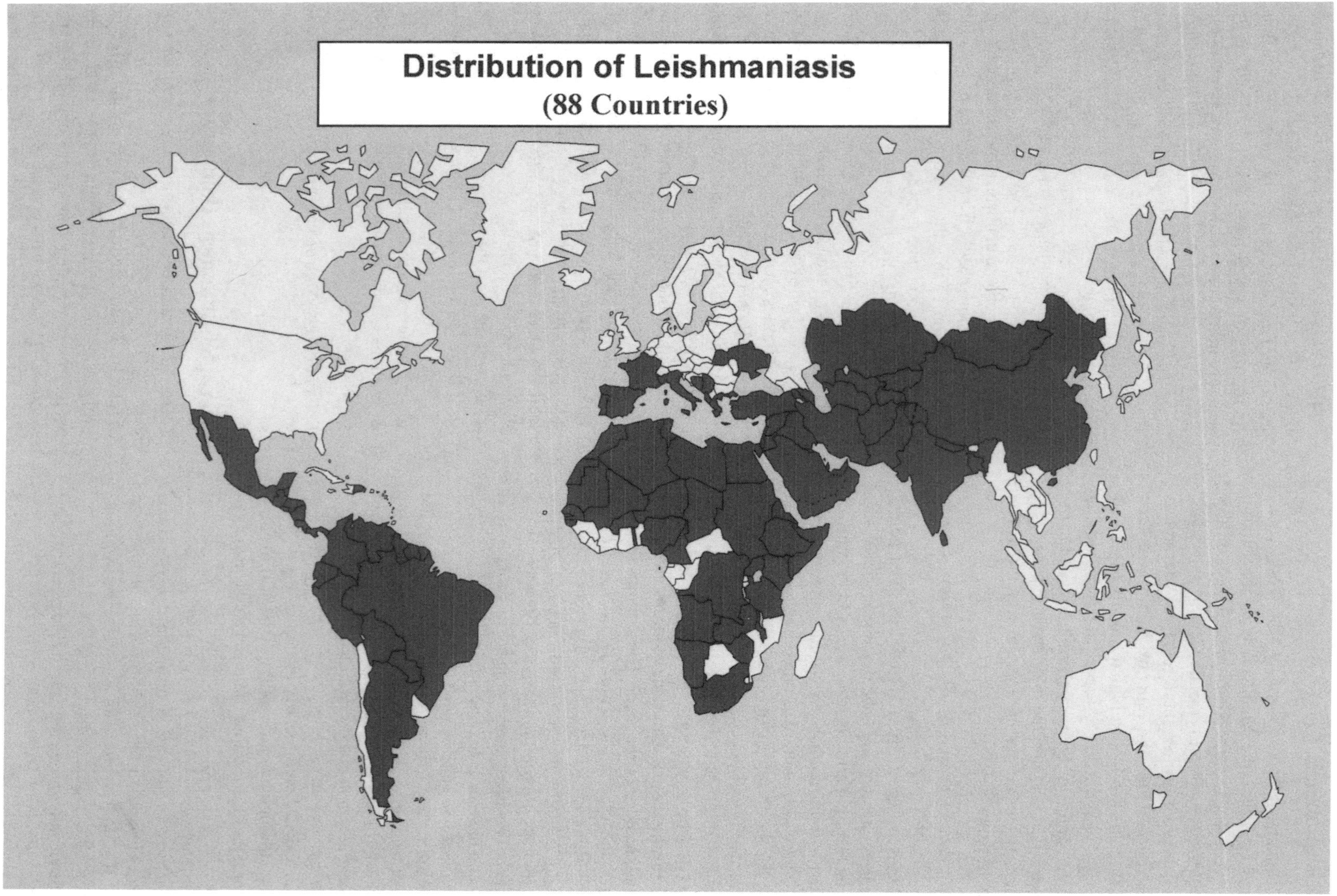

Distribution of Leishmaniasis
(88 Countries)

Figure 18.2A The distribution of leishmaniasis.
(Source: World Health Organization, WHO/CTD, 1998)

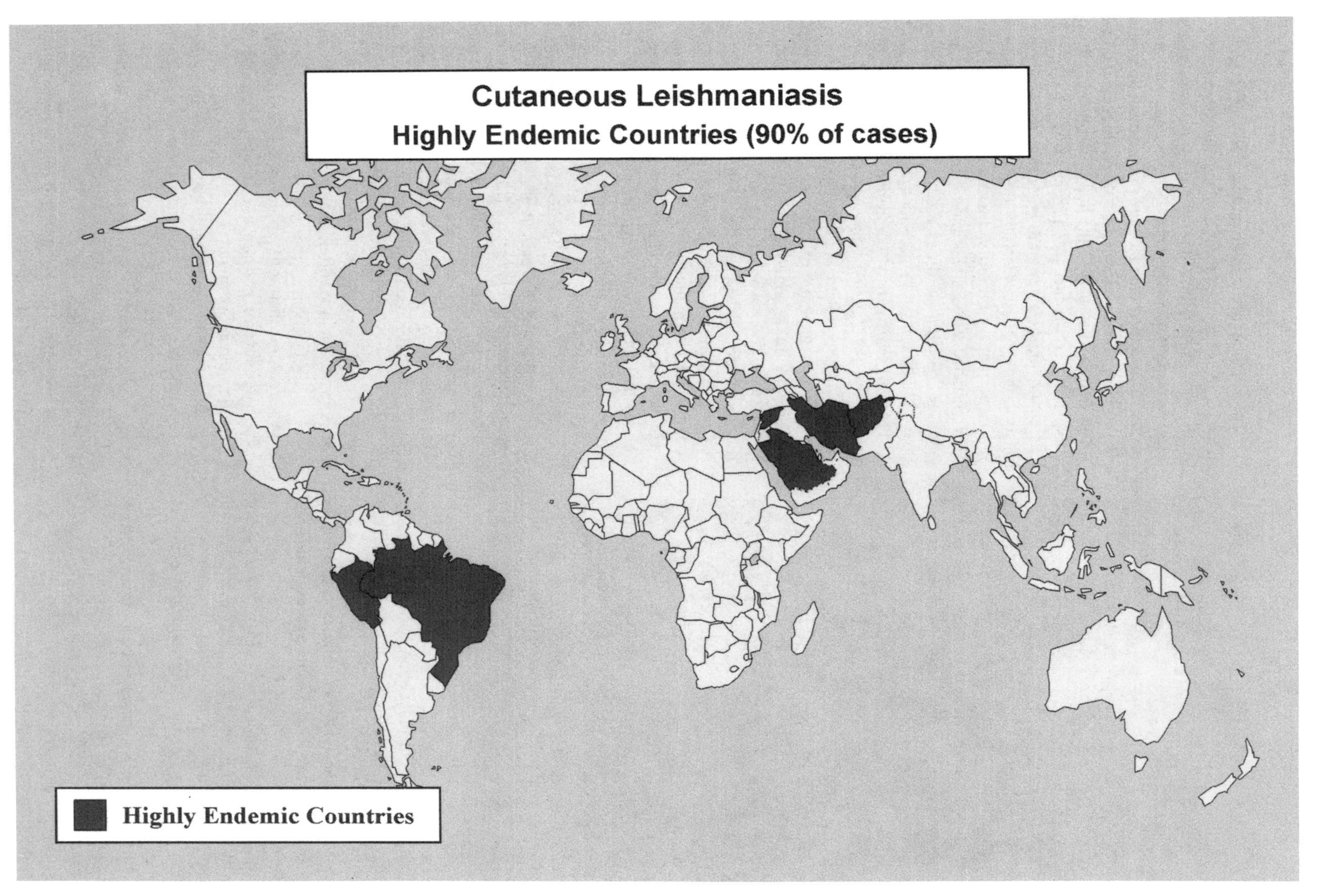

Figure 18.2B The distribution of skin leishmaniasis, and skin and mucous membrane leishmaniasis. (Source: World Health Organization, WHO/CTD, 1998)

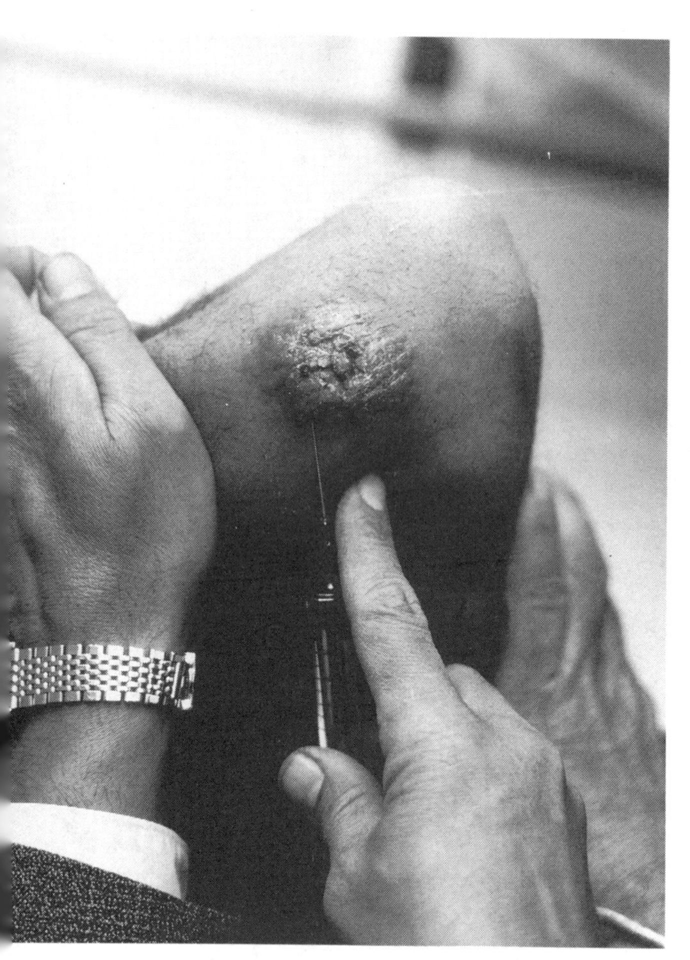

Figure 18.3 A typical skin lesion of skin leishmaniasis. Diagnosis will be confirmed by aspirating some fluid, putting it on a slide and examining it under a microscope for *Leishmania*.

become larger than normal. Some patient's cellular immunity may, however, control all signs of the infection.

In the Mediterranean region children and visitors are the ones mostly affected. In other areas, adults are affected too.

The illness starts with a fever. This is usually not severe at first and the patient continues his normal life. Sometimes however, the fever is severe. The fever may be worse in the afternoon and again at night.

The spleen soon becomes enlarged; and often becomes very enlarged (see Figure 18.5).

The liver becomes enlarged but not very enlarged.

The lymph nodes may become enlarged.

The patient becomes anaemic.

The patient may have repeated attacks of diarrhoea.

The patient becomes thin and wasted and often has a darkening of the colour of the face, hands and feet.

Dermal (skin) leishmaniasis may occur – often after treatment and when the patient is getting better (as the skin is then the place the organisms find it easiest to live). There are pale or reddish thickened areas of the skin on any part of the body. Lumps may form – especially on the face (see Figure 18.6).

Leishmaniasis may come back in a patient previously immune or successfully treated for the disease if the patient's immunity decreases, e.g. develops HIV infection/AIDS. Patients with HIV infection often get reactions to drugs used for treatment. They also often do not get better with treatment.

The *diagnosis* can be confirmed in the laboratory by finding the *Leishmania* organisms in a biopsy (best from the spleen but also bone marrow, liver, lymph nodes and skin, etc). Serology tests especially ELISA and direct agglutination test (DAT) are usually possible. When no laboratory is available the formaldehyde gel test can be used. Put 1 ml of the patient's serum in a test tube. Add one drop of 40% (commercial) formaldehyde (formalin). If the patient has kala azar the serum (1) becomes solid (so that if you tip the tube upside down the serum does not run out) *and* (2) the serum does not stay clear (but goes a milky or dirty colour). Both (1) and (2) are needed for the test to be positive. The test is not positive until a few months after the patient has been infected. and other infections can also give a (false) positive result.

Treatment is different in different parts of the world as the sensitivity of the organisms to drugs varies. Treatment is also by drugs with dangerous side effects. Unless you have been specially trained in the use of the best drugs for your area, transfer the patient for diagnosis and treatment to a Medical Officer.

Drugs will include (often in combination):

1. pentavalent antimony injections – sodium stibogluconate or sodium antimony gluconate or meglumine antimoniate;
2. aminosidine (paromomycin) may later be shown to be the best single drug but is best used in combination with 1;
3. aromatic diamidine injections – hydroxystilbamidine isethionate and pentamidine;
4. amphotericin B;
5. oral drugs are being tested and one such as miltefosine may be effective.

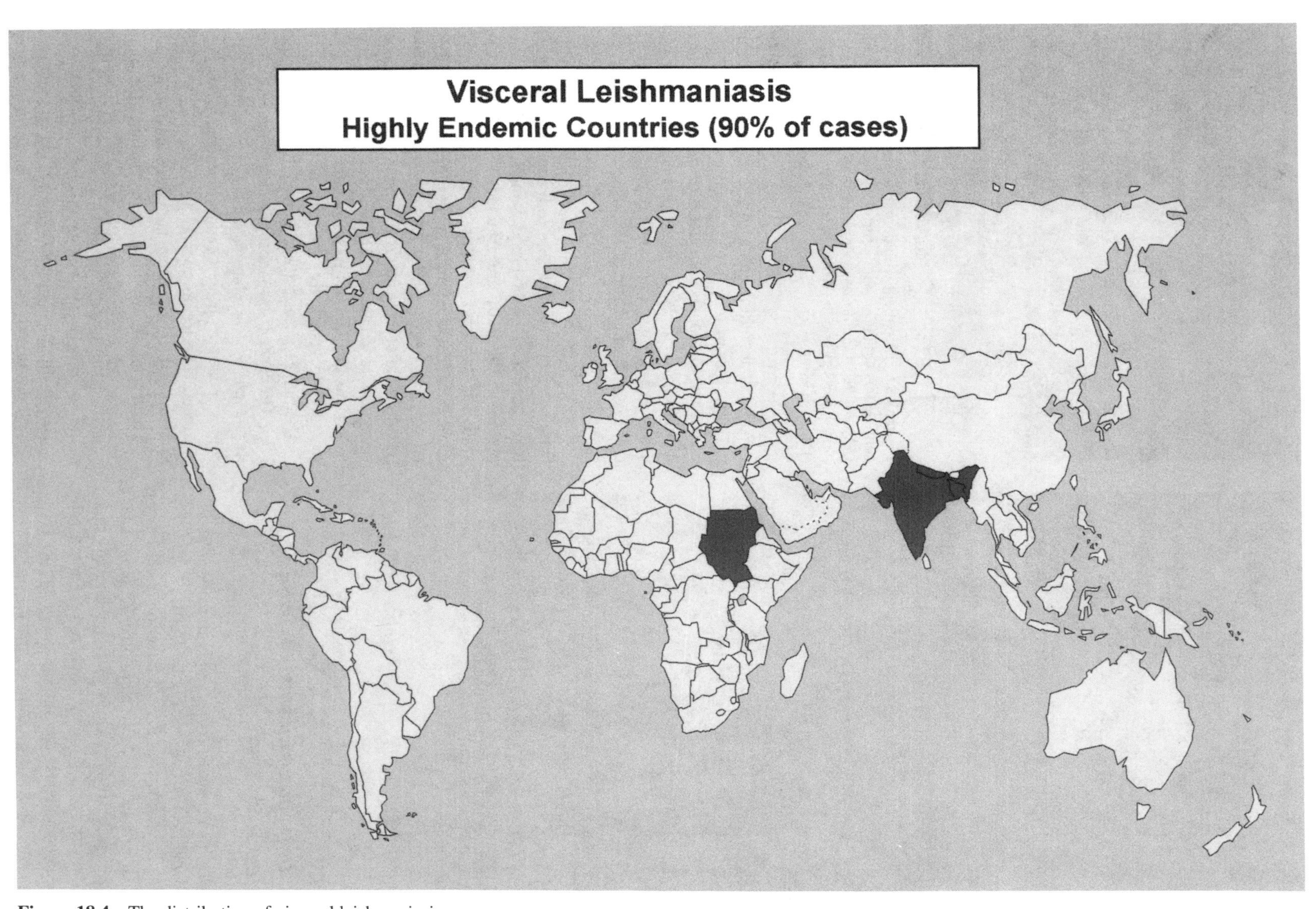

Figure 18.4 The distribution of visceral leishmaniasis.
(Source: World Health Organization, WHO/CTD, 1998)

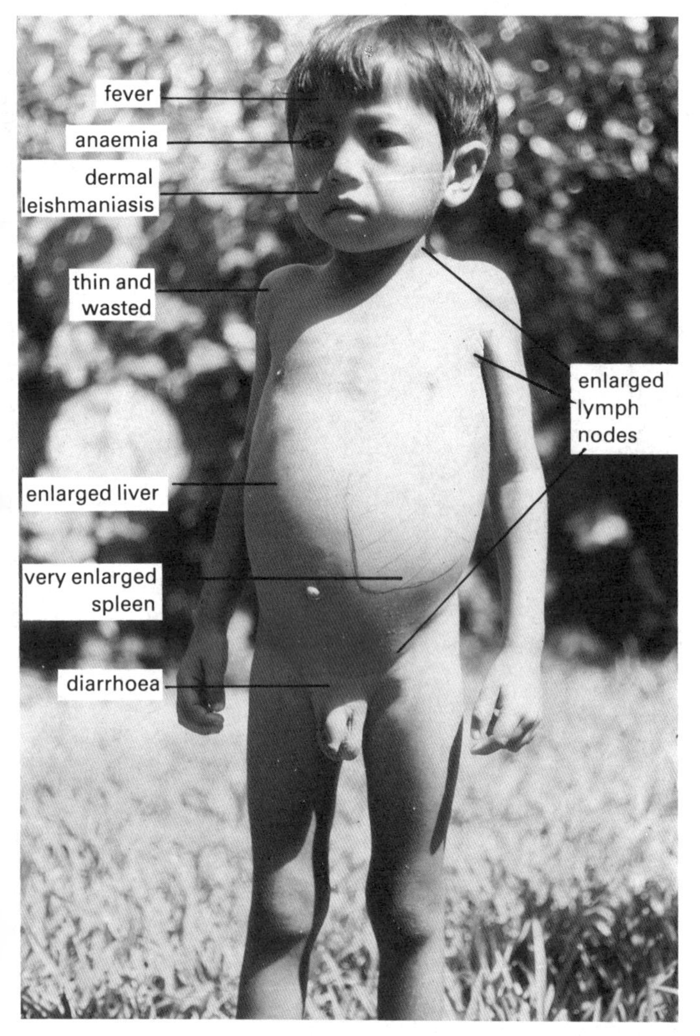

Figure 18.5 A patient with visceral leishmaniasis. Note the features of the disease listed above.

Epidemiology, *control* and *prevention* (See page 138)

African trypanosomiasis (sleeping sickness)

African trypanosomiasis occurs only in parts of West, Central and East Africa (see Figure 18.7).

African trypanosomiasis is an infection caused by a protozoal parasite called a trypanosome (*Trypanosoma brucei*). There are two kinds of trypanosomes that affect man. If a trypanosome is in blood or other fresh fluids examined under the microscope, it can be seen to swim with its tail (see Figure 18.8).

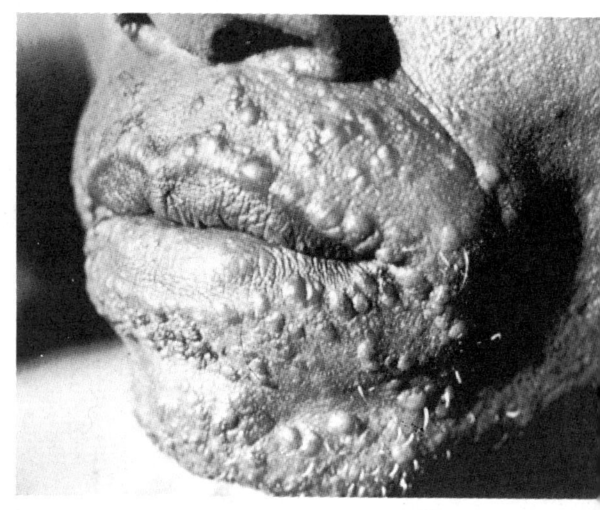

Figure 18.6 A patient with dermal leishmaniasis. Do not confuse this condition with leprosy. (Source: W. Peters and H.M. Gilles, *A colour atlas of tropical medicine and parasitology*, London, Wolfe Medical Publications 1981) (Dr D.M. Minter)

Animals including cattle and large game are affected as well as man.

The trypanosomes are carried from infected man or animals by the tsetse fly (see Figures 18.9 and 18.10). There are at least two kinds of fly which carry the disease and they have different breeding, living and biting habits.

The trypanosomes cause a chronic disease which causes death. At first a sore forms at the bite. Then a fever occurs when the blood, lymph glands and other organs of the body are affected. Later the nervous system is damaged and this nervous system damage is the usual cause of death. One type of trypanosome (*T. b. rhodesiense*) causes all of these things in a few months. The other type (*T. b. gambiense*) may take a year or more to cause death.

African trypanosomiasis occurs only in people who go into a tsetse fly infected area.

The bite of a tsetse fly is painful; but the pain soon goes. However if trypanosomes were injected by the fly, then 1–3 weeks later a reddish non-painful lump comes up at that place. It can form into an ulcer if it is scratched. The lesion goes away itself in 2–3 weeks. Sometimes the person does not notice the lesion.

The trypanosomes however then go into the blood and cause any of the following.

1. Fever with weakness, headache, etc. The fever may be there for a few days and then be gone for a few days over many months. However the fever

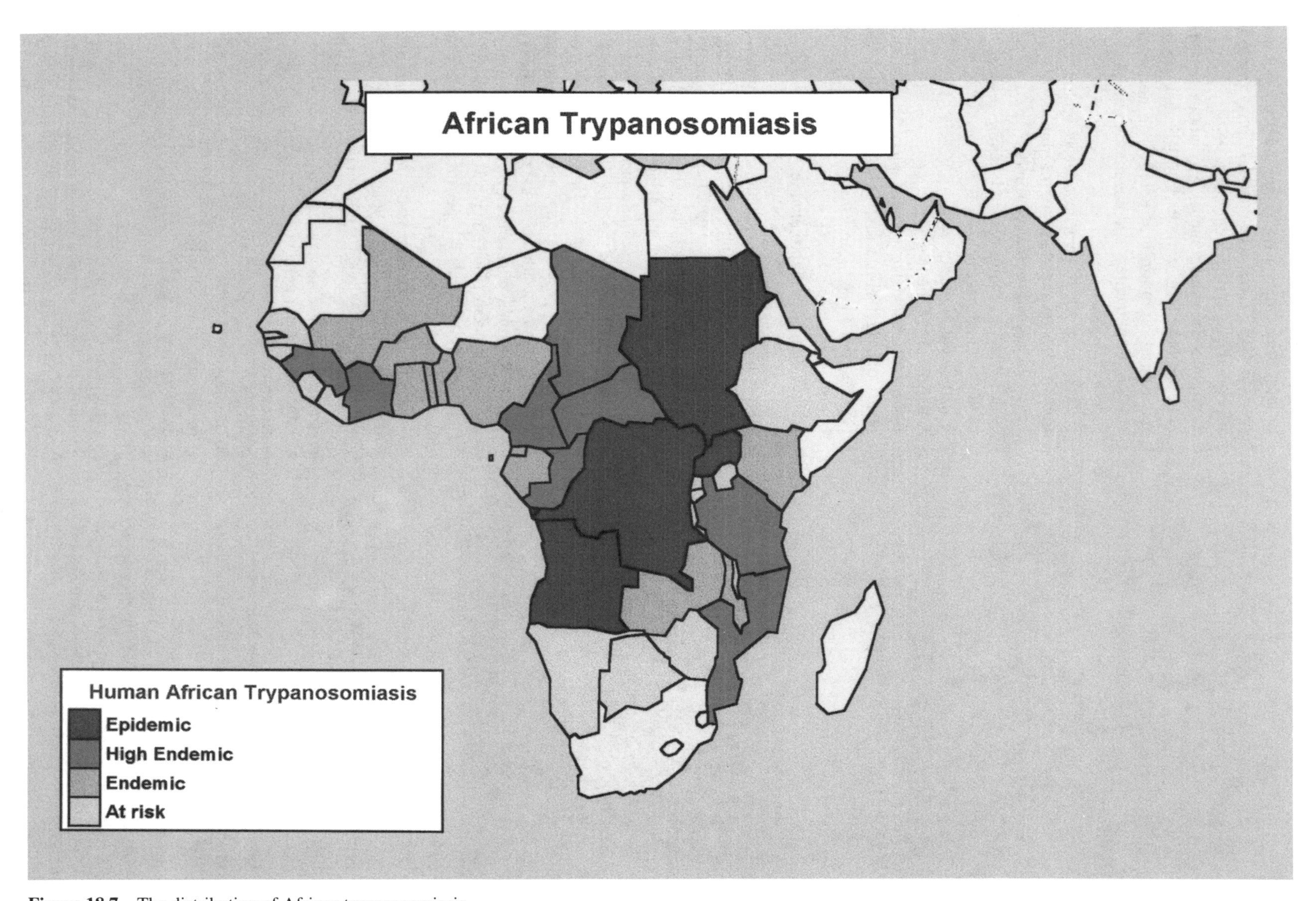

Figure 18.7 The distribution of African trypanosomiasis.
(Source: World Health Organization, WHO/CTD, 1998)

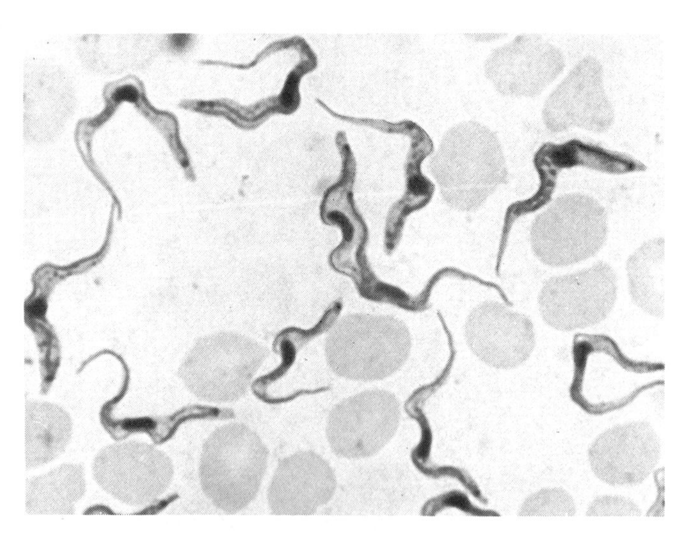

Figure 18.8 A trypanosome magnified many times.

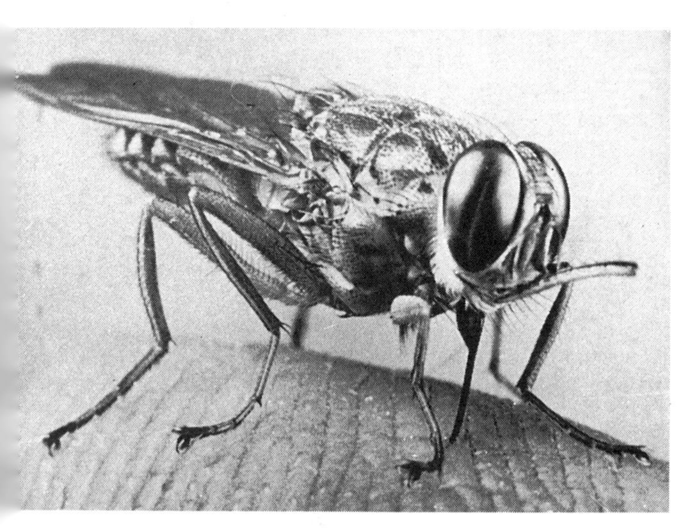

Figure 18.9 The appearance of a tsetse fly. The actual size is about 15 mm in length.

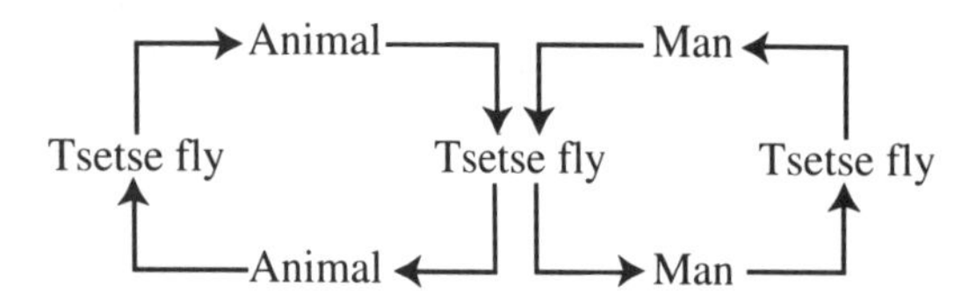

Figure 18.10 Diagram to show how the trypanosomes can be spread.

can be severe and present all the time. Everyone who has a fever in an area where trypanosomiasis occurs must be investigated for trypanosomiasis. Wet and also stained thick blood films must be examined for trypanosomes before any other diagnosis is made. The examination should be repeated at least three times if the patient does not get better. The CIATT test (see page 147) may prove to be a good easy quick diagnostic test.

2. Lymph node enlargement. Any nodes may be enlarged but those at the back of the neck are the ones most commonly affected. The nodes are smooth, firm, painless and not stuck to the skin or other structures.
   If in an area where trypanosomiasis occurs, aspirate fluid from the node with a fine needle and have it examined for trypanosomes.
3. Skin rashes or itchiness or thickening (especially of the face) may occur.
4. Enlargement of the spleen.
5. Enlargement of the liver.
6. Bone marrow damage with anaemia.
7. Heart damage with a fast pulse even when the fever is not present and later sometimes heart failure.
8. Kidney damage with proteinuria.

After some weeks or months the nervous system is affected. Signs of meningitis, encephalitis and organic psychosis then occur. (See Chapters 25 and 35.) The patient often has headache, abnormal behaviour, sleeps during the day but not at night, does not eat, shakes, becomes paralysed and passes into a coma and dies. Examination of the CSF shows an increase in the protein and in the cells. However, when there are no nervous system signs, a lumbar puncture should not be done just to see if the nervous system is involved. A lumbar puncture may cause infection of the nervous system from other parts of the body, if the nervous system was not yet infected, unless the patient is already on treatment.

If the patient is from or is in an area where trypanosomiasis occurs, then trypanosomiasis must be thought of and tests done for it in all cases of:

- fever,
- lymph-node enlargement,
- anaemia,
- wasting,
- sleepiness,
- meningitis,
- encephalitis,
- psychosis, and
- unconsciousness.

In any of these conditions, if another cause for the condition is not found and if the condition does not get better on the proper treatment for the diagnosis you made, then transfer the patient to a Medical Officer for the special tests to diagnose trypanomiasis.

Tests

Special tests which show who has the infection (even if there are no symptoms and signs) may soon be available. The card indirect agglutination test for trypanosomiasis (CIATT) is positive in almost all patients with symptoms and signs, and in infected people before symptoms and signs appear. It needs only blood from a finger prick. Other means of diagnosis need the trypanosomes to be seen under the microscope in body fluids, e.g.

- needle aspiration from the edge of the original sore,
- needle aspiration from enlarged lymph nodes,
- blood including wet films, thick films and use of special concentration methods,
- bone marrow aspiration,
- CSF obtained at lumbar puncture (which should not be done unless already on treatment).

Treatment

Treatment is more effective the earlier it is given. Early *gambiense* disease can be treated with IV pentamidine or suramin, but early *rhodesiense* disease can only be treated with IV suramin. These drugs kill only organisms in the body outside the brain. Once the brain has been infected, other drugs are also needed. Intravenous melarsoprol is the usual drug used for infection of the brain but it has very serious side effects and in fact up to 15% of patients treated may die from these side effects, mainly encephalitis. Before the patient is fit for treatment with melarsoprol he will need treatment with suramin and perhaps pentamadine, as well as treatment of any anaemia, malnutrition, etc. Do not do a lumbar puncture before the patient is on treatment with suramin or pentamadine as, if the brain is not infected, the needle going into the CSF may spread the infection to the spinal cord and brain. A new drug, eflornithine, is much safer and more effective treatment than melarsoprol; but it is effective only for gambiense infections and is very expensive at present. In view of the very serious side effects of most of these treatments and the great expense of the other drugs, if you suspect or diagnose a case of trypanosomiasis, then transfer the patient to Medical Officer care at a hospital (unless you have been specially trained to use the special drugs for your area).

Control and prevention

Control and prevention will depend on the advice of experts who will work out the best methods for your area. The usual methods are:

1. Kill the parasite in the body of the original host or reservoir.
   (a) Case finding and treatment is important in *T. b. gambiense* infections where man, not animals, is the chief reservoir.
   (b) Mass treatment may be considered in epidemics of either type but in *T. b. rhodesiense* infections in domestic animals may also need treatment. In *T. b. rhodesiense* infections where scattered cases are caused by bites from tsetse flies infected from game animals, this treatment of animals is not possible.
   If people are removed from an affected area and animals which can be infected are chased away from the area, tsetse flies will not be infected and the disease will tend to die out in that area.

2. Stop the means of spread.
   If tsetse flies can be removed from an area, the infection cannot continue.
   (a) In *T. b. gambiense* outbreaks, the tsetse flies which cause these breed in the shade along the river banks. They cannot however live and bite people at river crossings, washing or water collection places, etc. if trees are cut down for 20 metres on each side of the river for 200 m up- and downstream of where people are or go.
   (b) In *T. b. rhodesiense* areas in savannah and forest, the shade trees used by tsetse flies for breeding could all be cut down. This, however, may turn the area into a desert. If however tsetse flies are eradicated from an area, trees can be cut down around that area to create a 'tsetse barrier'. Any vehicles etc. crossing this barrier have to be sprayed to kill tsetse flies resting under the vehicle.
   (c) An area can be treated with insecticide to kill tsetse flies. This is best done by spraying from an aeroplane. It would need to be combined with the above.
   (d) Tsetse fly traps can be effective in catching or killing many flies especially in areas where there are many people.

3. Raise the resistance of the possible new hosts.
   Vaccines do not yet exist.

4. Prophylactic treatment.
   No safe cheap effective drugs are available for routine use, but in certain epidemic situations, all

people who have positive tests for infection could be treated.

American trypanosomiasis (Chagas' disease)

American trypanosomiasis occurs only in Central and South America (see Figure 18.11). The disease is caused by a protozoal parasite called a trypanosome

The trypanosomes live in dogs, cats and other animals as well as people.

These trypanosomes are spread from an infected animal or person to an uninfected person by the bite of an infected reduvid bug (see Figure 18.12). These bugs live in the cracks in ceilings and walls in the poorer houses in rural areas. The bugs bite the faces of people while they sleep at night.

The trypanosomes from the bug enter the body through the mucous membranes of the eye or the mouth or the skin of the face, where they cause a lesion. The organisms then travel in the blood to the lymph nodes, spleen and liver. They also enter the heart and nervous system and cause both acute and chronic disease in these places.

Transfusion of blood that contains the organisms will also cause infection and disease.

The acute disease affects children more often than adults.

A lesion appears where the organisms enter the body. This is usually on the face. There is often swelling of the eyelids of the eye on that side of the face; the lids are firm and red and swollen enough to close the eye. There can be a painful red swelling with much hard oedema around it on the skin. The nearby lymph nodes are enlarged. The swelling and the enlarged lymph nodes stay for some weeks.

One to three weeks after the infection, the patient develops a high fever and the liver, spleen and lymph nodes may be swollen. The pulse is often fast, even when the fever is not present, because by then the heart is also damaged. The organisms can often be found in the blood or the fluid aspirated from the swelling on the face or from an enlarged lymph gland, if it is examined under the microscope.

After some time the patient usually improves slowly; but the organisms stay in the body. They stay especially in the heart and in the nerves of the oesophagus and large intestine, which they slowly destroy.

After many years the patient may get heart failure or the patient may suddenly die because his heart stops. The muscles of the gastrointestinal tract may not contract properly and the patient may also develop difficulty in swallowing dry food; or aspirate (breathe in) food or drink, causing pneumonia. The patient may develop abdominal swelling and constipation. These things are due to the organisms causing chronic damage to the heart, to the nerves going to the heart and to the gastrointestinal tract.

Diagnosis

Diagnosis can be made by seeing the trypanosomes in the blood only during the first illness but not afterwards. Special laboratory culture methods are interesting and accurate but too expensive for routine use. Serology tests including CFT and IFAT can be used to tell who has been infected.

Treatment

Treatment is unsatisfactory. Drugs such as benznidazole if given early, seem to cure the patient and a new drug, with only a code name at present, D0870 made by the Zeneca Pharmaceutical Company may be more effective. However, at the late stage of the disease, no drugs can cure the damage to the heart, gastrointestinal tract, etc.

If therefore you suspect the disease, especially if it is early before incurable heart or gastrointestinal tract damage, send the patient to a Medical Officer for diagnosis and treatment, unless you have been specially trained in the use of methods for these.

Control and prevention

Control and prevention is as follows; but mostly by making better houses.

1. Kill the parasite in the body of the original host or reservoir.
   Kill dogs etc. that are known to be infected.
2. Stop the means of spread.
   The bug can be killed by various insecticides including gamma BHC applied to the house. This however is expensive and has to be repeated every few months. It may be cheaper, after the initial insecticide treatment, to use a special plaster which covers cracks and itself will not later crack. Best of all, but usually not possible, is to rebuild houses with smooth walls and non-thatched roofs which have no hiding places for bugs. Sleeping under a net will also stop bugs biting the face. However, new ways of using insecticides, e.g. fenithrothion which is put into paint which a family uses to paint inside the house; the use of tradi-

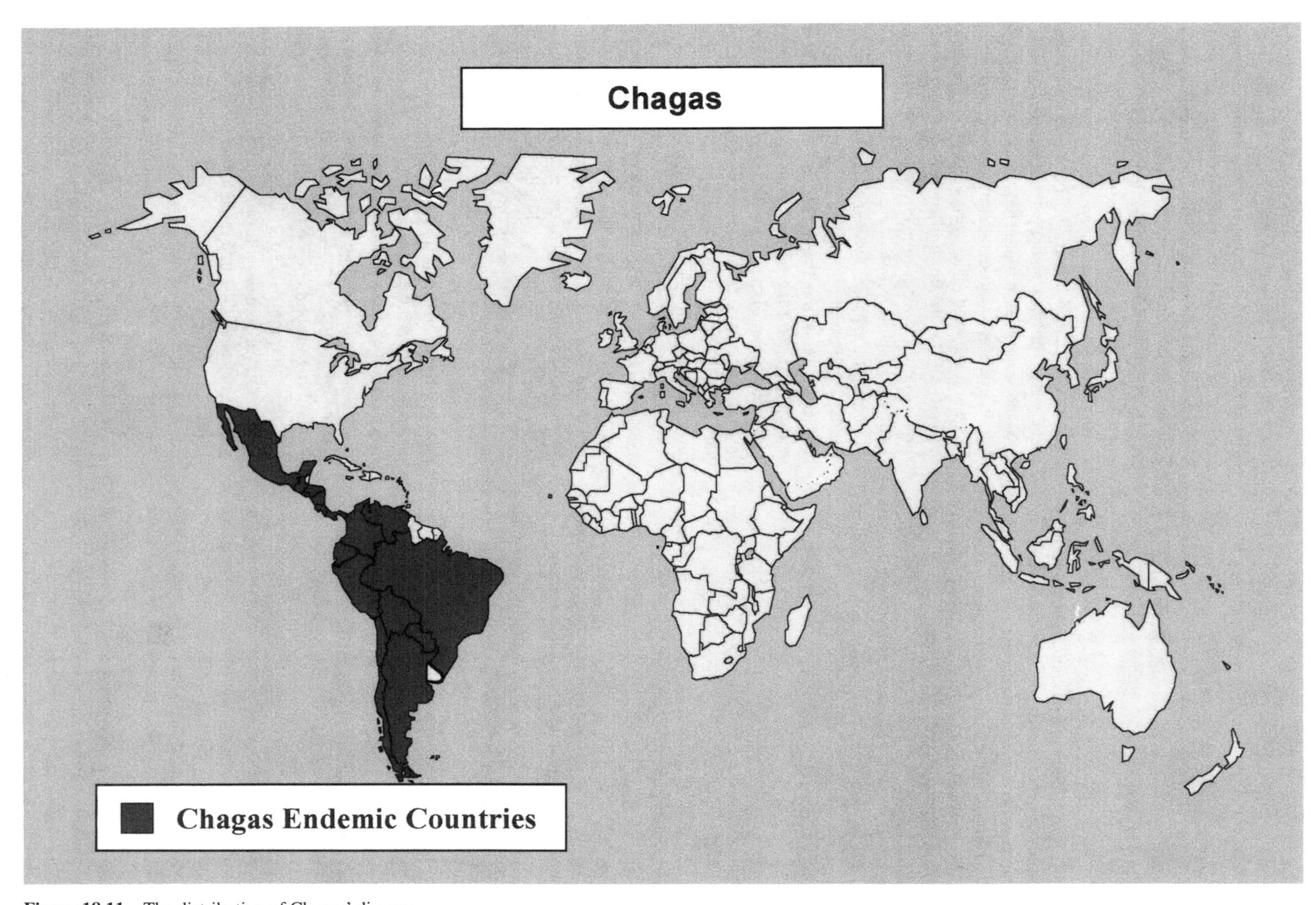

Figure 18.11 The distribution of Chagas' disease.
(Source: World Health Organization, WHO/CTD, 1998)

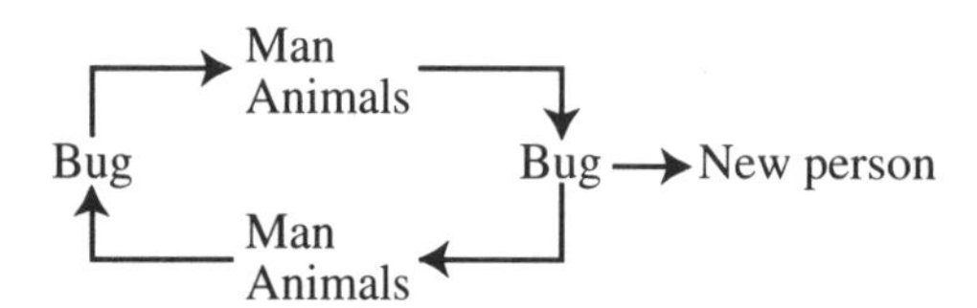

Figure 18.12 Diagram to show the means of spread of American trypanosomiasis.

tional insecticides outside the house; and also the use of insecticide-treated bedclothes and nets, have proved very effective.

All blood collected for transfusion should be tested for the parasite and not transfused if positive.

3. Raising the resistance of people is not yet possible.
4. Chemoprophylaxis is not yet possible.

Schistosomiasis (bilharziasis)

Definition and cause

Schistosomiasis is the disease caused by worms called schistosomes. These are small worms, like very short threads of cotton, which live in the veins of the pelvic organs. The female worm lays many eggs and these eggs damage the bladder, large intestine and liver.

Epidemiology

Three main types of schistosome affect people. Figure 18.13 shows the distribution of the different types.

1. *Schistosoma haematobium* and the less common *S. intercalatum* affect mainly the bladder of humans in Egypt, the Middle East and Africa only.
2. *S. mansoni* affects mainly the large bowel in people and baboons in Egypt, the Middle East, Africa, and South America.
3. *S. japonicum* (and the less common *S. mekongi*) affect the large and small bowel and other parts of people and many domestic and wild animals, in China, Japan, South-East Asia and the Philippines.

S. mansoni and *S. japonicum* live mainly in the pelvis in the veins which come from the bowel. The eggs cause marked chronic inflammation of and ulceration of the wall of the bowel. This causes diarrhoea and dysentery. It also allows the eggs to enter the bowel and be passed in the faeces. *S. haematobium* lives mainly in the pelvis in the veins which come from the bladder and the genital tract. The eggs cause marked chronic inflammation and ulceration of the wall of the bladder. This causes blood in the last part of the urine passed. It also allows the eggs to enter the bladder and be passed in the urine. Inflammation around the eggs also damages the urethra, bladder, ureters and kidneys). It also damages the female genital tract and this leads to infertility, ulcers and tumours.

If the eggs in the urine or the stool go into water, the eggs become worms, now called miracidia. These miracidia swim around until they find certain snails in which they can grow. Then the worms leave the snail and are called cercariae. These cercariae swim in the water until they find a person or a person swallows the water they are in. They can go through the skin of a person or through the mucous membrane of the person's mouth. The worms then travel around the body of the person until they enter the pelvic veins, where they develop into adult schistosome worms (see Figure 18.14).

Some of the eggs laid by the female do not enter the bladder or intestine. Some are carried away in the blood in the veins from the bladder and intestine. These veins join to form the portal vein which runs to the liver (see Chapter 24 page 304). The eggs then damage the liver. Some eggs can be carried to other parts of the body as well as to the liver – especially the lungs and the spinal cord and brain – and damage these parts too.

The body may very slowly develop antibodies and cellular immunity. At first this causes severe inflammation around the eggs laid in the venules with a lot of swelling around them. This swelling causes a lot of the symptoms. The inflammation lessens as better immunity develops in most adults. Also, the better immunity stops a lot of new worms developing from reinfections.

Symptoms and signs

1. A mild skin itch and rash may come where the cercariae go through the skin.
2. Several weeks later there may be fever, malaise, cough, abdominal pain and allergic-type symptoms and signs. These are caused by the worms travelling around the body to the pelvic veins. These symptoms last for 1–2 weeks. They are common only in *S. mansoni* and *S. japonicum* infections and in the first infection.
3. Then the patient is quite well until either urinary (see 4 below) or intestinal (see 5 below) schistosomiasis develops. Either urinary or intestinal schistosomiasis may be followed by other complications (see 6 below).
4. Urinary schistosomiasis is caused by *S. haematobium* laying eggs in the veins of the wall of the bladder. Inflammation in these areas causes the

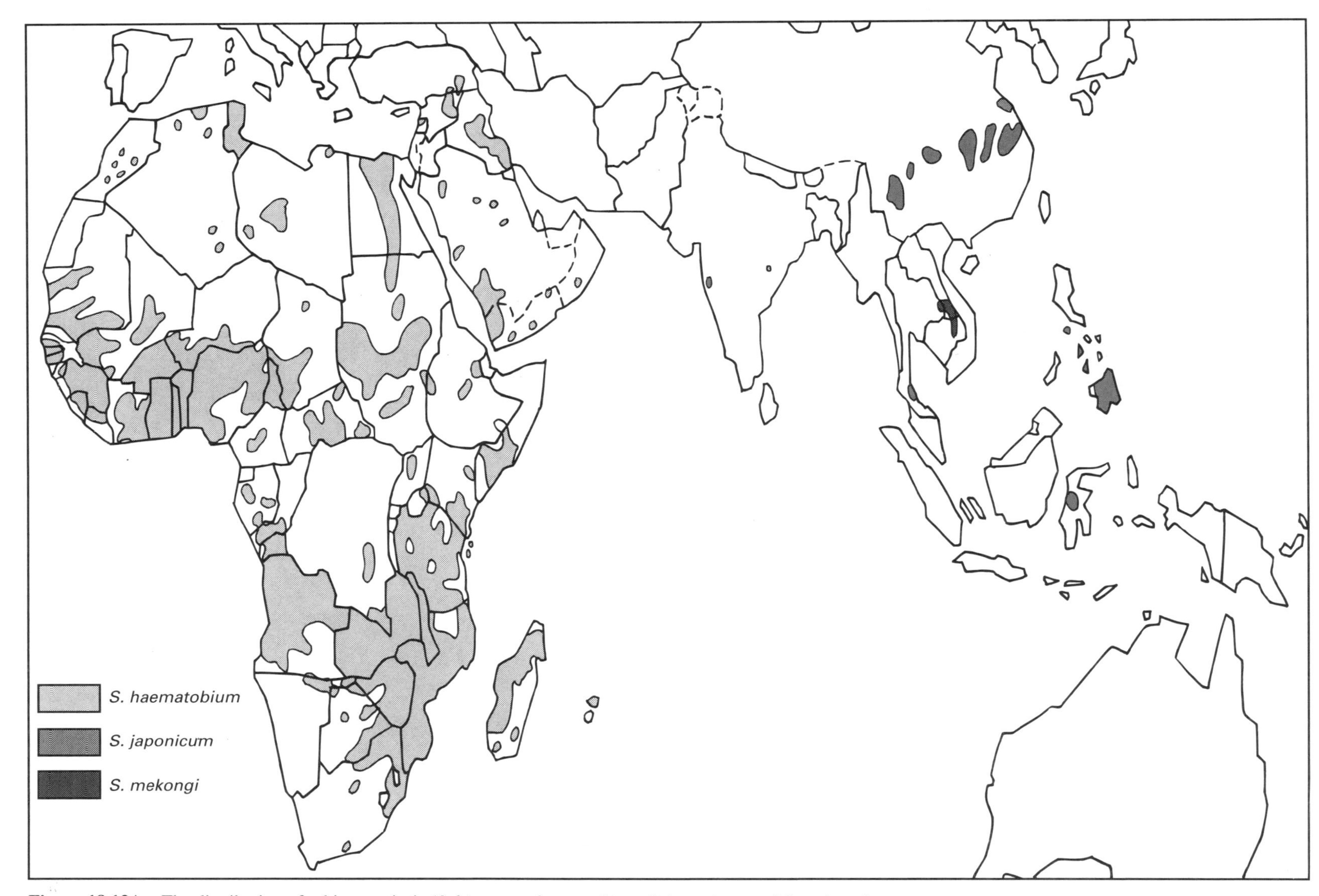

Figure 18.13A The distribution of schistosomiasis (*Schistosoma haematobium*, *S. japonicum* and *S. mekongi*).
(Source: *The control of schistosomiasis: second report of the WHO Expert Committee*. Geneva, WHO, 1993 (*WHO Technical Report Series* No. 830).

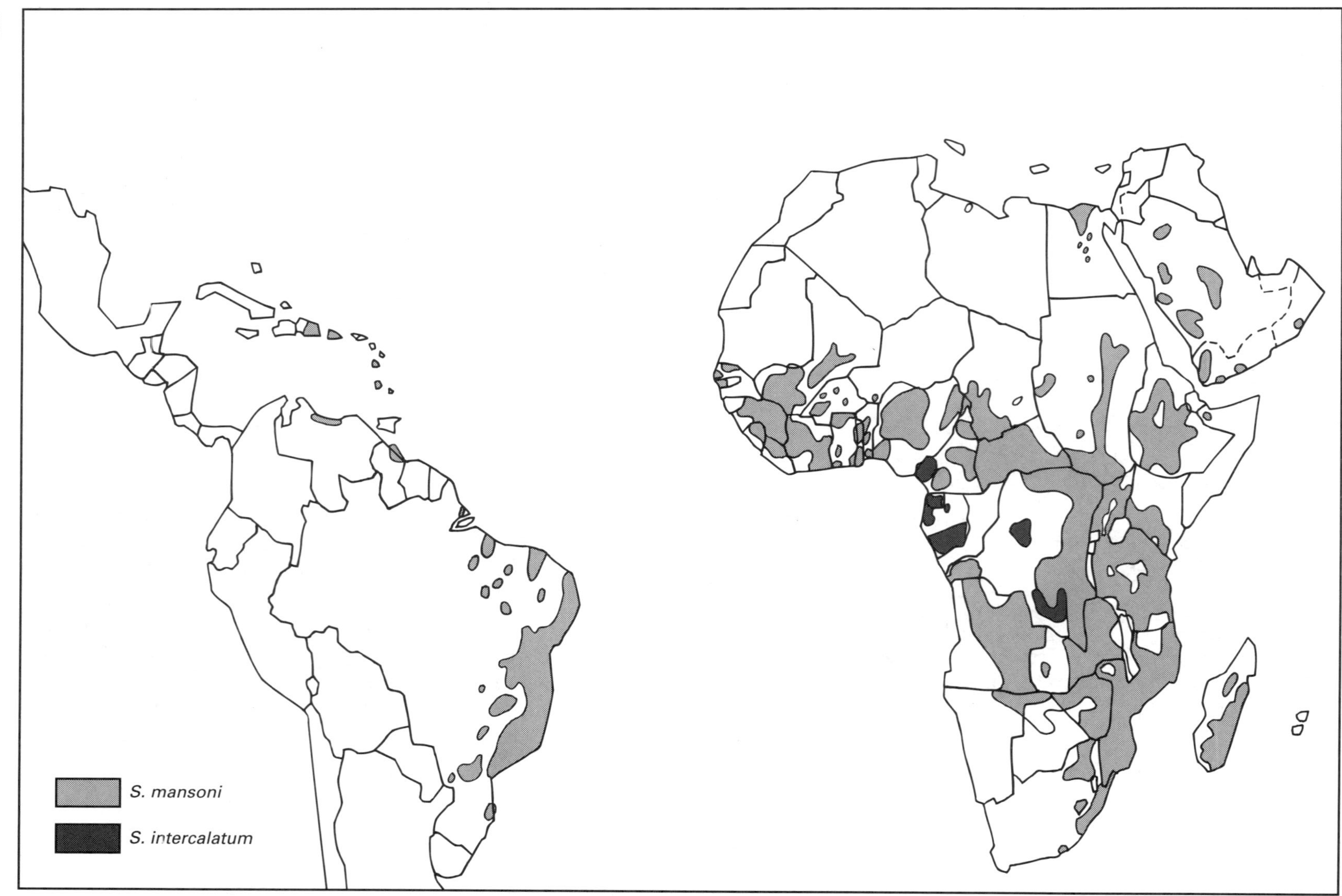

Figure 18.13B The distribution of schistosomiasis (*Schistosoma mansoni* and *S. intercalatum*).
(Source: *The control of schistosomiasis: second report of the WHO Expert Committee*. Geneva, WHO, 1993 (*WHO Technical Report Series* No. 830).

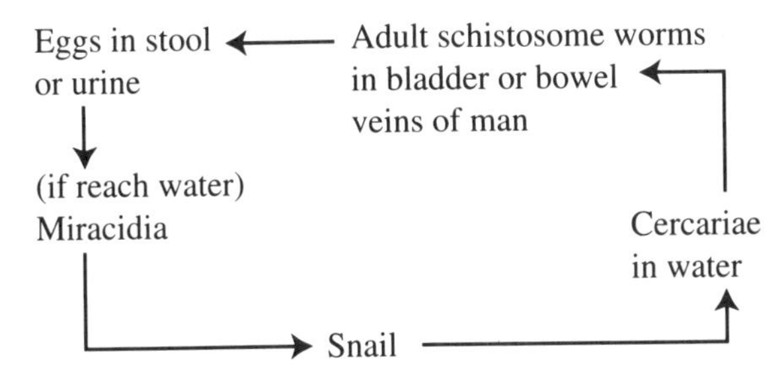

Figure 18.14 Diagram to show the life cycle of schistosomes.

bladder wall to be thick and ulcerated, and at times to bleed. Ulcers of the bladder wall cause blood in the urine. Usually the patient notices the blood in the urine when he has nearly finished passing urine. The patient also notices more blood after exercise. If there is a lot of blood in the urine, clots may form and there may be much pain (especially in boys). If there are not many worms the patient may slowly improve and have blood in the urine only sometimes. He may even get better. However if there are many worms and especially if the patient gets new infections, then other problems develop. The bladder cannot stretch and the patient has to pass urine often (urinary frequency). Bacterial urinary tract infection may develop (see Chapter 26 page 353). After years the ureters may become narrowed and cause chronic kidney failure (see Chapter 26 page 359). The urethra may become blocked and cause urinary retention (see Chapter 26 page 362). Cancer may grow in the damaged bladder. The female pelvic organs and the bowel can also be damaged. Ectopic pregnancy and infertility due to fallopian tube damage; ulcers and cancers of the cervix, vagina and vulva; and increased likelihood to get HIV infection if exposed to HIV all occur in infected women.

5. Intestinal schistosomiasis is caused by *S. mansoni* or *S. japonicum* laying eggs in the veins of the wall of the intestine. Inflammation in these areas causes the bowel wall to be thick and ulcerated and at times to bleed. This can cause abdominal pain, diarrhoea and dysentery (blood and pus in the faeces). If there are not many worms and no new infections there may be no symptoms or the symptoms caused may go away. If there are many worms or if there are new infections, the symptoms may be severe. Infected lumps on the inside of the bowel may prolapse (come out) through the anus.
6. Complications can develop if the eggs are carried in the blood to the liver, lungs or nervous system.

(a) The eggs can damage the blood vessels in the liver and cause portal hypertension (see Chapter 24 page 309). The liver becomes large at first; but later small. The spleen becomes very large. The patient can become anaemic. Fluid can collect in the abdomen (ascites) and in the legs and back (oedema). The patient can vomit so much blood that he becomes shocked and dies.
(b) The eggs damage the lung. The right side of the heart cannot pump the blood through the lungs and heart failure develops (see Chapter 27 page 373).
(c) The eggs can damage the brain or spinal cord. The patient can develop paralysis or epilepsy or blindness or coma, etc. (see Chapter 25). This is more frequent in *S. japonicum* infections.

It is usually only these patients who have many schistosome worms in their body and repeated infections as the original worms die, who develop significant symptoms and signs of disease. Even those with marked disease may however greatly improve with treatment, as many of the symptoms are due to the acute inflammation around new eggs that are laid, and if no new eggs are laid and the inflammation slowly goes away, the patient will improve.

Tests

1. Eggs may be seen through the microscope when the urine or stool is examined. The last part of the urine passed is the best to examine. A concentration method and repeat examinations may be needed for the stool.
2. If laboratory tests are not available at the health centre, add boiled then cooled water to a sample of urine or a sample of stool in a test-tube or bottle. Allow the urine to stand for 1 hour or the stool to stand for 1 night then examine the tube through a magnifying glass against a dark background. Miracidia may be seen swimming in the tube if eggs are present.

Differential diagnosis

1. Fever.
   See Chapter 36 page 482.
2. Blood in the urine.
   In an area where schistosomiasis is common, almost all cases of blood in the urine are due to schistosomiasis.
   If there are
   - no eggs (or miracidia) in the urine, or
   - other urinary symptoms present, or
   - symptoms present in other systems,

then transfer the patient to a Medical Officer for diagnosis of other causes and treatment. See also Chapter 26.

3. Diarrhoea/dysentery
   Bacillary and amoebic infections and cancer of the intestine also cause dysentery or large intestinal symptoms and signs.
   If eggs or miracidia are not present in the stool and if the dysentery continues or keeps on coming back and does not improve after treatment with metronidazole, and if available, an anti-schistosome drug, then refer or transfer the patient to a Medical Officer for diagnosis of other causes and treatment. See also Chapter 23 page 300.

Treatment

Do not spend a lot of time and money treating patients with mild infection and few symptoms of schistosomiasis if they are likely to become infected again soon. Give health education to these patients on how not to get more infections.

Also, many of the old drugs to treat schistosomiasis have serious side effects, which are more common if the patient has liver disease. Newer drugs are now available which are safer and easier to use but are expensive.

Also the best drug for your area depends on which type of schistosome worm is the most common in your area.

Praziquantel is effective against all schistosomes. The dose is 40 mg/kg once but for *S. japonicum* two doses of 30 mg/kg are needed – the second one 4–6 hours after the first, and given preferably after food in the evening. Tablets contain 600 mg, 500 mg, 200 mg or 150 mg. Side effects are mild – gastrointestinal upsets, dizziness, fever, skin rash. However, as mentioned, the drug is expensive. Not all worms may be killed with one dose.

Metriphonate 7.5–10 mg/kg body weight, given in three doses at intervals of 14 days, is effective treatment for *S. haematobium* only. It has very few side effects and is relatively cheap; but has the disadvantage of many people not taking the second and/or third doses.

Oxamniquine is given in doses that have to vary with the resistance of the schistosome worms in different areas. The doses vary from 15 mg/kg body weight as a single oral dose for adults and 10 mg/kg body weight for children with a second dose 4–6 hours later, up to 20 mg/ kg body weight for 3 days in a row. Oxamniquine has few side effects apart from occasional fitting and gastrointestinal symptoms but is effective against only *S. japonicum*.

You must therefore find out the Health Department policy for:

- which patients you should treat,
- which drugs you should use,
- the doses, side effects and precautions you should take for these drugs.

Refer patients who have urinary problems or rectal problems or gynaecological problems, which are not helped by the drugs, to the next visiting Medical Officer. Surgery may help some of these patients.

Control and prevention

You can use most of the normal methods of control and prevention. However experts need to study each area to find out which method is best. So again you must find out the Health Department policy for your area.

1. Kill the parasite in the bodies of the original host or reservoir.
   Patients with symptoms are treated. It is possible, after health education about methods of control of schistosomes, that the whole population will agree to co-operate in the programme. Only then can the community and health workers work out effective methods to distribute the drug (usually praziquantel) to all the population in the area.
2. Stop the means of spread of the parasite.
   (a) All people (including children) must use a toilet at all times. Proper toilets are needed for all people.
   (b) Control or eradicate the vector (the snail).
   Niclosamide poisoning is the main method used. There are many ways of doing this. Specialists will advise what way is best for your area.
   (c) Stop contact with water that has cercariae in it. Safe drinking water should be supplied. If water is left to stand in pots for 2–3 days before drinking, cercariae will die. No one should swim or wash in infected water.
   Houses would be best built away from water and safe water piped to the houses. Ideally safe swimming water should be supplied for children. People should not work in infected water – this is almost impossible for many farmers.
3. Raise the resistance of the people.
   Immunisation is not yet possible but vaccines are at present being developed.
4. Prophylactic treatment.
   This is used only in special circumstances.

19

Sexually Transmitted Diseases including HIV Infection

Anatomy

See Figures 19.1 and 19.2.

Pathology

Sexually Transmitted Diseases (STD) (also called venereal diseases (VD)) are *usually* spread by sexual intercourse. Sometimes they are spread by non-sexual means.

Sexually transmitted diseases, except HIV infection, *usually* show themselves in one of the following six ways:

1. Urethral discharge or pain.
2. Vaginal discharge or pain.
3. Sores or lumps or pain in the mucous membrane or skin of the genitalia.
4. Swelling of the inguinal lymph nodes near the genitalia (called a bubo) with or without a genital ulcer.
5. Scrotal swelling of sudden onset.
6. Lower abdominal pain in women.

Urethral discharge or pain in male

Urethral discharge which is caused by a sexually transmitted disease is usually caused by either:

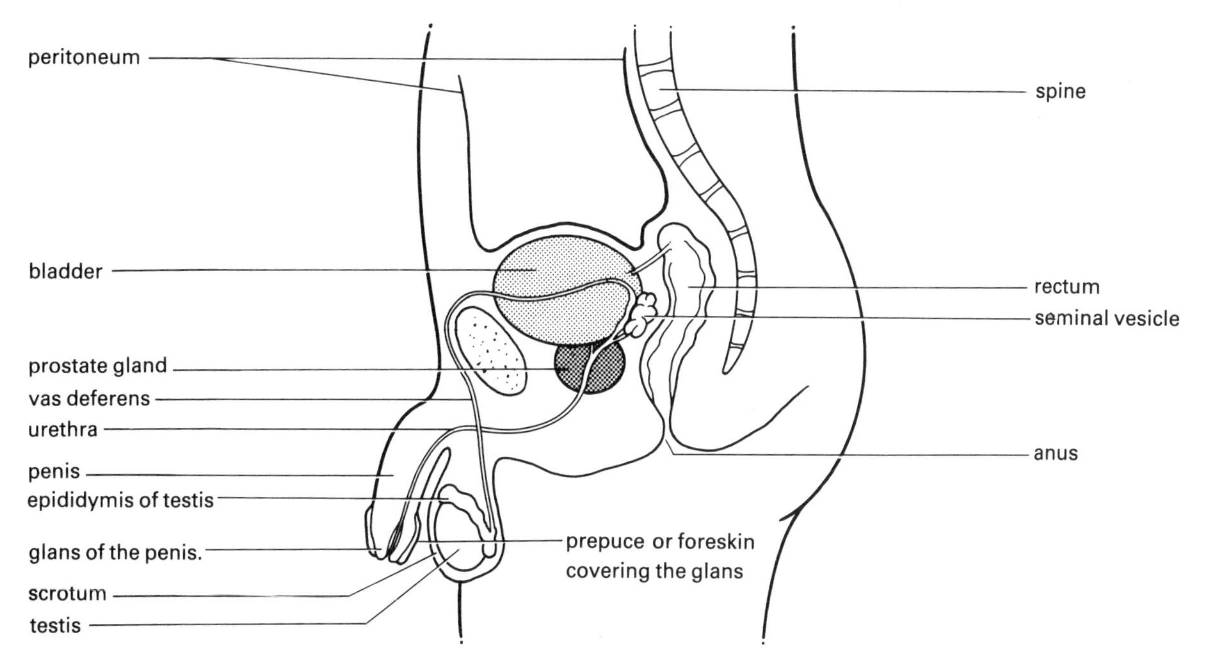

Figure 19.1 Diagram of the male reproductive system.

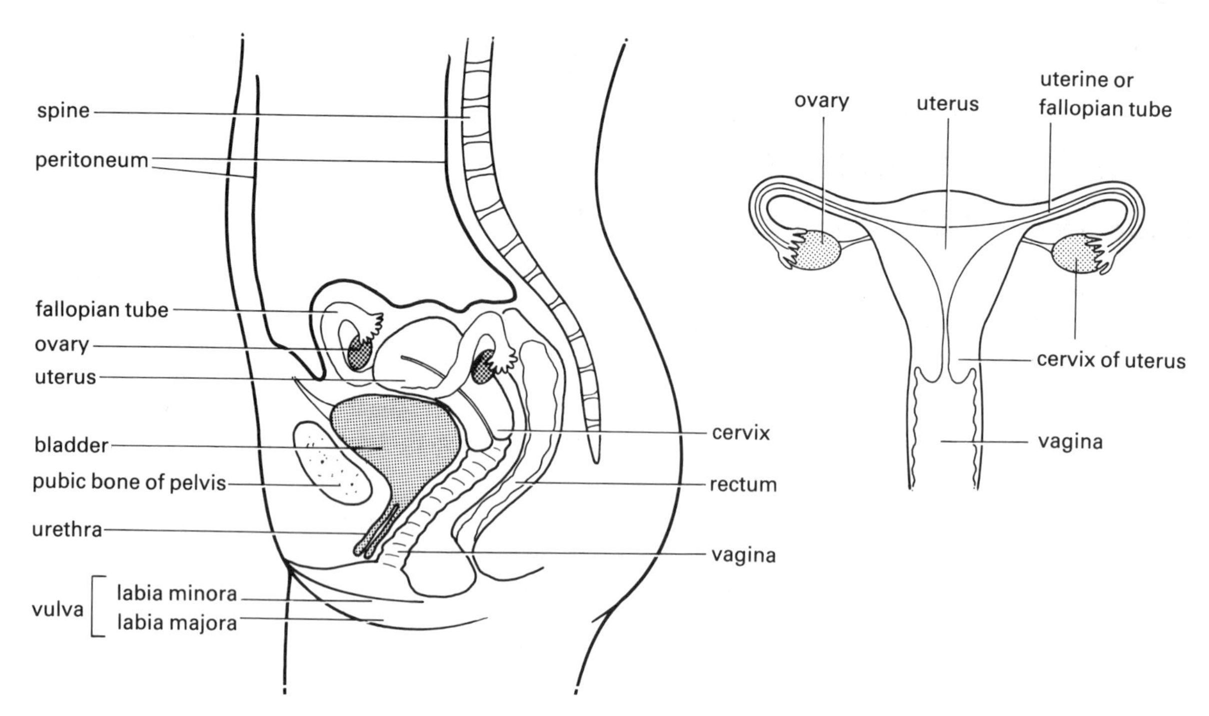

Figure 19.2 Diagram of the female reproductive system.

1. *Neisseria gonorrhoeae* also called the 'Gonooccus' which causes gonorrhoea, or
2. *Chlamydia trachomatis* infection.

However in up to 30% of patients there is more than one infection present. Treat for both.

Vaginal discharge or pain

Vaginal discharge due to STDs is abnormal in colour, smell or amount. The patient may also have itchiness or swelling of the vagina or vulva, pain on passing urine or lower abdominal or back pain.

STD causes of vaginal discharge

1. gonorrhoea causing cervicitis or urethritis;
2. *Chlamydia trachomatis* infection causing cervicitis;
3. *Trichomonas vaginalis* infection;
4. *Candida* (*Monilia* or thrush) infection;
5. bacterial vaginosis when the normal organisms of the vagina are replaced with other bacterial organisms (especially *Gardnerella vaginalis* and anaerobes);
6. conditions which cause sores or lumps in the vagina including syphilis, herpes genitalis, condyloma accuminata, etc. (see below).

Always treat gonorrhoea and chlamydia.

Non-STD causes of vaginal discharge include neoplasms and polyps, etc.

Non-pathological or normal vaginal discharge must not be considered abnormal and can occur at the times of ovulation or just before menstrual periods, when oral contraceptives are taken and after the insertion of an intra-uterine contraceptive device (IUD).

Genital sores or lumps or pain

Sores or lumps or pain in the mucous membrane or skin of the genitalia or in the skin near the genitalia are usually caused by:

1. syphilis (usually single painless ulcer),
2. chancroid (also called 'soft sore') (usually many tender ulcers).

Other causes could be:

3. granuloma inguinale (also called granuloma venereum or Donovanosis) (at first a single painless lesion like cut meat),
4. lymphogranuloma venereum (also called lymphogranuloma inguinale) (often no genital ulcer but only inflamed inguinal nodes),
5. herpes genitalis (usually many painful small ulcers),
6. condylomata accuminata (also called venereal warts) (wart like lesions),
7. amoebic ulcer (not always sexually transmitted),
8. pubic lice (not always sexually transmitted), and
9. scabies (not always sexually transmitted).

However many cases are not typical; and definite diagnosis by examination without special tests is not possible.

In view of this, therefore, *the two common important causes, syphilis and chancroid, are always treated first*; and then if the patient is not cured, the diagnosis of others considered later.

Swelling in the inguinal lymph nodes near the genitalia (inguinal bubo)

If there is also an ulcer of the genitalia, then the causes are usually the same two important ones:

1. syphilis,
2. chancroid,

and other causes are also as listed above.

If there is swelling of the inguinal lymph nodes near the genitalia without a genital ulcer, the most important cause is:

- lymphogranuloma venereum.

In both of the above situations, many cases are not typical and the definite diagnosis by examination is not possible. Always treat the most important causes as above. If the patient does not improve, then consider the possibility that other causes are present and then treat these causes.

Scrotal swelling of sudden onset

Scrotal swelling caused by an STD is usually due to inflammation of the epididymis and is of sudden onset and painful. There is also urethritis, or it has been present recently. The common causes are:

1. gonorrhoea,
2. *Chlamydia trachomatis.*

Other non-STD causes include:

1. acute torsion of the testis (twisting of the testis on its cord which blocks the blood vessels and needs urgent surgery or the testis will die);
2. trauma;
3. mumps;
4. urinary tract infection especially in older men with partial block of the urethra by the prostate;
5. tuberculosis;
6. tumours of the testis.

Lower abdominal pain in women due to 'pelvic inflammatory disease' (PID) i.e. inflammation of the uterus and/or fallopian tubes and/or ovaries and/or pelvic peritonitis.

The STD causes of PID are usually:

1. gonorrhoea,
2. *Chlamydia trachomatis.*

Always treat these two.

Pelvic infections not due to STDs can be due to:

1. postpartum or postabortion infections;
2. intra-uterine contraceptive devices – especially in the first month after insertion;
3. bowel infections such as appendicitis.

If pelvic inflammatory disease is not treated quickly, these infections can cause:

1. pelvic pain,
2. ectopic pregnancy,
3. infertility.

Non-sexually transmitted conditions often affect the genitalia. These include:

- traumatic sores,
- balanitis,
- cancer,
- amoebic ulcer,
- pubic lice,
- scabies, and
- many of the other skin conditions which can affect any part of the body.

History, examination and tests

When you see a patient with either a genital sore or lump or an urethral or vaginal discharge or other condition, which may be sexually transmitted, you should take a full history, do a full physical examination and do the necessary tests.

Remember:

1. One STD makes it more likely for the patient already to have other STDs and HIV infection.
2. STDs with ulcers or discharge make it more easy for the patient in future to be infected with HIV.

Details about the main STDs follow later in this chapter.

History (See Chapter 6 page 17)

In the history ask the patient who all the people are that he or she has had sexual intercourse with in the last few months. Also ask how long before the patient's complaints started it was that they had sexual intercourse with each of these persons.

Ask the date of the last normal menstrual period and about previous pregnancies and miscarriages. Ask about previous attacks of STD and hepatitis and if the patient has infection with HIV.

Physical examination (See Chapter 6 page 19)

Special things to note in the examination include:

All patients:

Wear disposable plastic gloves (which you throw away after seeing each patient) or reusable gloves (which you have sterilised before you use them again) to protect yourself.

Always ask yourself if there are any things to suggest HIV infection. (See Chapter 19 page 180.)

Male patients:

Look at the pubic hair for lice.

Examine the groin areas – for ulcers or lymph gland enlargement.

Look at the penis for sores or ulcers. Feel if a sore is hard or soft and if it is tender. If the patient is not circumcised, pull back the foreskin so that you can examine the glans too.

Squeeze the urethra gently to see if any discharge comes out of the urethra. If a laboratory is available, take a smear of any discharge.

Look at the scrotum for sores or ulcers. Gently feel the epididymides and testes for swelling, lumps or tenderness.

Put the patient onto his side and ask him to lift his knees so that you can look at the perianal region for sores or discharge. Do a pelvic examination through the rectum (PR). (See Chapter 26 page 351.)

Female patients:

If you are a male, ask a female assistant to be present.

Look at the pubic hair for lice.

Examine the groin areas for ulcers or lymph gland enlargement.

Examine the abdomen.

Examine the perineum and genitalia. Cover the abdomen down to the knees with a sheet. Ask the patient to lie on her back and bend her knees until the heels touch the buttocks. Ask the patient to let her knees go apart. You then have a good view of the external genitalia.

Examine the vulva for any sores, ulcers, swelling or discharge.

Examine the perianal region.

Examine the internal surface of the labia after gently separating them.

Feel if any sores are soft or hard and if they are tender.

Use a speculum to examine the vagina and cervix. If there is vaginal discharge use a swab on forceps to clean the cervix and then see if there is inflammation of the cervix or if pus is coming through the cervix.

If a laboratory is available, take a smear from the urethra and from inside the cervix.

Do a pelvic examination through the vagina (PV). (See Chapter 26 page 351.)

Tests

1. Take 10 ml of blood and send the serum to the laboratory with a request for the serological test for syphilis (VDRL or RPR; and if positive TPHA or FTA-Abs, which are more accurate, may be needed).
2. Make slides from swabs from the urethra and (in the female) inside the cervical canal for Gram stain and culture or put into a suitable culture material (e.g. Stuart's transport medium) to be sent to the laboratory for culture.
3. Test the urine (see Chapter 26 page 351).
4. Take blood for testing for HIV infection but only if the test is available and if pre-test counselling and consent is possible and where time and facilities for counselling and treatment would be available if the test were positive.

Control and prevention

If after the history and examination and tests you think that the patient has a disease which may have been sexually transmitted, then you should:

1. Start control and prevention of the spread of the disease which will almost always include treating the patient's contact – preferably at the same time as the patient, or soon after, and certainly before the contact has sexual intercourse again.

2. Treat the patient.

Kill the organism in the body of the original host or reservoir

All patients and all 'contacts' need to be found, investigated if possible and treated.

'Contacts' include the person who gave the patient the disease and anyone else the patient may have given the disease to, i.e. all persons the patient has had intercourse with before and after the symptoms started, as well as the patient's husband/wife. This may at times include people of the patient's same gender or sex. Many of these 'contacts' will have no symptoms but still have infection and be likely to spread the infection to the patient again and to other people, and may themselves develop complications.

Give health education to encourage all people who have the disease to come for treatment.

Health education should include:

1. how the diseases are spread;
2. the symptoms and signs of the diseases;
3. the serious results if no treatment is given, or if the person gets HIV infection; and
4. that the treatment is safe, and (except for HIV infection) effective, and free;
5. how not to get another infection, especially HIV infection (see page 194), and how to use condoms and have safe sex;
6. supply of condoms.

If you do not have enough money and staff to find contacts and offer them investigation and treatment, then you need to explain to the patient that he or she should:

1. bring contacts to you for treatment; or
2. give a 'contact card' (on which you write what treatment is needed and then give this to the patient) to each contact, so that the contact can bring the card to the health centre and he or she will immediately get correct treatment when this card is seen by the health worker;
3. at the very least, tell the contact that they may have the sexually transmitted disease and that they should come to the health centre to see you for treatment;
4. tell the contact not to have sexual intercourse until he or she has been treated.

If you have enough staff to do contact tracing, ask the patient for the names and addresses of ALL contacts as soon as STD is diagnosed. Write the names in the STD register.

Stop the means of spread

Give health education so that people know that:

1. The means of spread is intercourse (with an infected person).
2. The only real safe sexual practice for an uninfected person is to have sexual intercourse with only one other uninfected 'faithful' (that is, one who does not have sexual intercourse with any one else) partner. There is no way to tell from a person's appearance if they are infected or not. This can be done only by knowing the person and talking to them about it.

   A person who has many sexual partners is at high risk of an STD. A person who has sexual intercourse with just one person but that person has had many sexual partners is at high risk of an STD. To reduce the risk of STD, people need to reduce the number of their sexual partners, although there will always be a risk until sexual intercourse occurs only with one uninfected faithful partner.
3. If a person has sexual relations with more than one person or with a possibly infected person, some things will reduce the risk of getting STDs.

   (a) Change sexual activities from high risk to low risk activities. High risk activities are when semen or vaginal fluid comes into contact with the partner's oral (mouth), genital or anal (rectal) mucosa. Low risk practices are when these fluids come into contact only with skin which is not damaged (as unbroken skin is not able to be entered by most infections). This means that a low risk practice is when a man's penis does not enter the partner's vagina, anus or mouth.

   (b) Use of a condom will greatly reduce the risk of infected semen or vaginal fluid getting into the other person. It is important that people not only know this, but are shown how to use condoms properly and do have condoms available, and do actually use condoms each and every time they have sexual intercourse.

   (c) Washing with soap and water after removing the condom will reduce the chance of infection.

It is most important that patients with STDs are given the above information.

Health education about the above to groups at particular risk of STDs should be carried out whenever possible. These would include:

- prostitutes,
- people who visit prostitutes,
- STD patients,
- those who are away from their community and family, e.g. migrant workers, truck driver, sailors, etc.

Health education of special groups should be carried out whenever possible. These would include:

- school children,
- young people,
- groups of men,
- groups of women,
- those who can be reached by the mass media (radio, TV, newspapers).

If possible, some kind of measurement of the effects of these methods of health education should be carried out so that most effort can be put into those that are most effective.

Raise the resistance of susceptible people

Immunisation is not yet possible.

Prophylactic treatment

Give prophylactic treatment with the proper treatment dose for the disease to a person who has had sexual intercourse with a person who is known to have a sexually transmissible disease, even if they do not have symptoms and signs of the disease.

Summary of management of a patient with an STD

What you should and can do for patients with suspected STDs will depend on what part of the world you are in, what infections are common in your area, what antibiotics kill the organisms which cause STDs in your area, etc. It will also depend on what things you have available to examine a patient (e.g. vaginal speculum or not), and if you have a good laboratory service (e.g. to do smears for gonococci, serological tests for syphilis, examinations for Donovan bodies, etc.). It will also depend on what antibiotics are available for you to treat the patients.

In view of these things, your Health Department will probably have drawn up a number of policies and probably flow charts for your area, to tell you what you are to do. You must follow the advice of your Health Department.

If such policies and flow charts are not available, the WHO flow charts (Figure 19.3) should tell you what you should do if you choose the one which applies to your patient and the facilities you have. These flow charts and more details about STDs and their treatment are found in *WHO Model Prescribing Information: Drugs used in Sexually Transmitted Diseases and HIV Infection*, 1995, Geneva, WHO and *WHO Technical Report Series No. 810, Management of Patients with Sexually Transmitted Diseases*, 1991, Geneva, WHO.

Drug treatment of the patient and contacts (see box on page 96 first)

Urethral discharge

Urethral discharge is assumed to be due to *gonorrhoea* and *Chlamydia* if no tests are possible – *treat for both.*

Urethral discharge is assumed to be due to gonorrhoea and *Chlamydia* if smears from urethral discharge showed gonorrhoea (as there is no simple test for *Chlamydia*) – treat for both.

Urethral discharge is assumed to be due to *Chlamydia* if urethral discharge showed no gonococci – treat for *Chlamydia*.

Gonorrhoea

1. Give one of the following:
   - ciprofloxacin 500 mg by mouth once on an empty stomach *or*
   - ceftriaxone 250 mg by IMI once *or*
   - spectinomycin 2 g by IMI once
2. Only if the above are not available give:
   - sulphamethoxazole 4000 mg/trimethoprim 800 mg (co-trimoxazole) (10 single strength tablets or 5 double strength tablets) immediately and daily for 2 days more if available.
3. If the above are not available see Gonorrhoea page 169 for other possible treatments.

(a) Genital ulcers (laboratory support not available).

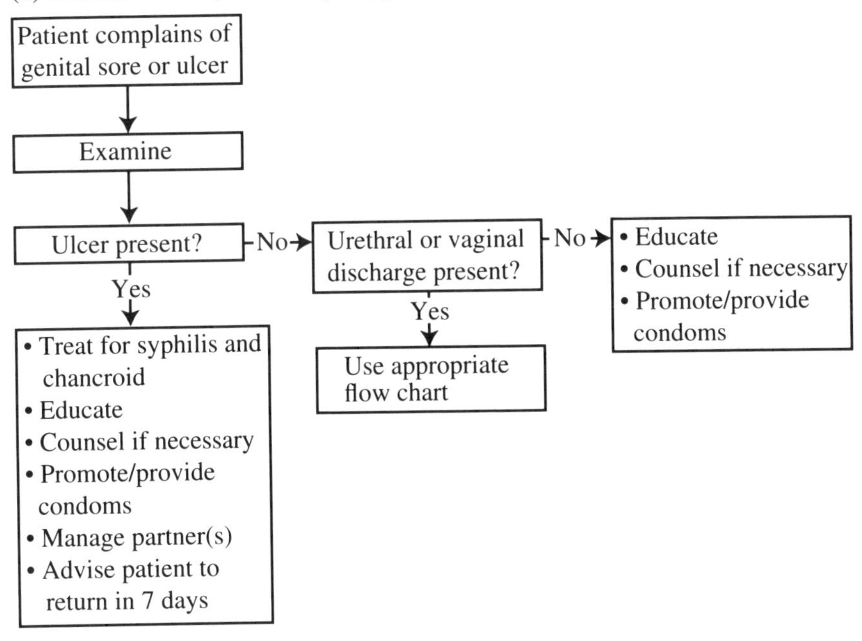

(b) Urethral discharge (laboratory support not available).

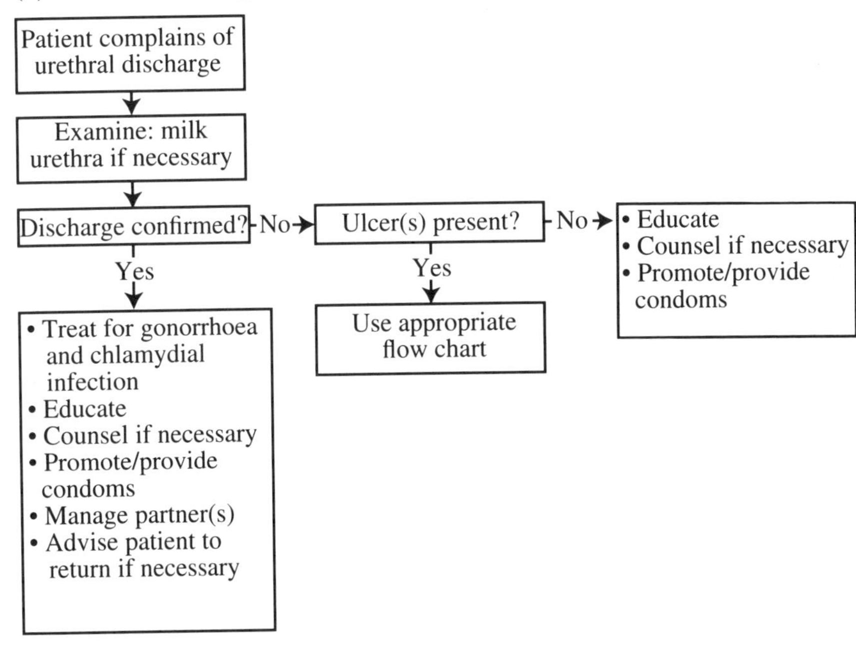

Figure 19.3 WHO flow charts for STD management.

(c) **Urethral discharge (microscope available).**

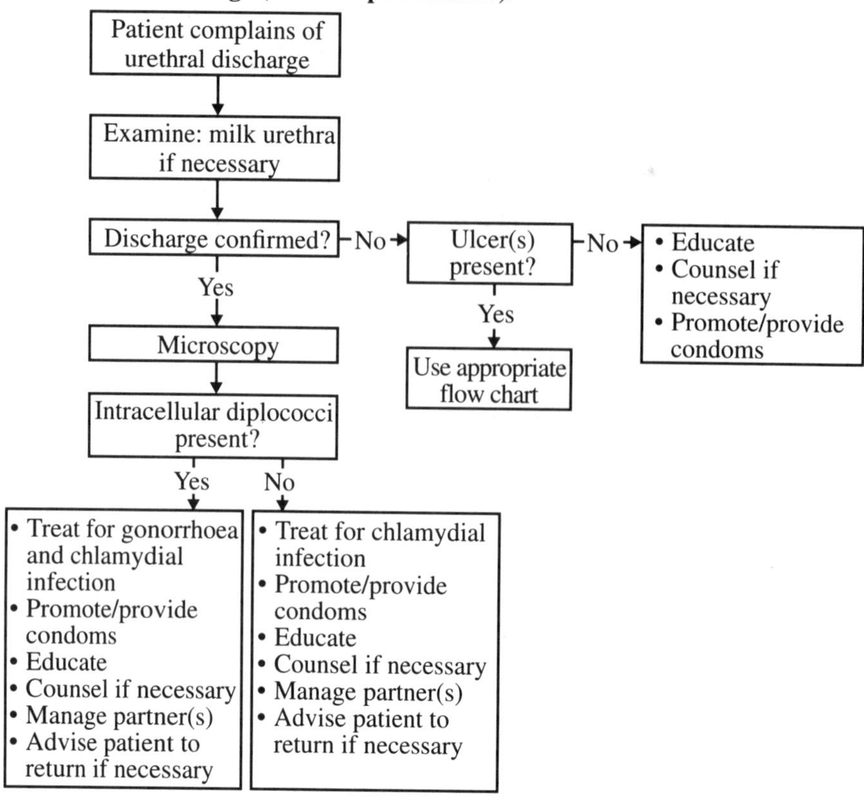

(d) **Vaginal discharge (vaginal examination and laboratory tests not possible).**

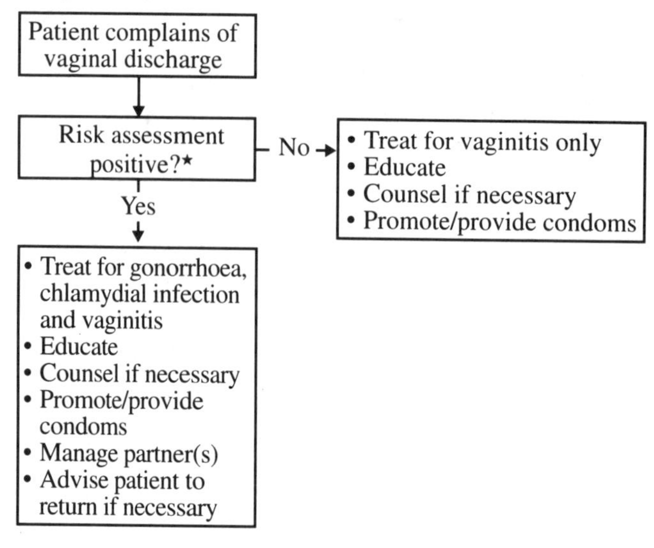

* The risk assessment is positive if the patient's partner is symptomatic or if any two of the following apply to the patient: age < 21 years; single; > 1 partner; new partner in the past 3 months.

Figure 19.3 (continued)

(e) Vaginal discharge (speculum available).

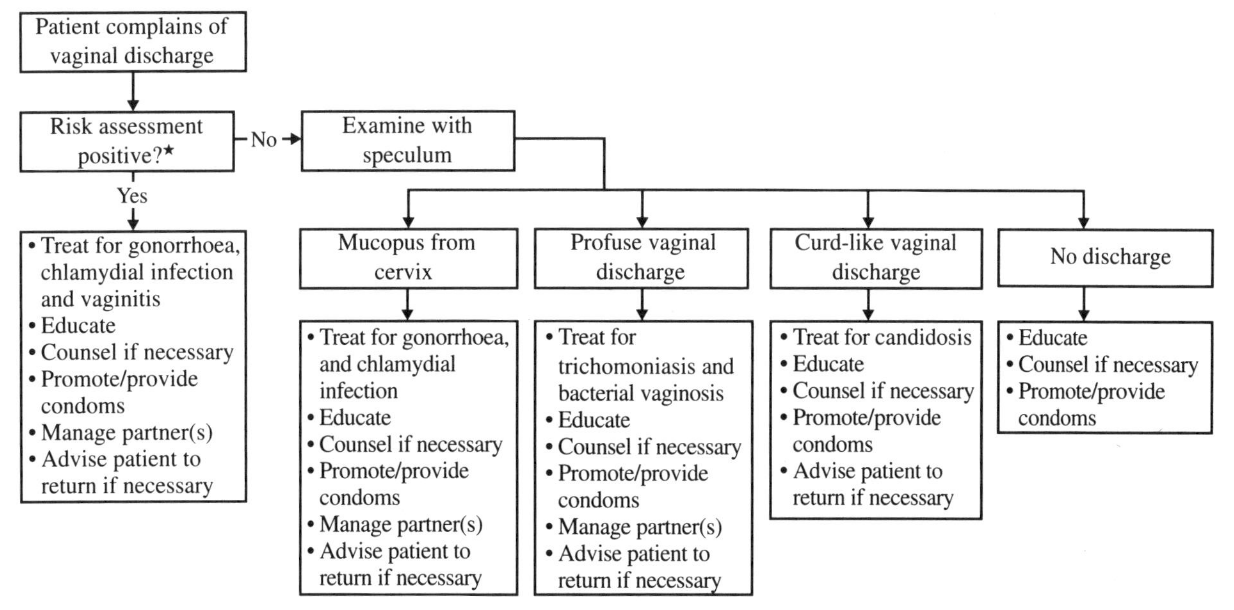

★ The risk assessment is positive if the patient's partner is symptomatic or if any two of the following apply to the patient: age < 21 years; single; > 1 partner; new partner in the past 3 months.

(f) Vaginal discharge (speculum and microscope available).

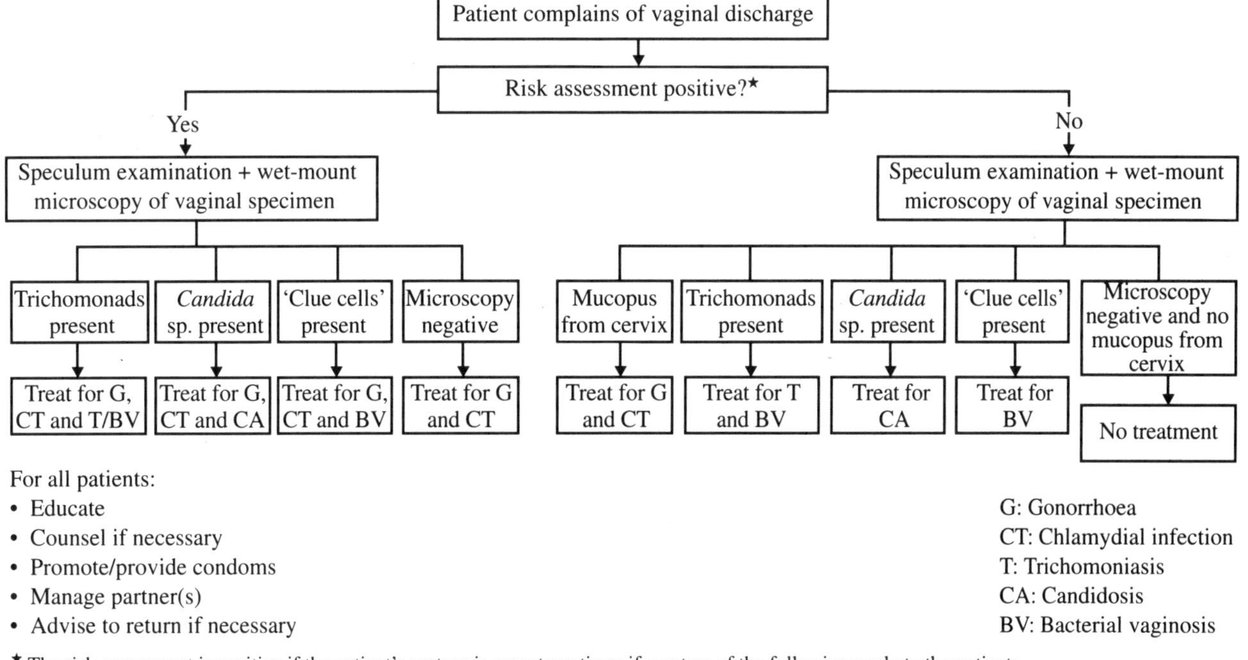

For all patients:

- Educate
- Counsel if necessary
- Promote/provide condoms
- Manage partner(s)
- Advise to return if necessary

G: Gonorrhoea
CT: Chlamydial infection
T: Trichomoniasis
CA: Candidosis
BV: Bacterial vaginosis

★ The risk assessment is positive if the patient's partner is symptomatic or if any two of the following apply to the patient: age < 21 years; single; > 1 partner; new partner in the past 3 months

Figure 19.3 (continued)

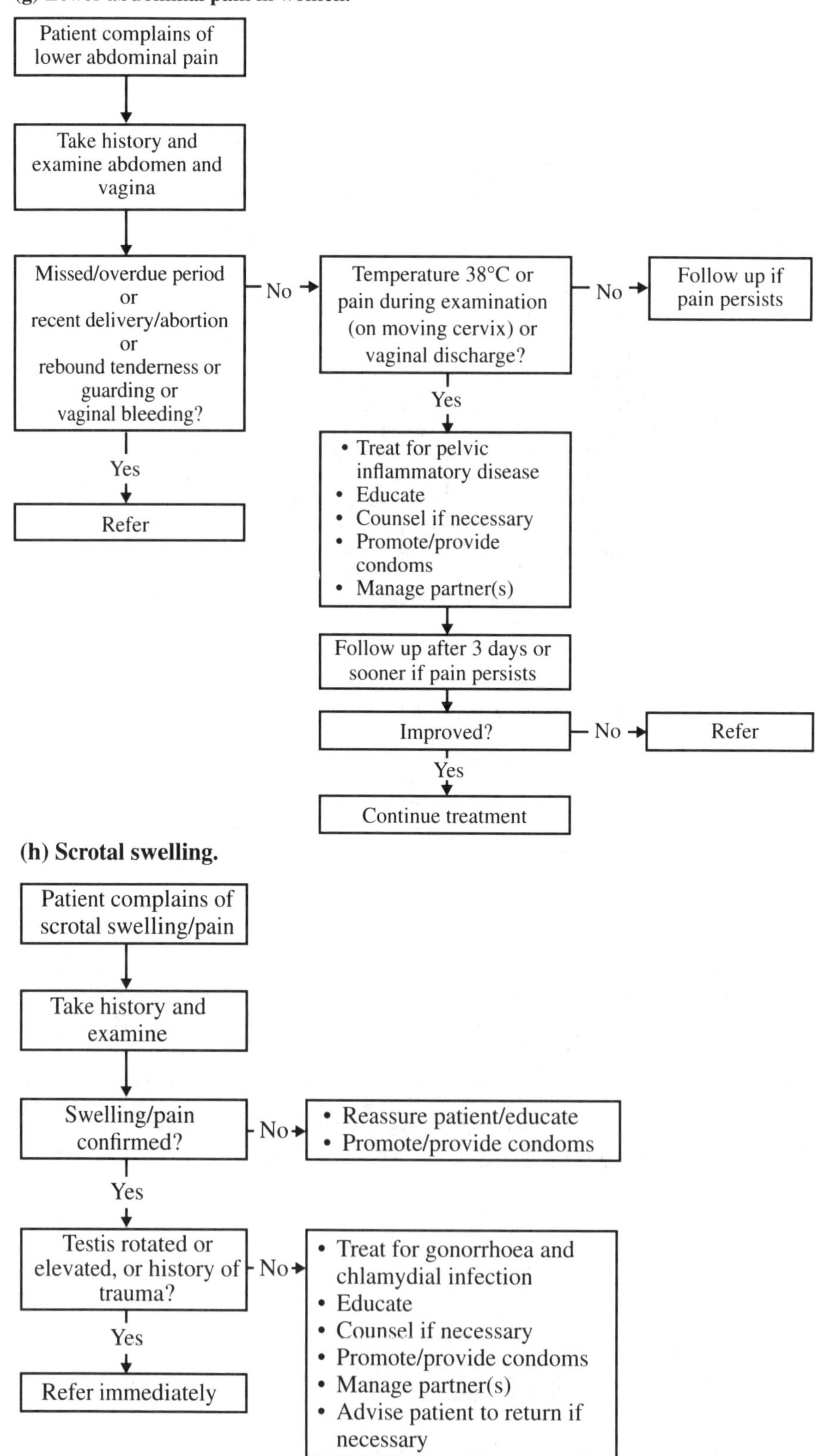

Figure 19.3 (continued)

(i) Inguinal bubo.

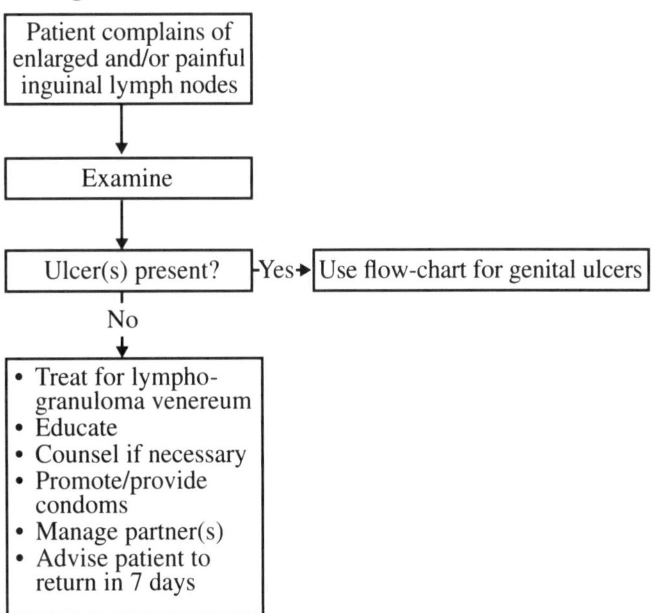

Figure 19.3 (continued)

Chlamydia trachomatis

1. Doxycycline 100 mg twice daily for 7–10 days but not if pregnant *or*
2. Tetracycline 500 mg four times a day for 7–10 days but not if pregnant *or*
3. Erythromycin 500 mg four times a day for 7–10 days if pregnant.

Genital ulcer (see box on page 196 first)

Genital ulcer is assumed to be due to *syphilis* or *chancroid* when first seen and treatment for *both* these given first. Treatment for other conditions may be added if they are thought more likely or if the treatment for syphilis and chancroid is not effective.

Syphilis

1. Benzathine penicillin 2.4 million units (1.2 million units each buttock) immediately once *or*
2. Procaine penicillin 1.2 million units IMI for 10 days (not recommended)

   or if allergic to penicillin:
   - doxycycline 100 mg twice daily for 15 days but not if pregnant *or*
   - tetracycline 500 mg four times a day for 15 days but not if pregnant *or*
   - erythromycin 500 mg four times a day for 15 days if pregnant.

Chancroid

1. Erythromycin 500 mg three times a day for 7 days *or*
2. Trimethoprim 160 mg/sulphamethoxazole 800 mg (co-trimoxazole) twice daily for 7 days.

Lymphogranuloma venereum

1. Doxycycline 100 mg twice daily for 14 days but not if pregnant *or*
2. Tetracycline 500 mg four times a day for 14 days but not if pregnant *or*
3. Erythromycin 500 mg daily for 14 days if pregnant.

Vaginal discharge due to cervicitis alone

Assumed to be due to gonorrhoea and *Chlamydia trachomatis* infections.

1. Gonorrhoea treatment (see above)
   and
2. *Chlamydia* treatment (see above)

Vaginal discharge and vaginitis as well as cervicitis or if examination not possible

Treat for all the usual causes:

1. Gonorrhoea treatment (see above)
   and

2. *Chlamydia* treatment (see above)
   and
3. Trichomonas vaginalis treatment:
   - metronidazole 2 g orally immediately once *or*
   - metronidazole 400–500 mg orally twice daily for 7 days

   and
4. Bacterial vaginosis treatment:
   - metronidazole 2 g orally immediately once *or*
   - metronidazole 400–500 mg orally twice daily for 7 days

   and
5. Candida infection treatment:
   - nystatin 100,000 unit pessaries 1–2 daily for 7–14 days *or*
   - miconazole or clotrimazole 200 mg pessaries 1 daily for 3 days *or*
   - clotrimazole 500 mg pessary 1 only immediately

Pelvic inflammatory disease

1. Treat for gonorrhoea with a once only dose of ceftriaxone 250 mg by IMI or alternatives (see Gonorrhoea, page 160).
2. Treat for *Chlamydia trachomatis* infection (if not pregnant) with doxycycline 100 mg twice daily or for 10 days or see page 165.
3. Treat for other organisms with metronidazole 400–500 mg three times a day for 10–14 days.
4. Remove any intrauterine contraceptive device once antibiotics have started but other contraceptives must be provided after this.

> Remember to always treat the patient's contacts at the same time or as soon after as possible and before the patient has intercourse with them again.

Common sexually transmitted diseases

Gonorrhoea

Gonorrhoea is a bacterial infection which usually causes urethritis in men and urethritis and cervicitis in women, but can cause infections of the rectum or throat or eyes. It can also spread within the genital organs causing more severe infections of them and through the blood to other parts of the body, causing serious disease there or septicaemia.

Gonorrhoea is common.

The cause is the gonorrhoea bacterium (*Neisseria gonorrhoeae*)

The original host is an infected person. Some infected people have symptoms and signs; but some men and many women are carriers with no symptoms.

The means of spread is direct contact. In adults this is almost always by sexual intercourse. It can infect the eyes of a child if the mother's cervix or urethra is infected at the time of birth. It can infect the throat if infected genitalia are kissed.

Infection does not give any immunity.

Symptoms and signs, course and complications in the male

Symptoms and signs usually develop within a week; but they can take longer or never develop.

There is an urethral discharge (Figure 19.4). It is usually white or yellow (pus) and often a large amount. Dysuria and urinary frequency occur. The symptoms slowly improve over weeks or months, although a little white discharge may continue to be present each morning. But the infection does not go.

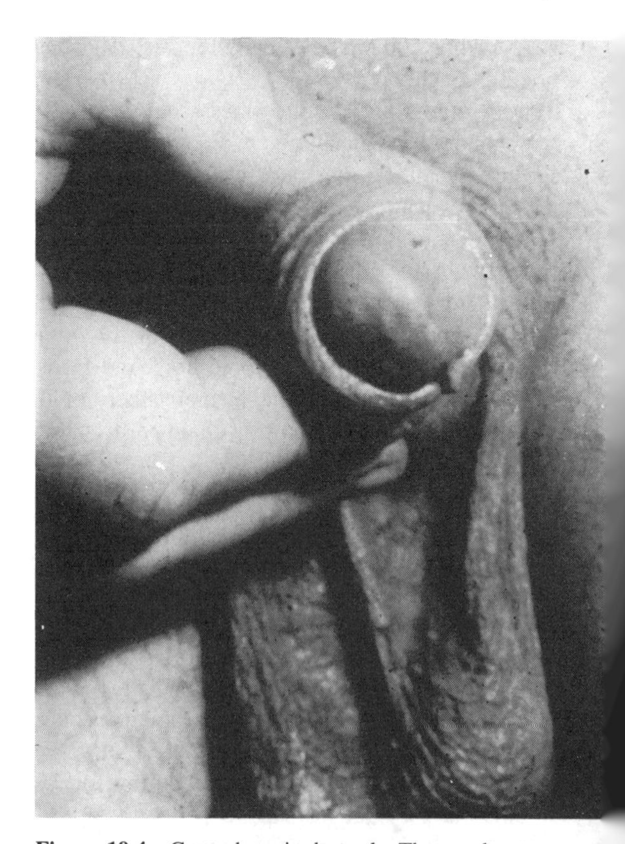

Figure 19.4 Gonorrhoea in the male. The usual symptom and sign of gonorrhoea – urethral discharge.

Complications include:

- abscess around urethra,
- inflammation of the epididymis and testis,
- sterility due to blocked epididymis and vas deferens,
- severe conjunctivitis and iritis (spread by fingers from the genitalia),
- bacteraemia with pustular skin rash,
- acute infective arthritis,
- septicaemia.

These complications usually occur soon after infection. Sterility will occur later. Urethral stricture (i.e. narrowing of the urethra due to scarring where there was previous infection around the urethra) causing difficulty in passing urine and distended bladder, occurs after many years.

Symptoms and signs, course and complications in the female

Symptoms and signs usually develop within a week; but they can take longer or never develop.

There is usually dysuria and urinary frequency and increase in vaginal discharge (Figure 19.5). This is often mistaken for an urinary tract infection. After treatment with sulphadimidine (which does not cure the infection), or after no treatment, the symptoms slowly improve over weeks or months. But the infection does not go.

Complications include:

- acute salpingitis,
- pelvic peritonitis,
- pelvic abscess,
- ectopic (tubal) pregnancies and/or sterility (due to blocked fallopian tubes),
- sterility (due to blocked fallopian tubes),
- severe acute conjunctivitis and iritis (spread by fingers),
- abscess in labia,
- bacteraemia with pustular skin rash,
- acute infective arthritis,
- septicaemia.

Tests

Smear some discharge from the urethra and (in the female) from inside the cervix (Figure 19.6), onto a glass slide, fix it by heat and send it to the hospital laboratory for examination for gonorrhoea bacteria. If available also collect a swab for culture, usually by putting it into a suitable transport medium such as Stuart's transport medium.

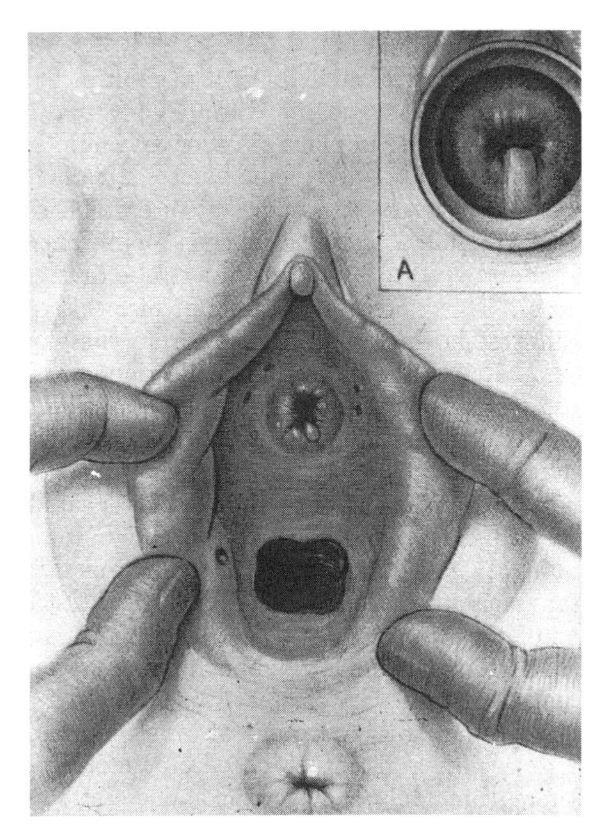

Figure 19.5 Gonorrhoea in the female. Urethral discharge may be seen. On speculum examination of the cervix, discharge may be seen (inset A). However, the patient will not complain of these. She may have symptoms of urinary tract infection or of a vaginal discharge.

Send also the serum from 10 ml of blood with a request for serological tests for syphilis (STS).

Diagnostic features

- Intercourse within previous week.
- Urinary pain and frequency.
- Urethral or vaginal discharge.

Differential diagnosis

Females:

1. Pelvic inflammatory disease after childbirth of miscarriage.
   - Recent childbirth or miscarriage.
   - Discharge yellow pus.
   - Pelvic tenderness and or masses.
   - Pus coming out of the cervix.
   - Pain when the cervix is moved during examination.
   - Possibly tenderness and guarding in lower abdomen.

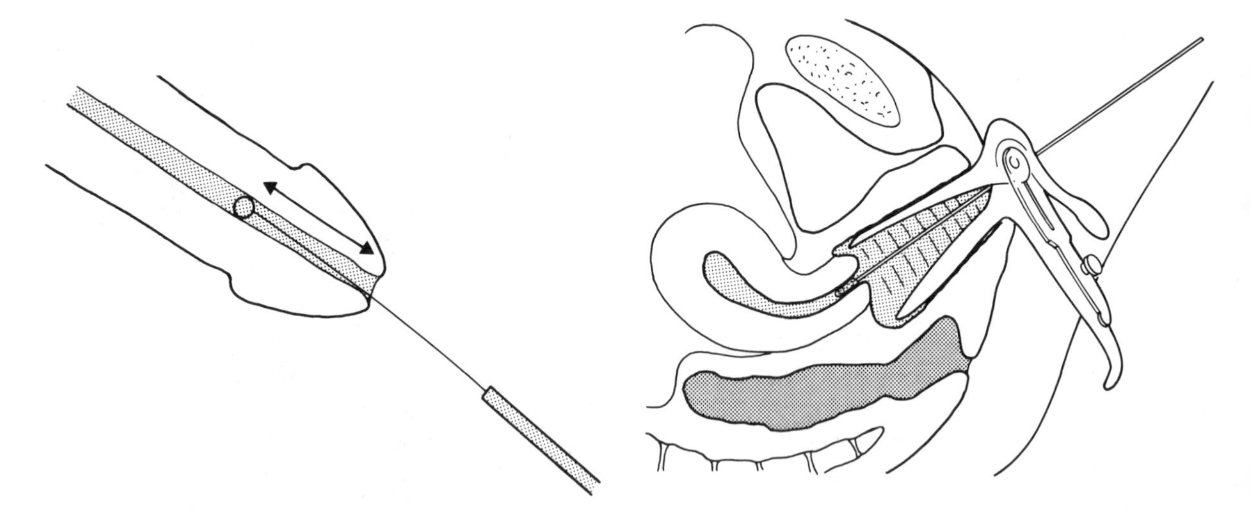

Figure 19.6 Methods of collecting specimens for examination in the laboratory for gonococci. Use a sterile swab to collect pus from the urethra. If there is not enough pus to be collected on a swab then use a 100L sterile bacteriological wire loop *but only if you have been trained how to use it.* Use a sterile swab to collect secretions from the inside of the cervix. If you have Stuart's transport medium, collect specimens and put them in the transport medium and send them to the laboratory for culture and sensitivity testing. However in a health centre all you can do yourself is to make a smear.

- Uterus enlarged and tender.
- General symptoms and signs of infection.

2. Trichomonal infection.
   - Vulval and vaginal itchiness.
   - Discharge yellow and frothy and smelly.
3. Bacterial vaginosis.
   - Similar to trichomonal infection.
4. *Monilia* (candida or thrush) infection.
   - Vulval and vaginal itchiness.
   - Discharge white, thick and lumpy.
5 *Chlamydia trachomatis* infections.
   - Symptoms or signs often mild or absent.
   - The symptoms and signs not diagnostic.
6. Other types of non-gonococcal infection not due to *Chlamydia trachomatis.*
7. Early pregnancy with increase in 'normal' vaginal discharge.
   - Period late or missed.
   - Uterus enlarged.
   - No pus or trichomonal or monilial discharge.
8. Others. See a gynaecology book.

Males:

1. *Chlamydia trachomatis* urethritis
   - Discharge often less and more watery than gonorrhoea.
   - Discharge often has come after apparently successful treatment of gonorrhoea.
   - Common.
2. Trichomonal urethritis
   - Rare.
3. Other types of non-gonococcal urethritis which are not due to *Chlamydia trachomatis* either.

In all patients:

Note that 30% of patients will have both gonococcal and chlamydial infections.

If no tests are possible, assume both infections are present and both infections need treatment.

If tests show gonococci, assume both infections are present and treat both infections.

If reliable tests from urethra and (in women) cervix show no gonococci, assume that chlamydial infection is present and treat only chlamydial infection.

Treatment

Treat for gonorrhoea *ALL* clinical cases of gonorrhoea including:

1. All persons with urethral discharges.
2. All persons with 'urinary tract infections' especially young adults if there is a possibility of gonorrhoea.
3. All persons with vaginal infections especially if cervicitis present and especially if the patient is a young woman and has had a recent change of sexual partner and especially if there is any other reason to suspect an STD.

Treat for chlamydial infection *ALL* clinical cases of urethritis.

Note that 30% of patients will have both gonococcal and chlamydial infections. In most cases it is therefore best to treat for both gonococcal and chlamydial infections. Treatment for chlamydia *alone* should only be given if you are sure the patient does not have gonorrhoea, i.e. urethral and cervical smears show pus cells and *no* gonococci when cultured in the laboratory.

Find out if there is or was also a sore on the genitalia or anus. If so, treat for syphilis too. Treatment for gonorrhoea is not adequate treatment for syphilis (see page 172).

> Treatment for gonorrhoea needs a high concentration of the antibiotic but for only a short time. Treatment for syphilis needs only a low concentration of the antibiotic but for a long time.

Treatment for gonorrhoea
Give if available one of the following:

1. Ciprofloxacin 500 mg by mouth once on an empty stomach; the side effects being nausea, headache, dizziness and hallucinations but being rare; *or*
2. Ceftriaxone 250 mg by IMI once; the side effects of this being very rare; *or*
3. Spectinomycin 2 g by IMI once; the side effects being very little.

Only if none of the above is available, give:

1. Sulphamethoxazole 400 mg/trimethoprim 80 mg (co-trimoxazole) 10 tablets or 800 mg/160 mg 5 tablets once daily every day for 3 days, the side effects being gastrointestinal or rash.
   Some gonococci are resistant to these drugs and the patient will not be cured. Some patients do not remember to take the tablets for 3 days and are not cured.
2. Gentamicin 240 mg IMI once, as well as the co-trimoxazole, if available.

If, however, your Health Department has determined the gonococci in your area are sensitive to penicillins, they may tell you to use the following:

1. Ampicillin or amoxycillin 3.5 g (7 of the 500 mg capsules or 14 of the 250 mg capsules) in one dose, once; *or*
   Procaine benzylpenicillin 4.8 g or 4,800,000 units (2.4 g or 2,400,000 units in each buttock) in one dose, once; *and*
2. Probenecid 1 g (2 tabs) once, 30 minutes before the ampicillin or the procaine penicillin.

Unfortunately, many gonococci are resistant to penicillins and if so, the patient will not be cured by the above treatment.

Treat sexual partners at the same time as the patient or as soon as possible afterwards, also treat all other recent sexual contacts.

If the patient is about to give birth or has given birth and may have gonorrhoea and has not been treated, as well as treating the patient, treat the baby, to prevent ophthalmia neonatorum with blindness, see also page 170 and give:

- ceftriaxone 50 mg/kg to a maximum of 125 mg, *or*
- spectinomycin 25 mg/kg to a maximum of 75 mg, *or*
- kanamycin 25 mg/kg to a maximum of 75 mg, *and*
- tetracycline 1% eye ointment each eye each hour for 1 day then each 8 hours for 10 days.

Treatment for chlamydia trachomatis infection
Give, if not pregnant, either

- doxycycline 100 mg twice daily for 7–10 days, *or*
- tetracycline 500 mg four times a day for 7–10 days.

Give, if pregnant, erythromycin 500 mg four times a day for 7–10 days instead of the above.

Treat the sexual partners at the same time as the patient or as soon after as possible, as well as treating all other sexual contacts.

Follow up
Ask the patient to come back to be checked for cure in 1 week, 3 weeks and 3 months. At the 3 month visit, also check the serological test for syphilis (STS) again.

If the patient is not cured, or if at first he or she seems to be cured but the condition comes back again, the three most likely possibilities are:

1. The 'contact' was not found and treated and the patient is still having intercourse with this infected person – this is the most likely.
2. The patient has gonococci resistant to the drugs used.
3. The patient has one of the other causes of urethritis (see 'Differential diagnoses' above).

Check the patient for all of these possibilities and take what action needed. Take another smear for gonococci.

Treat *Monilia* (*Candida* or thrush) vaginitis if present with nystatin (or other antifungal drug e.g., clotrimazole in the recommended dose) vaginal tablets or pessaries 1–2 each night for 2 weeks. If these or other antifungal vaginal tablets are not available, all that can be done is paint inside the vagina daily with 0.5% crystal violet solution in water.

Treat trichomonal infection with metronidazole 2000 mg in one dose or with 200 mg three times a day for a week. Give to both the patient and the patient's sexual partner.

Treat non-specific vaginitis with metronidazole as above.

Do not give tetracycline or metronidazole to a patient who is pregnant – refer or non-urgently transfer the patient to a Medical Officer.

Refer or non-urgently transfer patients who may have drug resistant infections.

Refer/transfer

Refer or non-urgently transfer to a Medical Officer:

1. patients not cured by the above management (first make sure their sexual partner/s has/have been treated); and
2. patients who cannot be managed by the above scheme.

Control and prevention

See page 158.

In gonorrhoea all sexual contacts for 2 weeks before the patient developed symptoms should be found, examined, if possible, but treated anyway (as not all infected people have symptoms).

Non-gonococcal infection usually urethritis (NGU) including *Chlamydial trachomatis* urethritis and non-specific urethritis

Urethritis and its complications are often due to gonorrhoea. However, many other causes do exist. Often these other causes do not produce as much urethral discharge as gonorrhoea, though most of the other complications of gonorrhoea can, and do, occur with these other infections. Pus may be seen in swabs taken of the urethral or other discharge, but gonococci are not seen.

About half of these cases are due to *Chlamydia trachomatis* which is usually sensitive to the tetracycline group of drugs. Others of these cases are due to other organisms, some of which are successfully treated by tetracyclines and some of which are not successfully treated by tetracyclines.

Some organisms causing non-gonococcal urethritis cause other complications such as Reiter's syndrome (urethritis and conjunctivitis and arthritis).

Treatment is by tetracycline 500 mg four times a day *or* doxycycline 100 mg twice daily if not pregnant *or* erythromycin 500 mg four times a day if pregnant for 1 week.

Treatment of the sexual partners with the same drugs before the patient has intercourse with them again is essential.

Treatment of other contacts with the above drugs is also necessary.

Children born to women who have untreated *Chlamydia trachomatis* infections may develop severe conjunctivitis and blindness or pneumonia. As well as treating the mother, the baby should be treated immediately as for gonococcal conjunctivitis or ophthalmia neonatorum (see page 169) and if there are still any eye symptoms or if the child develops pneumonia, then give erythromycin 12.5 mg/kg four times a day (50 mg/kg daily) for 2 weeks.

Syphilis

Syphilis is a bacterial infection which causes a sore where the organism enters the body. This sore heals without treatment. However, the bacteria spread all through the body and cause serious subacute and chronic disease of many organs.

Epidemiology

Syphilis is common especially among young adults. The cause is the syphilis bacterium (*Treponema pallidum*). The only host is man.

The disease usually spreads from an infectious lesion (chancre, mucous patch or condyloma) during sexual intercourse. The organisms can enter a new person through broken skin or normal unbroken mucous membrane of the genitalia or mouth. Infection can also occur through infected blood which is transfused, or through the placenta to an unborn baby from an infected pregnant women.

Previous infection with the similar yaws bacterium gives some immunity against syphilis.

Symptoms and signs, course and complications

Primary syphilis causes a chancre and enlarged lymph glands.

1. The chancre is the lesion at the site of infection (usually genitalia but can also be anus or mouth) (see Figures 19.7 and 19.8). First a painless lump develops. it soon ulcerates in the centre and clear fluid oozes from it. It is firm and hard, 'like a button' in the skin. It usually heals after 2–6 weeks, even without treatment. It may look different if secondary bacterial infection occurs.

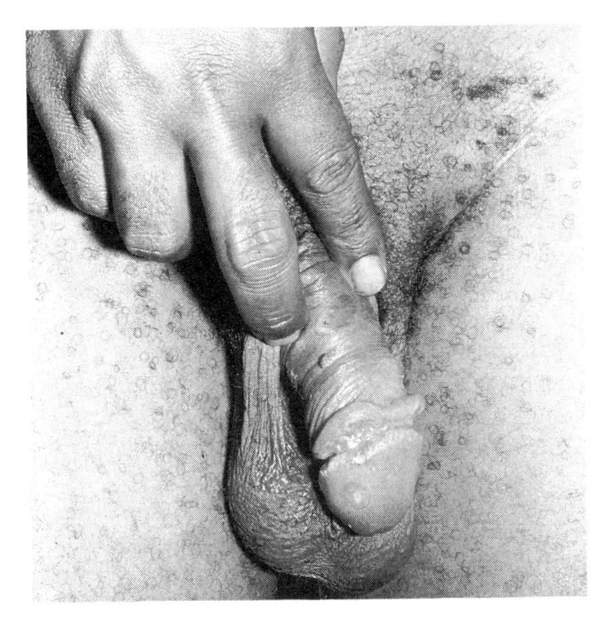

Figure 19.7 Primary syphilis. A chancre on the penis. Note however, that any ulcer on the genitalia is first treated as syphilis no matter what it looks like.

> Any ulcer of the genitalia is treated as syphilis no matter what it looks like.

A female patient may not know she has a chancre if occurs in the vagina or on the cervix.

2. The nearby lymph glands are usually hard but not tender.

Secondary syphilis usually comes about 6 weeks after the primary sore heals. (But it can be earlier or much later.) There may be any or all of these common lesions:

1. A skin rash with bilateral (on both sides) round, red, non-itchy flat patches 5–10 mm in diameter.
2. A skin rash with bilateral red, non-itchy lumps which may become scaly or turn into pustules.
3. A skin rash called condylomata lata in warm moist areas such as the perineum, vulva (see Figure 19.9), scrotum, inner thighs, under breasts, etc.

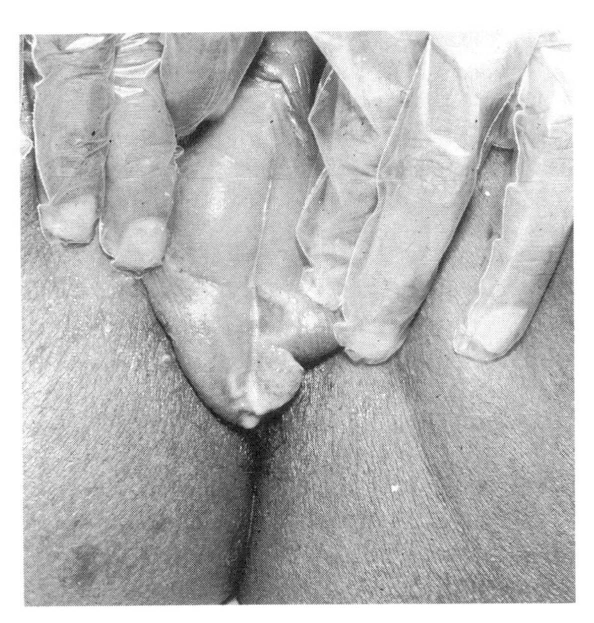

Figure 19.8 Primary syphilis. Chancre on the vulva. Note the fairly typical appearance (see text). However all ulcers in the genitalia are treated first for syphilis. Note also that in females the chancre may be in the vagina or on the cervix and not be noticed by the patient.

The above lumps here get bigger and the surface skin comes off to produce large painless raised moist grey areas. However, secondary infection may occur and change the appearance.

> Any wet skin lesions in groin, perineum, axilla, etc. must be suspected of being syphilis.

4. Mucous patches are painless, shallow grey ulcers with a narrow red margin (or edge). They occur on the lips or mouth, vulva, vagina, scrotum and penis.
5. Painless enlargement of all lymph nodes of the body.
6. General symptoms and signs of infection, e.g. malaise, fever, loss of appetite, loss of weight.

Any of these symptoms of the secondary stage are present for 2–6 weeks and then go away, even without treatment. But they may return again many times.

Tertiary syphilis occurs many years later, in one out of every two or three cases. 'Gumma' causing mostly non-inflamed ulcers on the skin as well as disease of the heart or disease of the brain can occur. (In some tropical developing countries there have only been a few cases of tertiary syphilis. This is probably because syphilis has not been common for very long, as infection with yaws used to give some immunity to syphilis.)

Congenital syphilis. A child may be infected through the placenta, if his mother has syphilis. The child may be born dead or develop any of the signs of secondary or tertiary syphilis.

Tests

Send the serum of 10 ml of blood to the laboratory with a request for a serological test for syphilis (STS). A VDRL or RPR test is usually done. Occasionally these tests are positive when the patient does not have syphilis. More accurate tests, e.g. TPHA or FTA-Abs may then be done.

The STS is positive in two out of three cases of primary syphilis but not until 3–4 weeks after the chancre comes.

The STS is positive in nearly all cases of secondary syphilis.

STS may remain positive for life. Re-treatment is needed only if the test is later about four times more positive (on titre testing) or the patient has exposure to further patients with infectious syphilis.

Diagnostic features

- Sexual contact about 3 weeks before.
- Hard, painless ulcerated sore on genitalia (or other area) with enlarged non-tender lymph nodes nearby. The sore heals after 2–6 weeks. However, you should suspect syphilis in all ulcers on the genitalia.
- Two to six weeks later, skin rashes, condylomata lata, mucous patches, general symptoms and signs, and possibly disease of other organs can occur.

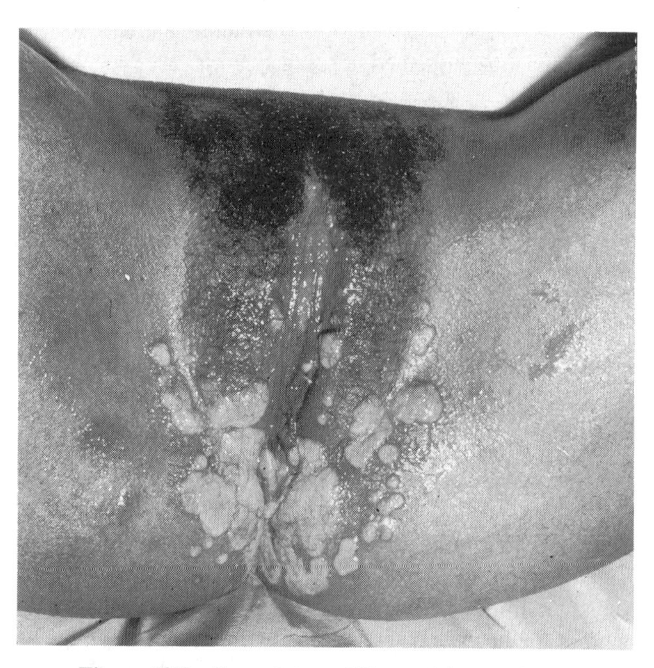

Figure 19.9 Secondary syphilis condylomata lata of vulva and perineum.

Treatment

1. Before giving treatment ask the patient about previous or present symptoms of gonorrhoea. If the patient has symptoms of gonorrhoea do tests and give treatment for gonorrhoea (see page 169) as well as the treatment for syphilis (which will not cure gonorrhoea).

> Treatment for syphilis needs only a low concentration of the antibiotic but for a long time. Treatment for gonorrhoea needs a high concentration of the antibiotic but for only a short time.

2. Treat also for chancroid. See page 176.
3. The best treatment for syphilis is an immediate injection of a long acting penicillin in case the patient does not come back. Give IMI benzathine penicillin 2,400,000 units (5 ml) immediately once. Divide the dose into $2\frac{1}{2}$ ml into each buttock. Repeat this each week for two more doses if later than primary syphilis.

If benzathine penicillin not available, *use* instead *either*:

1. Procaine benzylpenicillin 1.2 g or 1,200,000 units every day for 10 days; or if later than primary syphilis, for 14 days. *or*
2. Procaine penicillin in oil with 2% aluminium monosterate (PAM) 2,400,000 units (8 ml) immediately then 1,200,000 units (4 ml) 3 days later and again 6 days later, and if later than primary syphilis, for two more doses each 3 days.

If the patient is allergic to penicillin, give instead tetracycline 500 mg (2 capsules) four times a day for 15 days or doxycycline 100 mg (1 tablet) twice daily for 15 days but not to a pregnant woman.

If the patient is allergic to penicillin and is a pregnant woman, give instead erythromycin 500 mg four times a day for 15 days. After delivery the baby will need treatment with penicillin and the mother with tetracycline as erythromycin during pregnancy is not a very effective treatment for syphilis.

Ask the patient to return for another clinical examination in 2 weeks. If the patient is not cured, investigate and treat for the other likely causes (see page 156).

Even if the patient appears to be cured, ask him or her to return for another clinical examination and another STS in 3 months, 9 months and 2 years to make sure he or she is cured. If the patient is not cured, refer or transfer non-urgently to a Medical Officer.

Control and prevention

See 'Control and Prevention' page 158.

1. Before you give treatment, organise with the patient contact identification and treatment for all sexual contacts since the sore appeared and for 3 months before this.
2. Find and treat *all* the patient's contacts (most importantly the regular sexual partner). Also examine them, if possible.
3. If the sore is cured by treatment, you can assume the diagnosis to be syphilis. Confirm the diagnosis in the STD register.
4. You should examine and test all groups of people who have a high risk of being infected, and treat them if necessary. These groups include:
   (a) patients who think that they have STD,
   (b) industrial and plantation and other migration workers (every year),
   (c) prostitutes (every month), and
   (d) people in prisons and similar institutions.
5. In areas where yaws is uncommon and syphilis occurs, do an STS on all pregnant women. Treat the woman, if the STS is positive, to stop congenital syphilis in her baby.

Donovanosis or granuloma inguinale

Donovanosis is caused by a bacterial infection (*Calymmatobacterium* (or *Donovania*) *granulomatis*) but the organism is not very infectious. It is very common only in certain places including parts of the Pacific, Africa and India. The main sign is a red ulcer on the genitalia without toxaemia. The lymph glands are usually affected only later and only in some cases.

The first lesion is usually a lump on one part of the genitalia. The lump soon develops into an ulcer. The ulcer is usually raised and irregular at its edges and bright red, because it is full of granulation tissue or like cut meat ('beefy red') and is not covered with a crust. The ulcer is not painful. The ulcer only slowly (over many weeks) gets bigger towards the groin areas or anus usually in the folds of the skin (see Figure 19.10).

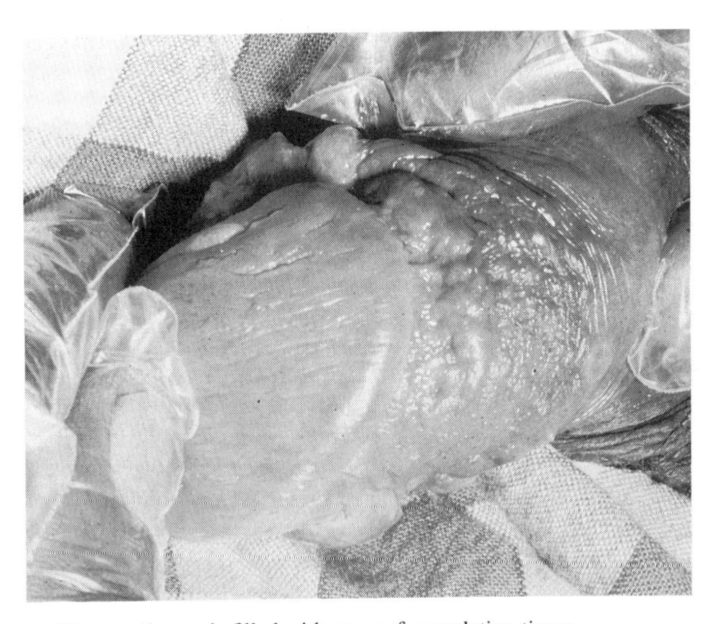

Figure 19.10 Donovanosis. Ulcer on the penis filled with areas of granulation tissue.

New lesions can appear on the genitalia; especially in places the first lesion touches.

Only if other infections are also present in the original ulcer do the lymph nodes in the groin areas become enlarged. However, the donovanosis organism can spread to the lymph nodes and cause an ulcer, similar to the one on the genitalia, which slowly gets bigger. (This is why the disease is called also granuloma inguinale – see Figure 19.11.)

If not treated, the lesions all slowly get bigger and destroy a lot of tissue. Occasionally the organism can spread to other parts of the body and start ulcers there too. After many years, if not treated, cancer can form in the edges of some lesions.

Diagnosis is often possible by a simple test which can be sent to the laboratory. Clean the sore with saline. Local anaesthetic is not needed. Cut a *small thin* slice from the top of the edge of the sore with a sterile scalpel or razor blade. Smear the cut side on a glass slide or crush it between two glass slides. Fix it with alcohol. Send it to the laboratory with a request for examination for 'Donovan bodies'. This is often positive if the disease is donovanosis. A proper biopsy would be diagnostic; but it is not usually needed.

For differential diagnosis and management see pages 156 and 165.

Treatment is by sulphamethoxazole 400 mg/ trimethoprim 80 mg (co-trimoxazole) (2 tabs) or 800 mg/160 mg (1 tab) twice daily, or if this is not effective, tetracycline 500 mg (2 caps) four times a day or doxycycline 100 mg (1 tab) twice daily, all of these for 2 weeks unless pregnant. If pregnant erythromycin 500 mg four times a day could be used although this is less effective. Treatment is usually needed for 2 weeks. Chloramphenicol may be needed in some countries where the organism is resistant to tetracycline. Streptomycin is effective but do not give streptomycin as you should keep it only for tuberculosis.

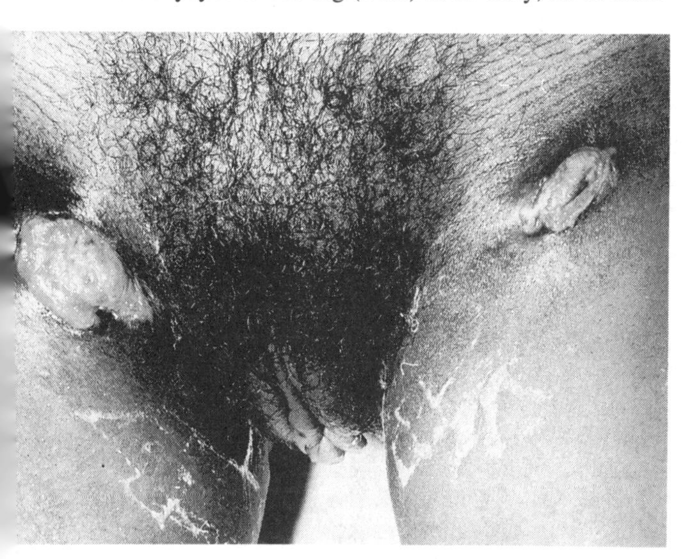

Figure 19.11 Donovanosis. Vulval ulcer and granulations with spread of the disease to the lymph glands in the groin, which have ulcerated.

Control and *prevention* – see page 158. You need only trace and examine the regular sexual partner, as the disease is not very infectious.

Amoebic ulceration of the genitalia

Amoebic ulcers are caused by a protozoal organism (*Entamoeba histolytica*) which normally lives in the bowel (see Chapter 23 page 294).

The lesion starts on or near the genitalia because of: direct spread of the organism from the anus; or anal intercourse; or intercourse with a person who has a genital amoebic ulcer.

The lesion is usually a fast growing (in days to weeks) painful ulcer which destroys much tissue. The ulcer is usually reddish in colour and covered with grey-white pus. If it is very acute, the discharge may be like watery blood. The lymph nodes nearby are usually enlarged and tender. (See Figure 19.12.)

Occasionally the lesion may grow more slowly and look like a cancer of the penis, vulva or cervix.

Diagnosis can be made by immediate microscopic examination of discharge from the edge of the ulcer for *Entamoeba histolytica*; but this is not usually possible in a health centre. A biopsy would be diagnostic, but is not usually needed.

Treat with metronidazole 800 mg three times a day for 5–10 days. If nausea occurs, reduce the dose of metronidazole to 400 mg three times a day but continue for 10 days. Warn the patient not to drink alcohol while taking metronidazole. Give tetracycline together with the metrondiazole if acute inflammation is present.

Lymphogranuloma venereum (inguinal bubo)

Lymphogranuloma venereum is caused by a type of bacterial infection (*Chlamydia trachomatis*). It is also called lymphogranuloma inguinale. The usual signs are no ulcer on the genitalia but very enlarged inflamed inguinal lymph nodes with toxaemia and then ulceration of the inguinal lymph nodes.

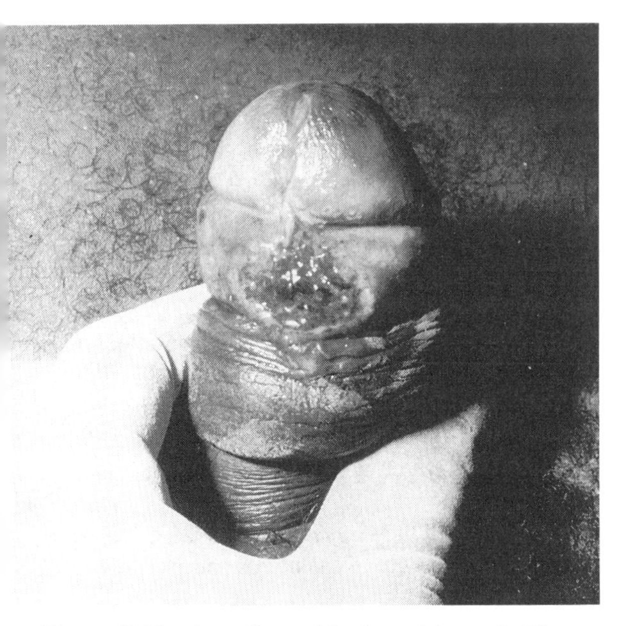

Figure 19.12 A small amoebic ulcer of the penis. The ulcer did not improve after penicillin or after tetracycline. The patient was therefore treated with metronidazole and was cured. (A smear taken from the edge of the ulcer before metronidazole was given and immediately examined under the microscope showed amoebae). Often amoebic ulcers are much larger than this ulcer.

One to three weeks after infection, a small blister or ulcer appears on the genitalia, and is usually not noticed. About 2–6 weeks later the lymph nodes in the groin become enlarged and inflamed. Pus forms in the lymph nodes which then burst. (See Figure 19.13.) As more nodes are affected, many abscesses discharging whitish fluid develop. Abscesses can join to make large ulcers. The area affected increases. Sometimes abscesses and ulcers form in the anal region.

During this time the patient may have general symptoms and signs of infection such as malaise, fever, etc.

After some months the ulcers usually get better. But there is often a lot of deformity left. There may be strictures (narrowing) of the rectum or urethra or vulva. There may also be chronic oedema of the genitalia.

Special tests for definite diagnosis are not usually done. Biopsy would also be diagnostic.

Treat for syphilis and chancroid if previous ulcer on genitalia.

Treat with either tetracycline 500 mg (2 caps) four times a day *or* doxycycline 100 mg twice daily, *or*, if pregnant, erythromycin 500 mg four times a day for 3 weeks. You should also aspirate any pus from lymph nodes before they burst, putting the needle through uninfected skin into the bubo and aspirating all the fluid before taking the needle out.

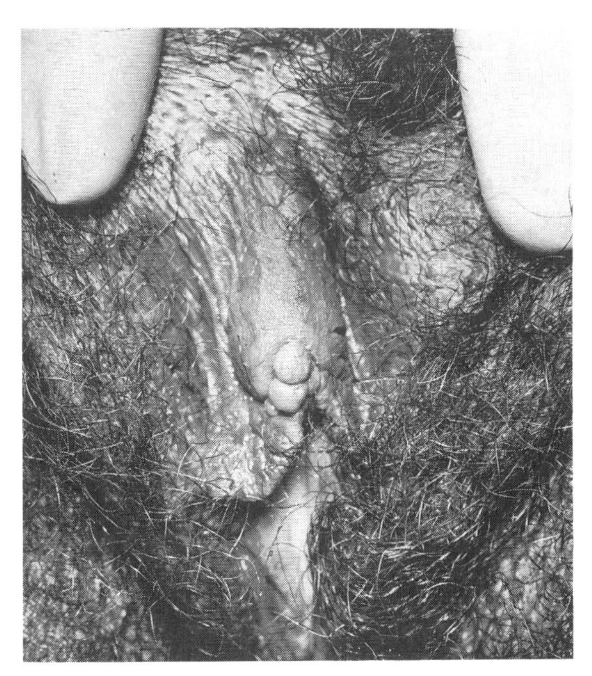

Figure 19.13 Lymphogranuloma venereum.

Control and *prevention* – see page 158.

Chancroid (soft sore)

Chancroid is an infection caused by special bacteria (*Haemophilus ducreyi*). The main signs are many tender ulcers on the genitalia and enlarged tender lymph nodes which can ulcerate. This infection seems to be becoming very frequent and in many areas is the most common cause of genital ulcer, especially in men and especially in HIV infected patients.

A small lump appears on the genitalia. The lump is on the surface of the skin or mucous membrane (different from syphilis, which is in the skin). The lump soon ulcerates. The edge of the ulcer is irregular and red, and it is covered with dirty pus (see Figure 19.14). The sore is very painful. Where the ulcer touches other parts of the body, new ulcers may appear. The ulcers are soft (again different from syphilis).

The lymph nodes in the groin on one or both sides become swollen, painful and tender. These inflamed lymph nodes often form a fluid-filled (fluctuant) mass which bursts to leave a large ulcer (again different from syphilis).

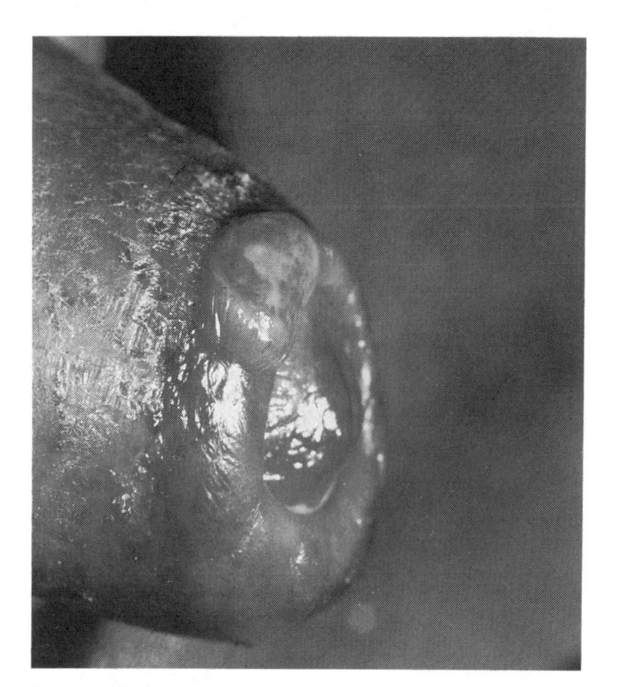

Figure 19.14 Chancroid (soft sore).

However, it is not possible to tell, by examination alone, if the condition is definitely due to chancroid or syphilis or due to other infection.

Diagnosis is possible in a laboratory by examining the discharge from an ulcer under the microscope. Also send blood for STS and HIV serology.

Treatment is with:

1. Sulphamethoxazole 800 mg/trimethoprim 160 mg (co-trimoxazole) twice daily or tetracycline 500 mg (2 caps) four times a day or doxycycline 100 mg (1 tab) twice daily may cure in 1–2 weeks. If not or if pregnant, give erythromycin 500 mg three to four times a day. It has also been found that the special antibiotics given for gonorrhoea are effective for chancroid.
2. Benzathine penicillin 2.4 million units IMI once in case syphilis is also present.
3. If lymph nodes look as if they will burst, then before this happens, aspirate (suck out) the pus through a needle put into the bubo through normal-looking nearby skin.

If the condition is not cured, consider both an antibiotic resistant organism, HIV infection or other conditions and refer to a Medical Officer.

Control and *prevention* – see page 158.

Venereal warts (condylomata accuminata)

Venereal warts are caused by one of the human papilloma viruses (HPV).

The warts are most common under the foreskin and on (and often around) the glans penis of the male. They are found on (and often around) the vulva and in the vagina and on the cervix of the female. They may also occur in the urethra and around the anus in both sexes.

The warts are soft pink fleshy growths like a cauliflower. There may be very many of them. They may grow very big (see Figures 19.15 and 19.16). Sometimes they look like warts on other parts of the body. They may get worse in pregnancy or if an HIV infection develops.

Infection with the virus may, years later, cause carcinoma of the cervix of the uterus and possibly other genital or anal carcinomas.

Always consider if the condition could be due to secondary syphilis or molluscum contagiosum. Always think of other STDs being present.

Treatment is difficult. Small warts may just go away themselves. You should treat any other STD, especially any genital discharge (see page 160). Regular washing with soap and water will help. Paint the warts with podophyllin 20% in tincture of benzoin

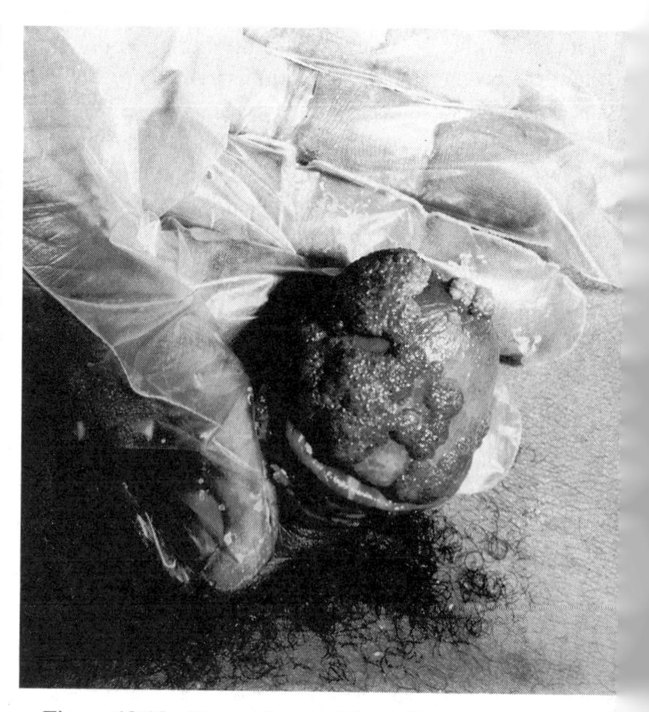

Figure 19.15 Venereal warts (also called condylomata accuminata) of the penis.

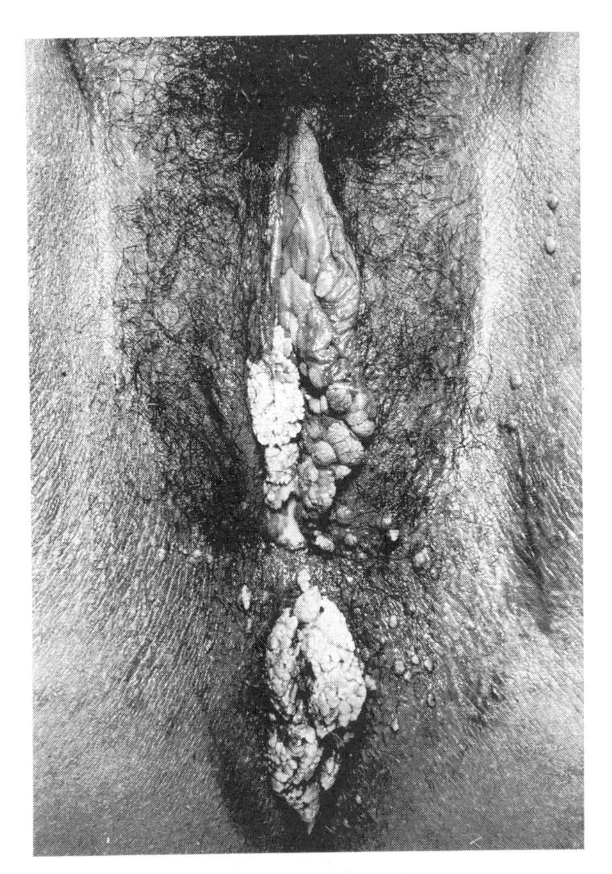

Figure 19.16 Venereal warts (also called condylomata accuminata) of the vulva and anus.

maximum dose 0.5 (1/2) ml or touch them with a silver nitrate stick. Do not use podophyllin during pregnancy. Do not put any podophyllin or silver nitrate on any normal part of the body. Wash off the podophyllin after 4 hours. Repeat the treatment each week until the warts are gone. Podophyllotoxin 0.5% liquid applied twice daily for 3 days each 7 days, is better but expensive; though patients may purchase this themselves. If the patient does not get better or warts are in the urethra or cervix or the patient is pregnant, refer them to the Medical Officer.

It may be that soon a vaccine at present under trial will be available to prevent this condition and the cancers (e.g. cervix) that may follow.

Control and *prevention* – see page 158.

Herpes genitalis

Herpes genitalis is an infection with herpes simplex virus.

Infection with herpes genitalis virus causes a number of small vesicles (blisters) to come up on the mucous membranes of the genitalia (glans penis, labia, cervix). The vesicles burst, and shallow ulcers develop (see Figure 19.17). Some ulcers join. The ulcers look like the 'cold sores' which appear on the lips during fever. The surface of the ulcer is green-grey or white. Near the ulcer the mucous membrane is red. The ulcers are very painful, especially if urine touches them. The ulcers may look different if they have secondary bacterial infection.

The lymph nodes in the groin are sometimes large, firm and tender.

During a first infection the patient may have the general symptoms and signs of infection – fever, malaise, etc.

The condition usually goes away after some weeks; but it may return many times for the rest of the patient's life. Tingling and other unusual feelings in the skin usually occur before another group of ulcers form. The patient is infectious any time ulcers are present, and should not have intercourse if the tingling or other feelings or ulcers are present.

It comes back more often and spreads further and lasts longer and in general is worse if the patient develops an HIV infection.

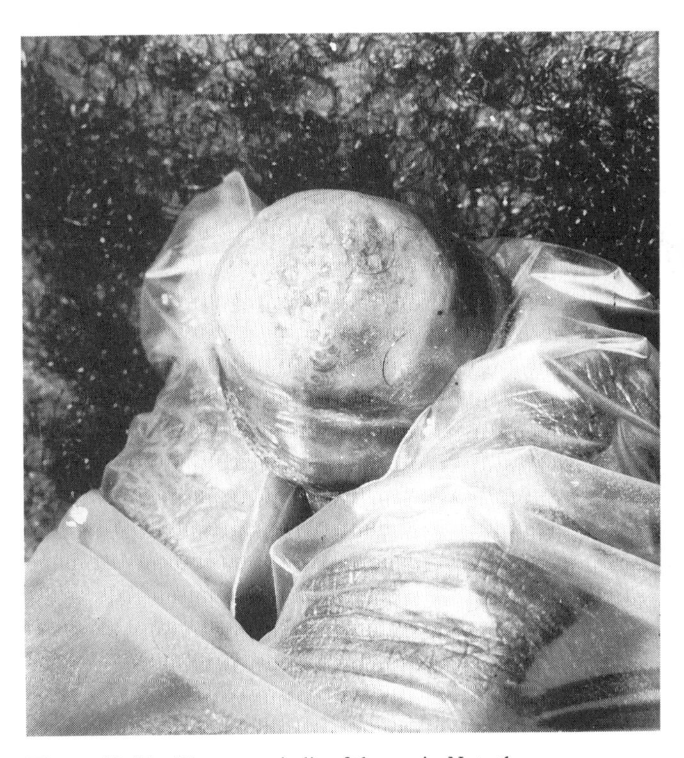

Figure 19.17 Herpes genitalis of the penis. Note the small vesicles on the glans. They soon burst to become ulcers and are very painful.

If a pregnant woman has the infection with ulcers on the genitalia at the time of birth, the child may be infected at birth and get a severe infection and die. Caesarean section may be needed. Discuss pregnant women with herpes with a Medical Officer.

No *treatment* available in health centres cures the condition. Special antiviral drugs such as aciclovir are very expensive and treatment does not cure the patient and does not stop the infection coming back. Keep the affected area clean and dry. You can give the patient crystal violet 0.5% in water solution to put on the ulcers.

Control and *prevention* – see page 158. As there is no treatment possible, it is not necessary to find contacts. The patient should not have sexual intercourse when infectious.

Other genital conditions

Balanitis

Balanitis is inflammation of the glans penis and the foreskin. it is more common in those who are uncircumcised, those who have phimosis, those who have diabetes and those who do not regularly wash under the foreskin. The inflammation can be caused by various types of organisms including bacteria, fungi and trichomonas.

The patient complains of a penile discharge; but on inspection the discharge is seen to come from under the foreskin and not the urethra. The glans penis is red, inflamed and sometimes ulcerated. The foreskin is inflamed and some times gangrenous.

Test the urine for sugar and refer or non-urgently transfer the patient for treatment, if he has diabetes.

Treatment includes benzathine penicillin 2,400,000 units (5 ml) IMI immediately in case it is syphilis.

The patient should wash the area regularly twice every day and apply gentian violet in water solution twice every day.

If the patient does not improve quickly give treatment with tetracycline and metronidazole (see page 174).

Prevention is by good personal hygiene.

The WHO flow chart is as shown in Figure 19.18.

Traumatic sores of penis or vulva

There are many causes for these, including small tears during intercourse.

Secondary bacterial infection can occur.

Give local treatment to the sore, e.g. 1% crystal violet in water solution twice daily after washing. As syphilis cannot usually be excluded, give 2,400,000 units (5 ml) of benzathine penicillin. See also page 160. Ask about previous or present symptoms of urethritis. See page 165 if there are symptoms.

Cancer of the penis or vulva

You should suspect cancer in elderly patients who have had an ulcer for some weeks or months. The ulcer is often full of growing tissues with raised, turned out edges (see Figure 19.19). If it has spread to the lymph nodes, they will be very hard like stones.

Any patient with a very suspicious ulcer should be transferred non-urgently for biopsy or biopsied and the biopsy sent for examination at the laboratory. While waiting for the result, you should treat the patient for amoebic infection as on page 174. If the disease is cancer the only treatment is non-urgent transfer for surgery.

Human immunodeficiency virus infection and AIDS

Dr Wendy Holmes and her collaborators at TALC have produced tape and slide sets on HIV infection from which all the photographs for this section were generously supplied. Some parts of the text are based on ideas from these sets.

Definition

The end result of human immunodeficiency virus (HIV) infection is acquired immuno-deficiency syndrome (AIDS). Infection occurs when the blood or body secretions from a person with HIV infection pass into the body of another person during unsafe sexual practices or pregnancy or from the injection of blood. HIV infection causes a progression of symptoms and signs. At first there are none. Then a seroconversion reaction may occur. Then again for many years there may be no symptoms or signs or just a persistent generalised lymphadenopathy. Then AIDS-related conditions occur. Some are due to the HIV itself. Some are due to infections with common oroganisms. The infections are more frequent or more severe than usual because of decreased immunity. At the end there

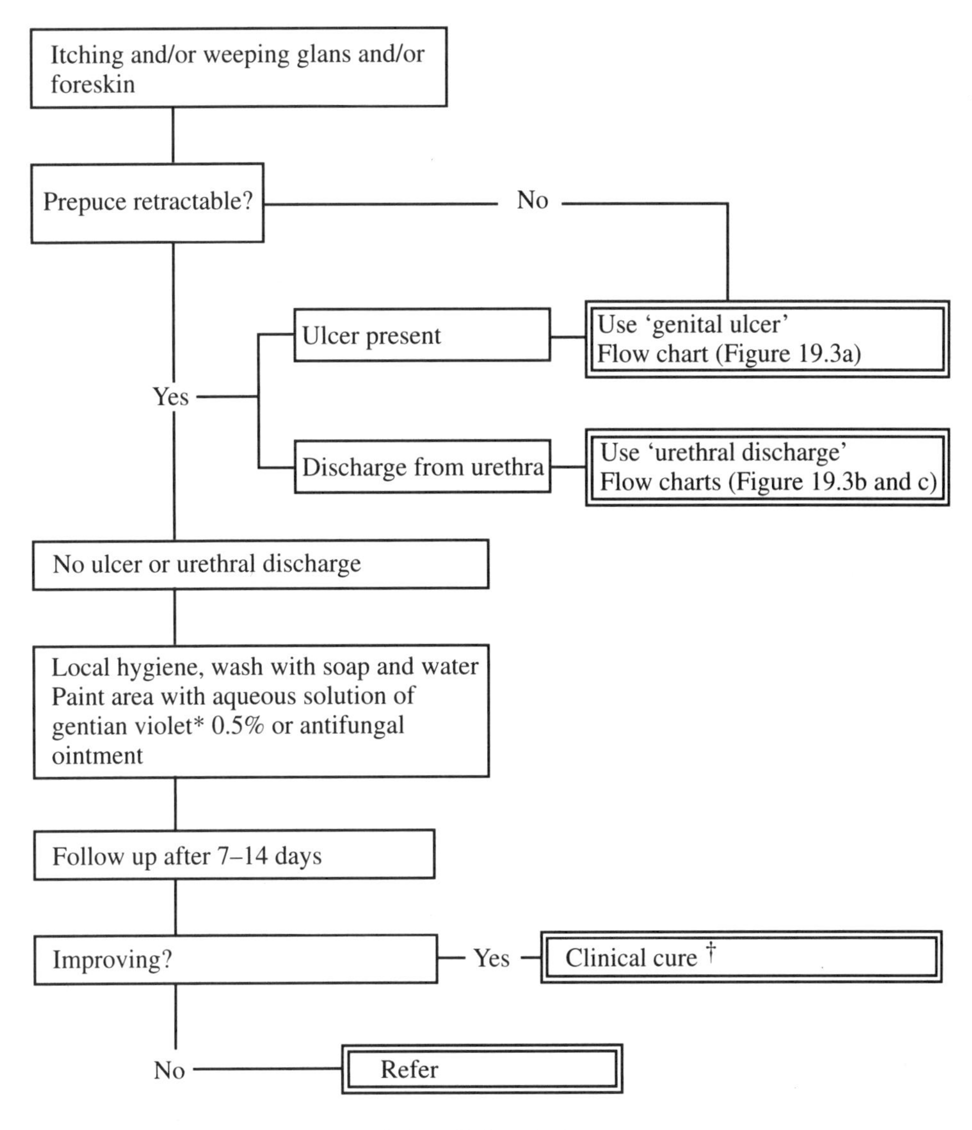

* International non-proprietary name: methylrosanilinium chloride.

† Treatment may have to be continued.

Figure 19.18 WHO flow chart for balanitis/balanoposthitis (From *WHO Technical Report Series* No. 810).

is AIDS with severe, often unusual and fatal infections or cancers. Although there is no cure for HIV infection, the other infections it allows to occur can be treated, and counselling and support can help patients and their families. Although there is no vaccine to prevent HIV infection, if practices that spread HIV are stopped, the infection can be prevented.

Epidemiology

HIV infection was first recognised in 1981. It is probably due to a new virus. The new HIV virus was probably made by a natural change in an old virus or a natural combination of parts of more than one old virus. HIV infection occurs only in humans.

The HIV is present in the blood of infected people who may be either apparently healthy carriers or be sick. The virus is also in some of the body secretions, mainly semen and vaginal secretions, but also discharges from wounds, milk and saliva. Infected blood, semen, vaginal secretions and possibly other infected secretions from a person infected with HIV may get into the body of another uninfected person by only a few special ways. By far the most common way for this to happen is through sexual intercourse

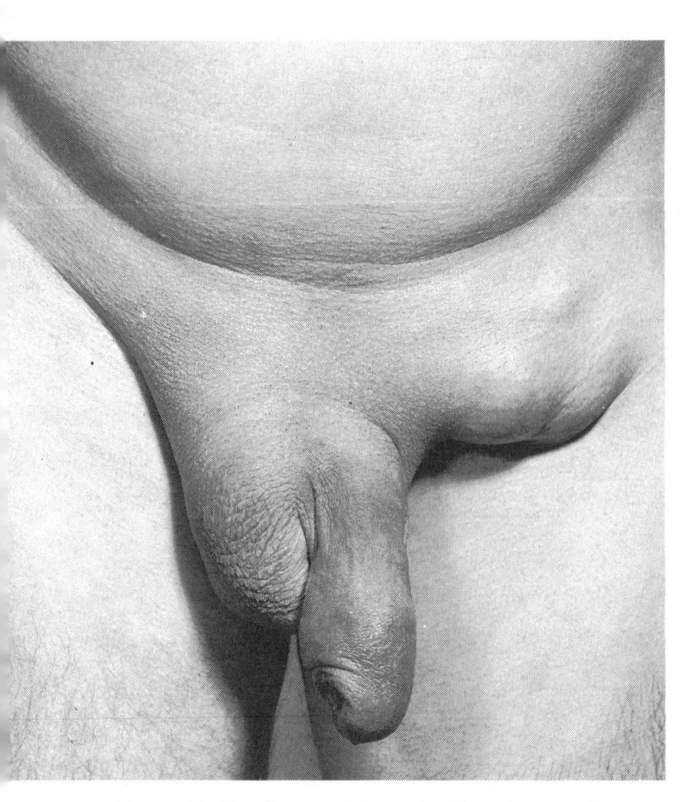

Figure 19.19 Cancer of the penis. Note that any ulcer which has recently formed and does not get better after treatment with penicillin and then tetracycline and if necessary metronidazole, as well as any chronic ulcer must be referred or transferred to a medical officer for a biopsy to see if it is a cancer.

(both normal heterosexual intercourse and even more easily by male homosexual intercourse). Transmission may result from other close physical contact, but only if both the infected person and also the uninfected person have open wounds or sores and the blood or secretions from the infected person gets into the wounds or sores of the uninfected person. Transmission of course occurs if infected blood is transfused or if the infected blood in needles or syringes is not properly cleaned out and sterilised after use and is then injected. This should never happen in health centres. However it does happen when drug addicts share needles and syringes and in some tattooing. Infected pregnant women pass the infection to their unborn children in about 30% of cases. Up to 15% of babies uninfected at birth can later be infected, probably from the infected mother's milk (but without breastfeeding even more than this 15% would die of malnutrition, infections, etc.; and breastfeeding therefore should continue).

It is not possible to be infected by caring for people infected by HIV (Figure 19.20) as long as their blood, semen or vaginal secretions, etc. do not enter the body of the carer by intercourse, injection or through wounds or sores. It is safe, therefore, to eat, drink, talk and play with infected people. It is safe to hug and even kiss (safest without contacting saliva) infected people. It would not be safe to use ungloved hands with cuts or sores on them to dress any open or bleeding wounds or sores. It would not be safe to share razors, toothbrushes or tooth-cleaning sticks which could go through the surface of the skin or mouth, etc. Any sexual intercourse, where the penis is placed in the vagina, anus or mouth, especially without a condom on it, would be likely to pass on infection.

HIV infection is common and quickly increasing. However the amount of HIV infection varies greatly from country to country and area to area (Table 19.1 and Figure 19.21). It can vary from below 1% in some rural areas to up to 30% among adults in some cities. It is as common in women as in men. It is most common in young adults. About half the people in some hospitals are there because of HIV infection. The commonest cause of death in adults in some areas is HIV infection. (This is different from industrialised countries where most sufferers are either homosexual males or drug addicts.)

Symptoms and signs

Some weeks to months after infection, a non-specific viral ('influenza'-like or 'glandular fever'-like) illness may occur. There may be fever, sweating, malaise, tiredness, loss of appetite, diarrhoea, pain in muscles or joints, headache, encephalitis, sore throat, enlargement of all the lymph nodes in the body, a flat vague reddish rash on the trunk, etc. The virus by then has spread all over the body. It is called the 'seroconversion reaction' as after it, the serum tests show antibodies to the HIV. There is no way, however, this illness can be clinically recognised as, or diagnosed as, HIV infection in the health centre.

Infants may not fully recover from the above illness and may 'fail to thrive' (not grow or gain weight) or within weeks or months they develop one or more of the complications below. However most adults seem to recover from the seroconversion reaction and stay apparently well for months to up to 5 (and at times 10) years. Nevertheless the virus is alive in the infected person's body and is able to infect others. The

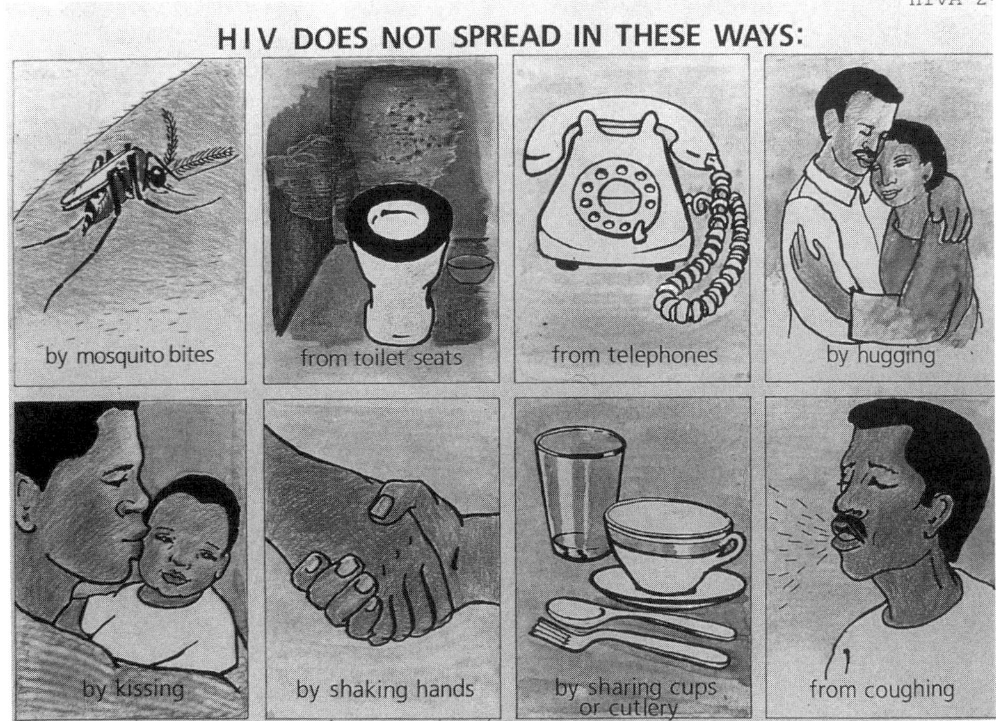

Figure 19.20 HIV does not spread in these ways.

Table 19.1 Global estimates of the HIV/AIDS epidemic as of the end of 1997.

People newly infected with HIV in 1997	Total Children <15 years	5,800,000 590,000
Number of people living with HIV/AIDS	Total Children <15 years	30,600,000 1,100,000
AIDS deaths in 1997	Total Children <15 years	2,300,000 460,000
Total number of AIDS deaths since the beginning of the epidemic	Total Children <15 years	11,700,000 2,700,000
Total number of AIDS orphans* since the beginning of the epidemic		8,200,000

* Children who lost their mother or both parents to AIDS when under the age of 15 years.
Data from *Report on the Global HIV/AIDS Epidemic June 1998.* Geneva, WHO.

virus is also slowly damaging special parts of the body, most importantly the immune system and also the nervous system but also the bowel walls, skin, etc. Most importantly, the lymphocytes (of the CD4 'helper' type) which are in the white blood cells and in lymph nodes and in the spleen and in other areas are damaged and their numbers become fewer. These CD4 lymphocytes are responsible for cellular immunity (which protects against viral, mycobacterial, fungal and protozoal infections) and also control B-lymphocyte cells to make antibodies in the correct amount. The patient's immunity, therefore, to infections and some special cancers becomes less.

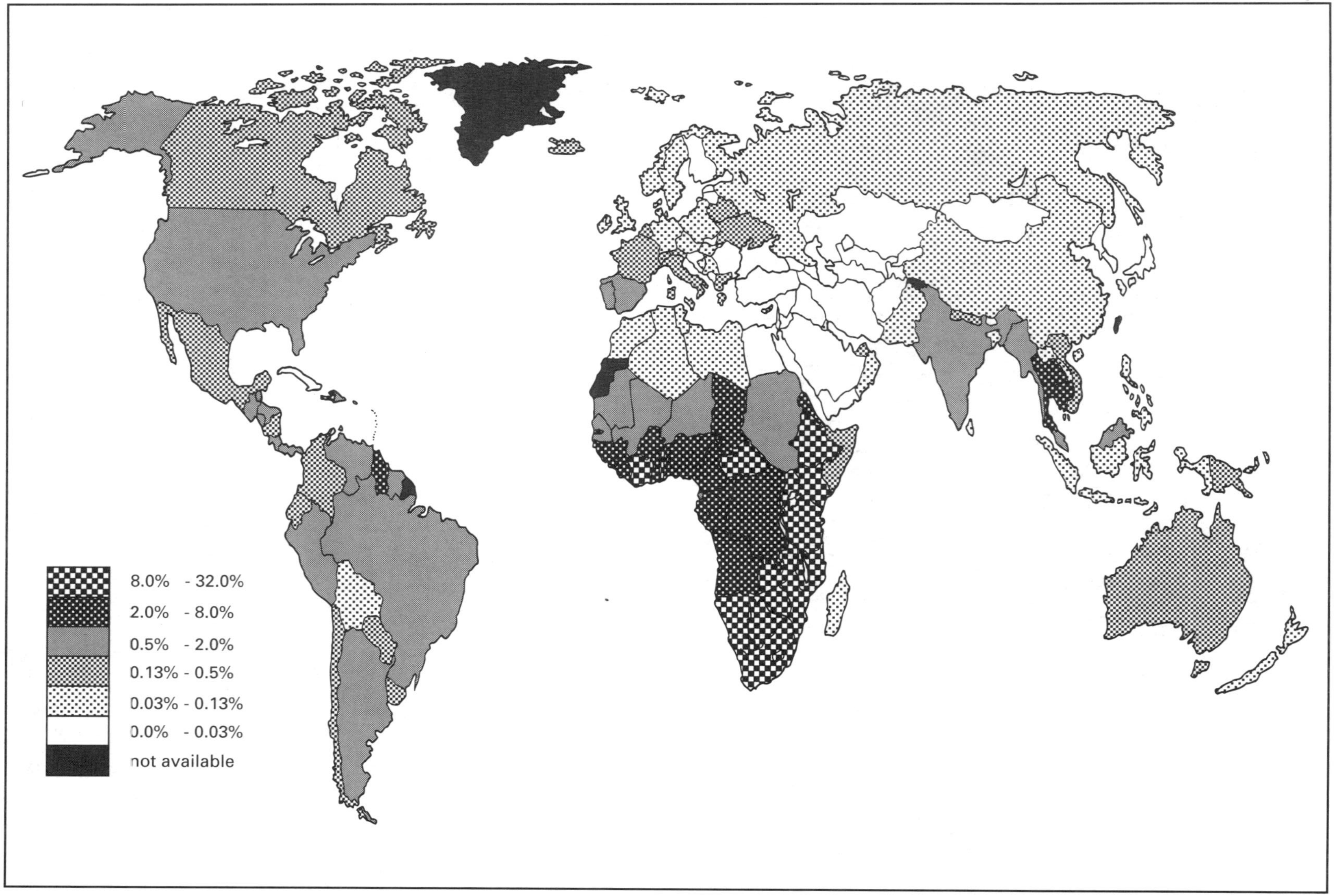

Figure 19.21 A global view of HIV infection (end of 1997). (Source: *Report on the global HIV/AIDS epidemic – June 1998*. Geneva, UNAIDS/WHO)

After some months or even 5 (to 10) years, symptoms and signs may develop due to:

1. Damage to some of the body's organs, especially the brain or lymph nodes or skin or bowel. This is caused by the virus.
2. More infections and more severe infections than usual. These infections are caused by the usual organisms causing the common infections in the community (such as those causing pneumonia and tuberculosis). These frequent and severe infections are caused or allowed by loss of immunity.
3. Unusual infections. These are allowed by severe loss of immunity. These infections are called 'opportunistic infections'. They are caused by organisms which normally do not grow in the healthy body and are killed or their growth mostly stopped by the healthy body's immunity. If however, the body's defence or immunity is decreased, then they can take this 'opportunity' to grow in the body and cause an unusual infection, or a much worse infection than usual for that organism.
4. Unusual tumours especially Kaposi's sarcoma or lymphoma but others also. Many of these tumours may be due to infection and be allowed by the loss of immunity.

Figure 19.22 (page 184) shows how HIV infection in a patient causes more and more loss of immunity as time goes by and what conditions are likely to be present at the different stages of loss of immunity.

HIV infection, may at times show no symptoms or signs, and may at other times cause one or more or all of the following:

1. *Persistent generalised lymphadenopathy* (PGL) (due to HIV itself) (Figure 19.23). There are enlarged lymph nodes without other symptoms in up to 50% of HIV infected people. (These are not inguinal or groin nodes which are often enlarged from chronic bacterial or filarial infections.)
   The enlarged lymph nodes are:
   - in more than one place and often symmetrical (the same on both sides),
   - larger than 1 cm but usually smaller than 3 cm and do not continue to get larger,
   - present for more than 3 months,
   - have no other cause obvious (e.g. syphilis, tuberculosis, etc.).

   Biopsy would be needed (as another diagnosis, especially tuberculosis, is more likely) if the lymph glands:
   - were present in only one place,
   - were large (more than 4 cm in diameter) and continue to get larger,
   - were tender or painful and there was no nearby infection,
   - had local signs of chronic infection, e.g. fluctuant or matted or a sinus nearby,
   - had other signs of infection including fever, night sweats, weight loss, etc.,
   - accompanied by a strongly positive tuberculin test.

   See Chapter 14 pages 82–3.
2. *Nervous system damage* (due to HIV itself).
   Encephalitis (see Chapter 25 page 327) or chronic organic psychosis (see Chapter 35, page 471). These are due to the virus. Chronic infections of the meninges or brain (see Chapter 25 pages 326–7) or an apparent tumour of the brain can all occur. They can occur at any time, but by the time the patient has clinical AIDS, the patient has usually already developed symptoms of these, e.g. becoming forgetful and having difficulty in walking, etc.
   Some infections (especially cryptococcus and toxoplasmosis) occur later in the disease and cause death by damaging the nervous system further.
   See Chapter 35 and Chapter 28 for management.
3. *Acute cough and fever/pneumonia* (due to infection with usual pneumonia organisms (e.g. *Pneumococcus*)).
   Pneumonia is much more common in patients with the decreased immunity in all stages of HIV infection. It has the usual symptoms and signs, etc. and is treated in the usual way (see Chapter 20 page 220).
   Note that pneumonia due to *Pneumocystis carinii* common in HIV patients in industrialised countries is rarely diagnosed in developing countries, but could be underdiagnosed. See page 192.
4. *Chronic cough and fever/tuberculosis* (due to infection with the usual *Mycobacterium tuberculosis* organisms).
   Tuberculosis is 5–10 times as likely if HIV infection is present than if it is not. In 1995, about a third of the 17 million HIV infected people in the world also had been infected with tuberculosis. About 50% of patients with both infections will develop tuberculosis disease; whereas without HIV infection only about 10% of tuberculosis-infected patients develop tuberculosis

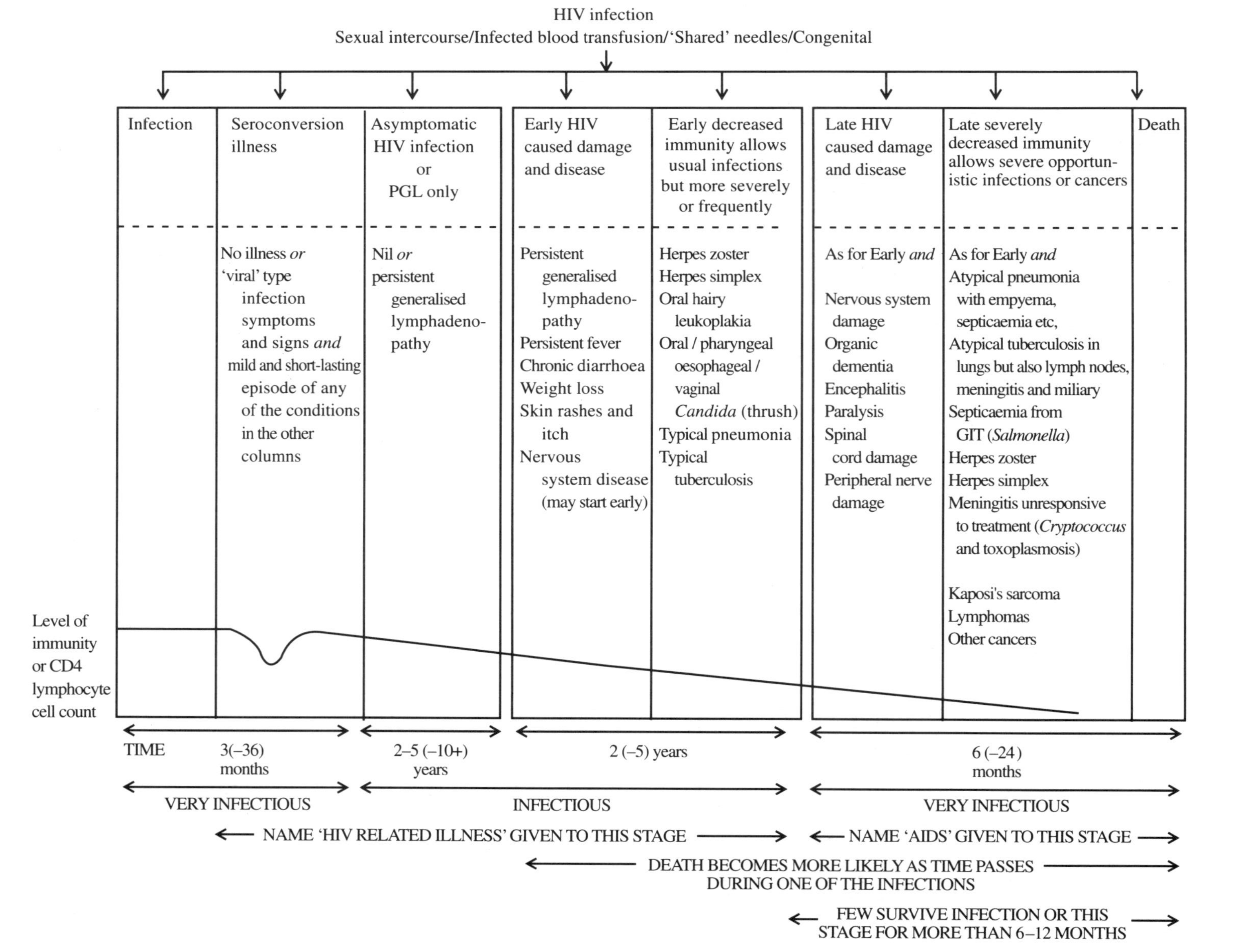

Figure 19.22 This shows the progress of HIV infection.

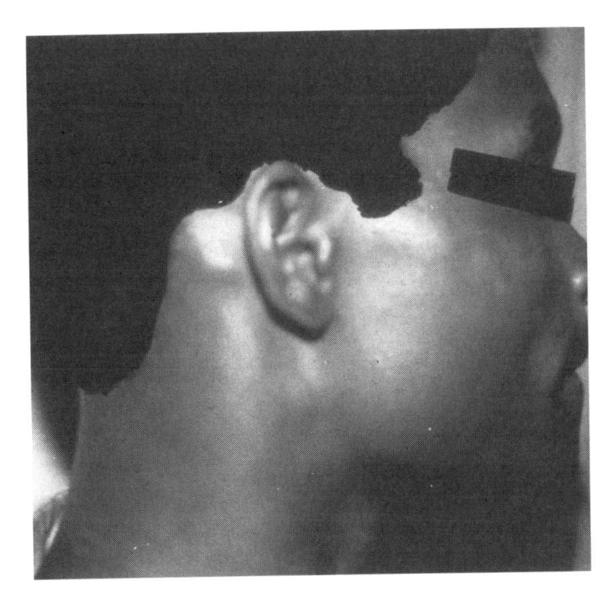

Figure 19.23 Persistent generalized lymphadenopathy (PGL) in HIV infection.

disease. Up to half of the people seen with tuberculosis, could also have HIV infection. In early HIV infection where there is reasonable immunity, the symptoms and signs of tuberculosis will be the same as for other people. However, later in the HIV infection, when there is little cellular immunity, tuberculosis may be unusual, e.g.

- lower not upper parts of lungs affected,
- pleural effusions more common,
- sputum tests positive for AFB less commonly,
- the tuberculin test (Mantoux) usually negative,
- lymph node, bowel, meningeal, and miliary tuberculosis more likely,
- unusual mycobacterial organisms which do not cause infection and could be resistant to the usual anti-tuberculosis drugs can infect patients (but this occurs usually only late in the course of HIV infections),
- reactions to anti-tuberculosis drugs especially thioacetazone are much more common and these reactions can be severe causing loss of most of the skin and mucous membranes and death.

Chronic cough and fever, if not due to pneumonia or empyema, which should be treated if present, are often due to tuberculosis. If this type of tuberculosis with HIV occurs in your area, find out from your Medical Officer if you should start antituberculosis treatment in these patients if the diagnosis is not proved by AFBs in the sputum. If antituberculosis drugs are started, they must be continued until the complete treatment is given, or resistant tuberculosis organisms will be produced. (See Chapter 14 page 83–91).

5. *Chronic diarrhoea and/or progressive weight loss and/or 'slim disease'* (due to HIV itself or infection with the usual gastroenteritis or diarrhoea organisms or due to 'opportunistic infections')

   Diarrhoea is often severe but can come and go. The bowel motions are often just watery without blood or mucus and the patient may have some colic around the umbilicus but it is usually mild and often absent. Weight loss keeps on occurring and is often severe, often more than 10 kg and up to 20% loss of the previous body weight (Figure 19.24). The cause of this may be one of the usual causes (see Chapter 23, page 282) and could be due to a tuberculosis infection including infection of the bowel wall; but if these are not present, it is probably due to the HIV infection itself damaging the bowel wall and stopping food being absorbed.

   For management see Chapter 23 page 282. Consider sending stool tests for AFBs. Treat with oral rehydration fluids and anti-diarrhoeal drugs (e.g. codeine phosphate 30 mg 4–6 hourly if needed). Always try treatment with sulphamethoxazole 800 mg/trimethoprim 160 mg (co-trimoxazole) twice daily for 10 days (for

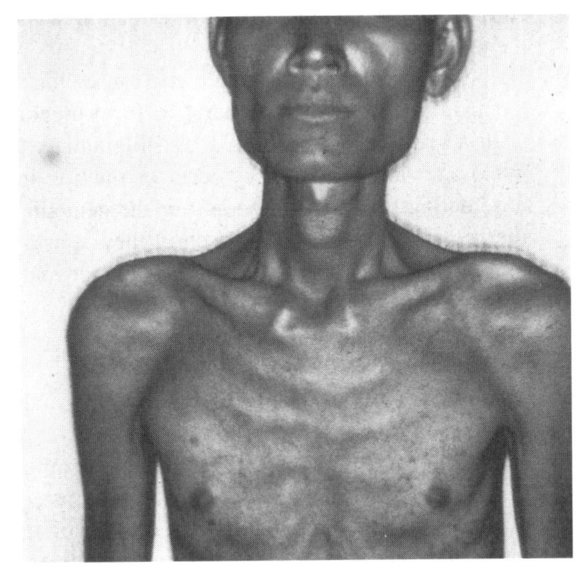

Figure 19.24 In parts of Africa this is called 'Slim Disease'.

Salmonella, Shigella and *Isospora belli*); then metronidazole 400 mg three times daily (for *Clostridium difficile* and *Microsporidia*); and chloramphenicol with the metronidazole if not improving by 5 days of metronidazole. However, do not continue giving of these drugs for more than 10 days for each. Most patients know the cause of the illness and that it will cause death soon and prefer to stay at home for treatment.

6. *Skin itching and rashes* (due to the HIV itself or infection).
   A chronic itchy maculopapular rash which may later become modular and darkly pigmented is very common. This may be due to the HIV virus itself. Sometimes a rash is due to scabies or to a fungal infection (one special kind is where it can be seen to cause inflammation around the hairs) or to secondary syphilis or to viral infections such as molluscum contagiosum or to a reaction to drugs given for treatment. Many of the non-infective skin conditions, such as seborrhoeic dermatitis or psoriasis, are worse during HIV infections.
   Make sure the rash does not need special treatment for scabies (Chapter 32 page 440) or fungus (Chapter 32 page 430) or syphilis (Chapter 19 page 165) or cessation of a drug (especially thiocetazone or sulphonamide). An antihistamine (e.g. promethazine or chlorpheniramine) and calamine lotion may help the itch of the HIV rash. See also page 192.
7. *Herpes simplex infection* (due to infection with the usual herpes simplex virus)
   Herpes simplex is a virus which can cause small but painful vesicles which burst to form ulcers with a grey base surrounded by inflamed red mucosa or skin. Usually they occur on the lips or nose during fevers ('cold sores') or the genitalia (herpes genitalis). In HIV infection they appear in other places, spread further, last longer and come back more frequently.
   See Chapter 19 page 177.
   See also Figure 19.27 page 187.
8. *Herpes zoster* (due to infection with the usual chickenpox virus)
   This is normally uncommon in young people unless they have HIV infection. If herpes zoster occurs in patients under 50 years of age, or if more than one nerve is affected, or if repeated attacks occur, always think of HIV infection.
   See Chapter 16 page 118.

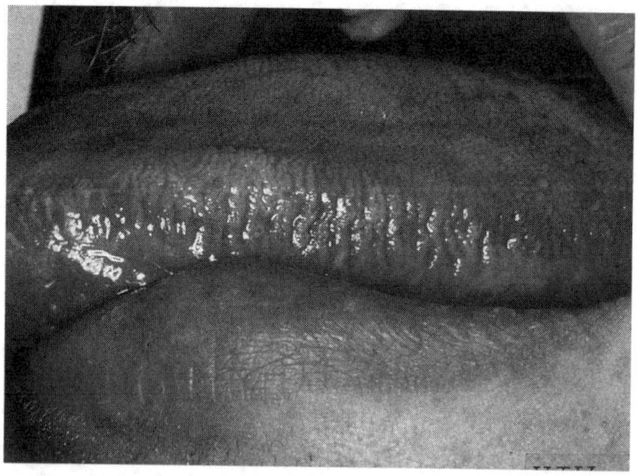

Figure 19.25 Oral hairy leukoplakia.

9. *Oral hairy leukoplakia* (probably due to EBV infection).
   Oral hairy leukoplakia (Figure 19.25) is probably caused by the Epstein–Barr virus (EBV). It causes patches of white material along the sides of the tongue. This white material is often in ridges or a series of lines. The material is stuck on and cannot be pushed off with a tongue depressor or spatula. It usually causes no symptoms and usually needs no treatment. Its main importance is that when you see it you should immediately ask yourself if this patient could have HIV infection.
10. *Candidiasis or moniliasis* (thrush infection in the mouth, throat and oesophagus; and in women, in the vagina) (due to infection with the usual (*Candida* or *Monilia* fungal organisms).
    Candida is a fungus which normally lives in all normal mouths and vaginas. An overgrowth of *Candida* occurs if other organisms in these areas are killed by antibiotics or if there is more than the usual amount of sugar present, i.e. diabetes mellitus, or if the patient is inhaling steroids for asthma, and at times in the mouth of normal babies. In all other conditions, the growth of enough *Candida* to be able to be seen in the mouth as white patches on top of red inflamed mucosa or there just being very red inflamed swollen mucosa, is very suggestive of HIV infection (Figure 19.26). The *Candida* overgrowth causes pain in the mouth, worse on eating or drinking. If the *Candida* also spreads to the oesophagus, then there is pain in the front of the chest on swallowing.
    Vaginal candidiasis (see Chapter 19 page 168) occurs more frequently in women who have HIV.

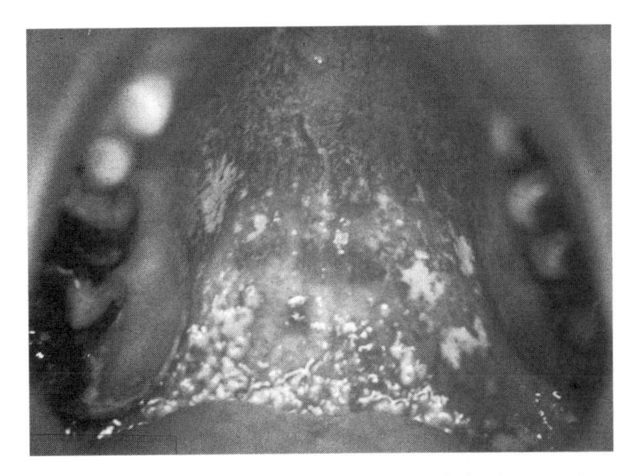

Figure 19.26 This appearance of *Candida* in the mouth should make you think of HIV infection if other conditions do not exist.

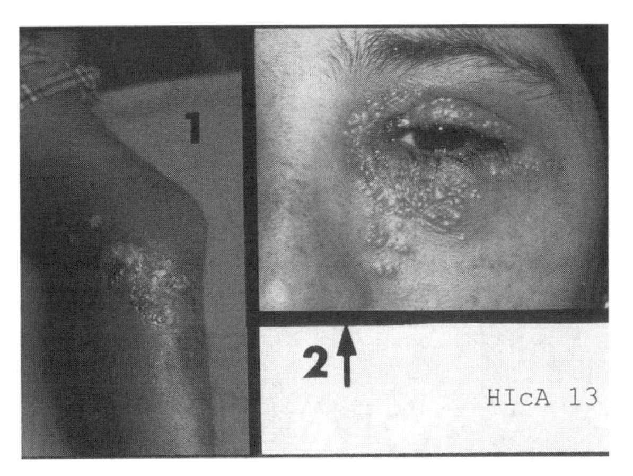

Figure 19.27 Photograph 1 shows an inflamed ulcerated area with a discharge of pus and blood. Some areas have healed. This patient had a chronic bacterial skin infection which improved with treatment but then came back. This was because of decreased body defence due to HIV infection. The treatment is more antibiotic and more dressings until it is fully healed.
Photograph 2 shows a patient with herpes simplex infection around the eye. Herpes in such an unusual place with so many vesicles should make you think of decreased immunity and HIV infection.

Treatment is with the special anti-candida drugs such as nystatin or natamycin or amphotericin mixtures or lozenges, or if these are not available, crystal violet 0.5% water solution, held in the mouth for as long as possible, then swallowed, 3 times a day after eating and before sleeping.

11. *Minor skin injuries and infections* which become quickly severe and at times cause septicaemia (due to infection with usual skin organism such as staphylococci).
    Always think of HIV infection as well as diabetes mellitus in such patients (Figure 19.27).
    See Chapter 32 page 439 and Chapter 12 page 53 for management.
12. *High fever (PUO)* (due to infection with the usual organisms causing infections).
    See Chapter 36 page 482 for diagnosis and management. This treatment will probably include antimalarials and, if needed, antibiotics (including chloramphenicol) for septicaemia (often for organisms from the bowel such as salmonellae) and, if needed, antituberculosis drugs (which must be continued until the full course is completed).
13. *Leishmaniasis (and other protozoal and tropical diseases)* (due to infection with the usual leishmaniasis organisms).
    Patients who were previously infected with leishmaniasis organisms but had immunity so good that no signs developed, and patients who had leishmaniasis previously and were successfully treated, may develop visceral leishmaniasis after they become infected with HIV. In patients infected with HIV, visceral leishmaniasis may not respond as well as expected to treatment and the patient may develop more rashes and other side effects to treatment than expected.
    See Chapter 18 page 142.
    As yet there is no proof that other protozoal and other tropical diseases (other than the above) become worse when HIV infection develops but it would be expected that more will be found.
14. *Kaposi's sarcoma* (due probably to infection with a special herpes organism).
    Kaposi's sarcoma is a cancer or tumour which is due to overgrowth of blood vessel lining cells. It is probably caused by a special herpes virus. Slow-growing Kaposi's tumours on the hands and feet in patients who are otherwise well have been present in Africa for years. However, in HIV infection, the lesions of Kaposi's sarcoma grow more quickly and more and more keep coming. They especially affect the roof of the mouth, tip of the nose, lower eye lid, penis and groin; but they can spread all over the body (Figure 19.28). They can look like a plaque or nodule. They can be red but become black. They can ulcerate. There is surrounding oedema. Lymph nodes, lungs, bowel and other organs can also be involved.

A

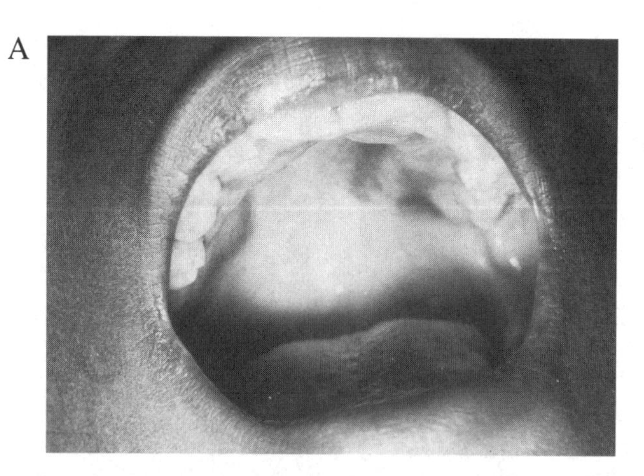

B

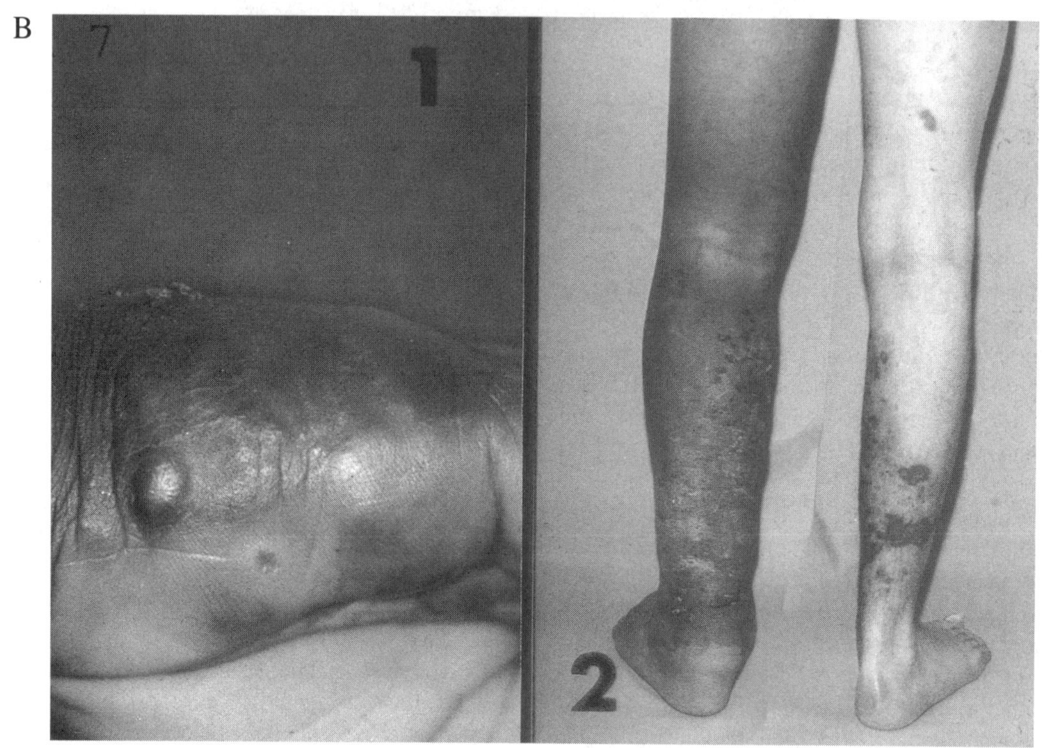

Figure 19.28 Kaposi's sarcoma of (A) mouth, (B) hand and legs.

Radiotherapy (and at times anticancer drugs) may help a little but are not usually available. No treatment, except of symptoms, is possible.

15. *Lymphomas*
    See Chapter 22 page 263.

Tests

There is no way of being absolutely certain in most health centres, whether a patient has an HIV infection or not. There is a blood test (at present in most places an ELISA test for HIV antibodies, or in some places a rapid immunobinding assay) available in some hospitals and health centres, but it is still expensive. As the antibodies do not kill the virus which is present in the body cells, most of the patients with a positive antibody test do have the infection and are infectious. Occasionally the test is falsely positive when the patient does not have the HIV infection. At times a second (or more complicated, expensive) test is needed (but usually cannot be afforded).

A blood test for HIV is needed only if it will change the management of the patient. In many rural areas the result will not change what can be done for the patient, and is not really needed.

The blood test for HIV is, however, needed in any hospital or health centre which gives blood transfusions; and the HIV serology test should be done and be negative on any blood before it is transfused.

It may take 3 or more months after infection before the blood test becomes positive so a negative blood test does not make it certain that the patient does not have HIV infection.

Pre-test counselling is needed before an HIV blood test is taken, to help the patient decide to have the test or not and to be prepared for the reseult.

The advantages of having the test include (if positive):

- no continuing worry about having or not having HIV infection,
- able to make better decisions for the future, e.g. getting pregnant,
- know to get early treatment of any infection.

The disadvantages of getting the test include (if positive):

- unable to get life insurance,
- unable sometimes to get visas to travel overseas,
- risk of loss of job,
- risk of loss of family support,
- risk of discrimination from the community.

Counselling should prepare patients for a positive result as, when told a positive result, patients do not often recall what is said to them. Counselling should also prepare them for a negative result so that they can use the relief that comes from this to reinforce preventive measures against possible future exposure to AIDS infection.

Differential diagnosis

The two conditions most likely to be confused with HIV infection are tuberculosis without HIV infection (see Chapter 14 page 75) and depression (see Chapter 35 page 474). Of course it is possible for patients with HIV infection to develop both of these conditions.

HIV infection can be diagnosed with certainty only by a positive blood test in a patient who may have HIV infection, especially if there are consistent symptoms or signs or other special tests available.

HIV, later in its course, is probable if there are (WHO clinical definition of AIDS):

1. any two of the following major signs:
   - weight loss more than 10%,
   - chronic diarrhoea for more than 1 month,
   - a fever, constant or intermittent, for more than 1 month, for which there is no obvious cause and no response to the usual treatment;

   and any one of the following minor signs:
   - chronic cough for more than 1 month,
   - generalised itchy rash,
   - herpes zoster which comes back,
   - *Candida* infection of the mouth,
   - herpes simplex which has spread over the body or is getting worse,
   - generalised lymphadenopathy,

   for which there is no obvious cause and no response to the usual treatment;

   or
2. disseminated Kaposi's sarcoma *or* meningitis due to *Cryptococcus* (i.e. a fungal meningitis not responsive to treatment with antibacterial and antituberculosis treatment);

in the absence of any known cause for loss of immunity, e.g. long-term high dose prednisolone or cortisone treatment, lymphoma or certain other cancers, chemotherapy drugs for cancer, etc.

Suspect HIV infection in a patient who has an infection which:

1. does not respond as usual to treatment, or
2. comes back unexpectedly after treatment appeared to cure it,
3. is an unusual infection,
4. is in a person who is from one of the risk groups for HIV infection, i.e.
   - prostitute,
   - patient with an STD,
   - someone who has spent a long time away from his family and community (e.g. immigrant worker or truck driver or sailor),
   - male homosexual,
   - drug addict.

Management

There is, at the time of writing, no cure for HIV infection. A number of drugs including zidovudine (or AZT) have shown some effect against the virus especially if they are used early in the infection and especially if a number of drugs are used together to slow the development of symptoms and signs. However, they also have marked side effects in the patient and are very very expensive. It may be that a new drug, not yet discovered, or a combination of drugs will kill the virus. However, this is not yet possible and when it is possible, it is likely that for many years the cost of these drugs will be far more than most people could ever afford.

Help, however, can be given to people with HIV infection, including the following:

1. Counselling or helping them decide how to cope with the disaster of their being HIV positive. Give them also the little good news that if they care for their health well, they may have 5 or more years after infection until severe disease develops.
2. Treatment of symptoms is possible. Make sure you always treat as above and for the following:
   - itch with, e.g. antihistamines,
   - nausea with, e.g. chlorpromazine,
   - diarrhoea with, e.g. codeine,
   - fever with aspirin or paracetamol and if needed, anti-malarials,
   - any infection with appropriate antibiotic and other treatment possible as this will help stop symptoms from the infection.

   However for details on diagnosis and treatment of symptoms see pages 191–4 and 183–8.

Counselling

Counselling is the major part of managing HIV infection. Counselling is not for the health worker to tell people what they should do (especially as this may make them just decide to do exactly what they are already doing). Counselling is to help people make their own decisions about what to do. Listen to what the patient says after encouraging them to talk about themselves, their circumstances, their problems and their feelings. Show them that you understand them and feel the same feelings that they feel. Give correct information about all the important things above, to help them make correct decisions. Help them to actually come to making a decision and try to not let them just stay as they are without a plan. Support them, and try to give them confidence in what they decide to do, and help them to do it.

Counselling needs privacy so that people can say and act how they really think and feel. Counselling needs to be done by people who are accepted and trusted by the patient and have the knowledge and the time to do the counselling properly. It is likely that it is best for a special couple of health workers, or if these are not available, religious or community or other leaders to be found, who can be given the knowledge and have the time to spend doing this counselling, as it cannot all be done by the officer in charge of the health centre.

Counselling will occur at many different times.

1. *Preventive counselling.*
   This is done at all times that the subject of sexual relations, drug addiction, etc. comes up; when advice is given how to prevent the transfer of AIDS infection.
2. *Pre-test counselling* is done before the HIV test See Chapter 19 page 188.
3. *Post-test counselling, if the HIV test is positive.*
   This takes time and privacy and the patient should be told only when both of these are available. See Figure 19.29.
   Some patients cry. They need to be allowed to do so. Some patients are so shocked that they understand nothing of what is said to them. They need to be made to talk and engage in conversation. Some patients become angry. It is important that the health worker also does not become angry. Some patients become agitated. It is important that the health worker should stay calm. Information on HIV infection should be supplied according to what the patient can understand. Literature for them to take home and read, if appropriate, should be supplied. Ask what the particular worries are going to be straight away and help them try to deal with these first. Discuss how the patient will tell his partner. Discuss which family members will help and how to get their help. Discuss what support groups are available and how to get their help.

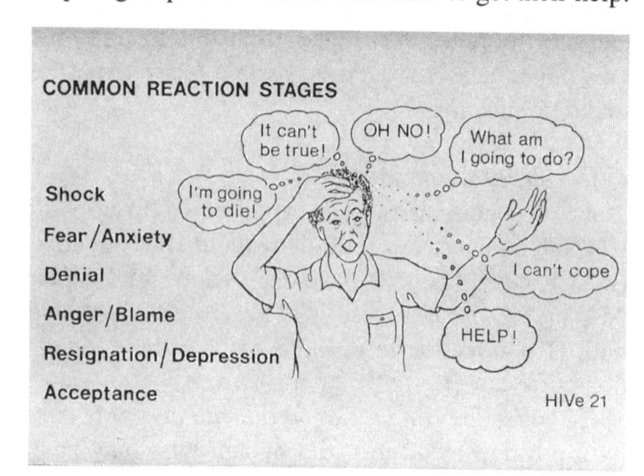

Figure 19.29 You must have time, privacy, knowledge, ability to help and you must show the patient you understand and care if you are going to properly counsel a patient who has a positive HIV test.

Discuss 'safe sex' and the precautions that should be taken (see Chapter 19 page 159). Discuss how care can be carried out at home (see Chapter 19 page 195).

4. *Crisis counselling* is given when a problem gets too much for the patient to cope with and they become distressed or agitated. This counselling is to help them get back control of the situation again.
5. *Post-test counselling, if the HIV test is negative.* Explain that the HIV test takes 3 months but occasionally up to 3 years to become positive after infection and this must be taken into account. Use the patient's happiness at the test's results to try to make sure that in future he lives and behaves in such a way that there will never be further worries about another HIV infection in that patient.

Although there is, at present, no drug or other treatment to cure the HIV infection, not all patients who have the infection will have developed any of the clinical conditions caused by the infection. The methods, including drugs, needed for treatment of most of the chest, bowel and others problems caused by the HIV, are available in health centres. Others, which may be tried and which you may read about in other books, are very expensive and often have severe side effects and need to be given in hospitals. However, many are not available even in many hospitals. As well as this, the condition often returns soon after treatment stops. In most health centres, most important treatment as outlined in the sections of this book, is all the treatment possible. As well as this, many patients may prefer to stay at home for their treatment and collect drugs for symptoms as needed, attending the health centre only for treatment of any severe infections etc. that occur.

Patients are usually treated in a normal health centre ward. However, all the precautions to prevent spread of the HIV as outlined below and as for hepatitis B (see Chapter 24 page 308) are carried out. Also do not put patients who have HIV infection together with patients who have or may have tuberculosis and have not been on proper antituberculosis treatment for at least 2 weeks as the HIV patients can easily be infected by tuberculosis organisms.

Notes on Diagnosis and Treatment of Common Symptoms in the Various Body Systems

1. Treat any other sexually transmitted diseases present

See Chapter 19 for details.

Urethral discharge

- see page 169; or *if unavailable* sulphamethoxazole 4000 mg/trimethoprim 800 mg in one dose for 3 days; *with*, if possible, gentamycin 240 mg IMI one dose, *and*
- doxycycline 200 mg daily for 7 days; but not *if pregnant*, when *give instead* erythromycin 500 mg four times a day for 7 days.

Vaginal discharge

- as above *and*
- metronidazole 2 g in one dose once orally *and*
- nystatin 100,000 unit pessaries or vaginal tablets 1–2 once daily for 2 weeks.

Genital ulcer with or without inguinal bubo

- benzathine penicillin 2.4 million units IMI once *and*
- sulphamethoxazole 800 mg/trimethoprim 160 mg (co-trimoxazole) twice daily for 7 days, *unless pregnant* when *give instead* (or if fails) erythromycin 500 mg three to four times daily for 7 days

Inguinal bubo without genital ulcer

- doxycycline 200 mg daily for 14 days, *unless pregnant* when *give instead* erythromycin 500 mg daily for 2 weeks

Anogenital warts

- 20% podophyllum applied to the lesions

2. Treat any skin problems present

See Chapter 32 for details.

Herpes simplex

- keep clean and dry.

Varicella zoster

- keep clean and dry and give analgesics as needed

Tinea

- benzoic acid compound ointment (Whitfield ointment) or salicyclic acid paint (Castellani's paint) *or*
- if available and not cured by the above, clotrimazole or miconazole to affected areas twice daily *or*, if necessary,
- griseofulvin by mouth

Candida

- nystatin ointment or cream, *or* if unavailable
- crystal (gentian) violet 0.5% in water twice daily

Impetigo/furuncles

- penicillin or other antibiotics – especially cloxacillin or erythromycin if does not respond
- wash all over with an antiseptic regularly
- dressings

Pyomyositis

- see Chapter 28 page 386

Papular folliculitis

- antihistamines
- calamine lotion
- antifungals such as clotrimazole or miconazole together with hydrocortisone or other adrenocorticosteroid cream

Seborrhoeic dermatitis

- see Chapter 32 page 448, and, if needed,
- shampoos containing zinc pyrathione or selenium sulphide, and, if needed,
- hydrocortisone 1% cream

Psoriasis

- strong coal tar 10% and salicylic acid 1–2% ointment twice daily

Scabies

- see Chapter 32 page 440 benzyl benzoate

Kaposi's sarcoma

- treatment of symptoms is the only thing possible apart from aspirin or if this is not effective,
- one of the newer non-steroidal anti-inflammatory drugs (e.g. naproxen, ibuprofen or indomethacin) may help.

3. Treat any mouth problems present

Candida infection

- amphotericin or nystatin or natamycin lozenges or mixtures *or*, if unavailable,
- crystal (gentian) violet 0.25% solution in water three times a day after meals and at night, held in the mouth as long as possible before swallowing.

Hairy leukoplakia

- no treatment possible but not usually needed

Mouth infections

- penicillin or
- metronidazole if penicillin ineffective

Mouth ulcers

- mouth washes with salty water, but if this and treatment of *Candida* not effective
- refer to Medical Officer

Kaposi's sarcoma

- treatment of symptoms is all that is possible
- aspirin if pain, or if this is not effective
- one of the newer non-steroidal anti-inflammatory drugs (e.g. naproxen, ibuprofen or indomethacin) may help

4. Treat any gastrointestinal problems present

Difficulty or pain on swallowing

- treat as for candidiasis of mouth (see above) and if does not settle
- refer to Medical Officer

Diarrhoea

- give rehydration if needed (see Chapter 23 page 285)
- send stool tests if possible for ova, cysts, parasites and for culture of ordinary organisms
- treat with sulfamethoxazole 800 mg/trimethoprim 160 mg (co-trimoxazole) twice daily for 10 days and *if not settled*, give
- metronidazole 400 mg three times a day for 10 days and *if by 5 days is not settling, add*
- chloramphenicol 1 g four times a day for 10 days
- codeine phosphate 30 mg each 4 hours if needed for diarrhoea if the above are not successful

5. Treat any respiratory problems present

Pneumonia

- penicillin or sulphamethoxazole/trimethoprim (co-trimoxazole) for 5–10 days – see Chapter 21 page 220 if not settling
- look for complications especially empyema or tuberculosis and treat with doxycycline or tetracycline
- if not settling, look for any complications especially empyema or tuberculosis needing treatment, otherwise chloramphenicol
- if still not settling, will need further sputum examination for AFB and referral to the Medical Officer
- if this is not possible, start the patient at this time on sulphamethoxazole 1600 mg/trimethoprim 320 mg (co-trimoxazole) three times a day for a small adult and four times a day for a large adult (treatment for *Pneumocystis carinii* pneumonia)

Tuberculosis (not getting better on treatment)

- send sputum for examination for AFB and if possible other organisms and parasites
- check that the patient is really swallowing his treatment

- check that the patient does not need treatment for non-tuberculous infection as well, i.e. pneumonia
- check that the patient does not have a complication such as empyema
- if none of these can be found or treated, refer to Medical Officer

6. Treat any neurological or mental problems present

Acute organic psychosis

See Chapter 35 page 471 and think especially of:

- malaria, pneumonia, meningitis, septicaemia
- low oxygen from anaemia, heart failure, pneumonia, pneumothorax
- dehydration
- drug reaction
- acute liver failure especially from reaction to drugs
- syphilis – send blood test
- chronic meningitis – do a lumbar puncture if any neck stiffness
- trypanosomiasis – do a blood test (but not a lumbar puncture) if this is possible

Treat *headache*

Think of:

- local causes – do examination for dental abscess, otitis media, sinusitis, etc.
- infections especially malaria, syphilis, trypanosomiasis – send blood tests for these
- meningitis especially chronic meningitis – do a lumbar puncture if there is a stiff neck, looking for bacterial meningitis, tuberculous meningitis and sending the CSF for examination for cryptococcus and other opportunistic infections
- cerebral tumours or abscesses especially with opportunistic infections

Refer to Medical Officer or if this is not possible, give both chloramphenicol 1 g four times a day and sulfadoxine 500 mg and pyrimethamine 25 mg twice daily for 6 weeks (for toxoplasmosis and *Nocardia* infections) and chloramphenicol 1 g four times a day for 2 weeks (for cerebral abscess).

Treat *difficulty walking*

- check for spinal tuberculosis or spinal bacterial abscess by examination and refer to Medical Officer for X-ray of any suspicious signs
- syphilis – send blood for serological test for syphilis
- schistosomiasis – if in an area where schistosomiasis occurs, give praziquantel 30 mg/kg one dose and a further dose 6 hours later
- vitamin B12 and folate deficiency – send blood for examination for macrocytosis
- side effects of isoniazid – give pyridoxine 100 mg daily

See Chapter 25 page 326. In almost all of these cases the patient will of course be transferred to a Medical Officer for investigation.

Treat *sight getting worse*

- if on ethambutol, stop ethambutol and replace with streptomycin

Treat *pain in or burning feeling in feet* (peripheral nerve damage)

- If on anti-tuberculosis treatment, give pyridoxine 100 mg daily and if available, also vitamin B compound

In other cases give:

- vitamin B compound if available
- amitriptyline 75 mg at night or *if this is ineffective*
- try an anti-convulsant such as phenytoin 100–300 mg at night *or* carbamazepine 100–200 mg twice daily

7. Treat any fever present

See Chapter 35 page 482.

- Think especially of malaria, pneumonia, septicaemia, tuberculosis and especially if rash, drug side effects.

8. Treat any anaemia present

See Chapter 21 page 240.

Consider the possibility of side effects of any drugs being given.

9. Treat any kidney disease present

See Chapter 26 page 360.

Note that HIV itself can cause nephrotic syndrome or kidney failure.

10. Treat any cardiovascular system problem present

Treat heart failure, see Chapter 27 page 371.

Note that HIV infection can also cause heart failure.

11. Treat any shock present

See Chapter 27 page 378.

Note that acute failure of the adrenal glands due to infections can cause shock and would need treatment with adrenocorticosteroids. See Chapter 30 page 408.

12. Treat any arthritis present
See Chapter 28 page 399.

- treat any bacterial arthritis in the usual way with aspiration and antibiotics
- if on any tuberculosis treatment, consider side effects of pyrazinamide and give aspirin
- for all cases give aspirin, or if ineffective, consider one of the newer non-steroidal anti-inflammatory drugs (e.g. naproxen, ibuprofen or indomethacin)

Control and prevention

1. Kill the organisms in the body of the original host or reservoir. This is as yet not possible.
2. Stop the means of spread. See below.
3. Increase the resistance of possible new hosts. This is as yet not possible. It is hoped, however, that soon a vaccine may be available to immunise against HIV infection.
4. Prophylactic treatment, drugs, vaccine, etc. for this are not yet available. When they do become available, treatment of any health worker possibly infected by needle stick or other such injury likely to cause infection, would be very important.

The following things are important in stopping the spread of the infection.

Ensure information about safe sexual practices is available to everyone
The only really safe sexual practice for an uninfected person is to have sexual intercourse with only one other uninfected 'faithful' partner (that is, one who does not have sexual intercourse with any one else). There is no way to tell from a person's appearance if they are infected or not. This can be done only by knowing the person and talking to them about it.

A person who has many sexual partners is at high risk of HIV infection. A person who has sexual intercourse with just one person but that person has had many sexual partners is at high risk for HIV infection. To reduce the risk of HIV infection, people need to reduce the number of their sexual partners; although there will always be a risk until sexual intercourse occurs only with one uninfected faithful partner.

If a person has sexual relations with more than one person or with a possibly infected person, some things will reduce the risk of getting HIV infection.

1. Change sexual activities from high risk to low risk activities. High risk activities are when semen or vaginal fluid comes into contact with the partner's oral (mouth), genital or anal (rectal) mucosa. Low risk practices are when these fluids come into contact only with skin which is not damaged (as unbroken skin is not able to be entered by the virus). This means that a low risk practice is when a man's penis does not enter the partner's vagina, anus or mouth; or a woman's vaginal fluid does not enter the partner's mouth.
2. Use of a condom will greatly reduce the risk of infected semen or vaginal fluid getting into the other person. It is important that people not only know this, but are shown how to use condoms properly and do have condoms available and do actually use condoms each and every time they have sexual intercourse.

It is most important that patients with AIDS are given the above information.

Health education for groups of particular risk of HIV infection to be carried out whenever possible. These would include:

- prostitutes,
- people who visit prostitutes,
- STD patients,
- those who are away from their community and family, e.g. migrant workers, truck drivers, sailors, etc.

Health education (see Figure 19.30) of special groups should be carried out whenever possible. These would include:

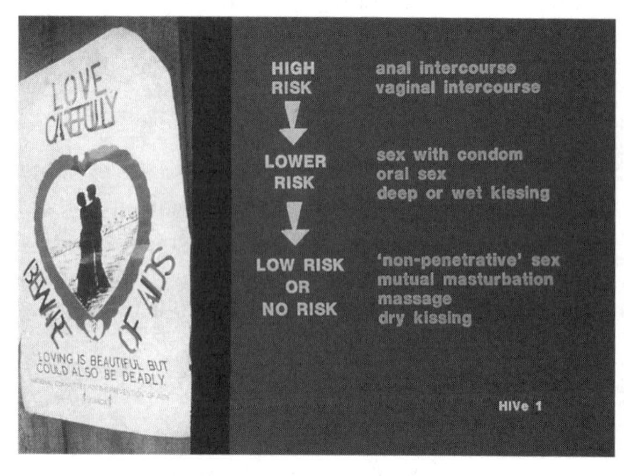

Figure 19.30 Posters and literature which are understood by the people in your area are needed to get them to understand how HIV infection is spread and how not to get the infection.

- school children,
- young people,
- groups of men,
- groups of women,
- those who can be reached by the mass media (radio, TV and newspapers).

If possible, some kind of measurement of the effects of these methods of health education should be carried out so that most effort can be put into those which are most effective.

Stop the spread by transfusion of infected blood

1. Do not transfuse anyone unless blood is really needed.
2. Do not transfuse blood unless the HIV test on that blood is negative before the blood is transfused.
3. Do not collect blood for transfusion from anyone who has any risk factors for HIV in the previous 3–6 months as they still could be infected but the HIV test not yet be positive.
4. Tell patients who have HIV infection they must not donate blood.

Stop spread of infection in the health centre

1. Do not allow health workers to get blood on them from patients in case the patient's blood is infected. Wear gloves and an apron or gown when doing dressings, etc. and use a 'no touch' technique. Use a mask which is waterproof and glasses or goggles if you are doing something which splashes droplets of blood or body fluid near your face. Use a mask for 'mouth to mouth' resuscitation. If blood does get on to a health worker, gently but completely wash off all this blood with soap and water.
2. Make sure health workers do not accidentally get injuries from needles and other sharp instruments. Do not put caps back on needles after the needle has been used. If possible use disposable needles which, together with other sharp disposable contaminated objects, are dropped into a 'sharps' plastic or cardboard strong container which, when full, is all burned then buried. If a needle-stick injury occurs, squeeze the wound to make it bleed and then wash it well with soap and water.
3. If you do artificial ventilation use a face mask or face shield (see Chapter 37 page 504).
4. Sterilise instruments, etc. correctly:
   - Soak for 30 minutes in disinfectant; then clean them carefully, wearing gloves, mask and eye protection, then sterilise by autoclaving or by steam or by boiling for 20 minutes or by dry heat at 170°C.
   - Suitable antiseptics include chlorine as in sodium hypochlorite solution (10,000 ppm chlorine) or household bleach diluted 1 in 10; gluteraldehyde 2% solution freshly prepared; formalin 4% solution; povidone iodide 2.5% (Betadine); hydrogen peroxide 6%. Note that alcohol and phenolic antiseptics (e.g. 'Dettol') are not adequate
5. Ensure all wounds etc. are covered.

Stop spread of HIV in the home

1. See Chapter 19 pages 179–80.
2. For the washing of plates, spoons, clothing, etc. use ordinary soap or detergent and water and if possible, use hot water or dry then in the sun.
3. Clothing, bedclothes, floors, etc. soiled with body fluids can be covered with household bleach diluted 1 in 10 for half an hour and then cleaned as usual.
4. The HIV patient must be told how he must not get his blood or body fluids into any one else's body. This will include safe sexual practices, not sharing sharp items such as razors, toothbrushes or tooth cleaning sticks, etc.

Stop the spread of HIV by drug addicts

1. Discourage people from becoming drug addicts.
2. Discourage drug addicts from using injected drugs.

If drug addicts do inject themselves, either get them to use a clean needle and syringe for each injection by using disposable needles and syringes or tell them how to clean the needles and syringes and sterilise them with a 1 in 10 solution of household bleach for half of an hour.

Stop the spread of HIV to unborn children

1. Advise any HIV patient against any pregnancy.
2. Supply contraceptive advice and condoms.
3. Do not stop HIV infected mothers breastfeeding their own child. The risk of this child contracting HIV from his mother's milk is less than the risk of the child dying from malnutriton or gastroenteritis, etc. if not breastfed. See page 180.

At the time of writing, the situation with HIV is different in different areas. What action the health worker should take will depend on how common HIV infection is in his area, how it is spread in that area and what facilities for diagnosis and treatment exist. These should therefore be discussed with the supervising Medical Officer. The action to be taken will depend on the above and should be written down under the headings in this book. Remember, however, that the situation and the correct thing to do will change as time goes by and the epidemiology of the disease and its treatment changes.

TREATMENT OF SEXUALLY TRANSMITTED DISEASES

Urethral discharge

1. Ciprofloxacin 500 mg by mouth once on an empty stomach
   or
   Ceftriaxone 250 mg IMI once
   or
   Spectinomycin 2 g IMI once
   or
   Sulfamethoxazole 4000 mg and trimethoprim 800 mg (co-trimoxazole) orally in 1 dose daily for 3 days
   and
   Gentamicin 240 mg IMI once if available

and

2. Doxycycline 100 mg orally twice daily for 7–10 days if not pregnant
   or
   Erythromycin 500 mg orally 4 times a day for 7–10 days if pregnant

and

3. Treatment for genital sore if present.

Genital sore

1. Benzathine penicillin 2.4 million units IMI once

and

2. Erythromycin 500 mg orally four times a day
   or
   Trimethoprim 160 mg and sulfamethoxazole 80 mg twice daily for 7 days if not pregnant

and

3. Treatment of urethral discharge if present.

20

Disorders of the Respiratory System

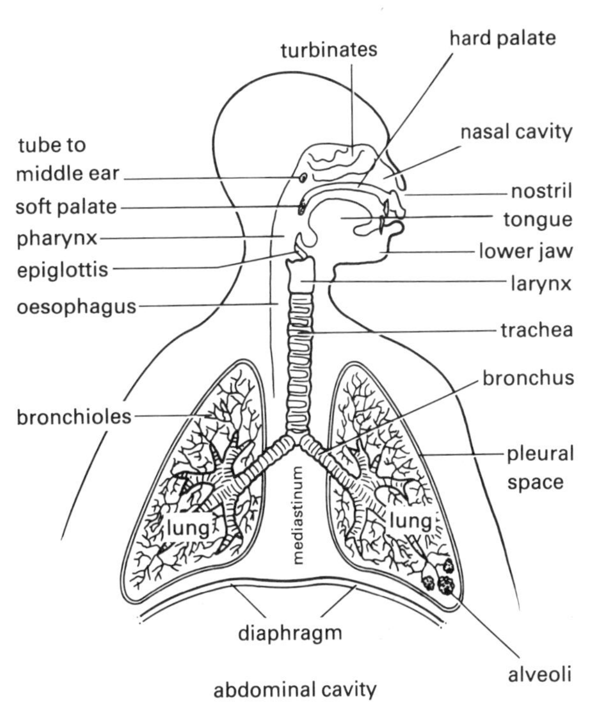

Figure 20.1 Anatomy of the upper and lower respiratory tracts.

Anatomy and physiology

All the cells of the body need oxygen. The cells make carbon dioxide while they work, which must be taken away. If the carbon dioxide is not taken away, it will poison the cells.

Air is about 20% oxygen, 80% nitrogen and much less than 1% carbon dioxide. The body cells take oxygen from the air and excrete carbon dioxide into the air (where it is used by plants which make it into oxygen again).

The oxygen and carbon dioxide are taken to and from the body cells in the blood. The respiratory system is where the body takes the oxygen from the air and puts it into the blood, and the carbon dioxide from the blood and puts it into the air. Taking air in and out of the respiratory system is called ventilation. Exchanging the oxygen and carbon dioxide is called respiration.

The respiratory system is in two parts – the upper respiratory tract and the lower respiratory tract (see Figure 20.1).

The upper respiratory tract is above the lowest part of the larynx or voice box. The work of the upper respiratory tract includes taking air to and from the lower respiratory tract, and warming, moistening, filtering and purifying the air; also speech, hearing and other things. The upper respiratory tract is often called the 'URT' or the ear, nose and throat 'ENT'. Figures 20.2, 20.3, 20.4 and 20.5 show the parts of the upper respiratory tract.

The lower respiratory tract consists of the trachea, bronchi and lungs (see Figure 20.1).

Air is taken to the lungs by air passages. Air enters the mouth or nose, goes through the larynx then down the trachea, which divides into two main bronchi. Each main bronchus divides into smaller and smaller bronchi (see Figures 20.1 and 20.6). The smallest bronchi end in little air bags or sacs known as alveoli. If the lungs are taken from a dead person, scissors can be used to cut along the bronchi, tracing each one, until they finally become so small that they cannot be seen. The appearance is something like the branches of a tree and the system of bronchi is often referred to as the bronchial tree. The smallest bronchi, called bronchioles, divide and lead into air sacs or alveoli (see Figure 20.11).

The lungs (see Figures 20.1, 20.7, 20.8) are inside the chest – one on each side. They are separated by the heart and the other structures of the mediastinum. The right lung consists of three smaller separate parts or lobes (upper, middle and lower lobes) and the left lung of two smaller separate parts or lobes (upper and lower lobes, although a part of the left upper lobe is called the lingular lobe). Each lobe has one bronchus bringing air to and from it.

Each lung is surrounded by a thin but strong air-tight membrane called the pleural membrane or the pleura. The pleura surrounding and fastened to each

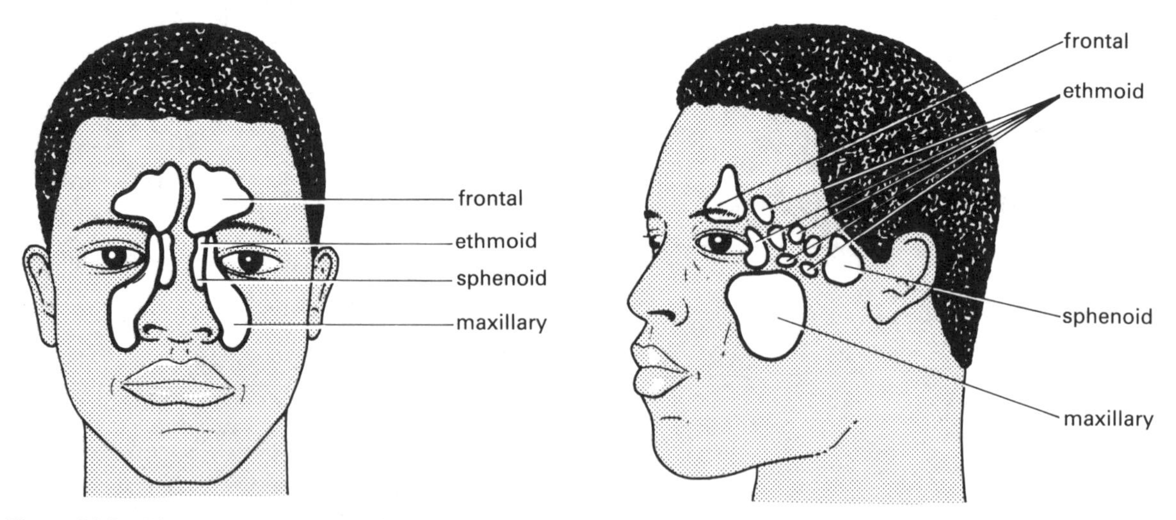

Figure 20.2 Diagrams to show the position of the paranasal sinuses.

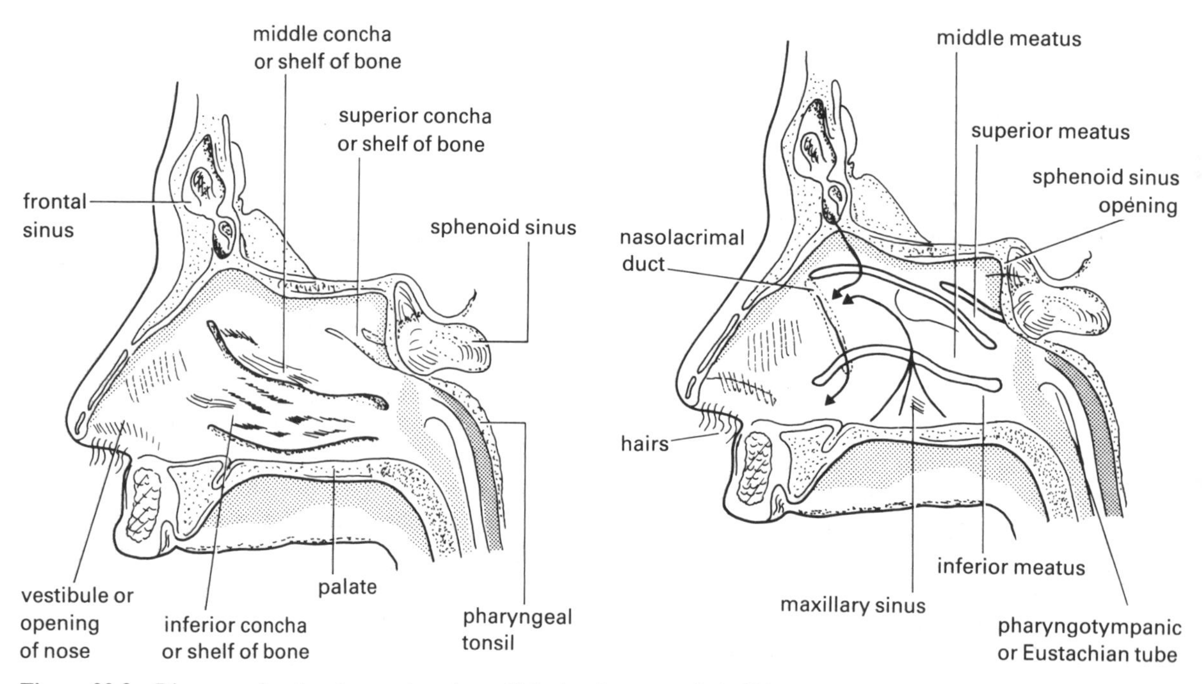

Figure 20.3 Diagrams showing the nasal cavity as if the head were cut in half from the front to back in the centre. The left diagram shows structures of the lateral (side) wall. In the right diagram parts of the conchae are removed to show the way the paranasal sinuses and naso-lacrimal duct (see Figure 31.1) drain into the nasal cavity.

lung is in turn surrounded by another layer of pleura which is on the inside of and fastened to the chest wall and the mediastinum. The two layers of pleura are not fastened to each other and so can easily move over each other. There is normally nothing between the two layers of pleura, except a thin layer of slippery fluid. (See Figure 20.9.)

Breathing is done by the muscles of the chest wall and the diaphragm (see Figure 20.10). During breathing in, the muscles pull the rib cage outwards and upwards and the diaphragm downwards. When the chest wall (with the outer layer of pleura) moves away, the lungs (with their inner layer of pleura) follow, and the lungs expand. The lungs expand because a negative pressure (or vacuum) is developed between the pleura lining the inside of the chest wall and the pleura lining the outside of the lungs when the chest and diaphragm start to move away from the

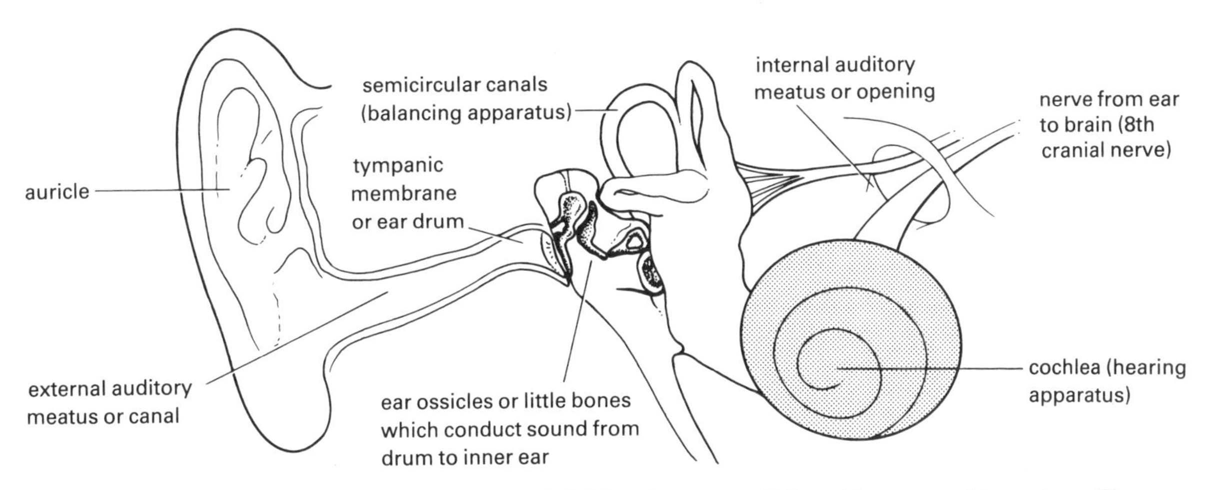

Figure 20.4 Diagram to show the ear especially its subdivisions into outer middle and inner ear and its anatomy. The middle ear is connected to the nasopharynx (back of the nose and throat) by means of the Eustachian or pharyngotympanic tube or canal.

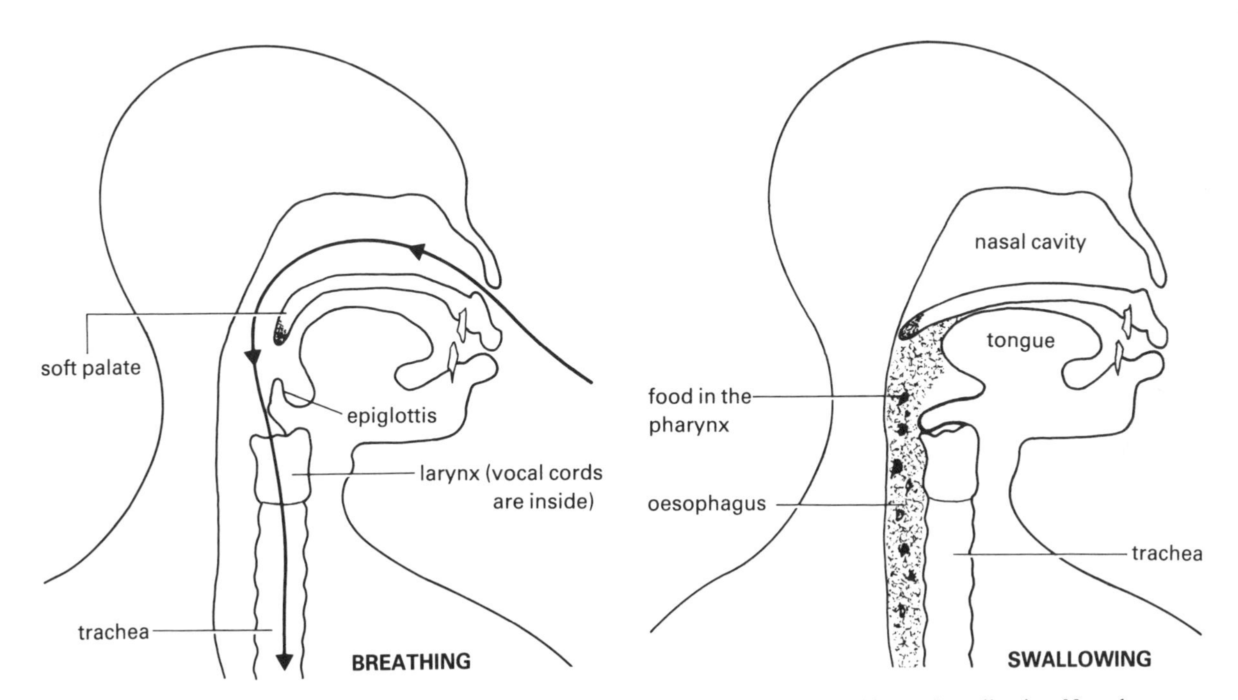

Figure 20.5 This diagram shows the changes in the upper respiratory tract during breathing and swallowing. Note the positions during swallowing of the soft palate (to stop food going into the nose) and of the epiglottis (to stop food going into the larynx and trachea, bronchi and lungs). This does not occur when the patient is deeply unconscious.

lungs. During breathing out, the muscles relax and the lungs which are somewhat elastic and stretched, contract and pull the chest wall and diaphragm with them – again because of the negative pressure between the pleura of the lungs and the pleura of the chest wall.

A system of blood vessels (called the pulmonary circulation) goes through the lungs. The pulmonary artery takes blood pumped by the right side of the heart. This blood is rather blue and is low in oxygen and high in carbon dioxide. The blood vessels divide into smaller and smaller vessels. When they are very small capillaries, exchange of oxygen and carbon dioxide occurs between their blood and the air in the alveoli. (See Figure 20.11.) The capillaries then join up to form veins. The blood in them is

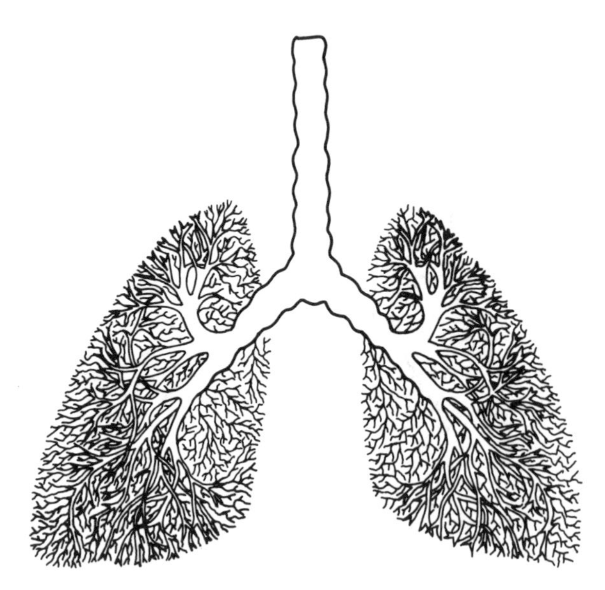

Figure 20.6 Diagram to show how the bronchi divide to form smaller and smaller bronchi (like branches of a tree). The smallest air passages lead into air sacs or alveoli (see Figure 20.11).

taken back to the left side of the heart by the pulmonary veins.

The blood in the pulmonary vein is more red, as it has a high content of oxygen and a low content of carbon dioxide.

The left-over air with high carbon dioxide content and low oxygen content is breathed out of the lungs through the bronchi, etc. and fresh air with high oxygen and low carbon dioxide content is breathed into the alveoli.

Pathology of the respiratory tract

Most diseases of the respiratory tract are caused by infection. These infections are usually caused by viral, bacterial or tuberculosis organisms; but there are others. HIV infection decreases immunity and has allowed respiratory infections to become much more common and severe. In the near future, diseases caused by smoking (especially COLD and lung cancer) are going to become more common as so many young people in developing countries have started to smoke tobacco. Some diseases are caused by allergy. Some are caused by dust and fumes in mines and factories. A few are caused by other things known and unknown.

Symptoms and signs of diseases of the respiratory tract

Symptoms of diseases of the upper respiratory tract

Ear

- pain in ear

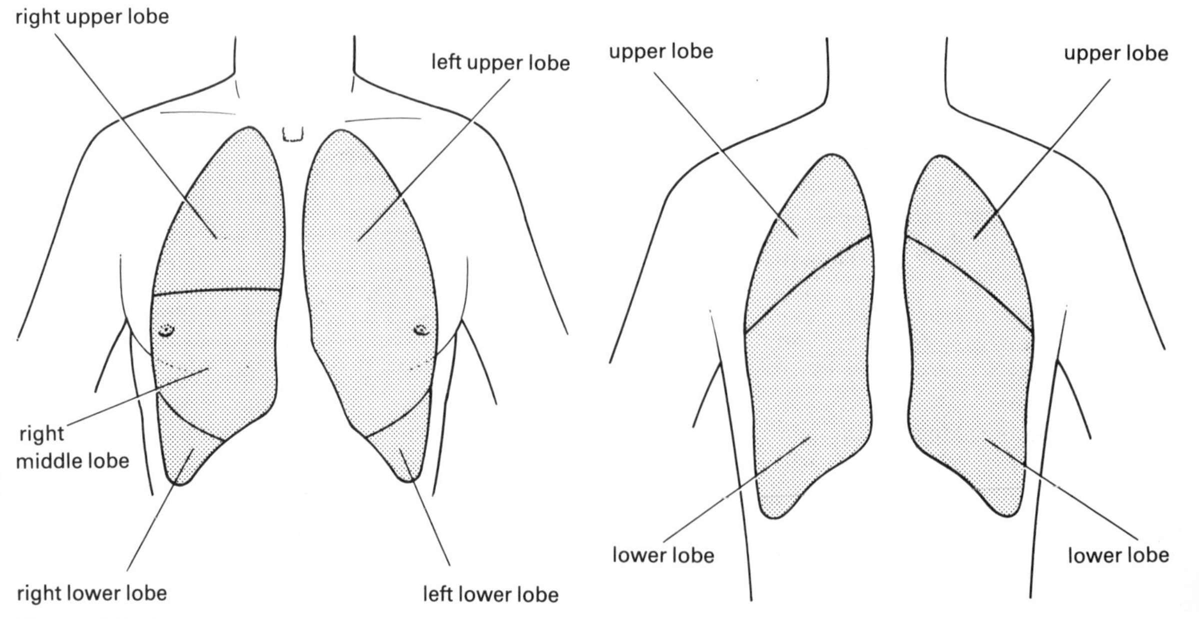

Figure 20.7 Diagrams to show the position of the lungs in the chest and to show which lobes of the lungs are affected when abnormal signs are found during examination of the front and back of the chest.

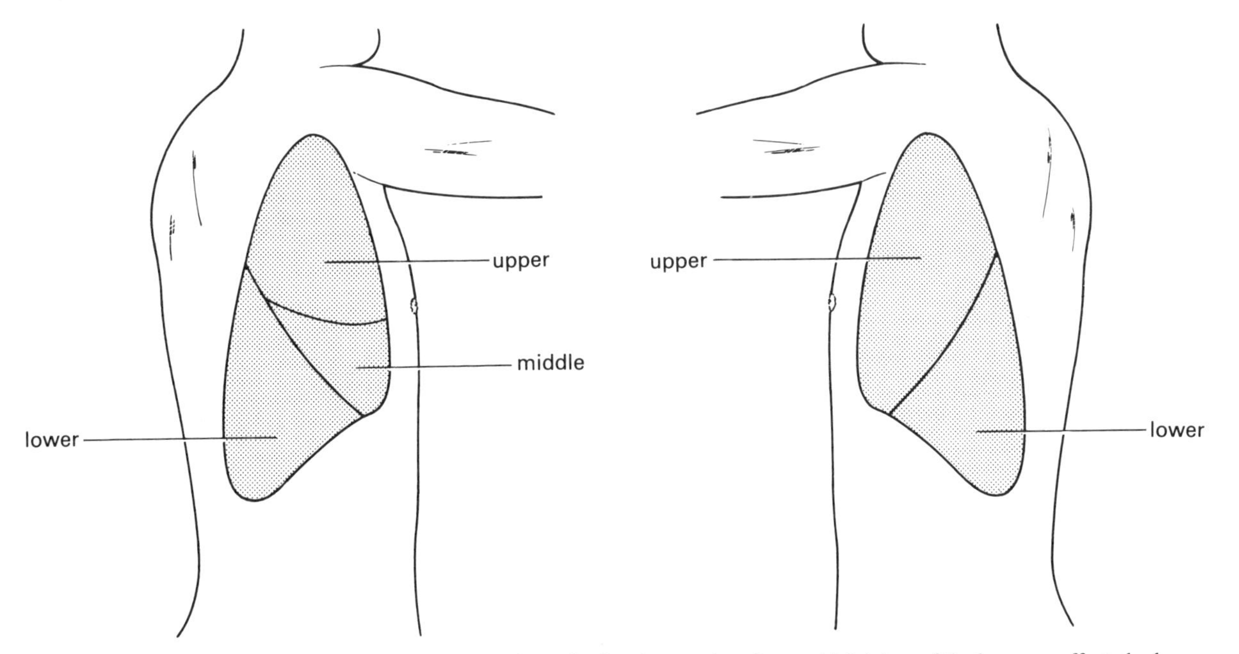

Figure 20.8 Diagram to show the position of the lungs in the chest and to show which lobes of the lung are affected when abnormal signs are found during examination of the lateral (side of the) chest.

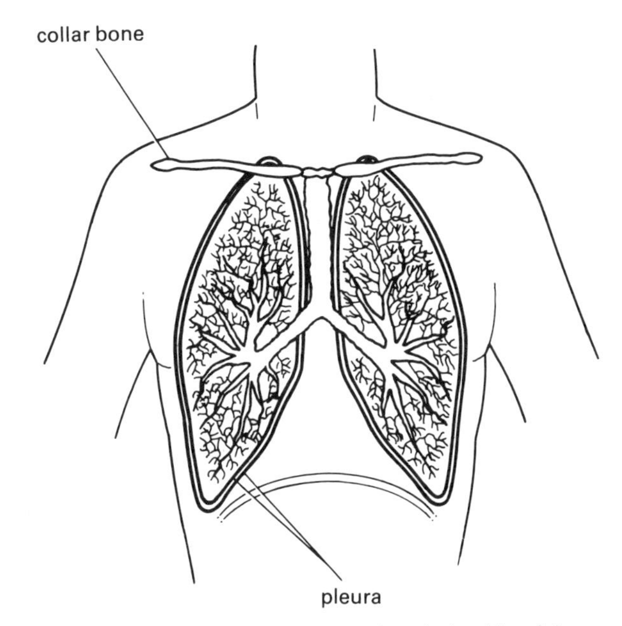

Figure 20.9 This diagram shows the relationship of the two layers of pleura to each other. (See also Figure 20.1.) There is normally no air and only a little fluid in each pleural space or cavity.

- discharge from ear
- deafness

Nose

- nasal discharge
  - clear fluid
  - pus
  - blood
- pain in face or forehead (over paranasal sinuses)

Throat

- sore throat
- hoarse voice or loss of voice

All

- cough

For causes and management of these symptoms, see page 211 onwards.

Signs of diseases of the upper respiratory tract

Ear

- external canal
  - discharge (clear fluid, pus, blood)
  - foreign body
  - injury
  - dermatitis
  - inflammation of the whole canal
  - furuncle (pimple or boil)
- drum
  - retraction (pulled in)
  - bulging (pushed out)
  - inflammation (dilated vessels, dull or red or yellow, loss of light reflex, red or yellow)

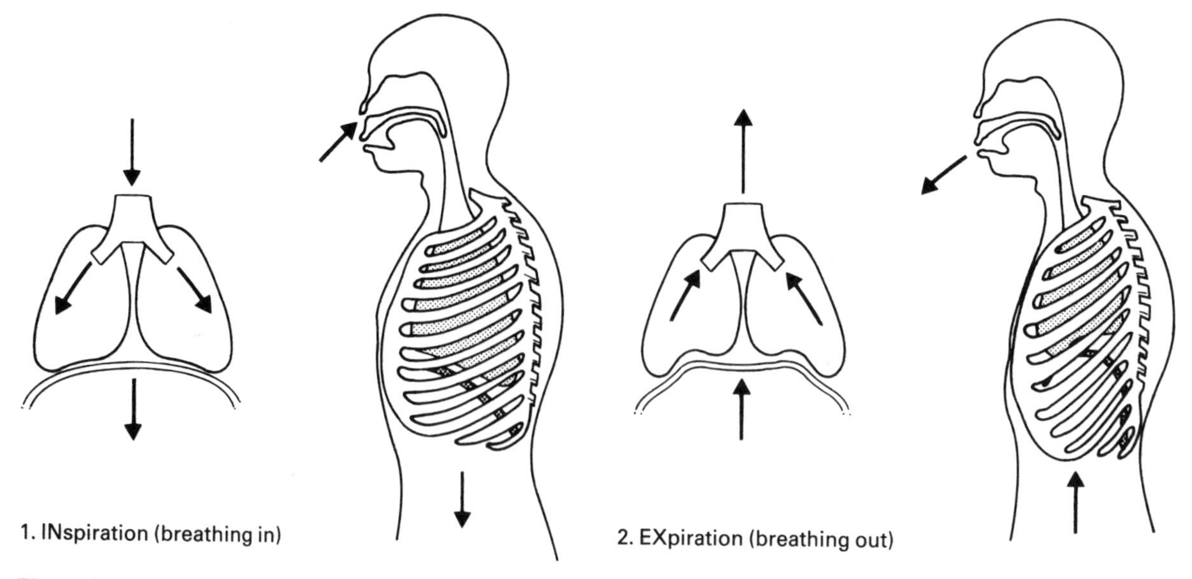

Figure 20.10 Diagram showing how the ribs and diaphragm are used to ventilate the lungs.

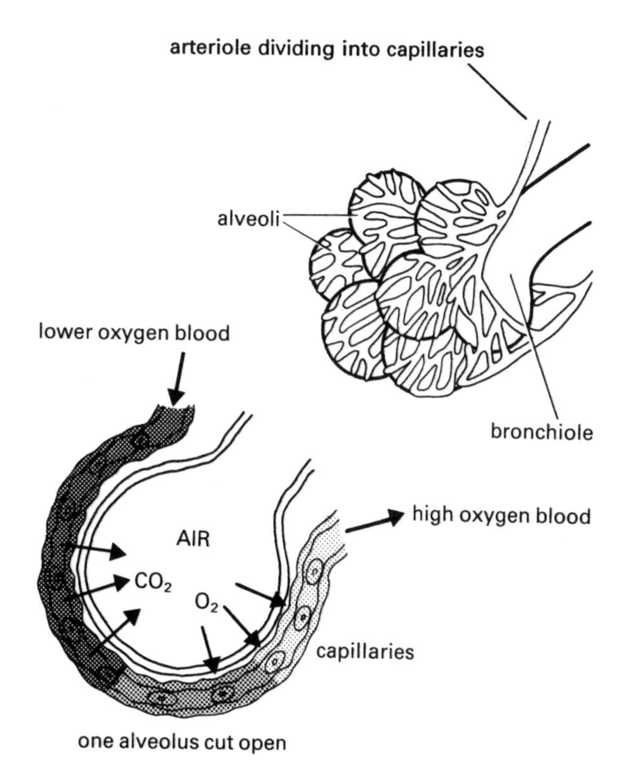

Figure 20.11 Diagrams showing anatomy and physiology of the small air sacs and blood vessels.

  - perforation (hole)
- hearing – all degrees of deafness

Nose

- discharge
  - watery fluid
  - pus
  - blood
- mucous membrane
  - inflammation
  - thickened blue-pink 'allergic' appearance

Mouth and throat

- inflammation of all or a part (especially tonsils)
- pus over a part (especially tonsils)
- post-nasal discharge

All

- cough

Use the auriscope to inspect the external ear canal and the ear drum like this:

Hold the auriscope in your right hand. Pull the pinna (outside ear) upwards and backwards with the finger and thumb of the left hand to straighten the external ear canal. Rest your right hand on the side of the patient's face. Then, if the patient suddenly moves, your hand will also move, and the auriscope cannot push into his ear and damage it. Use the largest speculum possible to push into the ear without hurting the patient much.

It may hurt the patient a little to push the speculum of the auriscope into the canal. There may be wax in the canal. Both of these things are normal.

Pain on moving the ear, swelling and redness of the skin lining the canal (either in one area or involving the whole canal), or pus in the canal itself, all suggest inflammation of the external canal (external ear inflammation)

The ear drum is normally white. It also reflects the light, in its lower part, as a bright white triangle called the 'light reflex' (Figure 20.12).

The ear drum may be retracted (pulled back) if the Eustachian tube is blocked.

The ear drum may be pink or red, small dilated blood vessels may be seen running in from the edge, the light reflex may not be present and fluid levels may be seen behind the drum in early acute inflammation of the middle ear.

A little later in acute middle ear inflammation the drum usually bulges (is pushed out). As it cannot bulge where it is held in the centre by a little bone, the drum then looks like the buttocks of a baby at a breech birth!

The drum may be perforated (broken) and pus may come out of the hole and even fill the ear canal in late acute middle ear inflammation.

If you cannot see the eardrum clearly because of wax or pus in the canal, gently clean the canal with a swab (or by syringing) until you can see the drum clearly.

To test the hearing of an ear

Block the other ear of the patient with one of your fingers which you keep moving in his ear (to make a noise so that he can hear nothing else with that ear); do not let him see your mouth; ask in a quiet voice

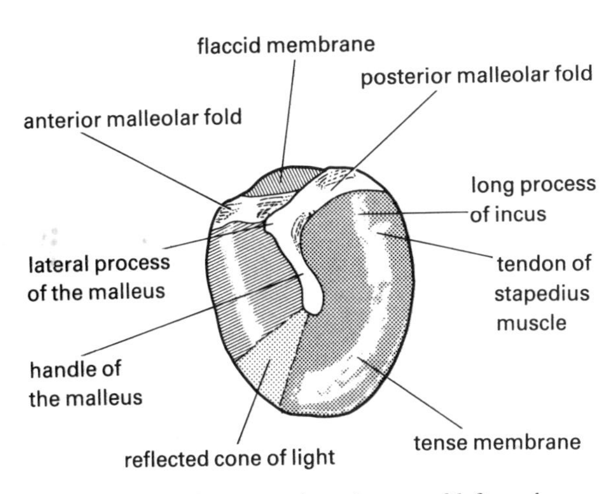

Figure 20.12 Diagram to show the normal left ear drum, also called tympanic membrane. The names of the parts of the membrane and of the small bones (see Figure 20.4) are not important. It is important to look at the ear drums of many normal as well as sick patients, so that you can recognise a normal ear drum.

questions which need answers that are more than just 'yes' or 'no'.

Examination of the nose using a torch or auriscope

Put the patient's head back and press gently on the end of his nose. This will open the nostrils and allow you to look in. If you have a large speculum for the auriscope, use this to look inside the nose – you will be able to see much better.

Red, swollen mucous membrane will be seen in acute rhinitis. If the infection is viral, you may see watery discharge on the mucous membrane. If the infection is bacterial, you may see pus on the mucous membrane.

A blue or pale, swollen, watery-looking mucous membrane suggests an allergic rhinitis or hay fever.

Tenderness of sinuses

Tenderness can be tested for by pressing firmly or tapping the bones containing the sinuses (above and below the eyes).

Examination of the mouth and throat, using a torch and tongue depressor

Examine the inside of the mouth, the tongue, the soft palate, the tonsils and the back of the throat for redness and swelling and pus from acute inflammation. You may need to press the tongue down and ask the patient to say 'Ah' to see the back of the throat wall. You may see pus from the nose running down the back of the throat (called post-nasal discharge or drip).

Symptoms of disease of the lower respiratory tract (lung)

- Cough
- Sputum
  - white (mucus)
  - yellow or green or brown (pus)
  - jellylike (mucus)
- Haemoptysis (blood in sputum)
- Pain in chest
  - tracheal (in the front of the neck or centre of the chest present only on coughing)
  - pleural (at the side of the chest more on breathing or coughing)
- Shortness of breath
  - on doing exercise (what ?) or on walking (how far?) or on climbing stairs (how many?)
  - at rest in the day sitting down

Table 20.1 Summary of the symptoms and signs of the common lung diseases

	Pneumo-thorax	*Fluid in pleural cavity*	*Lobar pneumonia*	*Broncho-pneumonia*	*Acute bronchitis*	*Asthma*	*Chronic bronchitis (COLD)†*	*Bronchiectasis*	*Laryngeal or tracheal obstruction*
Temperature	varies	varies	*raised	often raised	*often raised	*normal NOT raised	*normal	sometimes raised	varies
Sputum	varies	varies	*pus	pus	*pus sometimes	*thick mucus NOT pus	*mucus	*pus or mucus	varies
Respiration rate	sometimes fast	sometimes fast	*fast	often fast	sometimes fast	slow	usually normal	normal	slow
Respiration type	sometimes shallow	sometimes shallow	*shallow	often shallow	normal	deep	usually normal	normal	*deep stridor
Movement	*decreased	*decreased	*decreased	normal	normal	decreased	decreased	normal	normal or decreased
Percussion	very resonant	*very dull 'stony' dull	*dull	normal	normal	normal or more resonant	normal or more resonant	normal	normal
Breath sounds	*reduced or absent	*reduced or absent	*reduced	normal	normal	normal or reduced	normal or reduced	normal	normal or reduced
Type of breath sounds	varies or absent	varies or absent	*bronchial	normal	normal	normal	normal	normal	normal
Wheezes or rhonchi	none	none	none	none	usually present	*present	present	none	*stridor
Crackles or crepitations	none	none	*present	*present	usually absent	usually absent	usually absent	*present	none

* These are the important signs for this condition
† Chronic obstructive lung disease (COLD)

– at rest in the night in bed
- Wheezing

For causes and management of these symptoms, see page 217 onwards.

Table 20.1 summarises the symptoms and signs of the common lung diseases.

Signs of disease of the lower respiratory tract (LRT)

Examine for
- Rate of respiration (normal 16–20/minute)
- Type of respiration (deep or shallow, use of extra muscles, insuction, grunting, prolonged expiration, etc.)
- Deformity of chest or spine

Palpate for
- Decreased movement of (1) all of chest, (2) part or parts of chest

Percuss for
- Dullness or abnormal resonance of (1) all of chest or (2) part or parts of chest

Ausculate for

• Amount of breath sounds (normal or decreased) • Breath sounds (bronchial instead of normal) • Crackles (or crepitations) • Wheezes (or rhonchi) • Rubs	in	all of chest part or parts of chest

Ask the patient to cough. Listen to type of cough.
Examine any sputum (pus? mucus? blood?)

Examination of the rate and type of respiration (or breathing)

The normal rate is 16–20 breaths/minute. The type of respiration is often more important than the rate.

Is the patient distressed or not? Is the patient taking rapid shallow respirations which suggest pneumonia, or deep wheezing respirations which suggest asthma? Is there any indrawing of the soft tissues above and below the clavicle and between and below the ribs ('insuction') and dilation of the nostrils on breathing in? Is there grunting during breathing out? Insuction, dilation of the nose and grunting mean that the patient is having to do much extra work in order to breathe. This is common in pneumonia (especially in children), and in asthma and chronic respiratory disease (especially in the old).

Wheezing is when you hear the whistling noises of the air moving through the air passages without the stethoscope. The causes are the same as for rhonchi or wheezes heard with a stethoscope (see page 206).

Stridor is when you hear a loud whistling or crowing noise during breathing *in*. (Noisy breathing *out* is not as important.) It is caused by obstruction of the larynx or trachea. Stridor is always dangerous. Stridor is very dangerous if there is also insuction, rib recession (lower ribs moving *in* not *out* during breathing in), and the neck and abdominal muscles are being used for breathing.

Ask the patient to take a deep breath and look at the chest movement once again. Stand back from the patient when looking for these signs. See how well the chest moves. If he has great difficulty in moving the chest wall, it is said the chest wall is 'fixed'. This is a sign of chronic respiratory disease. Is one side moving and the other not moving? The side which does not move is the side with the disease in it.

Palpation of the chest (Figure 20.13)

Palpate the chest to find out if there is decreased movement of (1) all of the chest, or (2) part or parts of the chest.

You must find out from examining many normal people how much chest movement is normal – it is usually more than 1 cm on each side.

Disease affecting all of the lungs will cause decreased movement of all of the chest and the same amount of decrease on both sides. This decreased movement of all the chest is caused by chronic obstructive lung disease and acute asthma.

Disease of one part of the lung causes decreased movement of the chest on the same side. This decreased movement of one part of the chest is caused by lobar pneumonia, tuberculous pneumonia, pleural fluid, lung cancer and pneumothorax.

> The side of the chest which moves less is the abnormal side.

Percussion of the chest

Press the middle finger of the left hand firmly over the area you are percussing. Place the finger in the same line or direction as the ribs in that area and between the ribs (over the muscles between the ribs). Percuss or hit the middle of this finger in a light and

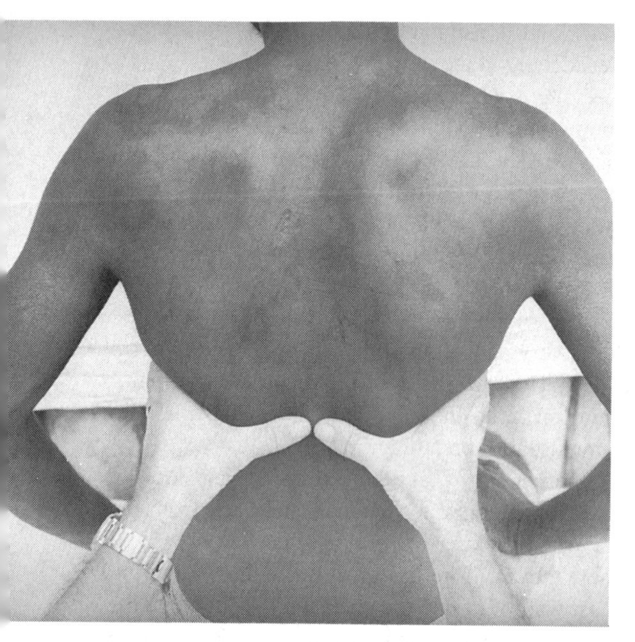
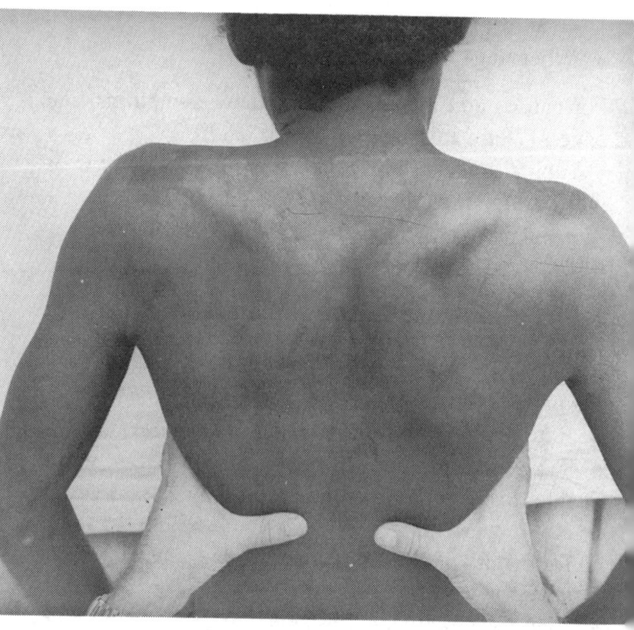

Figure 20.13 Photographs to show method of palpation of the chest for movement. Press your finger-tips firmly into the lateral chest wall so that they stay in the same place between the ribs. Put your finger-tips in such a position that when the patient breathes right out, then the ends of your thumbs just meet in the midline of the spine. (See left photograph.) Then get the patient to take slow deep breath in (and out). Let the palms of your hands and your thumbs slide over the skin; but do not let your finger-tips move. The movement of each side of the chest is shown by how far the ends of your thumbs move away from the spine in the midline. (See right photograph.)

loose fashion with the bent middle finger of the right hand.

Percuss the chest wall in a systematic fashion. Percuss the sides front and back of the chest wall (see Figure 20.14).

Percuss the *same* part of *each* side of the chest and decide if the percussion note is normal or not and equal or not on both sides before percussing another part.

Feel *and* listen for the type of percussion note. The percussion note may be either dull or resonant (hollow sounding).

Normally the chest over the lungs is resonant, but it may be a little dull if the person is very muscular or fat. The area of resonance moves down 2–5 cm during breathing in as the diaphragm moves down and the lungs expand.

Percussion over the heart, liver and large muscle masses in the shoulders will give a dull note.

Percussion over the air in the stomach will give a very resonant note (see Figure 20.15).

The percussion note will be dull if anything more solid than lung filled with air is underneath.

The percussion note will be dull over an area of pneumonia because there is a lot of fluid in the alveoli. The percussion note will be very dull when there is pleural fluid as no air is under the chest wall there.

In patients who are acutely ill with breathlessness and fever, see if the percussion causes pain. Pain on percussion is a sign of pleurisy usually due to pneumonia.

The percussion note will be very hollow if only air and not air and lung are underneath the chest wall, e.g. pneumothorax.

Auscultation of the chest

Listen in all areas including the axillae using a stethoscope (see Figure 20.14).

Listen in one place and then in the same place on the opposite side of the chest next. Decide if the breath sounds are present or not (air entry is normal or not), if they are normal or not, and if crackles or wheezes are present or not in the *same* places on *both* sides, before you listen to another place on the chest.

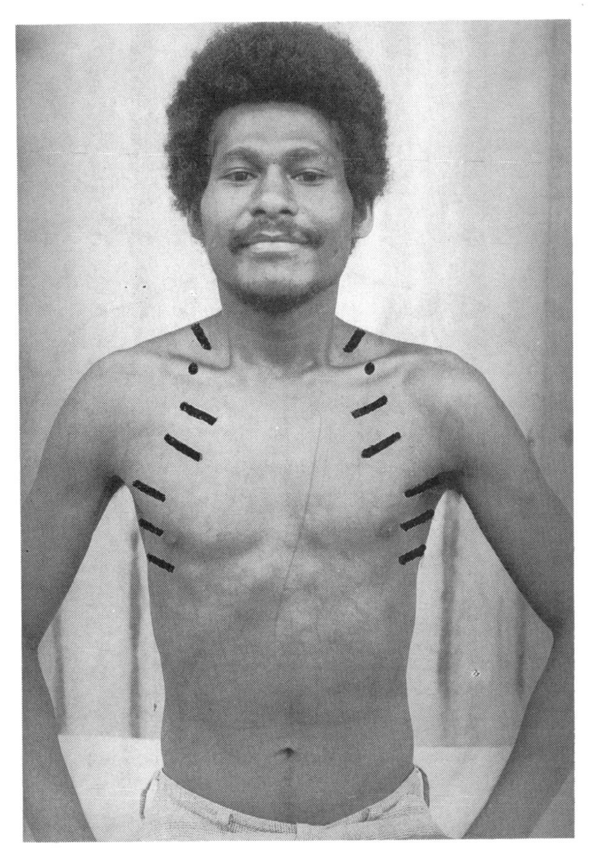

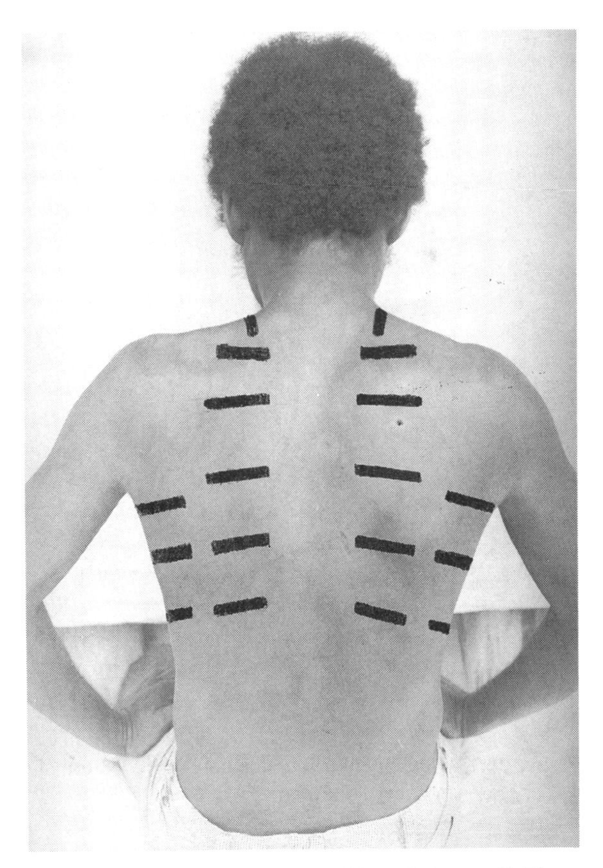

Figure 20.14 The left photograph shows sites for percussion and auscultation of the posterior and lateral chest wall. The right photograph shows sites for percussion and auscultation of the posterior and lateral chest wall.

It is better to use the bell of the stethoscope when you listen to the breath sounds. Do not press hard when you use the bell.

Listen for three things when you auscultate:

1. *The quantity of the breath sounds* (amount of air entry).
   Compare both sides of the chest and see if breath sounds are the same. The breath sounds may be loud, or soft, or absent. Breath sounds are softer or absent, if less air is entering that part of the lung under the stethoscope. Breath sounds may be softer (or less) over an area of pneumonia and may be softer or even absent over a collection of pleural fluid. Breath sounds may be soft in all areas if not much air is entering any part of the lung, e.g. severe chronic obstructive lung disease or very severe asthma.

2. *Quality of the breath sounds* (type of breath sounds).
   The breath sounds normally have a quality which is a bit like the sound of rubbing the hands together (or the rustling of leaves in a tree). These types of breath sounds are called 'vesicular'.
   Over the trachea the normal breath sounds you hear are louder, and sound something like blowing air over the top of a bottle. These types of breath sounds are called 'bronchial'. You hear bronchial breath sounds or bronchial breathing at the chest wall only if something solid *in the lung* (not in the pleura) conducts these breath sounds from the trachea to the chest wall.
   You hear bronchial breathing only over large areas of pneumonia or tumours (and very occasionally over very large tuberculous cavities, or at the upper level of plural fluid). You do not often hear bronchial breathing in diseases other than pneumonia. Bronchial breath sounds are not always easy to hear; but are very helpful if they are heard.

3. *Added sounds.*
   Added sounds are sounds which are not normally present. There are three kinds of added sounds which you may hear – 'crackles' which used to be

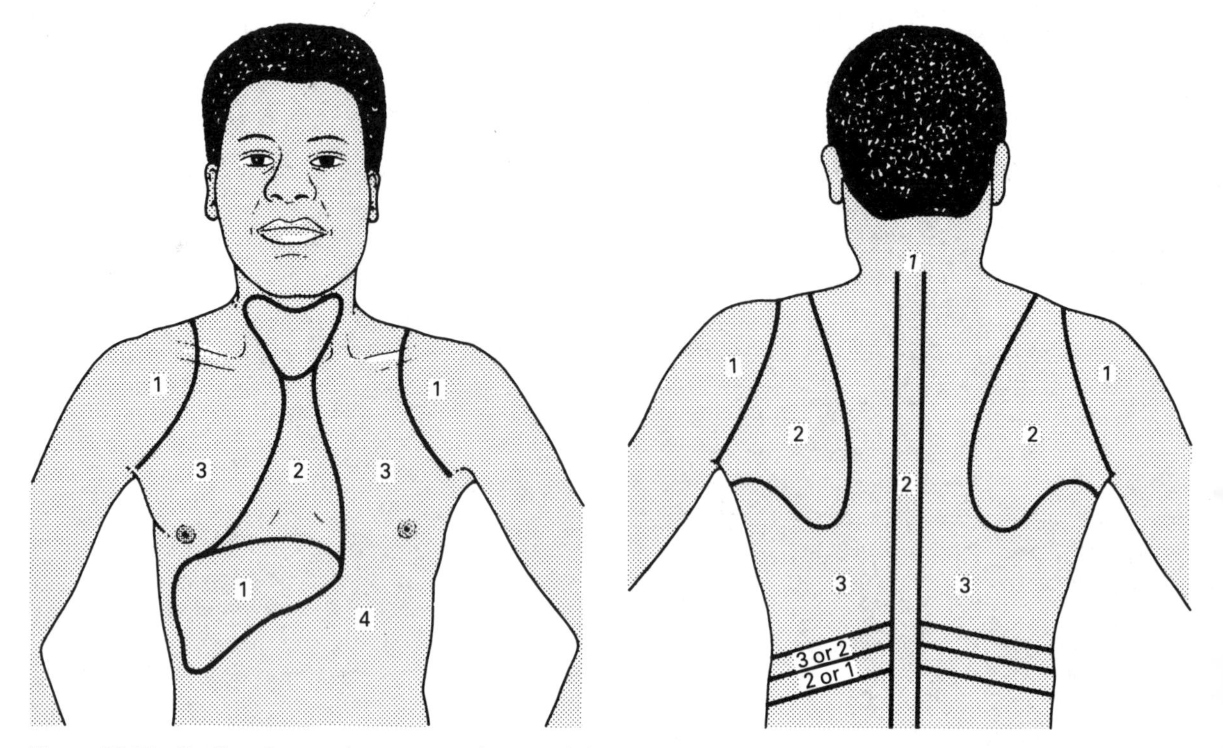

Figure 20.15 Quality of percussion note over the normal chest. 1. Flat or 'stony' dull. 2. Dull. 3. Resonant (hollow). 4. Very resonant (very hollow).

called 'crepitations' (crackling or bubbling sounds), 'wheezes' which used to be called 'rhonchi' (whistling sounds) and a 'pleural rub' (a rubbing or scraping sound). *Crackles* or *crepitations* are the crackling noises made by alveoli or bronchi which are closed but snap open and vibrate, and by air bubbling through fluid in bronchi.

Causes include:

(a) acute infections of the alveoli (lobar pneumonia, bronchopneumonia);

(b) chronic infections of the alveoli (tuberculosis);

(c) chronic damage to the bronchi with fluid in the bronchi (bronchiectasis);

(d) oedema of the lungs (left heart failure); and

(e) some cases of chronic obstructive lung disease, and after some attacks of asthma.

Wheezes, which used to be called *rhonchi*, are whistling sounds made by air going through narrowed bronchi. (These sounds are also called wheezing, when you do not need a stethoscope to hear them.) They are often louder during breathing out. Causes include:

(a) asthma,

(b) acute bronchitis, and

(c) chronic obstructive lung disease.

A *pleural rub* is a creaking, grating or rubbing noise usually heard in breathing in and out over one area. It is not changed by coughing (wheezes often are), but may be changed by pressing hard on the chest and thereby changing the position of the pleura. It is caused by pleural inflammation.

The important conditions that produce abnormal chest signs

1. Obstruction of the trachea or larynx, e.g.
   - foreign body inhaled,
   - infections, e.g. croup, acute bacterial epiglottitis, laryngotracheobronchitis, diphtheria
   - allergy (angio-oedema).
2. Obstruction of the bronchi, e.g.
   - pus, e.g. acute bronchitis,
   - mucus, e.g. chronic obstructive lung disease,
   - spasm of the muscles, e.g. asthma.
3. Fluid in the alveoli, e.g.
   - heart failure (left heart),
   - pneumonia (all types).
4. Solid lung (consolidation), e.g.
   - lobar pneumonia.
5. Fluid in the pleural cavity, e.g.

- water – effusion,
- pus – empyema,
- blood – haemothorax.

6. Air in the pleural cavity
   - pneumothorax.

Positions of lung lesions (see Figure 20.7)

Upper lobes or parts

- suspect tuberculosis

Lower lobes or parts

- suspect bacterial pneumonia
- suspect tuberculosis and HIV infection if it does not get better

Right middle lobe or lower front right side of chest

- suspect tuberculosis and inhaled foreign body as well as ordinary bacterial pneumonia

General symptoms that may be caused by respiratory disease

1. Fever
2. Weight loss
3. Malaise

General signs that may be caused by respiratory disease

1. The temperature may rise in any infective disease.
2. The pulse rate may increase in any infective disease, or any disease of the lungs that does not allow the body to receive enough oxygen.
3. The respiration rate and type of respiration may be abnormal (see page 205).
4. Cyanosis is the blue colour of the blood caused by low oxygen concentration in the haemoglobin of the blood.
   It is easiest to see cyanosis where blood is close to the surface of the body, and there is little or no pigment (e.g. the mucous membranes of the conjunctivae, the tongue and inside the mouth and under the finger nails and toe nails). Cyanosis is caused by haemoglobin that does not have oxygen. (Haemoglobin with oxygen is red. Haemoglobin without oxygen is blue.)
   There must be 1.5–5 g of haemoglobin without oxygen in each dl (100 ml) of blood to make the blood look blue. In a very severely anaemic person (with a haemoglobin of less than 5 g/dl) you may not see cyanosis, even if their haemoglobin does not have much oxygen. They may not have the necessary amount of haemoglobin without oxygen to show the blueness of cyanosis.
   If the blood in all parts of the body is blue, i.e. there is cyanosis of the tongue *and* the finger nails and toe nails, this may be caused by:
   (a) the patient not breathing enough (for any reason);
   (b) some diseases of the lungs, especially pneumonia;
   (c) some diseases of the heart;
   (d) some poisons in the blood which stop the haemoglobin combining with oxygen (e.g. sodium nitrite in 'anti-rust' tablets).
   If only part of the body is cyanosed and blue but the tongue is a normal pink, then the blood must be circulating slowly through the cyanosed area, and most of the oxygen is being taken out before the blood leaves that area.
   Be careful not to mistake the blue colour in the pigment or normal colouring of some person's mouths for cyanosis of the lips.
5. Clubbing of the nails. When clubbing occurs, the normal angle between the nail and the finger goes. Later on, the end of the finger may become swollen, and look like the head of a drumstick, (see Figure 20.16).
   Clubbing is usually caused by chronic respiratory diseases, but usually only those caused by chronic infection or cancer. It sometimes occurs in heart disease (some infective and congenital), chronic liver and bowel disease and other conditions. Very occasionally it is inherited.
   Do not confuse clubbing with curved finger nails (which are not important). With curved nails there is still a normal angle between the base (or back or top) of the nail and the back of the finger.
   Clubbing does not occur with usual chest infections (but sometimes does with tuberculosis) or with chronic obstructive lung disease or with asthma. If clubbing is present look for a serious chronic disease, especially chronic infection of the chest or lung cancer.

Tests in respiratory disorders

Chest X-ray

A chest X-ray is not possible in a health centre. It also takes a lot of training to be able to understand and use an X-ray properly. Fortunately most conditions can be accurately diagnosed and treated without the use of an X-ray.

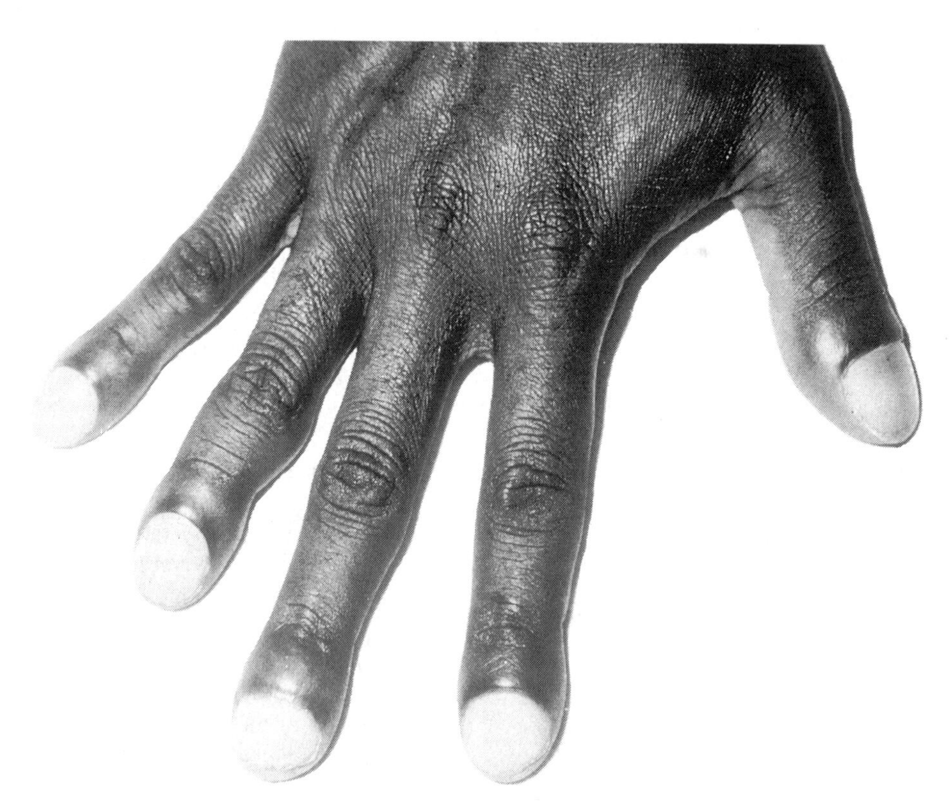

Figure 20.16 A patient's hands with severe clubbing of the nails. Note that there is no angle between the proximal (body) end of the thumb nail and the back of the thumb. In this severe clubbing the whole of the end of the finger is swollen. The finger nail does not seem to be firmly attached and seems to be floating (or be fluctuant) on top of the tissues at the end of the finger.

Sputum examination for AFB
See Chapter 14 page 81.

Summary of methods of treatment of respiratory diseases

1. Treat infections with antibiotics or, if tuberculosis, anti-tuberculosis drugs.
   Use penicillin first. It is usually effective. In some places where penicillin is not freely available, or where the common organism such as pneumococci may have developed high resistance to penicillin, other drugs such as co-trimoxazole (sulphamethoxazole/trimethoprim) are used first. One of the disadvantages of such treatment is that oral drugs may not be taken for the full course by the patient. Another disadvantage is that in some communities, there are a lot of reactions, especially of the skin, to co-trimoxazole. Another problem is that some organisms can quickly get resistant to co-trimoxazole. You need to find out from your health department what you should do and change the book as needed. Give chloramphenicol instead of penicillin if the infection is severe and may cause death. Use tetracycline or doxycycline if penicillin does not work and the patient is not likely to die soon from the infection and especially if he may need repeated courses of antibiotics. Do not use tetracycline if pregnant or a child. Use amoxycillin or ampicillin or erythromycin instead. Give chloramphenicol if penicillin and then tetracycline do not work; but look first for reasons why the antibiotics are not working. See Chapter 11 page 46.
   Give streptomycin *only* for tuberculosis. Do not use it for any other respiratory infection. Give at least two antituberculosis drugs to all cases of tuberculosis for every dose of the planned treatment. See Chapter 14 page 84.
2. Treat bronchial narrowing (causing wheezing and/or rhonchi) like this:
   (a) Treat the cause if possible (antibiotics if infection; stopping smoking if COLD etc.).

(b) Give adrenaline or salbutomol or terbutaline or orciprenaline or ephedrine (never more than one of these at a time). If these drugs are not effective *add*:

(c) Aminophylline or theophylline by tablet *or* suppository or IVI or IV drip.

3. Remove sputum or pus (if present) like this:
   (a) Encourage a patient to breathe deeply and cough sputum up.
   (b) Suck out the pharynx if the patient cannot cough.
   (c) Physiotherapy (see Chapter 21, page 218).
   (d) Postural drainage.
   (e) Postural sleeping (with head of bed down).
   But do not continue with any of these methods if less than 15 ml of sputum is produced.
4. Treat a cough like this:
   (a) Treat the cause.
   (b) Remove the sputum from the chest (See 3 above).
   (c) Do *not* give an effective anti-cough drug (e.g. codeine) if the patient has sputum.
   (d) Cough medicine ('Mist. tussi') does not help. Give it only if the patient wants medicine very much, and does not need effective drugs.
5. The patient should stop smoking.
   All of the lung conditions are made worse by smoking.
   Smoking causes chronic obstructive lung disease and lung cancer.
   It is very important that the patient does not start smoking again.
6. Treat low oxygen in the blood, which has caused cyanosis of the whole body including the tongue, with intra-nasal oxygen 1–4 litres/minute. Do not give more than 1–2 litres/minute if patient has COLD.
7. Treat swelling of the nasal mucous membrane with:
   (a) Ephedrine or other vasoconstrictor nasal drops, which narrow the blood vessels and make the swelling of the mucous membrane less.
   (b) Oral antihistamines (e.g. promethazine) if evidence of allergy.
8. Analgesics may be needed for pain. If the pain stops the patient coughing up sputum, give analgesics, but you *must* then make the patient cough up the sputum.
9. Rest and nursing are important for acute severe diseases.

Prevention of respiratory disease

The most important single thing you can do is to stop people smoking tobacco. In industrialised countries, smoking tobacco is *the most common* cause of preventable disease and death, but in some developing countries, more people are now smoking than in industrialised countries. Make sure you set an example to others by not smoking yourself. Use any chance you get to give health education to patients and to relatives as well as to the whole community on the dangers of smoking and why people should not start smoking, or stop smoking if they do.

Prevention of measles and whooping cough by vaccination will stop many people having damage done to their lungs when they are infants. Their lungs will then be less likely to have diseases such as bronchiectasis when they become adults.

Early and proper treatment of respiratory infections will cure them and not let them go on to cause chronic infections such as bronchiectasis and chronic sinusitis.

Tuberculosis is a very common cause of lung disease. It may be partly prevented by BCG vaccination. Early diagnosis and treatment will stop the infection destroying a lot of lung. The patient cannot, of course, grow new lung to replace damaged or destroyed lung.

Diseases of the respiratory system

The common cold

The common cold is an acute viral infection of the upper respiratory tract. It can be caused by one of many viruses.

Symptoms may include sneezing, watery nasal discharge, sore throat, cough, watery eyes, mild fever and malaise.

On examination there may be mild fever and red swollen watery mucous membranes of the upper respiratory tract.

There are no abnormal signs in the chest and there is no purulent sputum. There are no signs of severe general disease.

Complications can occur including acute otitis media, acute sinusitis, tonsillitis, acute bronchitis and pneumonia caused by bacteria. (These complications need treatment with antibiotics.)

Treatment

Examine all the respiratory tract to see if there is a complication which needs treatment (especially otitis media).

Treat as an outpatient.

Tell the patient to come back if a complication develops (especially pain in the ear or deafness; or shortness of breath or pus in the sputum).

You can only treat the symptoms:

1. Rest may be needed.
2. Give paracetamol 0.5–1 g or aspirin 300–600 mg (1–2 tablets) each 6 hours if needed for headache or aches and pains.
3. Give ephedrine or other nasal drops, which narrow the blood vessels, if the nose is blocked.
4. Cough mixture does not help. Give it only if the patient wants medicine.
5. Give antimalarials (usually chloroquine) if there is any fever. (See Chapter 13 page 61).

Influenza

Influenza is an acute viral infection of *all the respiratory tract*. It is caused by one of only a few (influenza) viruses:

Usually it is an epidemic disease.

Severe general symptoms and signs of infection occur:

- sudden start of the symptoms,
- fever,
- pains all over the body,
- loss of appetite, and
- feeling too sick to walk around.

But only mild respiratory tract infection symptoms and signs occur:

- cough (but no sputum)
- sore throat
- tracheal pain, and
- slight redness of the upper respiratory mucous membranes.

There is improvement after a few days; but the patient may not get better for two weeks.

The patient may get suddenly worse if he develops a complication, especially pneumonia or other bacterial infection of the respiratory tract. Pneumonia is more common in old people, or patients with chronic obstructive lung disease. Bacterial pneumonia is the usual cause of death in influenza epidemics.

Treatment

Examine all the respiratory tract, and look at any sputum. Find out if there is a complication (especially pneumonia) which needs treatment.

Treat as an outpatient.

Tell the patient to come back if any complication develops (especially bad cough, shortness of breath or pus in sputum).

Treat the symptoms as for a common cold (see this page); but rest, paracetamol or aspirin and antimalarial drugs will probably all be needed for some days.

Admit for inpatient treatment if any complications develop (especially pneumonia) and treat these complications in the usual way.

Notify the Health or Medical Officer if an epidemic occurs (e.g. more than 20 cases in 1 month).

Control and prevention are not possible in most places. During an epidemic you may be told to give procaine benzylpenicillin 1 g or 1,000,000 units daily to everyone who has a severe cough. This will help to reduce the number of deaths from secondary bacterial pneumonia.

Immunisation against influenza is possible, but it is expensive and difficult to organise and is usually not possible in most developing countries.

Acute middle ear inflammation (acute otitis media)

Acute middle ear inflammation is a common acute inflammation of the middle ear. It is often caused by bacteria and pus often forms in the middle ear.

Acute middle ear infection often develops with or after a viral or bacterial upper respiratory tract infection, especially if these block the eustachian tube.

Symptoms include:

- pain and a feeling of fullness in the ear,
- deafness,
- discharge from the ear, if the drum bursts, and
- general symptoms of infection sometimes, e.g. fever, malaise, gastroenteritis.

Signs (see Figure 20.17) can include:

- inflammation of the ear drum (the drum may be pink or red, there may be small blood vessels seen running in from the edge and the normal white colour and light reflex are not seen),
- fluid or pus seen behind the ear drum,
- bulging of the ear drum,

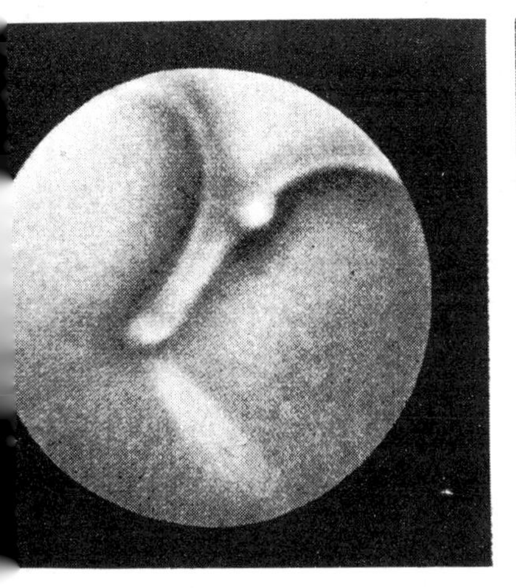
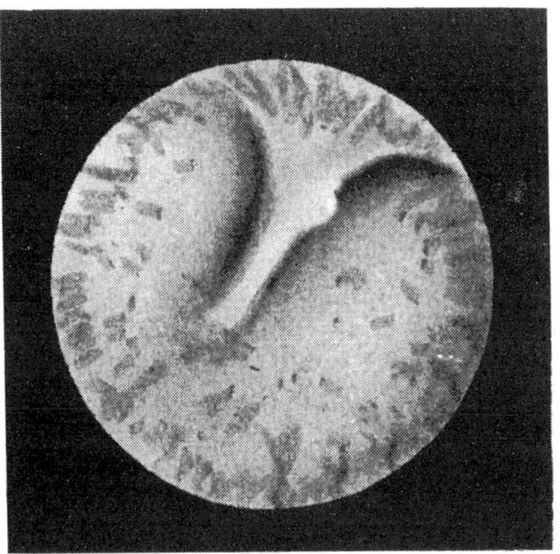
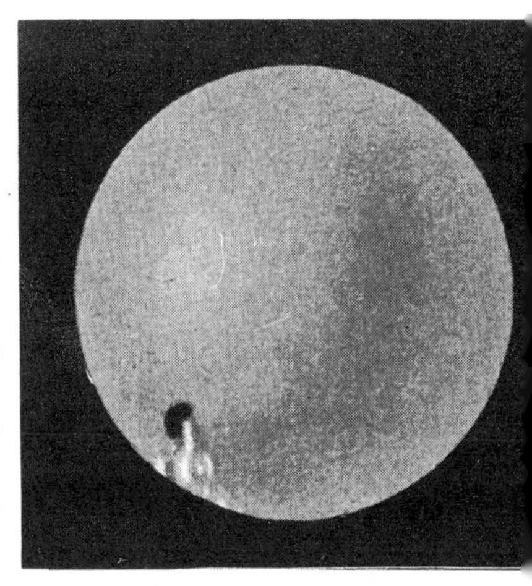

Figure 20.17 Left: normal ear drum. Middle: acute otitis media. Right: Otitis media with perforated drum.

- rupture of the ear drum, with a hole in the drum and pus in the external canal,
- deafness, and
- general signs of infection including raised temperature and pulse rate.

Many cases get better without treatment. Some cases develop complications. These include:

- 'glue ear' with partial deafness (the acute infection settles but thick fluid is left filling the middle ear),
- chronic otitis media (continuing infection in the ear that usually causes the ear drum to burst),
- acute mastoiditis (a tender swelling of the bone (not just the lymph node) behind the ear develops),
- meningitis,
- acute tonsillitis.

Treatment

Treat as an outpatient. Admit for inpatient treatment if there is discharge from the ear.

1. Give procaine benzylpenicillin 1 g or 1,000,000 units daily or sulphamethoxazole 800 mg/trimethoprim 160 mg (co-trimoxazole) orally twice daily until cured (6–10 days).
   If penicillin is not successful, use tetracycline or doxycycline; or, if pregnant, amoxycillin.
2. Give ephedrine or other vasoconstrictor nasal drops four times a day.
3. Tell the patient to blow his nose often (to try to open up the eustachian tube).
4. Give paracetamol 0.5–1 g or aspirin 300–600 mg (1–2 tablets) or codeine compound tablets (2 tablets) every 6 hours if needed for pain.
5. Give an antimalarial drug (such as chloroquine) if fever (see Chapter 13 page 61).
6. Do ear toilet and put in ear drops (see below) *if* the ear is discharging. Do this daily or more often if there is a lot of discharge. Continue the ear toilet and ear drops until the discharge stops.

Method for ear toilet

Cut the end off a clean size 8 feeding tube (or cut the needle off a scalp vein set) so that the tube is about 5 cm (2 inches) long. Put this on to a clean 5 ml or 10 ml syringe.

Draw up 2 ml of clean water (or better still normal saline made with $2\frac{1}{2}$ ml ($\frac{1}{2}$ teaspoonful) of salt in 200 ml (1 cup) of clean water).

Put the cut end of the feeding tube *gently* into the ear.

Do not put the tube deep into the ear or you will damage the ear.

Inject the water *slowly* into the ear. Then suck out the water and pus from the ear into the syringe. Throw away this dirty water. Refill the syringe with clean water again. Repeat the treatment until no more pus comes out.

Dry the ear like this – roll up a small piece of soft toilet paper into a spear shape, put it into the ear, leave it there for 1 minute, then take it out.

Look with an auriscope at the canal and drum. If there is still pus, etc., repeat the cleaning with the syringe and the drying with toilet paper. Continue until the drum is seen and the drum and canal are clean and dry.

After use, clean the syringe and feeding tube very well. Then soak them in antiseptic solution.

This method is very effective and not dangerous.

Another method of doing ear toilet

Clean inside the canal with a *small* piece of cotton wool wrapped around the end of a *very thin* swab stick. Do not push it into the drum. Use a new piece of cotton wool when the cotton wool on the stick becomes dirty or wet. Continue until you can see the canal and drum are clean and dry (through the auriscope). This method is harder for most health workers in health centres to do, and is also less effective.

After the ear toilet put 5 drops of boric acid 3% in alcohol or acetic acid 1% in alcohol ear drops into the ear.

Transfer

Transfer to Medical Officer care if:

1. the ear drum does not return to normal after 3 weeks of treatment (non-urgent), or
2. acute mastoiditis develops (urgent).

Chronic middle ear infection (chronic otitis media)

Chronic middle ear infection is a chronic infection of the middle ear by bacteria.

It is usually a complication of untreated or badly treated acute middle ear inflammation.

There are symptoms and signs of discharge of pus from the ear from time to time. The ear drum is perforated (has a hole in it) and does not heal. The patient is partly deaf.

Treatment

Treat as an outpatient. Admit for inpatient treatment, if necessary for ear toilet.

Ear toilet and drops daily as for acute middle ear inflammation (see above), until the discharge stops. If there is a lot of discharge, the ear toilet (or at least with toilet paper spears) followed by drops may be needed 2–4 times daily.

Treat as for acute middle ear inflammation (see above) if there has been evidence of acute otitis media in the last 6 weeks, or if the ear suddenly gets worse or if there is no improvement on the above treatment for 1 week. Tetracycline 250–500 mg (1–2 caps) four times a day or doxycycline 100 mg (1 tab) daily but not if pregnant when give amoxycillin 500 mg three times a day, may help if penicillin does not improve the acute infection. Antibiotics, however, will not help unless there has been a recent acute infection and antibiotics will not heal the eardrum.

Tell the patient that he must try to keep inside his ear dry (no swimming, care with washing, dry carefully if water does get inside, etc.).

Refer (do not normally transfer) the patient to the next visiting Medical Officer, as some cases need an operation.

External ear inflammation (otitis externa)

External ear inflammation is an acute or a chronic inflammation of the skin of the external canal of the ear. The inflammation is usually caused by an infection with bacteria and occasionally with fungi. This infection often complicates an injury or a chronic non-infective dermatitis (see Chapter 32 page 448) of the skin inside the ear. There may be inflammation of all of the skin of the canal, often with pus formation. At other times there is a furuncle (pimple or boil) (see Chapter 32 page 434) in one area.

Treatm3ent

Treat as an out-patient.

1. Ear toilet and ear drops daily or if needed 2–4 times a day (see page 213)
2. Use boric acid 3% in alcohol or acetic acid 1% in alcohol ear drops, 3–5 drops after the ear toilet. If this does not work, try crystal violet (methylrosanilinium chloride) 0.5–1% in alcohol solution 3–5 drops after the ear toilet.
3. If the condition is severe insert glycerine and ichthammol 10% on a gauze wick deep into the ear canal daily, until the condition is cured or improved enough to use ear drops.
4. Tell the patient to keep the ear dry (no swimming, care with washing) and to dry the inside of the ear carefully if water does get in.
5. Give paracetamol 0.5–1 g or aspirin 300–600 mg (1–2 tabs) or codeine compound tablets (1–2 tablets) if required every 6 hours for pain.
6. Antibiotics are not usually needed.

If the external ear inflammation returns many times, tell the patient to always keep the insidc of the ear dry (no swimming, care during washing, dry carefully if water does get inside, etc.) and to use boric acid 3% in alcohol ear drops or even just alcohol ear drops once or twice every week even when the ear seems to be well.

Foreign body in the ear

A foreign body in the ear may cause pain or discharge or no symptoms.

If the foreign body is an insect, put cooking oil into the ear; when the insect is dead, syringe the ear. You can syringe many other foreign bodies out of the ear. However do not put water into the ear if the foreign body is vegetable (e.g. dry bean) which may swell. Instead try sucking on it with the end of a small tube attached to a strong sucker. If you use forceps you can easily push the foreign body further into the ear and damage the ear drum. If the patient is unco-operative or has a lot of pain and you have to use forceps, give a general anaesthetic first.

Acute sinusitis

Acute sinusitis is an acute bacterial infection of one or more of the paranasal sinuses. (See Figures 20.2 and 20.3.)

There are often general symptoms and signs of infection – fever etc.

Local symptoms and signs of inflammation are almost always present as follows:

- Pain over the affected sinus. Sometimes there is also a general headache or pain in the nearby teeth or eye.
- Tenderness over the affected sinus.
- There is often nasal mucous membrane swelling, and pus in the nose and throat.

Treatment

1. Procaine benzylpenicillin 1 g or 1,000,000 units IMI daily or sulphamethoxazole 800 mg/trimethoprim 160 mg (co-trimoxazole) twice daily until cured.
2. Ephedrine or other vasoconstrictor nasal drops, 2–3 drops into each nostril four times a day.
3. Paracetamol 0.5–1 g or aspirin 300–600 mg (1–2 tablets) or codeine compound tablets (1–2 tablets) every 6 hours if required for pain.
4. Antimalarial drug (usually chloroquine), (see Chapter 13 page 61) if there is fever.
5. If these are not successful, get the patient to wash out the nose with saline once or twice daily (see page 230); add an antihistamine if there is any evidence of allergic rhinitis; change penicillin to tetracycline or doxycycline and metronidazole or, if pregnant, amoxycillin or erythromycin.

Foreign body in the nose

The most common symptom caused by a foreign body in the nose is a discharge of pus from one side of the nose.

> If a patient has discharge of pus from one side of the nose always look for a foreign body in the nose.

If you can see the foreign body remove it with forceps. Sometimes you will need general anaesthetic to see and remove the foreign body. If you cannot see the foreign body or if the foreign body is hard or round and you cannot easily hold it with forceps, then try to remove it with a probe. Gently push a thin round-ended metal probe along the floor of the nose (i.e. almost straight in; but pointed a little downwards as well as backwards) until it touches the back of the throat. Then press the end you are holding downwards until the end in the patient's throat hits the top of the back of the nose. The foreign body will then be on top of and in front of the probe. Slide the probe out, keeping your end gently pressed down as far as possible. The foreign body often comes out in front of the probe.

Bleeding nose (epistaxis)

Causes of a bleeding nose include:

1. a cause not found (common),
2. a small crusted area on septum (in the middle just inside the nose) which has cracked (common),
3. trauma,
4. strong nose blowing or sneezing,
5. others – snake bite, rare blood diseases, diphtheria etc.

Treatment

1. Treat any underlying cause found.
2. Sit the patient up.
   - Pinch his nose tightly together between finger and thumb.
   - Let the blood run out of his mouth into a dish.
   - Do this for 10 minutes by the clock. Do not stop before 10 minutes are over.

   If this does not stop the bleeding, then:
3. Put in anterior nasal pack. Soak a long strip of narrow gauze bandage in 1 in 10,000 solution of

adrenaline (epinephrine) (mix 9 ml of saline with 1 ml of the 1 in 1000 adrenaline solution used for injection). Use long narrow forceps to pack the gauze in layers into the nose. Start off by putting the first layer as far back as possible. (See a reference book for details.) If this does not stop the bleeding, remove this anterior nasal pack, put in a posterior nasal pack (see below) and then another anterior nasal pack, starting off as far back as possible and pressing it onto the posterior nasal pack.
4. A posterior nasal pack can be made with a Foley's urethral self-retaining balloon catheter. Push the catheter through the bleeding side of the nose until the tip can be seen at the back of the throat when the patient opens his mouth. Inflate the balloon of the catheter with 4–10 ml of air or saline. Make sure the balloon is not behind or below the tongue. Then pull the catheter forward as far as it will go until the balloon is stuck in the back of the nose. Fasten the catheter to the face with sticking plaster to keep the catheter pulled firmly forward so that it will press on any bleeding site at the back of the nose. Then put in an anterior nasal pack.
5. Treat for shock or anaemia if necessary. (See Chapter 27 page 378 and Chapter 21 page 240).
6. When the bleeding has stopped, gently put antibiotic compound ointment or white soft paraffin into the nose, three times a day for a few days, to soften and heal any hard cracked area.

Allergic rhinitis (hay fever)

An allergic reaction of the mucous membrane of the nose is called allergic rhinitis or 'hay-fever'. The allergic reaction often affects the eyes too (allergic conjunctivitis) and the throat.

The allergy is usually to something breathed in – often house dust or a pollen.

The nose (and eyes and throat) become itchy, watery and sore.

The patient often sneezes a lot and rubs his nose and eyes.

On examination the mucous membrane is thickened, bluish-pink and has watery material covering it. There is no pus in the nose and no fever.

The condition may continue for hours or days or weeks or months.

Try to discover what is causing the reaction. The patient must try to avoid this. But, this is not often possible.

Treat with an antihistamine, e.g. promethezine 10–25 mg at night; and if needed, but for no longer than 1 week, ephedrine nasal drops each 4 hours.

Acute tonsillitis and diphtheria

Acute tonsillitis is an acute bacterial or viral infection of the tonsils and surrounding area of the throat. This causes acute inflammation and usually pus formation in the throat and the general symptoms and signs of infection.

The patient complains of a sore throat worse on swallowing or turning the head, and headache and fever.

The patient may be quite sick with a high temperature and fast pulse. The tonsils and inside the throat are red and swollen and usually there are spots of white or yellow pus on the tonsils. The lymph glands in the neck are often swollen and tender.

Complications can occur including an abscess behind the tonsil or at the back of the throat or under the chin. Any of these can block the airway. After 1–3 weeks rheumatic fever (See Chapter 29 page 393) or an acute nephritic syndrome (acute glomerulonephritis) (see Chapter 26 page 358) can occur.

Diphtheria is a special kind of upper respiratory tract infection, although it can infect other areas including the skin. It usually causes tonsillitis but can cause infection of the larynx (voice box) or nose. It is caused by a special bacterium spread by droplet infection. It is much more common in children than adults. The diagnostic feature is a greyish covering or membrane over the affected area, usually the tonsils, which is firmly stuck on and cannot be pushed off with a tongue depressor as pus can be. Around the edge of the grey covering is an area of inflammation which sometimes bleeds. The illness can vary from mild to severe. In severe cases death can occur within the first couple of weeks from shock or from complete blockage of the larynx. Heart failure can occur in the next couple of weeks. Damage to nerves, which control muscles, can result in things swallowed coming back up the nose, difficulty seeing and even weakness of the arms and legs some weeks later.

Treatment

1. Procaine benzylpenicillin 1 g or 1,000,000 units IMI daily is preferable to sulphamethoxazole 800 mg/trimethoprim 160 mg (co-trimoxazole) twice daily.

2. Paracetamol 0.5–1 g or aspirin 300–600 mg (1–2 tablets) four times a day if needed for pain.
3. Antimalarials usually chloroquine (see Chapter 13 page 61).

If the patient has an acute severe infection, give benzyl (crystalline) penicillin.

If an abscess starts to block the airway see below.

If you think the patient has diphtheria, treat with benzyl penicillin but immediately contact the Medical Officer about the use of diphtheria antitoxin, examination or treatment of contacts and immunisation with toxoid. If there is difficulty in breathing or if stridor occurs arrange urgent transfer, as tracheostomy may be urgently needed. If the airway does become completely blocked, do an urgent laryngostomy (see Chapter 37 page 509). Diphtheria can be prevented by immunisation, especially DPT or triple antigen given during childhood.

Acute bacterial throat or laryngeal or tracheal infections

Acute bacterial infections in these structures can cause death by blocking the airway. This block may be caused by an abscess or infective swelling or membrane or secretion which can be seen; but sometimes one of these things is so far inside the throat or in the larynx or trachea that it cannot be seen.

Suspect possible block of the airway if:

1. You can see a swelling which could block the airway.
2. The patient has difficulty in breathing. Stridor means death may be close.
3. The patient looks very 'sick'.

If a block of the airway is possible, *treat* like this:

1. Immediately give antibiotics as for septicaemia (IVI chloramphenicol, see Chapter 12 page 53).
2. Nurse carefully (suck out when needed; give oxygen when needed; etc.) Observe carefully every 15 minutes.
3. Give adrenaline (epinephrine) and antihistamines if allergy is possible (see Chapter 10 page 40).
4. Transfer patient if he does not quickly improve.
5. Incise and let the pus out of any swelling that will cause death before transfer is possible; or do an emergency laryngostomy if incision is not possible. See Chapter 37 page 509.

Acute tracheitis and bronchitis

Acute bronchitis is a common acute inflammation of the mucous membrane lining the inside of the bronchi (see Figure 20.18). If the trachea is inflamed, acute tracheitis is also present.

Acute bronchitis is usually caused by an infection with bacteria; but viruses, chemicals and smoke can also cause the inflammation.

General symptoms and signs of infection may be present, including

- malaise and
- fever.

Symptoms of a chest infection may be present, including

- cough,
- tracheal pain (pain in the front and middle of the neck and upper chest during coughing),
- sputum made of pus, and
- shortness of breath and wheezing.

Signs of bronchial obstruction (wheezes) are usually present but there are no signs of pneumonia:

- chest movement unchanged,

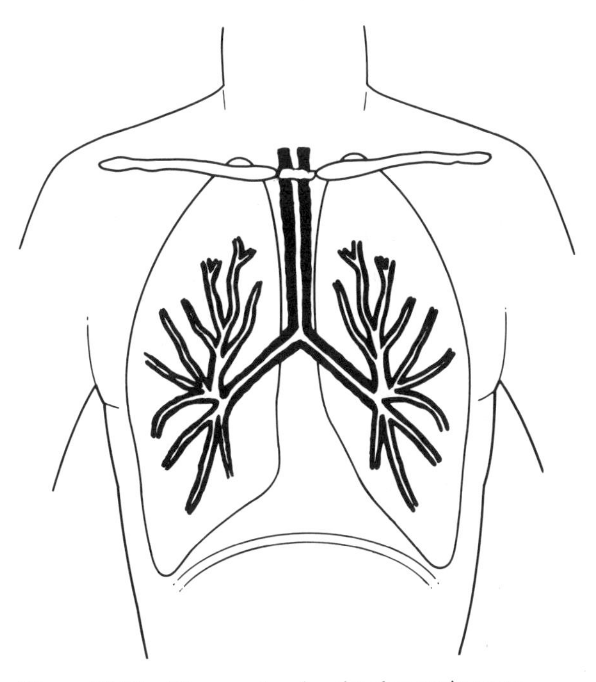

Figure 20.18 Diagram showing the changes in acute tracheitis and bronchitis. The mucous membrane lining all the air passages is inflamed and swollen and sometimes covered with pus. These things cause narrowing of all the airways to all parts of the lung. The alveoli themselves are normal.

- percussion note unchanged,
- air entry unchanged to all areas, but
- wheezes (and occasionally coarse creps) in all areas.

Treatment

Treat as an outpatient.

Tell the patient to return if shortness of breath gets worse (pneumonia or asthma).

1. Procaine benzylpenicillin 1 g or 1,000,000 units IMI daily or sulphamethoxazole 800 mg/trimethoprim 160 mg (co-trimoxazole) twice daily until cured (usually 5–7 days).
   Amoxycillin is the best oral treatment.
   Tetracycline or doxycycline are alternatives.
2. Paracetamol 0.5–1 g or aspirin 600 mg (2 tablets) every 6 hours if required for pain.
3. A 'bronchodilator', e.g. salbutamol 4 mg or terbutaline 5 mg or orciprenaline 20 mg (1 tablet) each 6 hours *if* wheezing present.
4. Inhalation (the breathing in) of steam (from a cup or tin of boiling water), for 5 minutes three or four times a day.
5. An antimalarial drug usually chloroquine (see Chapter 13 page 61) if there is fever.

Bronchopneumonia

Bronchopneumonia is an acute infection of groups of alveoli in the lungs (see Figure 20.19).

Bronchopneumonia is usually caused by bacteria.

Bronchopneumonia usually develops as a complication of another condition which has either:

1. stopped the patient moving around and breathing deeply and/or
2. has allowed bacteria to come into the lungs from the upper respiratory tract, e.g.
   - after anaesthetics, operations, accidents,
   - old or sick people lying in bed, or
   - measles or whooping cough.

There are the general symptoms and signs of infection:

- the patient has another condition but is not as well as he or she should be or is getting worse,
- fever (but not always),
- fast pulse etc.

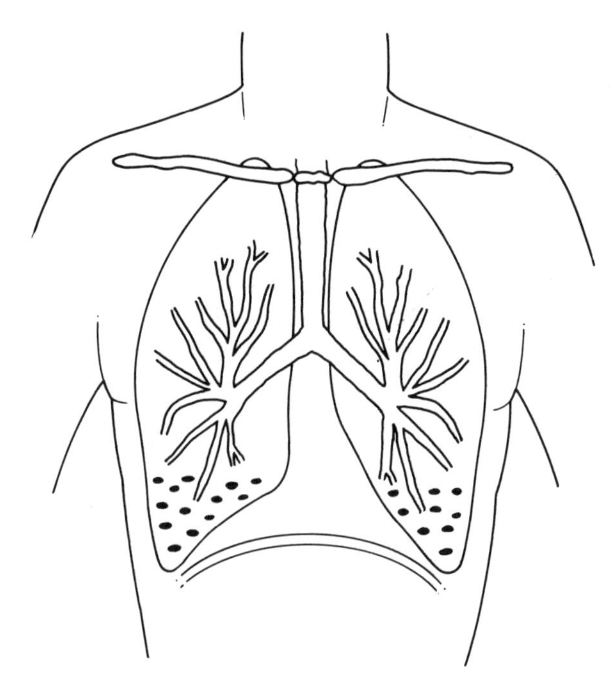

Figure 20.19 Diagram showing the changes in bronchopneumonia (in this case of both lower lobes – the most common places affected). Scattered groups of alveoli are involved. Bronchi are usually normal. However disease of the bronchi can also be present.

Symptoms of a chest infection are usually present (but not always):

- cough,
- sputum (made of pus), and
- shortness of breath.

Signs of the chest infection include:

- sputum made of pus,
- respiratory rate usually fast and shallow,
- normal movement, normal percussion note and normal air entry, but scattered crackles or crepitations throughout the lungs, often mostly low down at the back.

Treatment

1. Antibiotics – procaine benzylpenicillin 1 g or 1,000,000 units IMI daily or sulphamethoxazole 800 mg/trimethoprim 160 mg (co-trimoxazole) twice daily until cured. (See page 221 for details about other antibiotics.)
2. Physiotherapy twice daily (see Chapter 20 page 218).
3. Tell the patient to take 10 deep breaths and cough each hour when awake.

4. Tell the patient to move around in bed and if he is able, make him get out of bed and walk around.
5. Antimalarials, usually chloroquine if any fever. (See Chapter 13 page 61.)
6. Treat any underlying condition.

Prevention of bronchopneumonia is by encouraging activity in old, ill or postoperative patients.

Lobar pneumonia

Lobar pneumonia is a very common cause of sickness and death in the tropical and developing world.

Lobar pneumonia is an acute inflammation of all the alveoli in one lobe or one part of the lung. (See Figure 20.20.) The affected part of the lung becomes filled with organisms, plasma and blood cells and becomes 'solid' (often called 'consolidation').

The cause is usually one of the bacterial organisms *Streptococcus pneumoniae* (the pneumococcus) or *Haemophilus influenzae*; though viral, rickettsial, other bacteria (especially *Staphylococcus aureus*), mycobacterial and other organisms can cause pneumonia. If pneumonia does not improve on treatment as it should, always think of it possibly being due to tuberculosis. Inhaled chemicals (e.g. kerosene) or acid if gastro-oesophageal reflux, etc. are also causes.

Pneumonia is very common in patients with decreased defences against infections. The most common of these decreased defences is HIV infection. In all patients with pneumonia (especially if severe or repeated attacks), ask yourself if there is anything in the history or examination to suggest HIV infection (see Chapter 19 page 180).

Pneumonia is most likely to cause death in those who are young or old or have no spleen (including from sickle cell anaemia) or who have any chronic medical condition such as HIV infection, diabetes mellitus, heart condition, anaemia, etc., or if they have something else wrong with their lungs especially COLD or bronchiectasis.

Symptoms

- The start of the infection is usually sudden; but sometimes there has been an upper respiratory tract infection before.
- A rigor at first is common.
- Cough is almost always present.
- Sputum usually – rusty looking (from blood) or made of pus.

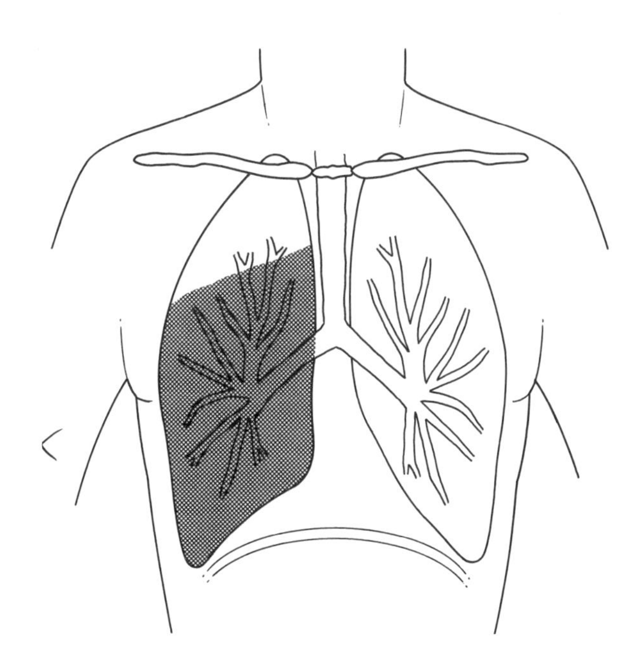

Figure 20.20 Diagram showing the changes in lobar pneumonia (in this case the right lower lobe). One whole lobe (or section) of lung is solid (bronchi and alveoli filled with organisms, fluid and blood cells). The solid lung extends from large central airways to the edge of the chest wall.

- Pleuritic chest pain (pain at the side of the chest but occasionally in the shoulder or in the upper abdomen, worse when the chest moves, for example on deep breathing or coughing and relieved by keeping the chest still, for example by holding or lying on the painful side).
- Shortness of breath

Signs

- High temperature.
- Fast pulse rate.
- Sometimes cyanosis.
- *Respiration fast and usually shallow*, sometimes irregular due to pain. This is probably *the most important sign to show pneumonia is present (when there is a chest infection) and to show how severe it is (if pneumonia is present).*
- Respiratory distress if severe – insuction and/or dilated nostrils on breathing in; grunting on breathing out.
- In the affected area of the chest
  – patient can often point to the place where the pleuritic pain is over area of pneumonia,
  – movement less,

– percussion note dull (percussion often causes pain),
– breath sounds or air entry less,
– bronchial breathing,
– crackles or crepitations.

The rate and type of respiration is a very good sign for the presence and severity of pneumonia. It is difficult for the chest muscles to stretch a 'solid' lung. And chest movement often causes pleuritic pain. So the patient often takes shallow breaths which do not exchange as much oxygen and carbon dioxide as normal respiration with normal lungs. So breathing is usually also fast when it is shallow.

If the pneumonia is more severe (and the patient has to do much extra work to breathe and his lungs do not exchange oxygen and carbon dioxide well and the body needs more oxygen than when it is not fighting an infection) there are signs of respiratory distress:

1. indrawing of the soft tissues between the ribs and below and above the clavicles when the patient breathes in, (called 'insuction');
2. use of neck and shoulder muscles when he breathes in;
3. dilation of the nostrils when he breathes in; and
4. grunting when he breathes out;
5. as well as fast respiratory rate.

The earliest signs in the chest are usually increase in the respiratory rate, decreased movement of the affected side and decreased breath sounds. Percussion at this stage often causes pain. At first there may be no, or only a few, crackles or crepitations. It is often a day or two before many crackles are heard. Not all the signs do develop in every case. If you give antibiotic treatment early fewer signs develop. Sometimes you can hear a pleural rub if inflammation of the pleura (pleurisy) has developed.

Complications

- Heart failure (see Chapter 27 page 371).
- Septicaemia sometimes with shock (see Chapter 12 page 53).
- Jaundice (see Chapter 24 page 314).
- Pleural effusion (see page 222).
- Empyema (see page 224).
- Pneumothorax (see page 223).
- Lung abscess.
- Infections in other organs especially meningitis (see Chapter 25 page 322) and arthritis (see Chapter 29 page 392).
- Others.

Tests

Tests are not usually necessary. But, always do sputum examinations for AFB in any case which is unusual (see Chapter 14 page 81). This is especially important if the pneumonia does not get better when it should.

Without treatment, 20–40% of severe cases result in death.

Treatment

Management includes:

1. Antibiotics until cured.
   - Procaine benzylpenicillin or sulphamethoxazole/trimethoprim (co-trimoxazole) if it is a mild case.
   - Benzyl (crystalline) penicillin, if it is a moderate case.
   - Tetracycline or doxycycline instead if benzyl penicillin does not cure but it is not a severe case.
   - Chloramphenicol, if it is a severe case, or if penicillin and tetracycline do not cure a moderate case.
2. Antimalarial drugs as indicated.
3. Treatment of symptoms, especially pain.
4. Oxygen, if necessary.
5. Physiotherapy, if very much sputum.
6. Look for and treat complications, especially
   - heart failure,
   - septicaemia/shock,
   - infections in other parts, especially meningitis and arthritis,
   - pleural fluid, and
   - pneumothorax.
7. Look for and treat other important conditions (e.g. severe anaemia).
8. Look for tuberculosis in unusual cases.
9. Transfer the patient if necessary.

Treat according to severity.

Mild

- no respiratory distress[1] and RR < 30 and < PR 100 and
- no cyanosis and
- no complications[2]
  See below.

Moderate
- respiratory distress[1] but not severe and RR < 40 and PR < 120 and/or
- cyanosis if present but not marked and
- no complications[2] except, if there is COLD, the patient may have heart failure. See below.

Severe
- respiratory distress[1] and RR > 40 and PR > 120 and/or
- cyanosis and/or
- complications[2]
  See below.

Mild case
Treat as an outpatient.

1. Procaine benzylpenicillin 1 g or 1,000,000 units IMI *or* sulphamethoxazole 800 mg/trimethoprim 160 mg (co-trimoxazole) orally twice daily until 4 days after fever and symptoms have gone (usually 5–7 days).
2. Antimalarial drug as indicated (see Chapter 13 page 61) usually chloroquine 450–600 mg (3–4 tabs) daily for 3 days.
3. Paracetamol 0.5–1 g or aspirin 300–600 mg (1–2 tabs) every 6 hours if necessary for pain.

If the patient is not much improved after 5 days, or if he gets worse, look for a complication especially a pleural effusion. If no complication that needs special treatment is found, then treat as a moderately severe case.

Moderate case
Admit for inpatient treatment.
1. Benzyl penicillin 600 mg or 1,000,000 units IMI every 6 hours until improved, then procaine benzylpenicillin 1 g or 1,000,000 units IMI daily until 4 days after all fever has gone.
2. Antimalarial drugs as indicated (Chapter 13 page 61) usually chloroquine 450–600 mg (3–4 tablets) daily for 3 days.
3. Aspirin 600–900 mg (2–3 tablets) or codeine compound tablets 2 tablets every 6 hours if necessary for pain.

If the patient is not much improved after 2–5 days, but is not worse and is not severely sick, then:

1. Change pencillin to tetracycline 500 mg (2 caps) every 6 hours, or doxycycline 100 mg (1 tab) twice daily but not if pregnant when use erythromycin 500 mg four times a day or amoxycillin 500 mg three times a day.
2. Send sputum for examination for AFB.

If the patient gets worse at any time treat as a severe case with chloramphenicol (see below).

Severe case
Use this treatment for severe cases (the patient will die soon if the treatment is not successful) and moderate cases not cured by treatment.

1. Chloramphenicol 2 g immediately, then 1 g every 6 hours until much improved, then 750 mg every 6 hours. Give chloramphenicol for 10 days or until cured – whichever is longer. If the patient has shock or is *very* sick or cannot swallow or is vomiting, give IV or IM chloramphenicol 2 g immediately and 1 g every 6 hours until he can take oral chloramphenicol (if shock, IV needed).
   In other cases give oral chloramphenicol 1 g (4 caps) immediately and 1 g (4 caps) every 6 hours until much improved; then 750 mg (3 caps) every 6 hours until cured.
2. Antimalarial drugs as indicated (see Chapter 13 page 61) usually chloroquine 450–600 mg (3–4 tablets) daily for 3 days. You should give quinine first to *very* sick patients (see Chapter 13 page 64).
3. Oxygen at 2 litres per minute by intranasal prongs or catheter, if the patient is cyanosed or very short of breath.
4. Paracetamol 0.5–1 g or aspirin 300–600 mg (2 tablets) every 6 hours for pain.
5. Look for complications (see page 220). Treat in the usual ways.
6. Look for other conditions that need treatment, especially severe anaemia. Treat in the usual ways (see index).

Look for tuberculosis in all cases of pneumonia
Send sputum for AFB if:

1. Previous chronic cough (ask *all* patients if they had a chronic cough before the present illness).

1 Respiratory distress is (1) indrawing of soft tissues between the ribs and below and above the clavicles when the patient breathes in (insuction); (2) use of neck and shoulder muscles when he breathes in; (3) dilation of the nose muscles when he breathes in; (4) grunting when he breathes out. It is not distress from pain during breathing.
2 Complications include: (1) heart failure, (2) shock/septicaemia, (3) infections in other organs, (4) pleural fluid, and (5) pneumothorax.

2. Pneumonia is in an upper lobe or in the (right) middle lobe.
3. Patient not as acutely sick as you would expect when he has marked chest signs.
4. Past or family history of tuberculosis, or other history that suggests tuberculosis.
5. Wasting or lymphadenopathy or other sign that suggests tuberculosis.
6. Patient does not get better as quickly as expected, or patient not cured after 2 weeks of proper treatment.

Send sputum for AFB (three smears) from these patients. If the smear is negative and you still suspect tuberculosis, send three more smears for AFB after 1–2 weeks of treatment with antibiotics.

Think of HIV infection in all cases of pneumonia

Ask for past history and look for signs which could suggest HIV infection (see Chapter 19 page 180).

Send blood if HIV test is indicated (see Chapter 19 page 188).

Transfer

Transfer these cases to Medical Officer care:

1. severe cases which do not improve, or get worse after 2 days chloramphenicol (urgent);
2. cases not cured or much improved after 2 weeks chloramphenicol (non-urgent);
3. those with complications that you cannot treat at the health centre (urgent).

Prevention

Pneumococcal vaccine, polyvalent, 0.5 ml injection gives good protection for about 5 years against pneumococci, which cause most cases of pneumonia. Ask if it is available for those in your population who are most at risk of dying from pneumonia – the young; the elderly; those with splenectomy or severe sickle cell disease; chronic obstructive lung disease; HIV infection; or any chronic medical condition such as heart condition, diabetes mellitus etc. Sometimes it is given to all children.

Pleural fluid

There are often no symptoms of fluid in the pleural cavity, but there may be shortness of breath and/or pleuritic pain. (See Figure 20.21.)

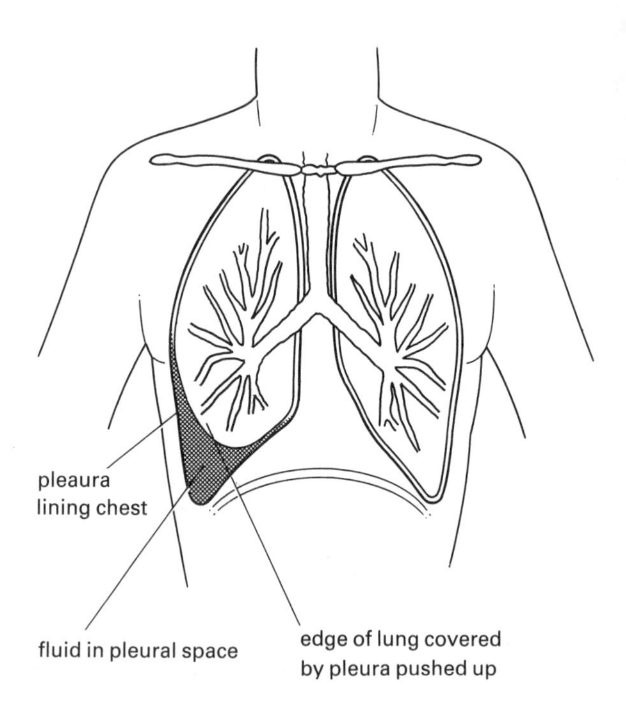

Figure 20.21 Diagram showing the changes with pleural fluid to the right in the standing position. The fluid in the pleural space pushes the lung up. The fluid can fill almost all the chest and squash (collapse) almost all of the lung so that no ventilation is possible.

Signs of fluid in the pleural cavity include (on the affected side):

- movement less,
- percussion note very dull ('stony dull'),
- breath sounds or air entry less (usually none), and
- no crackles or wheezes but occasionally a pleural rub.

There may *also* be symptoms and signs of the cause of the pleural fluid.

When you diagnose fluid in the pleural cavity:

1. *Always do a diagnostic pleural aspiration* to find out what kind of fluid it is, i.e.
   (a) Clear (usually yellow) fluid ('effusion'), but this can either be a transudate which is just watery fluid or an exudate which has a lot of protein in it.
   Stand a sample of fluid in a clear glass bottle for half an hour. If a web forms in it, it is likely to be an exudate.
   If a small capped bottle or a solution of 2.3 g of copper sulphate dried crystals ($CUSO_4\ 5H_2O$) dissolved in distilled water made up to 100 ml is kept and 1 drop of pleural fluid dropped into this bottle,

the drop will float if it is a transudate and will sink if it is an exudate.

If possible send a sample of the fluid to the laboratory with some in a bottle used for a blood count (which has anticoagulant in it) and some in a clear sterile bottle and ask for Gram and AFB stains, cell count, protein, sugar and specific gravity (SG).

(b) Pus ('empyema').

(c) Blood ('haemothorax')

> You must transfer all patients with pus or blood to a Medical Officer immediately for drainage of all the fluid and other treatment.

2. *Always find out the cause*

   (a) Pneumonia can cause an effusion (clear yellow fluid). If this is a transudate it will usually go away itself with treatment of the pneumonia. If it is an exudate or an empyema it all should be drained urgently and the patient needs urgent transfer to a Medical Officer.

   (b) Tuberculosis can cause an effusion (clear yellow fluid). This can be a transudate or an exudate. If the patient is put on anti-tuberculosis treatment, this will almost always clear itself.

   (c) Heart failure which will cause only an effusion (clear yellow fluid). This will be a transudate and go away with treatment of the heart failure.

   (d) Many other conditions can cause fluid, pus or blood in the pleural cavity, all of which need transfer to a Medical Officer for diagnosis and/or treatment.

> If the patient does not have
> - clear fluid which is a transudate and pneumonia or heart failure, or
> - clear fluid which is a transudate or exudate and sputum positive for AFB
>
> THEN you must transfer the patient to a Medical Officer for diagnosis and treatment (even if the effusion goes away – early tuberculosis often causes an effusion which goes away without treatment).

Pneumothorax

A pneumothorax is when there is air in the pleural cavity (see Figure 20.22).

Symptoms include shortness of breath and at times pleuritic pain.

Signs may include (on the affected side):

- movement less.
- percussion note very resonant or hollow (difficult to be sure of this), and
- breath sounds or air entry less.

There may also be symptoms and signs of the cause of the pneumothorax (NB tuberculosis).

Contact your Medical Officer urgently for management of any case you diagnose.

Transfer all cases urgently.

If there is severe shortness of breath, put a plastic cannula (or a needle) into the pleural cavity immediately. The best place is in the mid-clavicular line in the second intercostal space (i.e. 2–3 cm below the middle of the clavicle). Make a valve for the cannula or needle before you put it into the chest with part of a surgical rubber glove, like this:

1. Take a rubber surgical glove or, if unavailable, a plastic glove and cut a small 1 cm slit at the top of one of the glove fingers.
2. Then cut that glove finger from the glove, where it joins the palm of the glove.

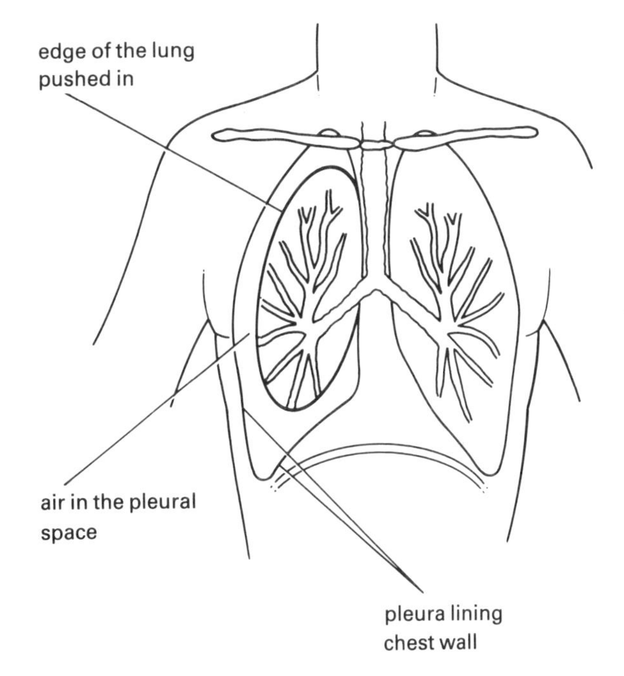

Figure 20.22 Diagram showing the changes in a pneumothorax. The air in the pleural space pushes the lung towards the trachea. The air can fill almost all the chest and completely collapse (squash) the lung so that no ventilation of that lung is possible.

3. Put the glove finger, where it joined the glove palm, around the hub of the cannula which is to go in the chest (i.e. where the needle can join onto a syringe).
4. Tightly tie the glove finger onto the cannula or needle with suture material or cotton around the hub of the needle.

This will allow air to go out of the chest, through the needle and the slit in the glove but it will not allow air to go back into the chest as the glove will be pushed into the end of the needle by the air and stop the air going in.

Asthma

Asthma is a condition of inflammation of the bronchi. This causes times when all of the bronchi are narrowed (see Figure 20.23) causing episodes of shortness of breath and wheezing called attacks of asthma. Between attacks, the bronchi may not be narrowed and there may be no symptoms or just cough.

You often cannot find the cause of a patient's asthma in a health centre. There may be a family history of asthma or allergies. There may be a history of attacks of shortness of breath; or of allergies (see Chapter 10 page 39) to things breathed in, or swallowed (including drugs), or touched; or cough. Often asthma is caused by allergy to dust (especially house dust) or pollens. Sometimes it is caused by reaction to organisms that cause respiratory infection or from gastro-oesophageal reflux. Make sure the asthma is not made worse if the patient takes aspirin tablets.

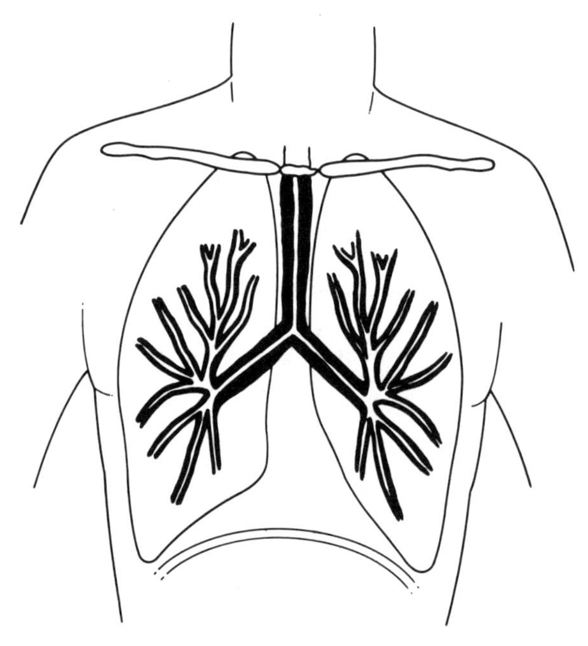

Figure 20.23 Diagram showing changes during an attack of asthma. All the bronchi going to all parts of the lung are narrowed by a thick layer of thick mucus, swelling of the mucous membrane, and contraction of the bronchial muscles. Between attacks the bronchi return to normal.

The bronchi have bronchial muscle spasm, swelling of the bronchial mucous membrane, and thick layer of jelly-like mucus on the bronchial walls. There is also shortness of breath, cough and sputum.

Symptoms include:

- sudden shortness of breath, most common at night or when the patient starts sudden exertion or if he goes into cold air,
- a feeling of tightness in the chest,
- wheezing,
- often repeated little coughs, and
- usually a history of previous attacks and being well in between attacks or cough only.

Signs include:

- temperature normal (no fever),
- respiration slow and deep with wheezing and sometimes coughing,
- pulse rate fast if a severe attack,
- jelly-like sputum (not pus),
- chest – rhonchi or wheezes in all areas especially when the patient breathes out.

There are two very important exceptions to the above:

1. In some patients the asthma does not ever go away completely (especially people who do not have the allergic type of asthma and whose asthma started when they were in middle or late adult life). These patients do have acute attacks of asthma. But between acute attacks they may have chronic shortness of breath and wheezes may be heard on examination of the chest. Some just have cough. This is called 'chronic asthma'.
2. Some patients have very severe attacks when almost no breath sounds or breathing in can be heard. In this case the patient is very anxious, has respiratory distress (see page 221), has very fast pulse rate, is cyanosed, has decreased breath sounds or air entry and few wheezes or rhonchi can therefore be heard. This patient is near death.

Treatment

Chronic asthma[1]

1. Give a bronchodilator,[2] e.g. salbutamol 4 mg *or* terbutaline 5 mg *or* orciprenaline 20 mg *or* ephedrine 30 mg (1 tab) when needed up to 4 times a day and at night.
   Reduce the dose if side effects occur (shaking, nervousness, sweating, giddiness or palpitations).
   Increase the dose slowly if no side effects but still asthma. Do not give more than 2 tablets four times a day. If the tablets are needed two or three or more times daily, add regular aminophylline and then give these bronchodilator[2] tablets only if needed.
2. Add aminophylline or theophylline if necessary if the patient is taking more than two or three doses of the above and this does not control the symptoms.
   Increase the dose until:
   - the asthma is controlled, or
   - there is nausea, or other side effects (then reduce dose a little), or
   - you are giving 400 mg (4 tablets) four times a day (do not give more).

   It would be best to give regular aminophylline or theophylline and only if needed doses of the bronchodilator drugs above, rather than the other way round.
3. Find and avoid or treat the cause if possible.
4. Treat any acute attacks which occur (see below).

Acute attack asthma

1. If infection of the respiratory tract is present (fever or pus in sputum) or likely (attack present for 2 or more days) give:
   - Procaine benzylpenicillin 1 g or 1,000,000 units IMI daily or sulphamethoxazole 800 mg/ trimethoprim 160 mg (co-trimoxazole) twice daily *or*
   - Tetracycline 250 mg (1 cap) four times a day or doxycycline 100 mg once daily but not if pregnant when give amoxycillin 500 mg three times a day
2. Give a bronchodilator[2] salbutamol 4 mg *or* terbutaline 5 mg *or* orciprenaline 20 mg *or* ephedrine 30 mg (1 tablet) immediately if it is a mild attack, *or* adrenaline tart. (epinephrine) 1:1000 solution 0.5 ml ($\frac{1}{2}$ ml) subcutaneous injection if it is a moderate or severe attack.

> DO NOT give both terbutaline or salbutamol (or similar drug) and adrenaline (epinephrine) at the same time or either within 4 hours of the other.

3. Give intra-nasal oxygen 2–4 litres/minute for a moderate or a severe attack.
4. Give aminophylline or theophylline orally or aminophylline IV for a moderate attack or IV for a severe attack. *Give IV slowly* – take 10 minutes by the clock.
   - Small adult (< 50 kg) 300 mg (3 tabs) orally *or* 250 mg (10 ml)IV
   - Large adult (< 50 kg) 400 mg (4 tabs) orally *or* 375 mg (15 ml) IV.

> Do not give this large dose of aminophylline or theophylline if the patient has taken regular oral aminophylline or theophylline or had a large oral dose in the last 12 hours. In these cases start an aminophylline drip (see below).

---

1 The best treatment in prevention or stopping attacks of asthma occurring is an anti-inflammatory drug which is inhaled through the mouth into the lungs. Sodium cromoglycate or cromoglycic acid and nedocromil are safe for all ages though less effective than beclomethasone, budesonide and fluticasone which can cause oral thrush, a hoarse voice and bruising of the skin. These anti-inflammatory drugs are far more expensive than the treatment drugs and at the moment are not likely to be available for use. If they are ever used, carefully read and follow the instructions and do not give more than correct dose. Only these help chronic cough caused by asthma.

2 These bronchodilator drugs would be much better inhaled through the mouth into the lungs, either as a powder or an aerosol. A much smaller dose is much more effective. Terbutaline as, e.g. Bricanyl powder from a Turbohaler or an aerosol can and salbutamol as, e.g. Ventolin powder from an Accuhaler or an aerosol can gives one dose when the patient breathes in. However patients have to be taught how to use these drugs and they are usually far too expensive for patients to buy. The dose of terbutaline is 250–1000 micrograms and for salbutamol 100–400 micrograms. Long 12-hour acting drugs including salmeterol and eformoterol are also now available.

These drugs can also be inhaled when a solution containing them is turned into a fine mist by a special mask when air or oxygen is pumped through the mask, i.e. nebulised. This can be used for treatment in the health centre. Masks must be disinfected properly if used for more than one patient. The dose for terbutaline is 5 mg and for salbutamol 2.5–5 mg.

5. Do *not* give morphine, pethidine or phenobarbitone. Instead, if mentally abnormal, treat as a severe attack; also look for other causes of mental abnormality (see Chapter 35 page 466).
6. If the attack is moderate or severe and the patient has been taking prednisone, prednisolone or other cortisone-like drug, urgently consult the Medical Officer. If the patient does not quickly improve, give 60 mg (12 of the 5 mg tablets) of his prednisolone (or 6–12 times his usual total daily dose of other cortisone-like drug) immediately and daily until you get further advice from the Medical Officer.
7. Find and avoid or treat the cause, if possible. Do not give aspirin (give paracetamol instead) unless you know aspirin does not cause an attack of asthma in this patient.

IF the symptoms and signs go within 2 hours THEN discharge on terbutaline 5 mg *or* orciprenaline 20 mg *or* salbutamol 4 mg (1 tab) four times a day for 5 days; then four times a day if necessary.
IF symptoms and signs do not all go in 2 hours
or
IF it is a severe attack from the start,
THEN immediately treat as follows (as well as 1–7).

8. Start an aminophylline drip
   Add aminophylline solution
   - 150 mg (6 ml) for a small adult (< 50 kg) *or*
   - 225 mg (9 ml) for a large adult (> 50 kg) to 1 litre of 4.3% dextrose in 0.18% sodium chloride. Use only half of these doses of aminophylline if the patient has heart failure or liver disease.

   Give 1 litre every 8 hours. Continue until the attack has completely gone.
   If the patient is a smoker *and* if the asthma does not improve *and* if there are no toxic effects, you can double the dose of aminophylline.
   If, however, there is continuous nausea or headache or any vomiting, then slow the drip to half ($\frac{1}{2}$) the rate, or (better) reduce the dose of aminophylline in each flask to half the previous dose and continue to run the drip at the same rate.
9. Give adrenaline (epinephrine) every 4–6 hours (see page 225).
10. Give antibiotics (see page 225).

When the patient improves:

1. Stop oxygen.
2. Change adrenaline (epinephrine) injections to salbutamol 4 mg or similar tablets (1 tablet) four times a day.
3. Change aminophylline drip to aminophylline or theophylline tablets four times a day. Start 100 mg (1 tablet) four times a day. Increase the dose if necessary.
4. Continue salbutamol and aminophylline until the attack is clinically cured and then for 5 days more.

When the patient is better he can go home, with a supply of:

1. salbutamol 4 mg or similar tablets, 1 tablet four times a day (or more) if necessary, *and*
2. aminophylline tablets *or* theophylline if necessary (see chronic attack page 225).

Transfer to Medical Officer care if there is:

1. Very severe asthma which does not improve, or is worse, after 8 hours of proper treatment for a severe case, i.e. if
   - PR 120 or more,
   - severe shortness of breath and respiration distress, or
   - cyanosis

   (urgent – emergency);
2. Severe asthma after 2 days of full treatment (urgent);
3. Repeated acute attacks needing repeated inpatient care during several months, (non-urgent).

Chronic obstructive lung disease

Chronic Obstructive Lung Disease (COLD) (also called Chronic Obstructive Airways Disease (COAD) or chronic bronchitis and emphysema) is a common chronic non-infective disease of the bronchi and lungs.

Mucous membrane lining the bronchi is thickened and covered by a layer of mucus. This narrows the bronchi and causes shortness of breath, cough and sputum. Walls of the bronchi are of irregular size and are weak. When the patient breathes out, many of the bronchi collapse before the air from the alveoli can go through them. This traps air inside the lung. Many alveoli are destroyed. This also causes shortness of breath. (See Figure 20.24.)

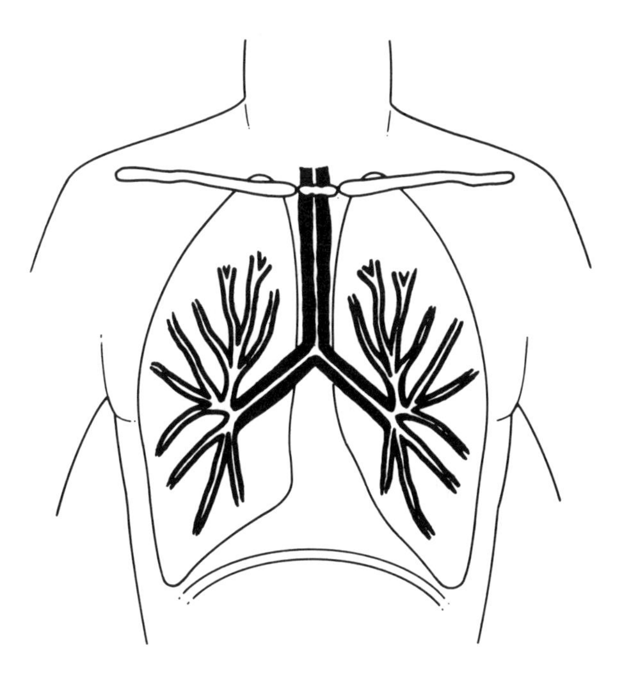

Figure 20.24 Diagram showing the changes in COLD. The bronchi going to all parts of the lung are narrowed by (1) a thick layer of mucus on the surface of the mucous membrane, (2) the mucous membrane itself is thickened and (3) the irregular size of many damaged bronchi, many of which collapse when the patient breathes out thus trapping air in the lungs.

COLD is caused by smoking tobacco or other things; smoke from fires in homes; some smoke or special dusts at work; or repeated attacks of lung infections.

Symptoms

- Chronic cough (on most days for at least 3 months of the year for at least 2 years).
- Sputum which is white or mucus (except if there is also acute chest infection).
- Shortness of breath – at first during exercise or respiratory infection, but later all the time.
- Wheezing at times.

Signs

- Middle aged or old person who has been a smoker or had repeated chest infections.
- Normal temperature.
- Normal pulse.
- Increased respiratory rate (if severe).
- Wasting (if severe).
- Chest – looks as if the patient is holding his breath in all of the time; abnormal use of neck and shoulder and abdominal muscles for breathing and indrawing of the skin and soft tissues above and below the clavicles and over the upper and lower chest during breathing in ('insuction') (if severe).
- Only a little but equal movement on both sides (the chest is almost fully expanded *all* the time).
- The percussion note often more resonant (hollow) than normal but on both sides.
- Breath sounds – air entry often decreased equally on both sides.
- Wheezes or rhonchi and sometimes crackles or crepitations – heard equally on both sides and more often low down in the chest.

Complications

- Acute bronchitis (see page 217) and pneumonia (see page 219) which occurs more and more often.
- Asthma (see page 224) is very common.
- Heart failure (see Chapter 27 page 370).

The patient usually gets worse slowly over years, and dies because of one of these complications.

Tests

Always send three sputum smears to the laboratory for examination for AFB. See Chapter 14 page 81.

Do not diagnose COLD until smears have been negative for AFB.

Treatment

Treat as an outpatient.

Admit for inpatient treatment only if a complication (pneumonia, moderate or severe asthma or heart failure) develops.

1. Tell the patient to stop smoking (or to at least smoke less).
2. If there is wheezing or rhonchi then supply:
   (a) aminophylline or theophylline tablets regularly (see page 225) if there is shortness of breath all the time; or as required (see page 225) if there are only attacks or shortness of breath.
   (b) terbutaline 5 mg *or* salbutamol 4 mg *or* similar tablets, one tablet three or four times a day if necessary for attacks (as well as (or)).
   See Asthma, page 224.
3. *Show* the patient how to look for pus in his sputum (yellow or green colour).
   Tell the patient to look every day and to come for antibiotics immediately if he sees pus.
   Treat any chest infection immediately, until there is no pus in the sputum (it is white again).

Treat as follows: procaine benzylpenicillin 1 g or 1,000,000 units IMI daily *or* sulphamethoxazole 800 mg/trimethoprim 160 mg (co-trimoxazole) twice daily for 5–10 days. If this fails give: tetracycline 250–500 mg (1–2 caps) four times a day or doxycycline 100 mg (1 tab) daily but not if pregnant, when use amoxycillin 500 mg three times a day.
Use chloramphenicol only for infections which threaten life.

4. Look for heart failure. If it is found start hydrochlorothiazide 50–100 mg (1–2 tablets) daily, and see 'Heart failure' (Chapter 27 page 374).
5. Do not give oxygen unless there is a complication (e.g. pneumonia). Do not give oxygen faster than 2 litres/minute intranasally. (Too much oxygen may make the COLD patient unconscious and cause death.)
6. Never give morphine, pethidine or phenobarbitone (as these may stop the COLD patient breathing and cause death).

Transfer to Medical Officer care is not necessary as no more treatment is possible at a hospital.

Control and prevention

1. Treat chest infections quickly and properly.
2. Tell everyone never to smoke tobacco.

Lung diseases caused by worms

A number of lung diseases can be caused by worms.

Bronchitis and pneumonia can be caused by the larvae of worms (e.g. hookworm or roundworm) as they travel through the lung.

Asthma and other chest pains and other symptoms can be caused by worm larvae (e.g. roundworm or hookworm) as they travel through the body, or by some of the filarial worms.

Chronic lung disease with heart failure can be caused by schistosomiasis but usually there are signs of portal hypertension also.

Haemoptysis, pneumonia or chronic lung disease or a condition like tuberculosis can be caused by lung flukes.

None of these conditions can be diagnosed without the help of a laboratory. Do not worry. If one of these conditions is very common in your area, you will be taught about it. Otherwise the condition will be diagnosed when you refer or transfer the patient to a Medical Officer (usually when the patient does not get better with your treatment).

Bronchiectasis

Bronchiectasis is a condition when there is permanent damage to the bronchi of part of the lung. The bronchi are permanently dilated (widened) and do not work properly. They often become infected and finally become just like tubes or bags of pus, (see Figure 20.25).

Bronchiectasis is caused by obstruction and infection of bronchi which are not treated and cured quickly. This infection and obstruction may be caused by tuberculosis or pneumonia or bronchitis (especially attacks complicating measles or whooping cough which are not treated quickly or properly).

Symptoms include:

- Chronic cough that is present every day and worse after waking in the morning or after exercise.

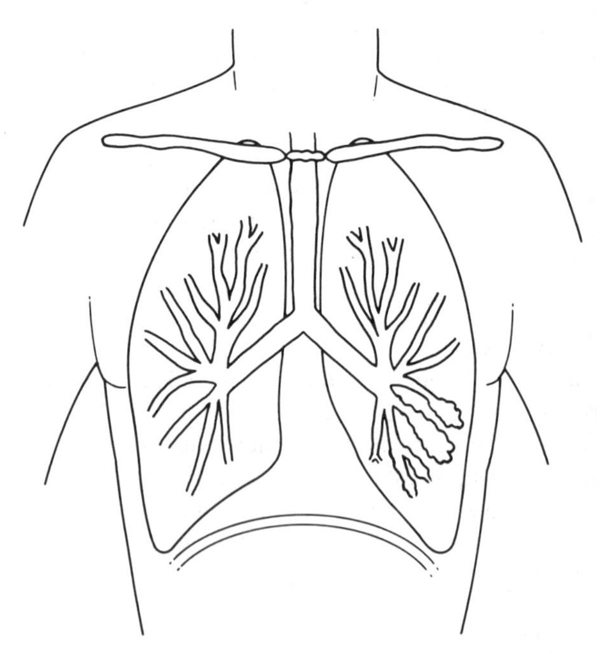

Figure 20.25 Diagram to show the changes in bronchiectasis affecting some of the bronchi of the left lower lobe. The bronchial walls have been weakened or destroyed. The bronchi therefore became irregular in size and shape. The bronchial mucous membrane has been destroyed. The bronchi therefore cannot move secretions out through the bronchial tree. The bronchi therefore become filled with secretions. The bronchial secretions often become infected and form pus.

- Sputum in large amounts (e.g. 20–200 ml or more daily) which is often made of pus (e.g. green or yellow or brown and often smells bad).
- Sometimes blood in the sputum.
- Shortness of breath; but only late in the disease.

Signs of bronchiectasis are few early in the disease. Often there is only one sign – crackles or crepitations in the affected part of the lung which stay there after deep breathing and coughing and are always in the same place every time the patient is examined.

Signs which come later include: wasting, anaemia, and clubbing of the fingers.

The symptoms and signs of attacks of acute bronchitis and pneumonia are common.

Send sputum for AFB to check the patient does not have tuberculosis.

Treatment includes:

1. Postural drainage and physiotherapy for 15–30 minutes once or twice *every* day of the patient's life. Most patients will not do this; but without this, any other treatment is of no real help. Show the patient how to raise the foot of a straight bed by using blocks of something about 0.2–0.5 m high; lie on this with the head on the low end of the bed and the affected part of his lung (i.e. where the crackles are heard) upwards (i.e. on the roof side); then take deep breaths and cough up the sputum as he (or someone else) hits the affected part of the lung with the palm of the hand. Tell the patient to do this for 15–30 minutes each morning and also if possible each evening. Also tell the patient to sleep on a straight bed if possible; even better sleep with the foot of the bed raised.
2. Antibiotics as for pneumonia if there is an acute bacterial infection (but do not continue the antibiotic if it does not cure the infection).
3. Surgery to cut out the whole part of the lung which has bronchiectasis in it, can help only very occasionally.

Discuss treatment of the patient with the next visiting Medical Officer.

Pulmonary tuberculosis

See Chapter 14 page 75.

Lung flukes

Paragonimus westermani and some other small worms about 10 mm long normally live in the lungs of dogs, cats, pigs and other animals in Asia, parts of the Pacific and West Africa. Their eggs are coughed up or passed in the stool and if they reach fresh water, develop in crayfish and crabs, ending up in their muscles. When animals eat these crabs, etc. the worms travel from the bowel to the lung where they live by destroying part of the lung and making little 'nests' about 1 cm in diameter. These cause cough, sputum, haemoptysis, chest pain, fever, etc.

Man can become infected by eating uncooked freshwater crayfish and crabs. The symptoms in man are the same as for animals and very similar to those of tuberculosis. Diagnosis can be made by finding the eggs in the sputum or stool.

The main problem is making the diagnosis. If a patient appears to have tuberculosis and repeated tests do not demonstrate AFB in the sputum, it is worthwhile requesting sputum and stool examination for eggs of *Paragonimus* if this parasite is known to occur in the area.

Treatment is with praziquantel 25 mg/kg three times a day for 3 days.

Prevention is of course not eating uncooked crabs or crayfish even if they are pickled.

Some problems of diagnosis and management

Deafness

Causes include:

1. any condition blocking the external ear canal, including wax, foreign body or external ear inflammation;
2. any condition damaging the middle ear, including blocked eustachian tube and acute and chronic middle ear infection;
3. any condition damaging the inner ear, the nerve to the ear or the brain, including side effects of streptomycin and trauma of the head;
4. others. If the cause is not one of these, see a specialist book.

Always look in the ear with an auriscope. Do ear toilet or syringing until you can see the ear drum. Treat any condition in the usual way (see index).

Ear pain

Causes include:

1. external ear infection (otitis externa);
2. foreign body in the external ear canal;
3. middle ear inflammation (otitis media), acute or chronic;
4. mastoiditis;
5. acute parotitis – mumps or acute bacterial;
6. infection of teeth;
7. others. If the cause is not one of these see a specialist book.

Always look in the ear with an auriscope. Do ear toilet and syringing until you can see the ear drum. Examine behind the ear (mastoid) in front of the ear (parotid) and below the ear (in the mouth).

Treat any condition in the usual way (see index).

Ear discharge

Causes include:

1. external ear inflammation (otitis externa);
2. foreign body in external ear canal;
3. middle ear infection (otitis media), acute (with perforated ear drum) or chronic;
4. others. If the cause is not one of these see a specialist book.

Always look in the ear with an auriscope.

Do ear toilet or syringing until you can see the ear drum. Treat any condition in the usual way. See Index.

Nasal discharge – both sides

Causes include:

1. virus infections of the upper respiratory tract including measles (watery discharge);
2. bacterial infections of the upper respiratory tract, e.g. sinusitis (pus);
3. foreign body in the nose (pus or blood);
4. allergy ('hay fever') (watery discharge);
5. irritation by dust, smoke etc. (watery discharge);
6. others. If the cause is not one of these see a specialist book.

Treat any condition in the usual way (see index). You can sometimes improve chronic infections by washing out the nose twice daily with normal saline solution ($2\frac{1}{2}$ ml or $\frac{1}{2}$ teaspoon of salt in 200 ml or 1 cup of clear water). Tell the patient to sniff up or squirt in with a 20 ml syringe (without a needle) or pour in the saline through the nose; then blow it out or let it run into the mouth then spit it out. This thins the pus and washes it away.

Nasal discharge – from one side only

Always look for a foreign body in the nose.

See also nasal discharge both sides (above).

Acute loss of voice or hoarse voice (present for less than 4 weeks)

Causes include:

1. shouting, singing or talking too much;
2. smoking too much;
3. acute viral throat/larynx/tracheal/bronchial infections (the patient is usually not 'sick');
4. acute bacterial throat/larynx/tracheal/bronchial infections (the patient is usually 'sick');
5. others. If the cause is not one of these see a specialist book.

Treat any condition found in the usual way. See index.

Chronic loss of voice or hoarse voice (present for more than 4 weeks)

Causes include:

1. tuberculosis of lung and larynx;
2. cancer of neck, lung or larynx;
3. others.

You must transfer all patients with this so that the Medical Officer can examine the patient's larynx, except patients with sputum-positive tuberculosis (who you will treat for tuberculosis at the health centre).

Sore throat

Causes include:

1. common cold, and other viral upper respiratory tract infections;
2. acute tonsillitis, and other bacterial upper respiratory tract infections;
3. one of the causes of a painful ear (see page 229).

Always look in the mouth and throat with a tongue depressor and light, and in the ear with an auriscope.

If these conditions are not present see a specialist book. Treat any condition found in the usual way (see index).

Cough

The cause is usually obvious from the history and examination.

Do full history and examination (see Chapter 6).

Look at sputum (? mucus ?pus ?blood).

Always ask how long the cough has been present see below. If it has been present for more than 3 weeks send sputum for examination for AFB.

Cough present for less than 3 weeks

Upper respiratory tract infection

- No other chest symptoms.
- Respiratory rate normal and no respiratory distress (see page 221).
- No chest signs.

Asthma

- Shortness of breath. Episodes of coughing often without sputum. Previous similar attacks.
- Sputum, if any, not made of pus, i.e. not yellow or rusty.
- Wheezes or rhonchi in chest.
- No fever.

Acute bronchitis or pneumonia

- Fever
- Sputum is pus or of rusty colour.
- Respiratory rate fast.
- Respiratory distress may be present.
- Other chest signs.

Cough present for more than 3 weeks

Where tuberculosis OR HIV infection is common

Make three sputum smears for examination for AFB – specimen 'A' collected immediately; specimen 'B' collected by the patient the next morning as soon as he wakes; specimen 'C' collected when the patient returns with 'B'.

Where tuberculosis AND HIV infection are not common

- Treat for 1 week with procaine benzylpenicillin 1 g or 1,000,000 units daily IMI.
- If the cough is not cured treat for 1 week with tetracycline 250 mg (1 cap) *or* doxycycline 100 mg (1 tab) daily but not if pregnant when use amoxycillin or ampicillin three or four times a day.
- If the cough is still present continue the tetracycline and send three sputum specimens for examination for AFB.

If one or more sputum examinations positive for AFB

Tuberculosis. See Chapter 14 page 75.

If all sputum examinations negative for AFB

1. Repeat sputum for AFB × 3 again if:
   (a) past or family history of tuberculosis or other history suggests tuberculosis or HIV infection;
   (b) there is wasting or lymphadenopathy or other signs of tuberculosis or HIV infection.
2. Otherwise, and if repeat sputum examinations negative for AFB, check for:
   (a) Chronic Obstructive Lung Disease, smoking still;
   (b) asthma with cough;
   (c) repeated upper respiratory tract infections, acute bronchitis or pneumonia;
   (d) chronic sinusitis with post nasal discharge;
   (e) empyema or lung abscess;
   (f) whooping cough (whoop rare in adults);
   (g) bronchiectasis;
   (h) gastro-oesophageal reflux of stomach acid;
   (i) lung fluke infections;
   (j) tuberculosis with sputum negative for AFB. If you still suspect tuberculosis transfer non-urgently to Medical Officer.

Treatment of cough

1. Treat the cause (see index).
2. Stop the patient smoking.
3. Physiotherapy often helps; but only if it causes the patient to cough up more than 30 ml sputum every time. See page 229.
4. Cough medicines do not help.

Sputum

See causes of cough for causes of sputum.

Always find the answers to these three things:

1. Is the sputum from the lower respiratory tract (which is often serious) or from the upper respiratory tract (which is not as serious)?
2. What is the colour of the sputum?
   - Coloured sputum (yellow, green or brown) usually means bacterial infection, e.g. acute bronchitis, bronchopneumonia, lobar pneumonia, bronchiectasis, sinusitis, tuberculosis, etc.
   - White or mucoid sputum occurs in viral infections (if there is no bacterial infection as well).
   - White or mucoid sputum is also common from smoking, chronic bronchitis (COLD), asthma and some cases of chronic sinusitis.
   - Bacterial infection needs treatment with antibiotics. Antibiotics will not help other conditions.

3. Is there blood in the sputum (haemoptysis)? If there is blood in the sputum see below.

Blood coughed up – haemoptysis

1. Always check that it is *blood* that is coughed up. Always examine what is coughed up.
2. Always check that the blood was *coughed up*.
   - Check that the blood was not vomited up.
   - Check that the blood was not just from the upper respiratory tract (especially the nose).
3. Always find out *how much* blood was coughed up – if more than one cup, it is an emergency and you must start an IV drip.
4. Always find out the *cause*. Causes include:
   - Tuberculosis. Send sputum for AFB in all cases.
   - Lung fluke infection in some areas.
   - Any acute lower respiratory tract infection.
   - Bronchiectasis or lung abscess.
   - Chest injury.
   - Others. If the cause is not one of these see a specialist book. Causes such as pulmonary embolus and cancer of the lung are not common in the rural areas of tropical and developing countries but may be common in the towns and cities.

Tuberculosis is the most common and important cause of haemoptysis.

If you cannot diagnose the cause at the health centre, transfer the patient for investigation.

Treatment of haemoptysis

1. Treat the cause.
2. If there is shock or anaemia, give routine treatment for these (see Chapter 27 page 378 and Chapter 21, page 340).
3. If the patient has difficulty in breathing (because blood is filling the bronchi)
   - put the patient on his side, with the diseased part of the chest down or on his underside,
   - tip the head of the bed down,
   - suck out the pharynx and larynx if necessary,
   - give morphine 10 mg (1 ml) by slow IVI or IMI or IVI diazepam 5–10 mg (1–2 ml) 1 mg/minute or (*but* only if does *not* have COLD),
   - give intranasal oxygen,
   - transfer as soon as possible to Medical Officer care.
4. Wear protective clothing, goggles, etc. so that blood does not get into staff member's eyes, mouth, etc.

Shortness of breath

Do a full history and examination (see Chapter 6).

Look at any sputum (?pus ?blood).

Test the urine for protein and sugar.

See page 12 for classification

Look at the following 7 headings (pages 232–3) to see which paragraph will apply to your patient.

1. With stridor (loud noise breathing in)

Block of throat, larynx or trachea by foreign body, acute allergic reaction or acute bacterial or viral infection.

- Emergency. Act immediately.
- If inhaled foreign body or vomit is possible, pull these out of throat. If not successful, lay the patient face down, lift up his hips and abdomen and hit *very hard* between the shoulder blades. See Chapter 37 page 503.
- If acute allergic reaction is possible, give IM adrenaline (epinephrine) 0.5 ml ($\frac{1}{2}$ ml) and IV promethazine 50 mg (2 ml) immediately. See page 40.
- If infection is possible, give IV (or IM) chloramphenicol 2 g immediately, then 1 g each 6 hours.
- Give intranasal oxygen 4 litres/minute.
- If stops breathing see Chapter 37 page 506.
- Transfer urgently (emergency) unless the patient is cured immediately.

2. With pallor and/or shock (fast PR, low BP, cold hands and feet).

Anaemia ± blood loss.

- If shock or severe blood loss see Chapter 27 page 378.
- Give routine anaemia treatment to other cases (see Chapter 21 page 240).

3. With fever

Chest infections (cough, sputum made of pus or rusty, crackles or other signs in chest); septicaemia

- Give penicillin or chloramphenicol (see page 220).
- Send sputum for AFB if cough present for more than 3 weeks. See Chapter 14 page 81.

Malaria if there is no evidence of chest infection.

- Give antimalarials (see Chapter 13, page 61).

4. With wheezing and rhonchi

Asthma; COLD; acute bronchitis

- Give adrenaline (epinephrine) or salbutamol *and*, if needed, aminophylline orally or by IVI. (See page 225).
- Send sputum for AFB of cough present for more than 3 weeks. See Chapter 14 page 81.

5. With oedema, large liver, raised neck veins

Heart failure.

- Give diuretics – IV frusemide 40 mg (4 ml) immediately if severe or oral hydrochlorothiazide 50–100 mg (1–2 tabs) if not severe and see Chapter 27 page 374.
- Treat the cause (see Chapter 27 page 371).

6. And 'sick' but not distressed by shortness of breath

Dehydration usually from gastroenteritis

- Give IV fluids (see Chapter 23 page 285).

Meningitis or septicaemia.

- Give chloramphenicol by IVI or IMI (see Chapter 12 page 53).

Diabetes mellitus.

- Give IV rehydration. See Chapter 23 page 285.
- Transfer to Medical Officer urgently.

Chronic kidney failure

- See Chapter 26 page 259.

7. And very worried by shortness of breath but no abnormalities found on examination

The patient feels as if he cannot get enough air into the lungs – anxiety.

Obvious 'over-breathing' often with dizziness and strange feeling around mouth and in hands and feet – 'acting out'.

See Chapter 36 page 480.

Classification

Here is one classification of the causes of shortness of breath.

Shortness of breath is normal after strong exercise or in high areas (on mountains).

Diseases causing shortness of breath include:

1. Respiratory diseases
   (a) of alveoli
   pneumonia including severe or advanced tuberculous pneumonia – shallow quick breathing
   (b) of bronchi
   acute bronchitis, asthma (deep slow breathing), COLD } sometimes wheezing
   (c) of throat/larynx/trachea/bronchi,
   acute bacterial infections, acute viral infections (e.g. 'croup'), allergy, foreign body } often stridor
   (d) of pleura
   effusion or empyema, pneumothorax } shallow quick breathing
2. Cardiovascular
   (a) heart failure – shallow quick breathing
   (b) shock – gasping breathing.
3. Anaemia – deep fast breathing.
4. Kidney failure, Diabetes mellitus } deep slow breathing; but no distress
5. Anxiety – the patient feels as if he can't get enough air into his lungs; but on examination no abnormalities are found.
   'Acting out' – obvious overbreathing.
6. Others.

Stridor

Stridor is noisy breathing *in*. (Noisy breathing *out* is not as important.) Stridor is usually a crowing noise; but sometimes it is more like snoring.

> Noisy breathing is obstructed breathing. Immediately relieve the obstruction.

Stridor is always serious. Stridor is very dangerous if there is rib recession (insuction) during breathing in, and/or if the patient uses his neck and abdominal muscles to keep breathing.

Always think of these things and treat any present like this:

1. If the patient is weak or not fully conscious (often like 'snoring'):
   (a) lay the patient on his side,
   (b) tip his head back,
   (c) pull his jaw forward,
   (d) suck out his throat.
   } See Chapter 35 page 332
2. Infection of throat and/or epiglottis and/or larynx and/or trachea and/or bronchi
   (a) IVI (or IMI) chloramphenicol urgently for septicaemia (see Chapter 12 page 53).
   (b) if allergy possible, treat (see 4)

(c) Make the patient breathe moist air by boiling water near him if the air is cool and/or dry.
(d) Nurse him carefully (suck out if necessary).
(e) Give intranasal oxygen 4 litres/minute.
(f) Observe him carefully. Transfer urgently (emergency) if he does not quickly improve.

3. Foreign body
(a) Tip the patient with head and neck down; hit his back very hard between shoulder blades or try abdominal thrust. See Chapter 37 page 503.
(b) Transfer urgently if he does not cough up the foreign body.
4. Allergy
(a) IVI antihistamine, e.g. promethazine 50 mg (2 ml).
(b) IMI adrenaline (epinephrine) (1:1000 solution) 0.5 ml ($\frac{1}{2}$ ml)
5. Laryngostomy if breathing stops. See Chapter 37 page 509.

Chest pain

Do a full history (see Chapter 6).
Find out all about the pain:

1. Is it 'pleuritic'? i.e.
   - in the chest wall at the side of the chest,
   - worse on coughing or deep breathing,
   - helped by holding that side of the chest or lying on the side of pain.

   See this page.
2. Is it tracheal? i.e.
   - in the neck and front of centre of chest,
   - present only when coughs.

   See this page.
3. Is it spinal? i.e.
   - also in the back,
   - worse on bending or lifting,
   - tenderness of spine.

   See Chapter 29 page 400.
4. Is it cardiac (due to heart or pericardium or blood vessels)?
   - constant in the anterior chest, or
   - crushing type pain like a band around the chest,
   - may also be felt in arm or arms or jaw,
   - not made better or worse by anything; or angina,
   - middle-aged or elderly person or known high BP, heart trouble or kidney trouble,
   - may have irregular, slow or fast pulse or shock or heart failure.

   See page 235.
5. Is it constant and in the lower chest, and are abdominal symptoms or signs also present?
   See Chapter 36 page 489.
6. Is it in the lower chest and comes or goes with eating food?
   See Chapter 23 page 275.
7. Has it been present for more than 3 weeks, and has cough also been present for 3 weeks?
   See page 235.

Do a full examination (see Chapter 6).

- Ask the patient to cough.
- Listen to the cough.
- Observe if coughing causes pain (pleuritic or tracheal pain).
- Examine any sputum (?pus ?blood).

Diagnose and manage according to the seven types of pain (see above) that the patient has, like this:

Pain is pleuritic

1. *If* ± cough ± sputum (pus or rusty colour) ± shortness of breath ± fever ± fast pulse ± crepitations in chest, *then* pneumonia. See page 220.
2. *If* history of injury to chest, tender place on chest, *then* fracture of rib.
3. If short of breath ± cough ± haemoptysis ± recent other illness or operation or childbirth or even pregnancy ± a recent long trip where the legs were still ± a swollen, tender leg, then ? pulmonary embolus (clot of blood from leg or pelvic veins gone up to the lungs and blocking part of the pulmonary arteries). Exclude pneumonia and pneumothorax. Transfer to Medical Officer urgently.
4. *If* no abnormality found, *then* chest wall pain. Observe the patient daily for a few days.

Pain is tracheal

1. *If* cough ± sputum ± shortness of breath ± fever ± rhonchi in chest, *then* tracheitis/bronchitis. See page 217.
2. *If* no abnormality found, *then* viral upper respiratory tract infection or too much smoking or shouting etc. See page 217.

Pain is spinal

1. *If* pain gets worse over weeks, *then* ?tuberculosis, transfer urgently to Medical Officer.
2. *If* pain is sometimes present and sometimes not present, *then* ?osteoarthrosis. See Chapter 29.

3. *If* spinal tenderness on percussion or stiffness (will not bend properly) especially if lump, *then* ?tuberculosis. Transfer non-urgently to Medical Officer.
4. *If* weakness of legs, not able to pass urine properly, *then* ?tuberculosis, ?fracture. ?cancer. Transfer urgently to Medical Officer

Pain is cardiac

1. Give oxygen.
2. Give aspirin 300 mg 1 tablet immediately
3. Put a glyceryl trinitrate 0.5 or 0.6 mg or isosorbide dinitrate 5 mg tablet under the tongue and let it dissolve there; repeat in 5 minutes if pain still present and blood pressure above 100.
4. If pain still present, dilute 10 mg of morphine with 9 ml of saline and give 2 ml (2 mg of morphine) IVI each 5 minutes until the pain stops.
5. Give metoclopramide 10 mg IVI if nausea.
6. Treat any heart failure present in the usual way, including oxygen, diuretics and digoxin (see page 375).
7. If the pulse rate and heart rate (listening at the heart apex with the stethoscope) is 40 beats per minute or less, then (a) lift up the legs (feet above the hips) and tilt the head end of the bed down and (b) give atropine 0.6 mg (1 ml) IVI then repeat if still needed in 5 minutes and can be repeated in 1 hour and then each few hours to a maximum of 3 mg in 24 hours to try, if possible, to get the heart rate above 60.
8. If the pulse is irregular and fast (over 140) start digoxin (see page 375) and propranolol 40 mg or atenelol 25 mg.
9. If the patient's heart and breathing stop, give cardiopulmonary resuscitation for 5–10 minutes. See Chapter 37 page 504.

As soon as possible, you should have contacted the Medical Officer to ask for advice. Most deaths from myocardial infarctions occur within the first hour and if the patient survives the first hour after the pain starts, the most dangerous period is over.

Pain is constant in lower chest and there is tenderness or mass in upper abdomen

Then abdominal condition with referred pain. See Chapter 36 page 489.

Pain in lower chest that comes or goes with eating

Then peptic ulcer. See Chapter 23 page 275.

Pain and cough present for more than 3 weeks

Then ?tuberculosis. See Chapter 14 page 75.

21

Disorders of the Blood and the Blood Forming Organs

Anatomy

Blood is made of many cells, called blood cells, and a liquid, called plasma. There are two kinds of blood cell – red blood cells (RBCs) and white blood cells (WBCs). Platelets are detached (broken off) parts of special cells which stay in the bone marrow. (See Figure 21.1.) The blood cells are suspended (or 'float') in the plasma. The plasma is made of water which carries many things (some dissolved) in it.

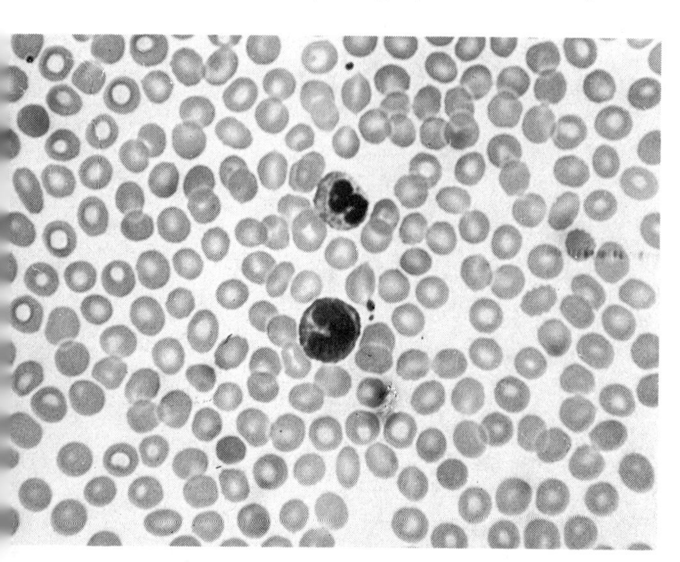

Figure 21.1 A blood slide as seen through a microscope. The blood was smeared on the slide, dried, fixed and stained. The plasma cannot be seen. You can see many RBCs, two WBCs and some platelets.

Proteins, sugars, fats and salts are all carried in the plasma.

Blood is made in the following parts of the body.

1. Bone marrow – the red marrow in the ends of the long bones and in the flat bones (e.g. sternum and pelvis) is most important for making blood. RBCs and most WBCs and platelets are made in the marrow.
2. Spleen.
3. Liver.
4. Lymph nodes.

The bone marrow needs iron, folic acid, vitamin B_{12}, protein and other things to make blood. These things are all in a good diet which includes protein foods (meat, fish, eggs, milk, peanuts etc.) and protective foods (dark green leafy vegetables, fruit etc.). Without enough iron and folic acid and protein in the diet, even a normal bone marrow cannot make enough blood.

Physiology

The body circulates blood to all its organs. The blood keeps the cells of these organs alive and functioning properly. Blood takes food and oxygen and hormones to the cells. Blood takes used and waste material and carbon dioxide away from the cells. Blood contains many parts of the body's defence system against infection. Different parts of the blood have different functions:

1. Red blood cells (RBCs) containing haemoglobin (Hb) – carry oxygen.
2. White blood cells (WBCs) – fight infection.
3. Platelets – make the blood clot to stop bleeding.
4. Serum proteins
   - antibodies – fight infection,
   - albumin – keeps water inside the blood vessels,
   - clotting proteins – make the blood clot to stop bleeding,
   - body building and repair proteins – build and repair the body.
5. Sugar (glucose) – for body nutrition and energy.
6. Fats – for body nutrition and energy.
7. Hormones – carry messages from one part of the body to another part.
8. Salts
9. Water
   – contain the other parts of the blood and also make up the main volume of the blood.

Pathology

Disease may make the blood have too much or too little of one of its parts. Too much or too little of parts of the blood may cause these conditions:

- too few RBCs or low Hb – anaemia
- too few WBCs – infection
- too few platelets – bleeding
- too little antibody protein – infection
- too little albumin protein – oedema
- too little clotting protein – bleeding
- too little body building and repair protein – wasting (body becomes thin)
- too much sugar – diabetes mellitus (see Chapter 30 page 406)
- too little sugar – hypoglycaemia – weakness and unconsciousness
- too little fat – wasting
- too much water and salt – oedema, heart failure
- too little water and salt – dehydration, shock

Most of the conditions affecting the blood are caused by:

1. not enough food to eat or not enough of the food eaten absorbed (taken into the body) so that materials for making blood are not available;
2. pathology in the organs which make and destroy the blood (i.e. marrow, spleen and liver);
3. damage to parts of the blood or loss of parts of the blood or whole blood from the circulation or body.

Conditions which affect the organs which make and destroy the blood

1. *The marrow*
   The marrow may not make enough blood cells or may make abnormal blood cells because:
   (a) The marrow was abnormal from birth (i.e. the patient inherited an abnormal marrow, e.g. thalassaemia).
   (b) The marrow does not get enough 'food' to function, e.g. iron deficiency anaemia, folate deficiency.
   (c) The marrow has been affected by disease or drugs, e.g. infection, kidney failure, chloramphenicol.
2. *The spleen*
   If the spleen gets larger than normal for any reason, it may destroy normal blood cells.
3. *The liver*
   If disease (e.g. cirrhosis) affects the liver, the liver may not be able to use and store the food absorbed from the intestine properly. This can affect the protein, sugar, fat, salt and water in the blood.

History and examination

The most important disease abnormality of the blood is anaemia (see page 238). Look for anaemia in *all* patients you see.

Symptoms of anaemia include:

1. shortness of breath,
2. weakness and tiredness,
3. dizziness.

The sign of anaemia is 'pallor' (i.e. paleness or whiteness). This may be obvious in the skin even in darkly pigmented skins – especially if there is also low protein in the blood (as occurs with hookworm infestations). But, also look for pallor in those parts of the body which are normally pink or red because you can see the red colour of the blood there. However, even in these places there are problems (as follows). However, always look in all of these five places for pallor (Figure 21.2):

1. the conjunctiva under the lower eye lid (but there may be inflammation from conjunctivitis);
2. the mucous membrane behind the lower lip (but the patient may have normal pigment here or have red staining from chewing betel nut);
3. the blood vessels under the finger nails (but the patient may have normal pigment here or might have white nails from liver disease);
4. the palms of the hands including the skin creases (but some patients can get very dark pigmentation of the palms in certain types of anaemia and the skin may be very thick from hard work);
5. the colour of the whole skin.

Test the level of the haemoglobin. Tests needed to find the exact cause of anaemia if the routine treatment does not work are listed in Appendixes 1 and 2 pages 248–50.

Another important abnormality of the blood is not enough white cells to fight infection. Infection can be anywhere in the body and of all types – depending on which white cells are low in number and which infections are common in the area. If someone has an unusual infection or repeated infections or infection not getting better on powerful antibiotic treatment, and especially a severe throat infection not getting better on treatment, send a blood smear for a full blood count; and the white cell count (total and differential) will show how many of what kind of white cells are present.

Another important abnormality of the blood is not enough platelets or not enough clotting proteins to stop bleeding. Bleeding is usually from the nose (epistaxis), mouth, lungs (haemoptysis), upper gastrointestinal tract (haematemesis and melaena), lower gastrointestinal tract, urinary tract (haematuria), skin (pinpoint spots – purpura, larger areas – ecchymoses), conjunctiva, muscles and soft tissues (haematoma), joints (haemarthrosis), etc. The platelets can be looked at on the thin blood smear but special blood tests are needed to tell if other things are wrong with the platelets or the clotting proteins. If you think the patient is having more bleeding than normal or bleeds for a longer time than normal, then ask the laboratory what blood needs to be sent for screening tests for platelet and clotting abnormalities.

If you suspect anaemia or any other disease of the blood examine very carefully the parts of the body where the blood is made:

1. The bones (which, of course, are around the bone marrow). Look for lumps.
   Feel gently for tenderness. Examine the sternum carefully.
2. The spleen. See Figure 22.10.
3. The liver. See Figure 24.14.
4. The lymph nodes. See Chapter 22 page 255.

Tests

1. *Examination of haemoglobin using a comparator (or haemoglobinometer)*
   If you do not have a laboratory worker to do it, you must do this test yourself. For methods see Appendix 1 and Appendix 2 at the end of this chapter.
2. *Examination of a thin blood film* – full blood count (FBC)
   This test must be done in a laboratory by a trained laboratory worker. If you do not have a laboratory worker to do it, you must make the blood film yourself and then send the blood film to a laboratory with a letter. The letter must state patient's problem and your diagnosis, and ask for both a report and an explanation of the results.
   See Chapter 6 page 22 for the method of making a thin blood film.

Disorders

Anaemia

Anaemia is said to be present when there is not enough RBC Hb (red blood cell haemoglobin) in the blood.[1] Normally there is more than 10 g haemoglobin in each decilitre (or 100 ml) of blood (written as 10 g/dl or 10 g/100 ml or 10 g% or 100 g/l).

Anaemia is very severe if the Hb is less than 2.5 g/dl.

Anaemia is severe if the Hb is less than 5 g/dl but more than 2.5 g/dl.

Anaemia is moderate if the Hb is less than 7.5 g/dl but more than 5 g/dl.

Anaemia is mild if the Hb is less than 10 g/dl[1] but more than 7.5 g/dl.

Anaemia is very common especially in hot wet tropical places where malaria and hookworm are common, where malnutrition is common, in women of childbearing age, and in children.

Pathology

The common causes of anaemia include:

1. Not enough haemoglobin to fill the red blood cells has been made by the bone marrow because:
   (a) Not enough iron is in or is absorbed from the food.
   (b) Not enough folic acid or other vitamins are in or are absorbed from the food.
   (c) Not enough protein is in or is absorbed from the food.
   (d) Diseases or drugs or chemicals have stopped the bone marrow functioning properly. The most common cause of this is chronic kidney failure (see Chapter 26 page 259); but there are others.
   (e) The patient was born with abnormal bone marrow which cannot make *enough* normal haemoglobin, i.e. thalassaemia (see page 247).

1 In countries that have good public health services, anaemia is diagnosed if the Hb is less than the following:
men 13 g/dl
non-pregnant women 12 g/dl
pregnant women 11 g/dl

2. Red blood cells are destroyed before they are worn out. This is called 'haemolysis'. When red blood cells are destroyed more quickly than new ones are made, this causes anaemia.
   Reasons for this include:
   (a) Malaria – acute attack.
   (b) Malaria – chronic.
   (c) Malaria – tropical splenomegaly syndrome or hyperreactive malarious splenomegaly.
   (d) Any cause of a very big spleen as well as malaria, e.g. schistosomiasis, kala azar.
   (e) Certain drugs or chemicals especially in patients who were born without enough G6PD (a special part of the red blood cells).
   (f) Sickle cell anaemia – the patient was born with an abnormal bone marrow, which makes an abnormal haemoglobin which causes the red blood cells to become an abnormal sickle shape (called 'sickling') and the abnormal red cells are destroyed quickly by the spleen. See page 244.
3. Red blood cells are lost from the body during bleeding. Reasons for this include:
   (a) Gastrointestinal tract bleeding. This is usually caused by hookworm in the small bowel sucking the patient's blood (see Chapter 23 page 228). This is sometimes due to bleeding from a peptic ulcer (see Chapter 23 page 275). This can be from bleeding veins in the oesophagus from chronic liver disease or schistosomiasis (see Chapter 24 page 308). This can be due to a cancer in the stomach or colon or elsewhere in the gastrointestinal tract.
   (b) Genital tract bleeding in the female. This is usually caused by an ante-partum or post-partum haemorrhage. But it can be caused by having pregnancies close together.

> The common causes of anaemia are:
> 1. not enough iron, folic acid and protein in the diet,
> 2. hookworm,
> 3. malaria,
> 4. repeated pregnancy,
> 5. sickle cell anaemia – in Africa and people of African descent only.
>
> You must find out the epidemiology of anaemia in your area. If other causes are common in your area, then change this list.

When you take the history of a patient with anaemia, find out if this patient has any of these common causes of anaemia. Ask about a family history of blood diseases. Ask about a past history of the common causes.

When anaemia is present there is not enough haemoglobin the blood to carry enough oxygen to any part of the body. No part of the body, therefore, functions properly. The heart pumps the blood through the lungs and through the body more quickly than normal to use the small amount of haemoglobin in the blood to carry oxygen more often – palpitations (feeling the heart beat more quickly or strongly than normal) occur. The patient breathes more deeply or quickly than normal – shortness of breath occurs. Muscles do not get enough oxygen – tiredness and weakness occur. The brain does not get enough oxygen – dizziness or headaches occur. The heart, which is also doing more work than normal, does not get enough oxygen – heart failure can happen.

Symptoms and signs

Symptoms of anaemia include:

1. weakness or tiredness,
2. dizziness,
3. shortness of breath.

Signs of anaemia include pallor (or paleness or whiteness) of:

1. the mucous membrane of the mouth inside the lips,
2. conjunctivae under the lower eye lids,
3. finger nail beds,
4. palms of hands,
5. all the skin.

See details and exceptions about this Chapter 21 page 238.

Symptoms and signs of (1) the cause of the anaemia, or (2) heart failure (see Chapter 27 page 371) can also be present.

Haemoglobin estimation (see pages 248–50) should always be made. This:

1. confirms the diagnosis of anaemia,
2. confirms how severe the anaemia is, and
3. gives a starting point to measure the success of treatment.

Management and treatment

Treatment of anaemia will usually cure the anaemia. However, treatment cannot increase the haemoglobin by more than 1 g/dl each week. Often the Hb rises by only 0.5 g/dl each week. As the haemoglobin estimation is often as much as 2 g/dl above or below the real level of the haemoglobin, you cannot tell for at least 4 weeks if the treatment is working (i.e. 0.5 g/dl × 4 weeks = rise of 2 g/dl). After 4 weeks the haemoglobin should have risen by at least 2 g/dl.

However, if the cause of the anaemia is not stopped the anaemia will usually return when the treatment is stopped. Therefore you must always try to *find out the cause of the anaemia and stop this cause*.

Blood transfusion is not the treatment of anaemia. Blood transfusion does not help the body make more blood, or stop blood being destroyed, or stop bleeding. Blood transfusion does not stop the cause of anaemia. Blood transfusion is used only if it is needed to keep the patient alive while the cause of the anaemia is found and stopped and the treatment of the anaemia is given time to work.

Management of anaemia in the health centre is by:

1. Treating the common causes of anaemia correctly.
2. If the anaemia does not get better or if it quickly returns, the diagnosis and/or treatment must be incorrect and the patient needs referring to a Medical Officer for investigation for correct diagnosis and treatment.
3. Do not continue with treatment and particularly do not continue with iron if the patient's anaemia is not cured by the treatment.

Admission for treatment is not needed for many patients. Admit for inpatient treatment *if*:

1. very pale or Hb less than 5 g/dl (until Hb 5 g/dl); *or*
2. a lot of dizziness, shortness of breath, weakness, etc.; *or*
3. heart failure (oedema, etc.); *or*
4. patient may get quickly worse (e.g. acute malaria, recent gastrointestinal bleeding, late pregnancy, etc.); *or*
5. time of stress for patient (e.g. infection, postpartum state etc.).

1. Give these six routine treatments for the common causes to all anaemic patients:
   - antimalarials,
   - iron,
   - folic acid,
   - nutrition education if needed,
   - anti-hookworm drug,
   - advice about family planning and antenatal care if needed.

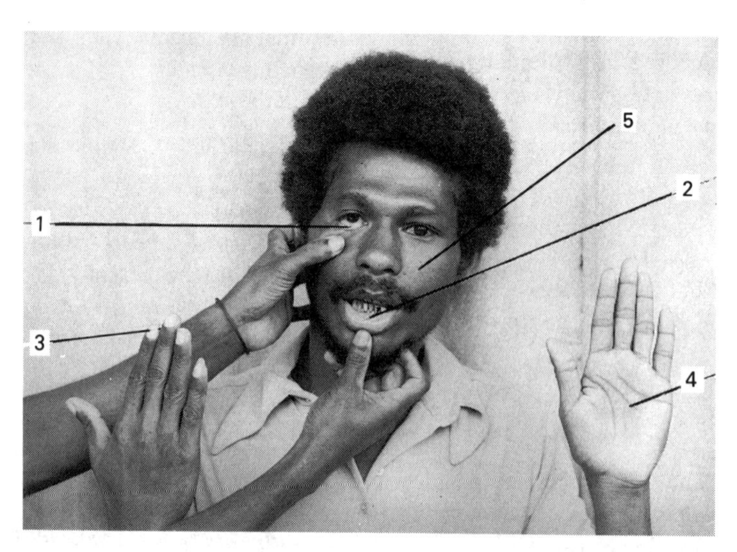

Figure 21.2 Photograph showing the *five* places of the body where pallor *must* be looked for in *all* patients. (1) The conjunctivae under the lower eyelid. (2) The mucous membrane inside the lower lip. (3) The fingernail beds. (4) The palms of the hands. Also (5) the colour of the skin. If the skin is very pale, think of hookworm disease as the hookworm makes the patient short of protein as well as haemoglobin and this makes the skin even more pale.

2. Look for other causes. Treat any other cause you find.
3. Blood transfusion; but only if special reasons for it.
4. See the patient and repeat the Hb each 4 weeks until Hb is 10 g/dl.
5. If the Hb does not rise by 2 g in 1 month and eventually reach 10 g/dl (except hyperreactive malarious splenomegaly (HMS) or tropical splenomegaly syndrome (TSS)
   - send special tests with an explanation to your Medical Officer or
   - send non-urgently or refer the patient to the Medical Officer for special tests.[1]

DO NOT CONTINUE IRON TREATMENT IF THE PATIENT'S Hb IS NOT RISING.

Give the six routine treatments for the common causes

1. *Antimalarial drug*
   Chloroquine 450–600 mg (3–4 tablets) daily for 3 days; *then* if the patient is in a malarious area: Chloroquine 300 mg (2 tabs) weekly until the Hb is above 10 g/dl (usually 6–12 weeks but up to 2 or more years if hyperreactive malarious splenomegaly (supply 8 tabs each 4 weeks); *then*: Chloroquine to be taken 450–600 mg (3–4 tabs) daily for 3 days if the patient gets any attack of fever. (Supply 9–12 tabs to the patient to keep at home.)
   If in chloroquine resistant malaria area use special anti-malarial drugs (see Chapter 13 page 64).
2. *Iron*
   Give ferrous sulphate (200 mg tablets) or ferrous gluconate (300 mg tablets)
   if:
   (a) anaemia not severe (Hb > 7.5 g/dl if pregnant *or* Hb > 5 g/dl in other persons), *and*
   (b) you think the patient will swallow 3 tablets a day for 3 months.
   Give 1 tab three times a day for whole of pregnancy or for 3 months to other patients.
   Give IMI iron dextran (any brand) to
   (a) all other cases *and*
   (b) if Hb does not rise by 2 g/dl after iron tablets given for 4 weeks.
   But see Appendix 3 at the end of this chapter, *before* giving IMI iron dextran, for contra-indications to giving IMI iron dextan and for method of giving IMI iron dextran. *Give* 5 ml daily for:
   - 6 days if weight < 40 kg,
   - 10 days if weight > 40 kg, and
   - 2 days extra if pregnant.

   Give IV iron dextran (only preparations not containing phenol) infusion if
   (a) treatment needs to be completed quickly (e.g. outpatient treatment) *or*
   (b) patient has little muscle for IM injections.
   The total dose required is the one infusion (TDI). *But* see Appendix 4 at the end of this chapter for contra-indications to giving IV iron dextran infusion and method of giving IV iron dextran infusion *before* giving it.

Give only half $\frac{1}{2}$ of these doses of iron if the Hb is 7.5 g/dl or above.

Do NOT give oral iron for more than 3 months unless pregnant or told to do so by the Medical Officer.

Do NOT give a course of iron by injections more than once in any 12-month period.

Do NOT give iron injection (IM or IV) while a patient is very sick or has a fever (above 37.5°C).

Wait until malaria, infections and fever have been successfully treated and then give iron injections.

3. *Folic acid*
   5 mg (1 tab) daily for 1 week *then* 5 mg (1 tab) weekly for 12 weeks.
4. *Diet*
   Educate to eat enough protein foods (e.g. meat, fish, eggs, peanuts) and protective foods (e.g. dark green leafy vegetables, fruit) daily.
5. *Hookworm treatment*
   Give pyrantel 20 mg/kg (maximum dose 750 mg) in one dose orally once or whatever is your usual drug for hookworm (see Chapter 23 page 278).
6. *Offer family planning and/or antenatal care advice if required.*

Treat also any other underlying cause found .

Arrange transfer for blood transfusion but only for the following patients

1. *If* the haemoglobin is 7.5 g/dl or less
   and
   if the patient is more than 36 weeks pregnant (postpartum haemorrhage possible) *or if* the anaemia is

1 See Appendix 6 for preliminary tests for anaemia not responding to treatment for iron deficiency and malaria.

due to haemorrhage which may occur again (e.g. recent haematemesis, melaena, or haemoptysis).

2. *If* the haemoglobin is less than 5 g/dl
   and
   if there is also
   - acute malaria (fever), *or*
   - heart failure (oedema, etc.), *or*
   - severe symptoms of anaemia (dizziness, shortness of breath, severe weakness, etc.), *or*
   - pregnancy at any stage, *or*
   - a severe infection or other illness, *or*
   - other time of stress such as the post-partum state.

Repeat Hb estimation each 4 weeks until Hb is 10 g/dl

Send special blood tests or refer to the Medical Officer if the Hb does not rise
The haemoglobin should rise by 2–4 g/dl in 4 weeks. However this is not true for hyperreactive malarious splenomegaly (HMS) previously called tropical splenomegaly syndrome (TSS) (see page 243 in which it may take 2 years to rise to 10 g/dl.

If the haemoglobin does not rise by at least 2 g/dl, give fully supervised treatment for another 4 weeks including iron by injection and you yourself watching the antimalarial tablets being swallowed and checking for drug resistant malaria.

If the haemoglobin does rise by at least 2 g/dl continue treatment and arrange special blood tests or referral or non-urgent transfer to a Medical Officer to find out what the real cause of the anaemia is and what the management should be.

Do not just continue treatment if it is not curing the anaemia. This would allow the cause of the anaemia to get worse and the anaemia to get worse. Incorrect treatment may also make the patient develop a new condition, e.g. iron may cause heart failure if the patient has thalassaemia.

Transfer to Medical Officer care if needed

1. If the haemoglobin does not rise by 2 g/dl after 4 weeks of correct, fully supervised treatment of the common causes (except hyperreactive malarious splenomegaly), the diagnoses and treatment are wrong. Correct diagnosis and treatment are needed (non-urgent).
2. If blood transfusion is needed (see this page) (urgent – sometimes emergency).
3. If anaemia has returned after full treatment (see page 240) and if necessary adequate treatment of malaria, before 1 year has gone (non-urgent).
4. If the haemoglobin does not rise by 2 g/dl and the spleen decrease in size by 2 cm in 6 months when the patient has hyperreactive malarious splenomegaly and has had correct prophylactic antimalarial drugs regularly (see page 243) (non-urgent).
5. If the patient has hyperreactive malarious splenomegaly and becomes pregnant (discuss with Medical Officer first) (non-urgent).

Prevention

Prevention of anaemia is the prevention and treatment of the common causes of anaemia. This includes:

1. Control and treatment of malaria (see Chapter 13 page 55).
2. Control and treatment of hookworm (see Chapter 23 page 277).
3. Good diet with enough iron folic and protein, etc. in it. The diet should be a mixed one which has in it protein foods (meat, fish, eggs, peanuts etc.) and protective foods (dark green leafy vegetables, fruit, etc.)
4. Good obstetrical advice and care. Advice and help with family planning. Antenatal care including iron, folic acid and anti-malarials for all women during pregnancy. Prevention of post-partum haemorrhage.

Hyperreactive malarious splenomegaly (or tropical splenomegaly syndrome)

Hyperreactive malarious splenomegaly (HMS) previously called tropical splenomegaly syndrome (TSS) is an abnormal reaction of the body to chronic malarial infection. It is present when a person who has had chronic malaria for years has a very big spleen, anaemia, wasting and repeated attacks of haemolysis (see below), and these things are not improving but are worsening.

Pathology

When a non-immune person starts to live in an area where there is malaria, first he gets acute malaria and then he gets chronic malaria. (See Chapter 13 page 58.) A person with chronic malaria has a big spleen, anaemia, wasting (or poor growth if a child) and repeated attacks of acute malaria and other infections. If the person does not die from acute or chronic malaria, he develops antibodies against malaria. After about 4–10 years he develops semi-immunity to malaria. Then his spleen becomes smaller, his haemoglobin rises, his wasting gets less (and he grows better if he is a child) and there are fewer attacks of acute malaria and other infections. However, a few people with chronic malaria do not develop normal antibodies and normal immunity to malaria. These people develop abnormal antibodies (of IgM type) and abnormal immunity to malaria. This causes hyperreactive malarious splenomegaly.

In these people who develop an abnormal immune reaction to malaria, the big spleen stays big and may get bigger. The big spleen (for no other reason than that it is big) destroys red and white blood cells more quickly than the bone marrow can make enough new ones.

This causes severe chronic anaemia, low resistance to infections, wasting and chronic ill health. At times the big spleen may suddenly destroy many more red blood cells than it usually does. This causes acute very severe anaemia (acute haemolysis) and fever and splenic pain.

Clinical features

The patient is usually a young adult from a malarious area. The condition happens more commonly in certain places and certain families.

Symptoms include those of:

- anaemia (malaise, inability to work, weakness, dizziness, shortness of breath);
- enlarged spleen (swelling of abdomen, abdominal discomfort); and
- episodes of acute haemolysis (severe weakness etc. often with fever and sometimes with pain in the abdomen over the spleen).

Signs include (see Figure 21.3):

- anaemia,
- wasting (thin muscles, little fat),
- spleen very enlarged, firm and usually non-tender,
- liver usually enlarged,
- episodes of fever, jaundice and tender spleen during which the patient is more anaemic than before (acute haemolytic episodes).

The patient has chronic ill health. He becomes worse from time to time because of haemolytic episodes. The condition does not improve by itself while the patient stays in a malarious area. Death usually occurs from acute malaria or acute severe bacterial infection or an haemolytic episode.

Management

You are not able to change the patient's abnormal reaction to malaria parasites to normal. You can, however, stop this abnormal reaction, by curing the patient of malaria and then giving him malaria prophylaxis so that no more malarial parasites are in his body. The patient must take the malarial prophylaxis until all the symptoms and signs of HMS are gone – this usually takes at least 2 years. After this, he will have to take malarial prophylaxis for life if the condition starts to return when he stops the prophylaxis. Details of the management of a patient with HMS are set out below.

Do a haemoglobin estimation (see page 248). Write down the result. Do this each time you see the patient.

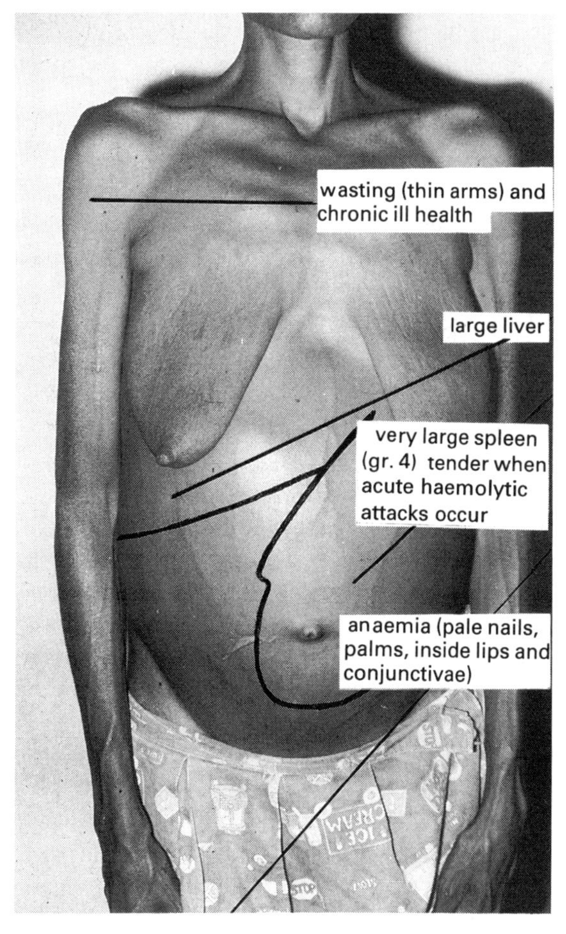

Figure 21.3 Hyperreactive malarious splenomegaly (previously called tropical splenomegaly syndrome). Note the features in an adult who has lived all her life in an area where malaria is always present.

Send a thin blood smear (and if possible 4 ml of blood in an EDTA bottle and enough blood on blotting or filter paper to cover a thumb nail) to the hospital laboratory and ask them to look for sickle cell anaemia, chronic leukaemia, thalassaemia and other rare blood diseases. (Result is not urgent).

Measure the size of the spleen before starting treatment. Write down the size. Do this again each time you see the patient.

Admit for inpatient treatment if

- the haemoglobin is less than 5 g/dl, or
- the patient has had recent acute haemolytic episode, or
- the patient is sick, or
- the patient is pregnant.

Give routine treatment for anaemia with chloroquine, iron, folic acid, pyrantel, or other anti-hookworm drug, education about diet, and family planning (see anaemia page 240). However, do not give total dose infusion of iron during pregnancy if the patient has HMS.

Give explanations and health education about the need for regular treatment for many years. Give chloroquine 300 mg (2 tabs) weekly or 125 mg ($\frac{1}{2}$ tab) daily (or other drugs if in an area where chloroquine resistant malaria) for at least 2 years and probably for life.

Give quick, effective treatment for any acute attacks of bacterial infections or malaria as they occur.

Transfer to Medical Officer care the following patients:

1. If the patient has a severe haemolytic episode at any time, but especially during pregnancy (i.e. sudden increase in anaemia often with fever, increased weakness, and possibly jaundice and spleen pain). Transfer for blood transfusion and prednisolone (urgent – at times emergency).
2. If a patient with HMS becomes pregnant. (First discuss with Medical Officer the need for transfer – non-urgent).
3. If after 6–8 months of treatment the Hb has not risen by 2 g/dl and the spleen has not decreased in size by 1 grade or 5 cm. (Transfer for investigation for other diseases – non-urgent).

Sickle cell anaemia

Sickle cell anaemia is a severe inherited disease which causes chronic anaemia, episodes of severe pain and tenderness of bones and other parts of the body, and often death.

Sickle cell anaemia is common only in people from parts of Africa and people of African descent. It occurs also in a few parts of the Middle East and India.

Pathology

Sickle cell anaemia is due to a large amount of an abnormal haemoglobin called Hb S, in the red blood cells (instead of normal adult haemoglobin). This abnormality must be partly present in both parents for a child to get the severe abnormality. A small amount of Hb S helps protect a person against malaria. A large amount of Hb S does not protect against malaria but does cause sickle cell anaemia. As the abnormality that makes Hb S (instead of normal haemoglobin) is inherited, there is no cure for the disease.

When a red blood cell that has a lot of Hb S in it gives up its oxygen, it changes to an abnormal long thin 'sickle' shape (see Figure 21.4). If the sickled cell is quickly given oxygen again, it goes back to the normal shape. If the sickled cell is not given oxygen for more than a couple of minutes, it cannot ever go back to the normal shape.

Sickling of red blood cells causes two groups of problems.

1. The abnormal red blood cells are destroyed in the body (mostly in the spleen) more quickly than normal red blood cells (called chronic haemolysis). This causes chronic anaemia and a big spleen.
   From time to time, sometimes because of an infection, but often for no obvious reason, the spleen may destroy many more red cells than normal. The anaemia becomes much worse with jaundice and the spleen becomes even larger. This is called a haemolytic crisis. The bone marrow makes as many red cells as it can to replace the ones being destroyed by the spleen. The marrow in the bones gets bigger. This may make the bones get bigger and give an unusual appearance to the bones of the skull and face. The bone marrow often needs more folic acid than it can get to make all the extra blood. All the body then becomes short of folic acid. This shortage of folic acid may stop the patient growing and stop puberty (a child developing into a man or woman).
2. The red blood cells become sickled as they give up their oxygen in the capillaries of the body tissues. The sickled cells can then get stuck in the capillaries and cannot then return to the lungs to

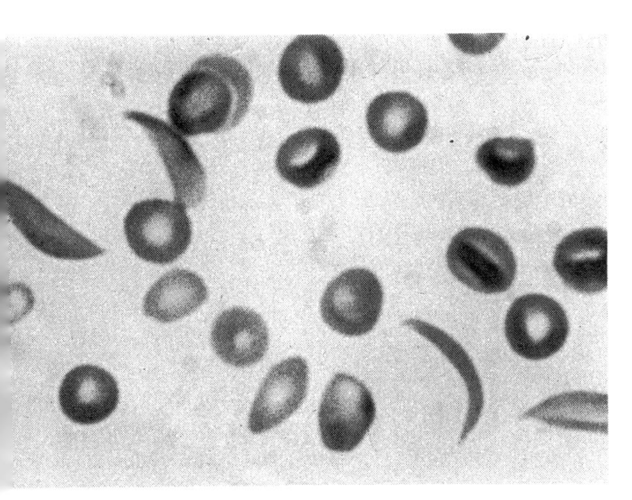

Figure 21.4 Photograph of normal red blood cells and sickle cells.

get more oxygen. The blocked capillaries stop other red cells passing through them and these other red cells give up their oxygen and then sickle. The blood then often clots in the blocked blood vessels. The part of the body, which the blocked blood vessels usually supply, gets no oxygen and so becomes inflamed and dies. Death of part of the body like this is called an 'infarction'. The process just described is often called an 'infarction crisis'.
The things which make an infarction crisis more likely are:
(a) infections (bacterial and malarial);
(b) dehydration;
(c) if less oxygen is breathed in than usual, e.g.
- during an operation,
- going high in an aeroplane which is not properly pressurised;

(d) if part or all of the body becomes cold and the blood circulation slows down;
(e) if the blood flow to part of the body is stopped, e.g. putting on a torniquet or tight bandage.
However, many infarction crises happen for no reason that can be found.
Some patients have many attacks of infarction – 1 or 2 each week. Some patients have few attacks – 1 or 2 each year.
The parts of the body most often affected by infarction crises are the bones. In infants, the fingers and toes are the most often affected. In older people, any bone or any other part of the body can be affected. If the spleen has many infarctions, it may become small.

The parts of the body which have been affected by infarction may be infected by bacteria which cause osteomyelitis, etc.

In pregnancy the above other severe complications can result in death.

Symptoms and signs

Anaemia and related conditions

The usual symptoms and signs of anaemia are present (see pages 239–40).

The haemoglobin is usually about 8 g/dl. (If a patient's haemoglobin is normal (and the patient is not dehydrated) the patient probably does not have sickle cell anaemia).

The patient may be mildly jaundiced.

The spleen and liver are usually large; though the spleen may become small.

Sometimes the anaemia may become much worse (haemolytic crisis).

The skull and face bones may have an unusual shape.

Growth and puberty may be slow.

Sometimes there are leg ulcers.

Infarction crises

Sudden severe pain and tenderness (and often fever) start in a bone or the spleen or another part of the body. With proper treatment, the pain usually greatly improves within 2 days and goes within 7–9 days.

The bones are affected more often than other parts of the body. Any bone can be affected, but often the fingers and toes are most affected. The infected bone becomes painful and tender.

Old bone infarctions may have made the fingers short and thick with narrow ends. Also the patient may not be very tall, because the trunk of the body is short.

If a joint is affected, acute arthritis occurs.

If the kidney is affected, there is often blood in the urine.

If the spleen is affected, there is a tender swelling in the left upper abdomen.

If the intestine is affected there may be acute abdominal pain and tenderness and vomiting.

If the brain is affected, there may be paralysis etc.

Infections

If pain and tenderness and fever in an area of infarction do not become much better after 2 days of proper treatment, and is not nearly gone after 7–9 days of treatment, then that part of the body probably has developed a secondary bacterial infection. Salmonella infections of bone are common.

Tests

Haemoglobin

The Hb is usually about 8 g/dl.

Sickling test

If you have a laboratory with a microscope, then you can do a simple test for sickling of the blood with sodium metabisulphate.

On one slide a drop of patient's blood is mixed with a drop of freshly prepared 2% sodium metabisulphate solution and placed under a cover slip. The same test is done with normal blood on another slide. Both are examined 20 minutes later. If the patient's blood but not the normal blood shows sickle-shaped or long curved red blood cells, then the patient *has* Hb S in his blood.

People who have only a *little* Hb S in their blood and do not have sickle cell anaemia *can* still have a positive sickling test.

If the sickling test is *negative*, it is almost certain that the patient does *not* have sickle cell anaemia.

The only *certain* way to diagnose that *the disease* is present is to send the blood to a laboratory where they do a special test for Hb S.

Thin blood smear

You can diagnose sickle cell anaemia fairly certainly in most cases if there is (1) anaemia and (2) a typical thin blood smear for sickle cell anaemia.

White cell count

The white cell count is often high (often twice the normal levels) even when there is no infection.

Treatment

There is no cure.

Treat the anaemia

1. Give regular prophylactic antimalarial drugs for life (if in a malarial area) (see Chapter 13 page 61).
2. Give folic acid 5 mg (1 tab) daily for life.
3. Do not give blood transfusion unless the Hb suddenly falls to very low levels or before operations etc.
4. Do not give iron after the first course as it is not usually needed. However ask the laboratory or Medical Officer to do tests to see if iron is needed if you suspect iron deficiency.

Tell the patient how to avoid infarction crises

1. Take prophylactic antimalarials for life (see Chapter 13 page 61).
2. Avoid infections and treat infections quickly.
3. Avoid dehydration – always drink enough to pass a lot of urine (especially if he or she has vomiting or diarrhoea or it is very hot). Never take (and health workers never order) diuretics (e.g. hydrochlorothiazide, frusemide (furosemide) etc.) even for heart failure or high blood pressure etc.)
4. Avoid becoming cold.
5. Avoid tight clothes on the limbs.
6. Do not go on unpressurised aircraft.

Treat infarction crises

1. Give aspirin or paracetamol or codeine as needed (see Chapter 7 pages 29–31). Do not give pethidine or morphine (unless told to do so by Medical Officer) as the patient may become addicted.
2. The patient must be fully hydrated. Use an IV drip in severe cases (see Chapter 23 page 286).
3. Make the patient rest.

Treat any infection quickly

If pain from an infarction crisis has not improved in 2 days and has not nearly gone in 7–9 days, there is an infection which you must treat with antibiotics (see Chapter 11 pages 46–52). Osteomyelitis, which could be due to *Salmonella* and may occur again and again, and may need repeated long courses of antibiotics (not safe for chloramphenicol), should be urgently discussed with the Medical Officer.

Transfer

Transfer patients who need an operation

The condition may be because of infarction crisis.

The operation may cause an infarction crisis.

The anaesthetic needs high concentrations of oxygen and may need a pre-operative blood transfusion.

No tourniquets can be used.

Do not operate on patients who have sickle cell anaemia yourself. Transfer all patients with sickle cell anaemia who seem to need an operation to a Medical Officer.

Transfer pregnant patients
Transfer all patients with sickle cell anaemia who become pregnant to a Medical Officer.

Prognosis

Without treatment most patients would die before they were adults. If proper treatment is given patients may have a reasonable life although they may have many attacks of the problems described.

Thalassaemia

Thalassaemia is an inherited disease in which the bone marrow cannot make enough haemoglobin and the patient becomes anaemic.

Thalassaemia is common around the Mediterranean Sea; but it can occur in all parts of the world.

Thalassaemia must be present, even if only mildly so, in both parents for a child to get severe thalassaemia.

Mild thalassaemia (called 'thalassaemia minor') causes only a few symptoms and signs. There is a mild anaemia which is like iron deficiency anaemia but which does not improve on routine anaemia treatment (see page 240). If blood tests are sent to the hospital laboratory (a thin blood smear, 4 ml blood in EDTA bottle and blood about 1 cm across on filter or blotting paper) or if the patient is referred or transferred non-urgently to the Medical Officer, the condition can be diagnosed by tests. Treat mild thalassaemia patients with regular prophylactic antimalarials if in a malarious area (see Chapter 13 page 61) for life and with folic acid 5 g (1 tab) daily for life. DO NOT GIVE IRON after the first course unless the Medical Officer tells you that the patient also has iron deficiency, as may occur in girls on vegetarian diets, women with many pregnancies etc. Iron treatment will otherwise damage the heart and other organs and may lead to death.

Severe thalassaemia (called 'thalassaemia major') affects children. They have very severe anaemia which does not improve on any treatment. The spleen becomes larger and eventually very large, also the skull and face bones are large and unusual to look at. You can only keep the patient alive by repeated blood transfusions and treatment as for mild thalassaemia. The iron from the blood transfusions and the food damages the heart and other organs and can cause death, if death is not caused by a complication of the anaemia (usually before adult life is reached).

Appendix 1 Haemoglobin estimation using a comparator

Principle

This is a method for estimating haemoglobin using the eyes.

The test solution is compared with a series of coloured glass standards that show the amount of haemoglobin.

Materials

- Haemoglobin comparator with standards to cover the range 3–13 g of haemoglobin per decilitre (g/dl)
- Two comparator tubes
- 0.05 ml (50 mm^3 or 50 μl) pipettes
- A rubber bulb or a syringe with a rubber or plastic tube attached. Use this to draw the blood into the pipette and to blow it out.
- Haemoglobin diluting fluid. This is made by adding 0.4 ml of strong ammonia solution to 1 litre of distilled water.

Method

1. Fill a test tube with 10 ml of the diluting fluid.

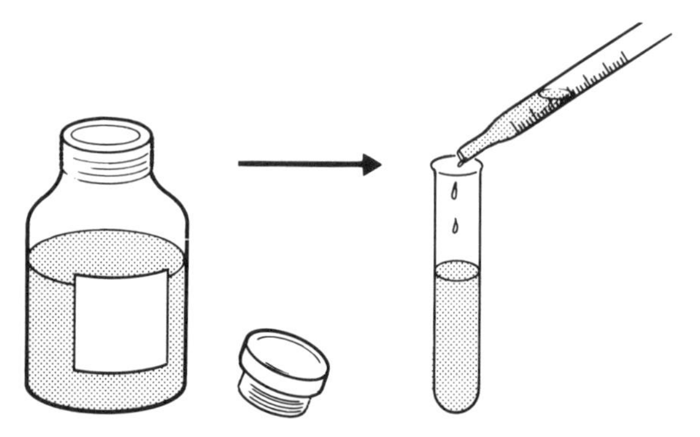

2. Draw venous or capillary blood to the 0.05 ml (or 50 mm^3 or 50 μl) mark of the blood pipette. Do not allow air bubbles to enter. If blood from a bottle is being tested, make sure that it is well mixed by tipping the bottle containing it and the anticoagulant repeatedly for about 1 minute immediately before pipetting it.
3. Wipe the outside of the pipette so that no blood is on the outside, check that the blood is still on the mark, and blow the blood into the 10 ml of diluting fluid. Wash the inside of the pipette 2–3 times with the solution containing the blood.

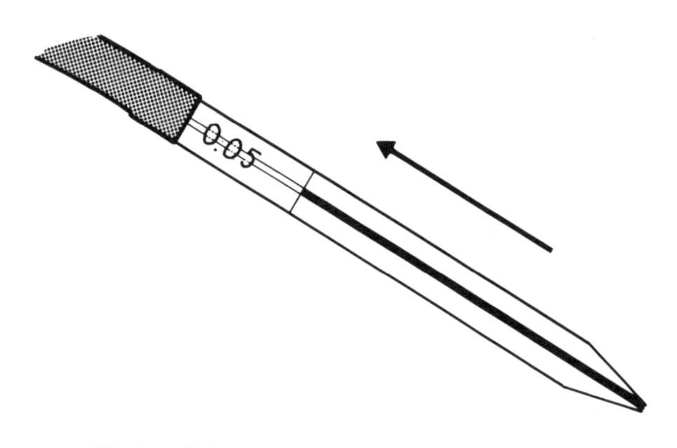

4. Mix the contents of the tube. The fluid will become a clear red as the red cells are haemolysed. The colour of the solution will not fade for a few hours.
5. Fill one of the comparator tubes to the mark with the fluid. Lift the lid of the comparator and place the tube in the right-hand side of the comparator.

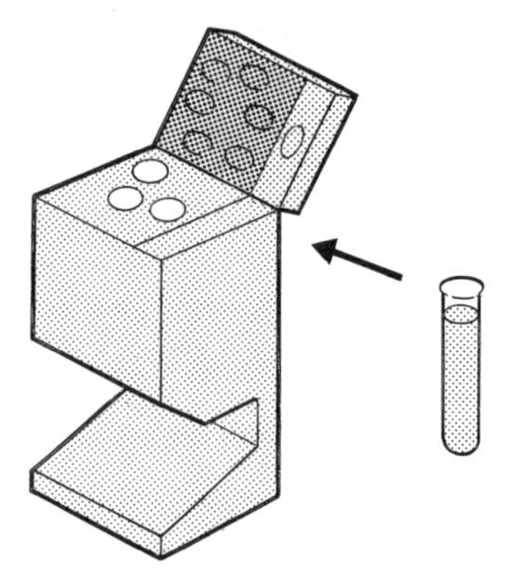

6. Fill the other comparator tube to the mark with the diluting fluid and place this in the left-hand side of the comparator. Close the lid.
7. Holding the equipment with the front of the comparator directed towards the daylight, look down through the viewing aperture, (as in the picture).

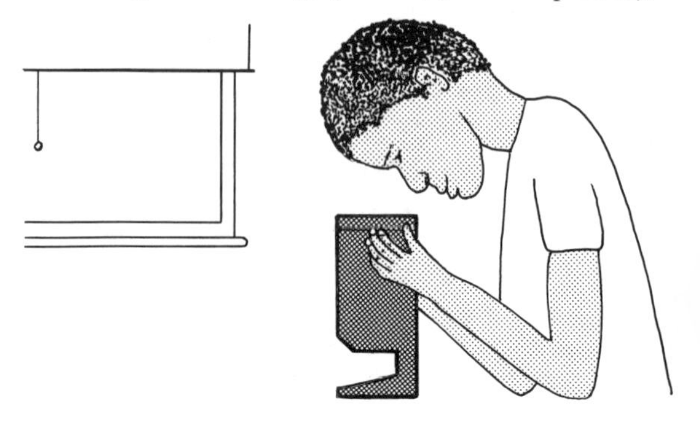

8. Daylight must be used, but do not hold the comparator in direct sunlight.
9. Starting with the pale-coloured standards, compare each with the colour of the test solution, as seen in the left-hand side of the viewing aperture. When the colours are matched as closely as possible, make a final check by comparing with the standard on each side of the one thought to match best.
10. Read the haemoglobin value in grams per decilitre (g/dl) as shown on the disc used to rotate the standards.

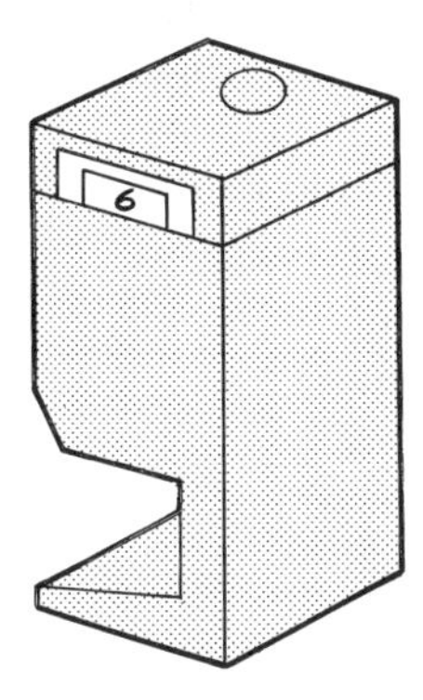

11. When the colour of the test lies between two standards, make an estimate between the two values.

Appendix 2 Haemoglobin estimation by Sahli method

Principle

The blood is diluted in an acid solution, converting the haemoglobin to acid haematin. The test solution is matched against a coloured glass reference. The Sahli method is not an accurate way of estimating haemoglobulin.

Materials

- Sahli haemoglobinometer
- Sahli pipette (graduated to 20 mm^3, i.e. 0.02 ml, or 20 μl)
- Small glass rod
- Dropping pipette
- Absorbent paper
- 0.1 mol/l (0.1 N) hydrochloric acid (HCl)

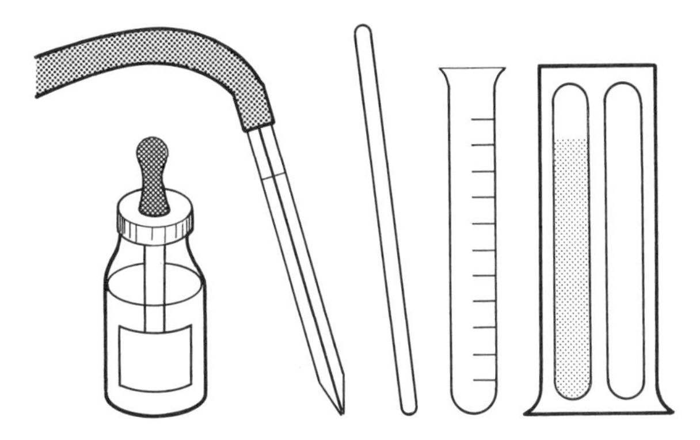

Method

1. Fill the graduated tube to the 20 mark (or the mark 3 g/100 ml) with 0.1 mol/l HCl.

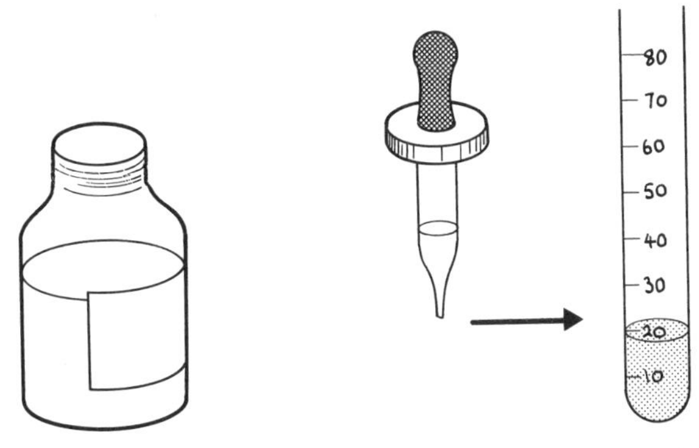

2. Draw venous or capillary blood to the 0.02 ml mark of the Sahli pipette. Do not allow air bubbles

to enter. If blood from a bottle is being tested, make sure that it is well mixed by tipping the bottle containing it and the anticoagulant repeatedly for about 1 minute immediately before pipetting it.

3. Wipe the outside of the pipette with absorbent paper to remove all blood. Check that the blood is still on the mark.

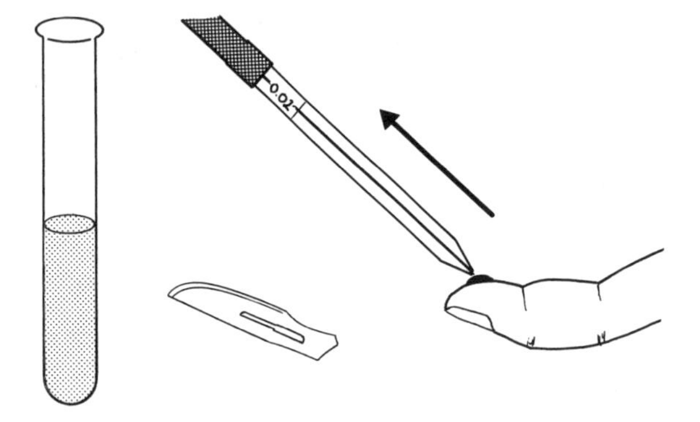

4. Blow the blood from the pipette into the graduated tube of the acid solution.
   Rinse the pipette by drawing in and blowing out the acid solution 3 times.
   The mixture of blood and acid gives a brownish colour.
   Allow to stand for 5 minutes.

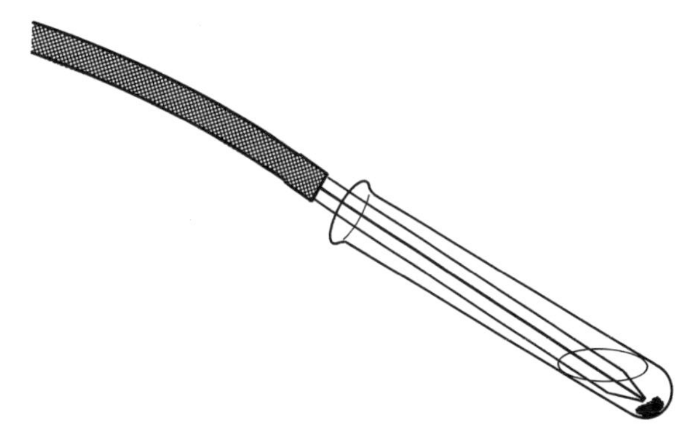

5. Place the graduated tube in the haemoglobinometer. Stand facing a window.
   Compare the colour of the tube containing diluted blood with the colour of the reference tube.
   If the colour is the same as or lighter than that of the reference tube the haemoglobin value is 4 g/dl or less.
6. If the colour is darker than that of the reference tube continue to dilute by adding 0.1 mol/l HCl drop by drop.

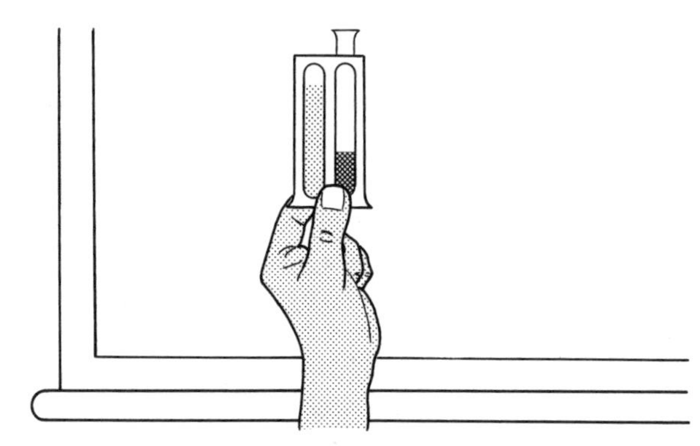

Stir with the glass rod after adding each drop.
Remove the rod and compare the colours of the two tubes.
Stop when the colours match.

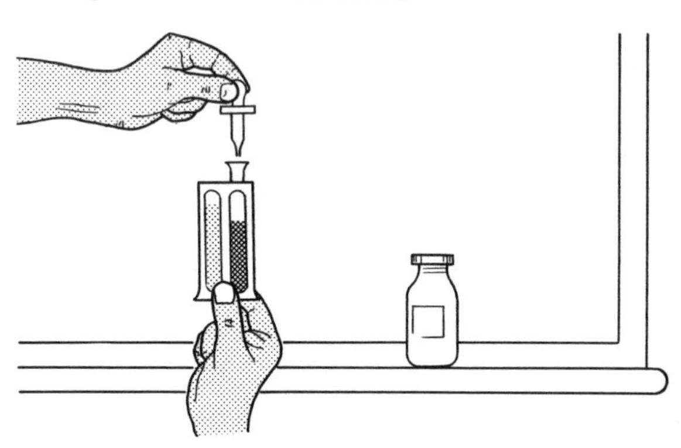

7. Note the mark reached. Depending on the type of haemoglobinometer, this gives the haemoglobin concentration either in g/100 ml (i.e. g/dl) or as a percentage of 'normal'. To convert percentages to g/dl, multiply by 0.146.

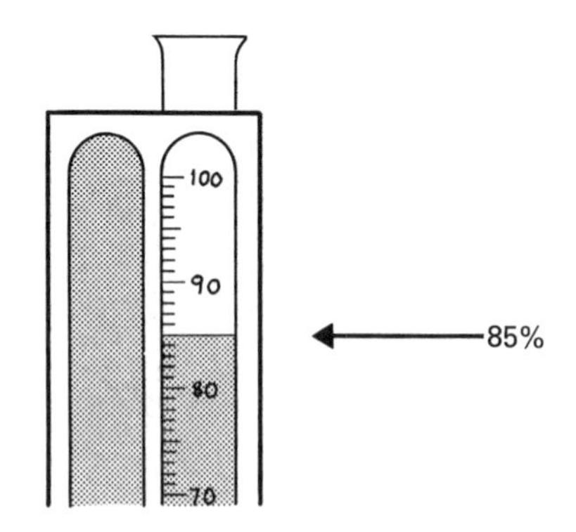

Appendix 3 Method of giving iron dextran by IMI

- Inject only into upper, outer buttock (see Figure 21.5A).
- Use a 19 or 20 gauge needle
- First, with the fingers of one hand, slide the skin and underlying tissue over the upper, outer buttock away from this area (see Figure 21.5B).
- Insert the needle through the stretched skin (from another area) into the upper, outer buttock (see Figure 21.5C).
- If blood comes back along or through the needle withdraw it and try again.
- Inject slowly.
- Wait 10 seconds after the injection is finished and then withdraw the needle.
- Allow the skin to slide back to its proper place (see Figure 21.5D).
- Make the patient walk around or move the leg.
- Do not rub the site of the injection.

> Do not give iron by injection until malaria, infections and fever have been successfully treated.
> Do not give more than one course of iron by injection in any one 12-month period.

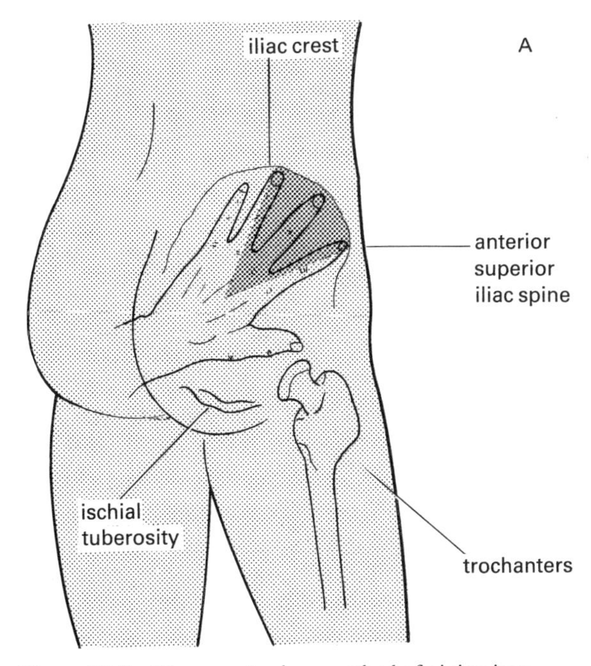

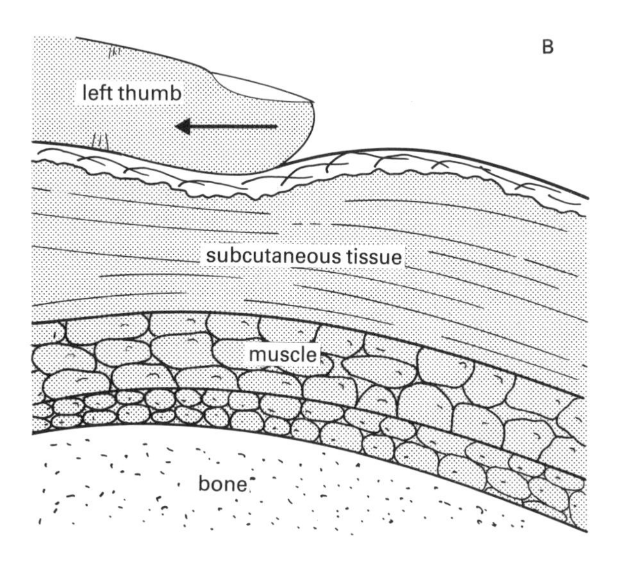

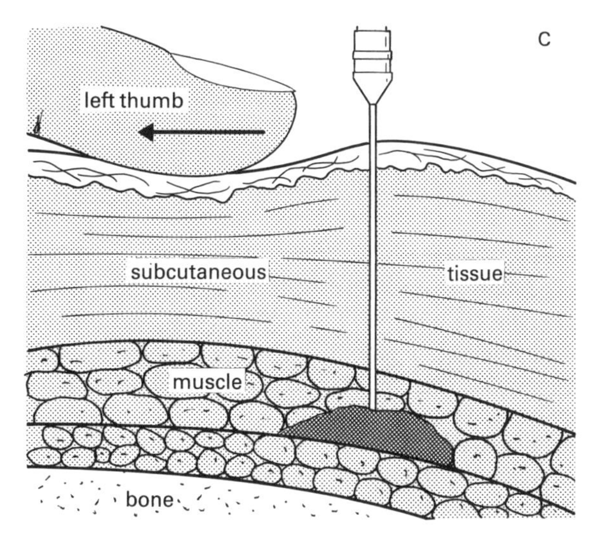

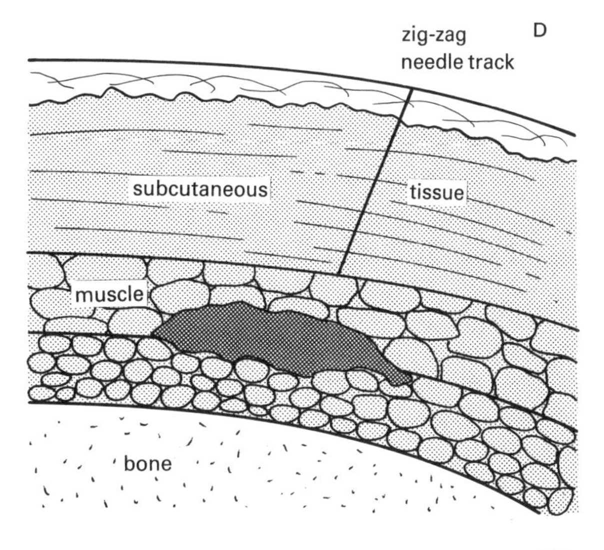

Figure 21.5 Diagrams to show method of giving iron dextran by IMI. See text for details.

Appendix 4 Method of total dose iron dextran by IV drip

Use only preparations that *do not* contain phenol. Preparations that contain phenol can be used only for intramuscular injections. Check with your Health Department which preparations are safe for you to give by IV as well as IM methods.

Give only if the patient (1) is past childhood, (2) has no history of allergy or asthma, (3) has no fever or infection and is not sick.

Record pulse rate and blood pressure.

Give promethazine 50 mg (2 ml) IMI first.

Insert the drip – 1 litre of dextrose 4.3% in sodium chloride 0.18% (or $\frac{1}{2}$ – 1 litre of 0.9% sodium chloride; but only if no heart failure).

Add only one ampoule of the iron dextran to the 1 litre of IV fluid.

Start the drip at 5 drops per minute. Check pulse and blood pressure after 5 minutes and again after 10 minutes.

If

- blood pressure falls more than 15 mm systolic,

or

- pulse rises more than 15 beats per minute, *or*
- patient becomes restless or breathless or coughs, or has chest pains, sweating, nausea or vomiting;

then immediately stop the drip, change both flask and drip set and treat for shock (Chapter 27 page 378).

Give adrenaline (epinephrine) 1:1000 solution 0.5 ml ($\frac{1}{2}$ ml) IMI.

Give promethazine 50 mg (2 ml) IVI if needed.

Also change to IM iron dextran (after patient has fully recovered).

If none of the above signs come, then add the rest of the total dose of iron dextran to the flask. Then observe the patient for another 10 minutes as above. Treat as above if signs of shock or allergy occur.

If none of the signs of shock or allergy (above) come, increase the drip rate to 40–60 drops/minute. Check PR and BP each 15 minutes. The drip should finish in 4–6 hours.

Appendix 5 Notes on blood transfusion

Refer to these notes and any other instructions you have been given on blood transfusion before giving blood.

1. One unit of blood usually raises the Hb in an adult by 1–1.5 g%.
2. Transfuse until Hb over 5 g/dl – all patients described on page 242. Transfuse till Hb over 7.5 g/dl – (a) patients who may bleed and bleeding could be difficult to control (after 36 weeks of pregnancy, recent gastrointestinal bleeding etc.) and (b) patients who have severe infections.
3. Use blood only if both the HIV test (see Chapter 19 page 188) and the HBV test (see Chapter 24 page 308) have been done and are negative. If from an area where *Trypanosoma cruzi* occurs, the test for this must have been done and be negative before blood is given.
4. Only use blood which has been properly grouped and cross-matched.
5. Make certain the *correct* bag of blood is given to the patient. The labels, etc. must be checked by two senior health workers.
6. Remove a bag of blood from Blood Bank refrigerator only when you can start transfusing it immediately.
7. Never transfuse blood that has been out of the refrigerator for more than 6 hours.
8. Take the temperature, pulse rate, blood pressure and respiration rate:
   - before the transfusion is started,
   - 15 minutes after the transfusion is started,

   and
   - each hour after the transfusion is started.

   A responsible health worker must stay with the patient all the time for the first 15 minutes.
   Observe the patient carefully for any kind of reaction (including low BP, fast PR, back pain, breathlessness, fever, restlessness, skin rash, etc.).
9. If the patient develops any kind of reaction (as above):
   - stop blood transfusion,
   - give promethazine 25 mg (1 ml) IV and 25 mg (1 ml) IM,
   - consult Medical Officer immediately,
   - see Chapter 27 page 378 if shock.

Appendix 6

Laboratory tests for anaemia needed by Medical Officer (other tests including bone marrow and further blood tests may be needed later).

1. Haemoglobin (Hb), packed cell volume (PCV), mean corpuscular haemoglobin concentration (MCHC) and if available mean cell volume (MCV).
2. Full blood count (FBC) including examination of red blood cells (RBC) for hypochromia, target cells, anisocytosis and poikilocytosis and of neutrophils for hypersegmentation.
3. Reticulocyte count and reticulocyte index.
4. Malaria smears.
5. Urea/creatinine.
6. Urine microscopy, culture and if needed AFB examination.
7. Tests for any other illnesses, acute and chronic, suggested by examination.

The tests will answer the following questions:

1. Is the anaemia:
   (a) hypochromic (MCHC less than 30–32% and later hypochromic appearance of the RBCs on film)? – see 2, *or*
   (b) normochromic? – see 3.
2. If hypochromic:
   (a) are there numerous target cells and a lot of anisocytosis and poikilocytosis? If so – thalassaemia,
   (b) if not – iron deficiency anaemia or if no response to treatment of this – anaemia of chronic disease.
3. If normochromic (RBCs on blood film normal and MCHC 32–36%)
   (a) is it normocytic (RBCs normal on blood film and MCV 80–100 fl)? – see 4, *or*
   (b) macrocytic (RBCs on films and MCV above 100 fl) – see 5.
4. If normocytic, what is the reticulocyte index?
   (a) if reticulocyte index low (less than 2%) and normocytic normochromic then –
   - bone marrow depression especially drug induced,
   - chronic disease,

   (b) if reticulocyte index high (greater than 2%) and normochromic normocytic then –
   - acute blood loss, *or*
   - haemolysis (including malaria, sickle cell, thalassaemia, GPD deficiency, immune type haemolysis, mechanical, drugs etc.).
5. If macrocytic, is the marrow:
   (a) megaloblastic (more than 30% of the polymorphs with 5 or more lobes)? or
   (b) not megaloblastic?
   - if megaloblastic macrocytic normochromic, then folate or vitamin B_{12} deficiency and needs trial of a test dose of only 50 micrograms of vitamin B_{12} (this one small dose will not cause acute spinal cord lesion) or only 200 micrograms folinic acid (no more) and then reticulocyte counts to determine which,
   - if not megaloblastic but macrocytic normochromic then consider – alcohol abuse, liver disease, haemolysis, myxoedema, marrow suppression, etc.

22

Disorders of the Lymphatic System and Spleen

The lymphatic system

Anatomy, physiology and pathology

The lymphatic system goes through most of the body. The important parts of it are:

- the lymph vessels,
- the lymph nodes (sometimes called 'lymph-glands' or just 'glands'),
- the spleen,
- the tonsils,
- the appendix, and
- collections of 'patches' of lymphoid tissue scattered throughout the gastrointestinal tract and the appendix.

A body fluid called lymph flows through the lymph vessels and lymph glands. The lymph system is connected to the blood circulation system (see Figure 22.1).

Lymph vessels are tubes like the blood capillaries and veins. There is a network of very small lymph capillaries over almost all of the body (see Figure 22.2).

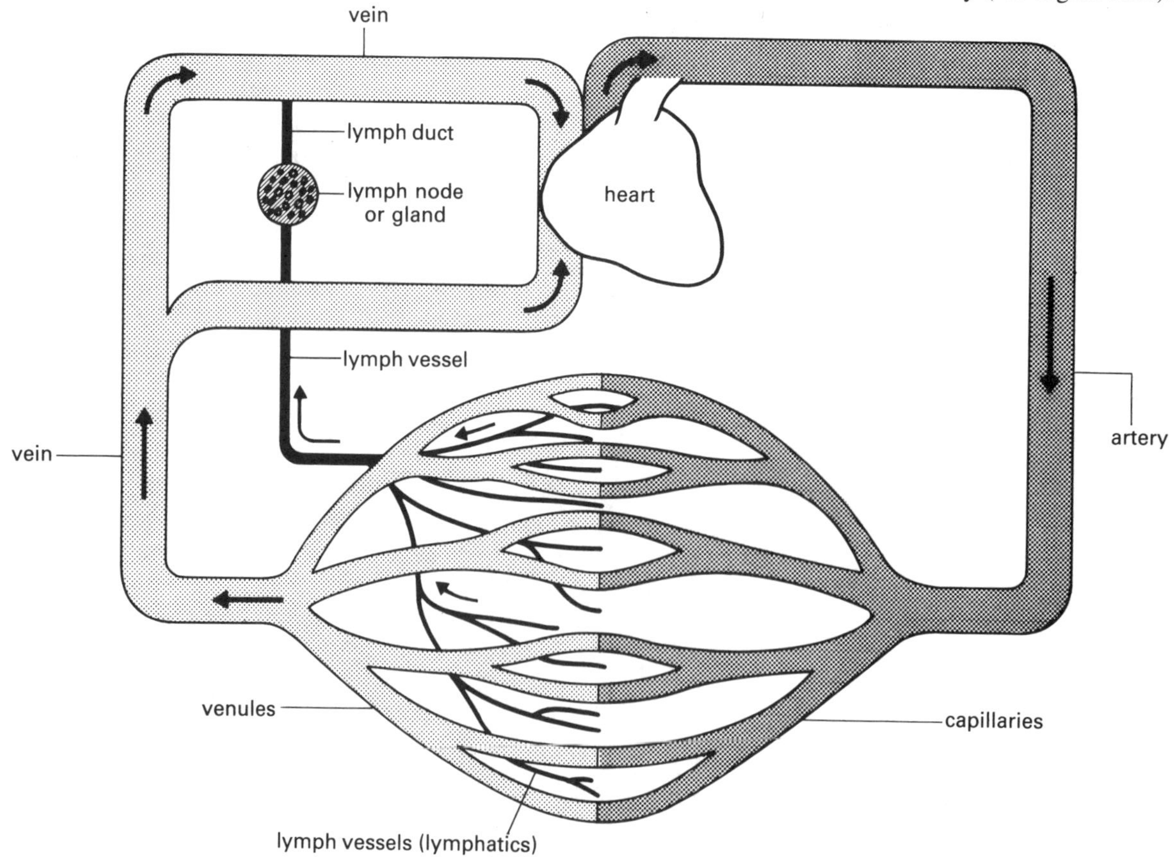

Figure 22.1 Diagram to show the relationship of the lymphatic system to the circulation of the blood.

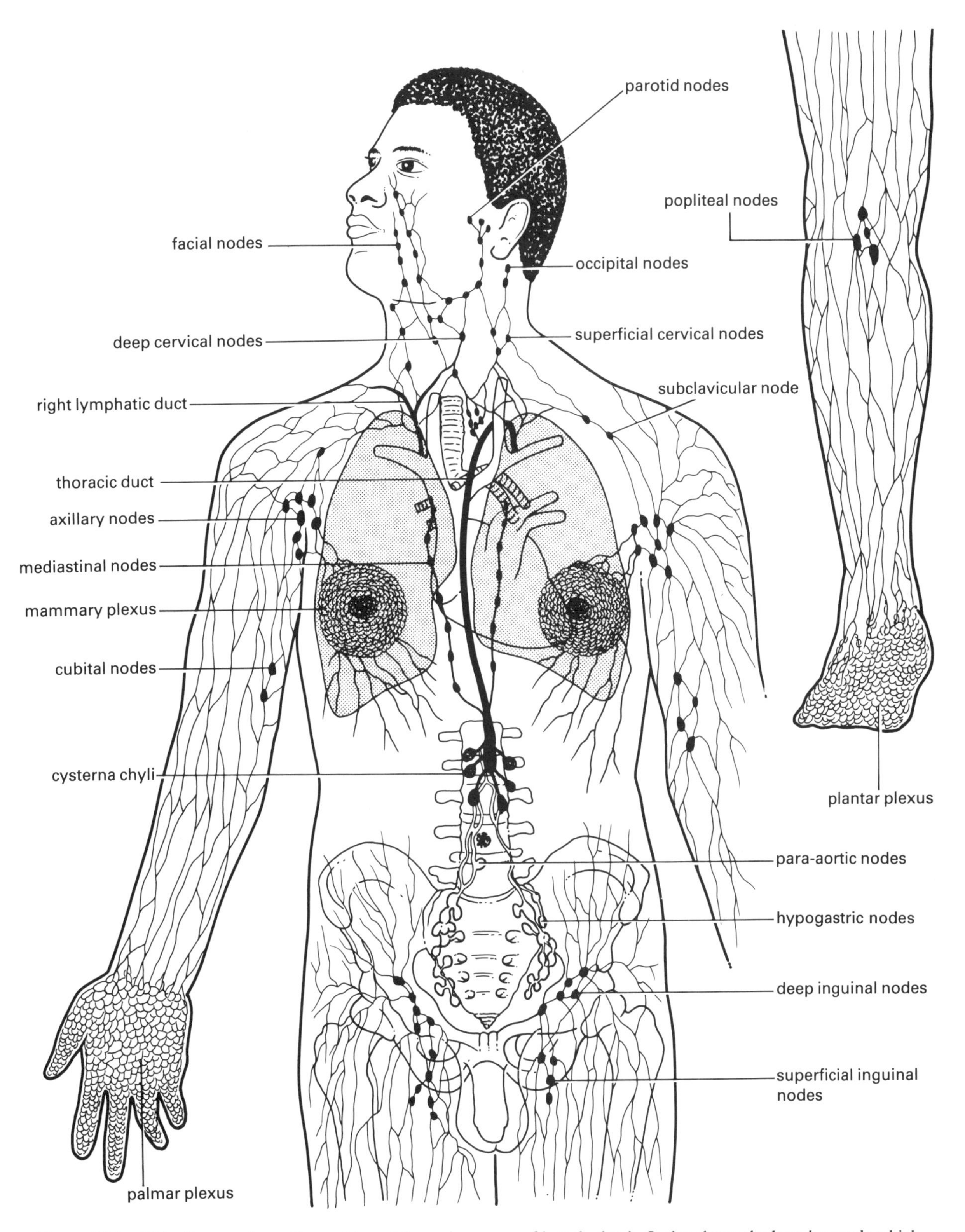

Figure 22.2 This diagram shows the position of the main groups of lymph glands. It also shows the lymph vessels which carry lymph into the glands. It also shows the lymph glands draining into lymphatic ducts. The largest lymphatic ducts then drain into the large veins.

These capillaries join to make larger lymph vessels as the vessels go towards the centre of the body.

Lymph nodes are collections of lymphatic tissue along the course of the lymph vessels.

Lymph vessels collect fluid from the capillaries and tissues in the same way as veins. But lymph vessels also collect larger things (such as large proteins and organisms) which veins cannot collect. These proteins and organisms are taken to the lymph nodes, where, if necessary, the lymphatic system cells make antibodies etc. against the protein or organism. (See Chapter 10 page 36).

The protein or organisms travelling in the lymphatic system can sometimes cause inflammation of parts of the lymphatic system. Inflammation of the lymph vessels is called *lymphangitis*. Inflammation of the lymph nodes is called *lymphadenitis*. If the infection is severe, pus may form in the lymph nodes.

If the lymph nodes are inflamed or destroyed and cannot take fluid and protein from the tissues in the normal way, then the extra fluid and protein in the tissues causes swelling. This is called *lymphoedema*. Lymphoedema is like ordinary oedema except that the fluid has much protein in it, so the oedema does not get a hollow in it, or 'pit', when you press on the area, as easily as ordinary oedema.

History and examination

If you suspect disease of the lymphatic system you must:

1. Examine the lymph nodes in the neck (see Figure 22.3), and axilla (see Figure 22.4), and groin.
   Examine the lymph nodes in the neck and axilla when you examine the head and neck, ENT and thyroid.
   Examine the lymph nodes in the groin when you examine the abdomen for herniae and lymph nodes.
   You cannot examine the lymph nodes in the chest or abdomen in a routine physical examination.

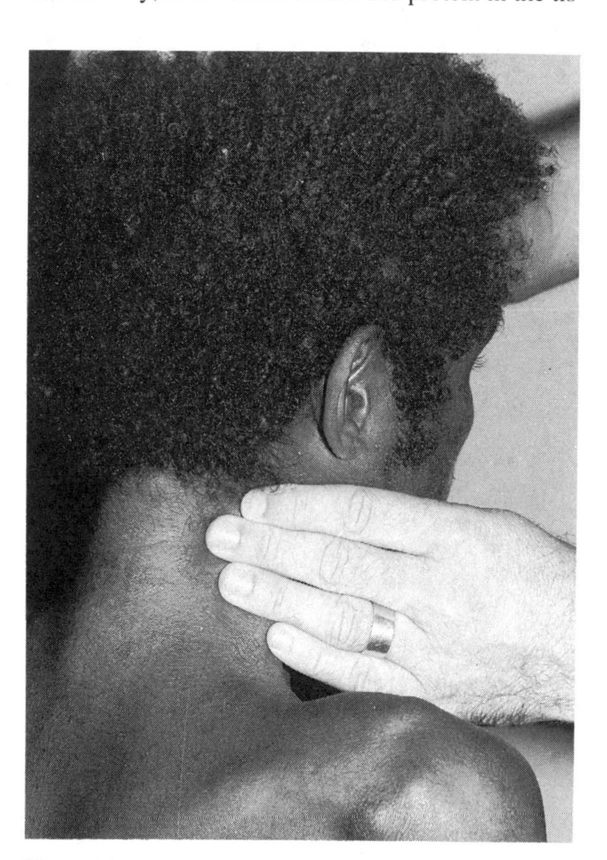
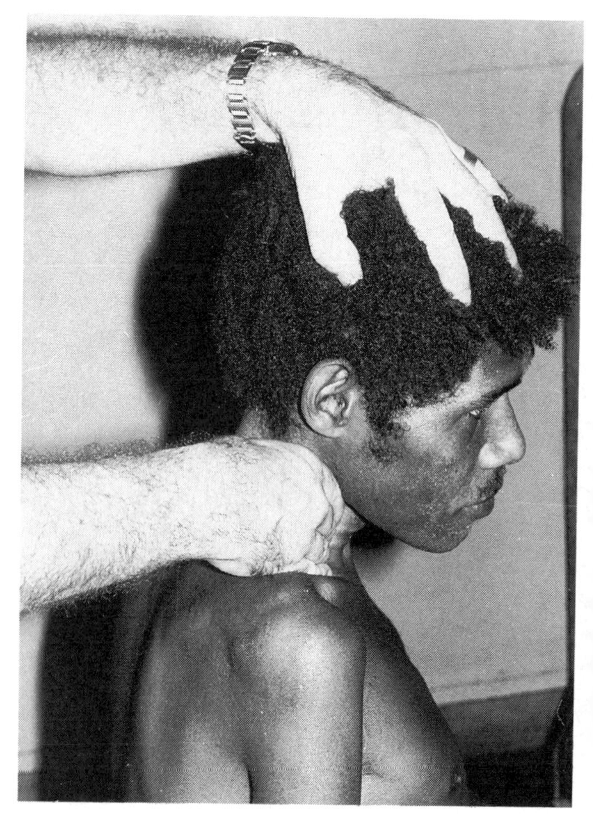

Figure 22.3 Method of examination of the lymph glands in the neck. The left photograph shows examination of the lymph glands at the back of the neck – from in front of the patient. The right photograph shows examination of the lymph glands at the front of the neck – from behind the patient with the patient's head tipped to the side you are examining to make the muscles relax.

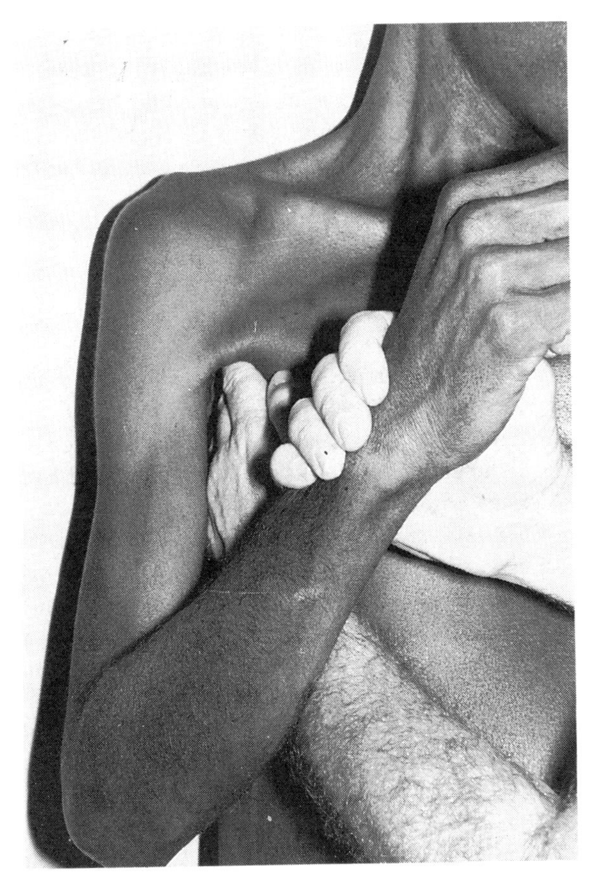

Figure 22.4 Method of examination of the lymph glands in the axilla. Note that the patient must not hold his arms out so that you can feel under them. That makes the muscles tight and you cannot feel the lymph glands under the muscles. The patient's arm must be at his side as in this photograph.

2. Examine the related organs:
   - liver (see Chapter 24 page 306),
   - spleen (see this chapter page 267),
   - bone (see Chapter 28 page 384), and
   - blood for anaemia, bleeding or infection (see Chapter 21 pages 237–8).
3. Examine the areas drained by any abnormal lymph nodes for lymphoedema, infections and cancer.

Common clinical conditions of the lymphatic system

Acute infective lymphangitis and lymphadenitis

Acute infection anywhere in the body may enlarge lymph nodes which drain the area. This may be because the nodes are making antibodies etc. (see Chapter 10 page 36).

But in some infections, the organisms defeat the body defences, and then these organisms may grow and multiply in the lymph vessels and/or lymph nodes, and cause inflammation.

In inflammation of the lymph vessels there is a red, hot, tender, swelling in a thin line between the place where the infection started and the lymph nodes. This is called *acute lymphangitis*.

In inflammation of the lymph nodes the nodes are enlarged and tender (and if they are close to the skin, they may be hot and red). This is called *acute lymphadenitis*.

In severe acute lymphadenitis, pus may form and the nodes become fluctuant.

In acute infections of the lymph vessels or lymph nodes, the patient will develop malaise, fever, fast pulse, and the other signs of toxaemia.

Most cases of acute lymphangitis and acute lymphadenitis are caused by bacterial infections. Sometimes they are caused by filarial infection (see page 258) and other causes.

Treatment includes:

1. Antibiotics – usually penicillin (see Chapter 10 page 46–52).
2. If there is pus and fluctuation, aspirate (suck out) the pus through a needle, or incise and drain (if aspiration is not successful).

Bubonic plague

See Chapter 17 page 125.

Inguinal bubo (lymphogranuloma venereum)

See Chapter 19 page 174.

Chronic infective lymphadenitis

Chronic lymphadenitis can be caused by repeated attacks of acute bacterial infection or by chronic infection.

These can cause (1) enlargement of the lymph nodes and/or (2) block of the lymph vessels and the lymph passages in the lymph nodes.

This block of the flow of the lymph can cause lymphoedema. Lymphoedema is swelling of the area drained by the affected vessels and nodes caused by oedema (see Figure 22.7).

Elephantiasis – chronic severe swelling of the affected body parts with thickening and folding of the skin (see Figure 22.7) – can develop if lymphoedema is present for many years. Lymphoedema and elephantiasis are particularly common in the leg and the scrotum.

Tuberculous lymphadenitis

Tuberculous lymphadenitis is a chronic infection of lymph nodes caused by the tuberculosis bacteria. Always think of tuberculous lymphadenitis if patient is like this:

1. He is a child or young adult (but can be any age).
2. His neck glands are affected (but can be glands in any other area).
3. He has only one symptom – a lump which does not go away but gets bigger.
4. His only signs are enlarged lymph nodes joined or matted together which are not tender or red or hot. Sometimes there is also a sinus (hole) discharging pus over the top of the nodes.
5. There is no obvious cause of the enlarged nodes (unless other signs of tuberculosis are present) (see Chapter 14 pages 77–80).
6. He has a positive tuberculin test (see Chapter 14 page 82).
7. Antibiotic treatment does not cure the infection even if continued for 3 weeks.

> Any chronic cervical gland enlargement with no obvious cause (e.g. infection in the ENT or head) which does not improve after 3 weeks' treatment with antibiotics must be aspirated or biopsied (see Chapter 14 page 82 to find out if it is caused by tuberculosis, especially if the tuberculin test is positive).

If an aspiration or a biopsy is not possible, and after 6 weeks the condition is still getting worse, a trial of antituberculosis treatment could be started. The full length of treatment must be completed even if the patient quickly improves. Always try at least an aspiration.

See Chapter 14 pages 84–91 for management.

Filariasis

Filariasis is a disease caused by infestation with small filarial worms (*Wuchereria bancrofti* or *Brugia malayi*). These worms live in the lymphatic vessels and lymph nodes and cause inflammation, and later block the flow of lymph through them.

Filariasis is common in only some areas in the tropical and coastal and island areas of Africa, Asia, the Pacific and the Americas (see Figure 22.6). However, about 120 million people in the world are infected. Also, WHO classifies filariasis as the world's number 2 cause of disability.

The adult filaria worms produce larvae called microfilaria. Microfilaria are carried around in the blood near the skin only at the time when certain mosquitoes in that area usually bite people. This is often at night between 10 p.m. and 2 a.m. but about midday in some areas of the Pacific. If these mosquitoes take up the microfilaria in their blood meal, the microfilaria then develop in the mosquitoes. These mosquitoes later pass on the filaria larvae, which are infective to people they bite (see Figure 22.5).

The adult filarial worms live in and irritate the lymph vessels and lymph nodes. This causes repeated acute inflammation, acute lymphangitis and acute lymphadenitis and eventually also chronic inflammation, chronic lymphangitis and chronic lymphadenitis. After a long time the lymph vessels and glands become so scarred that lymph cannot flow through them. It has now been found that these patients have also repeated bacterial infections and that these

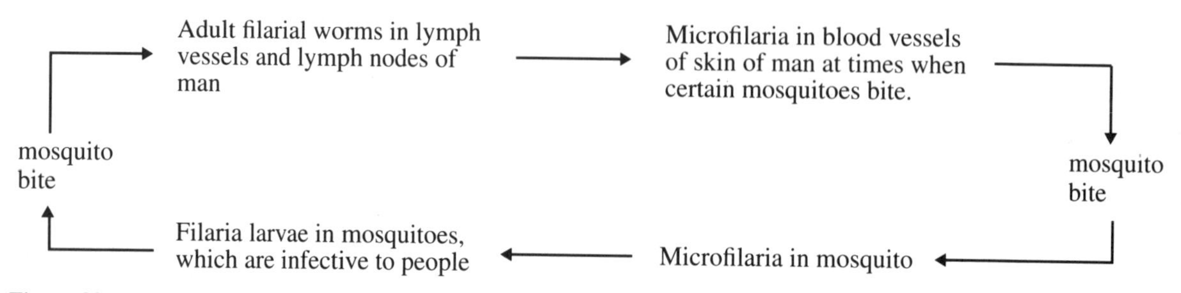

Figure 22.5 Diagram to illustrate the life cycle of filarial worms.

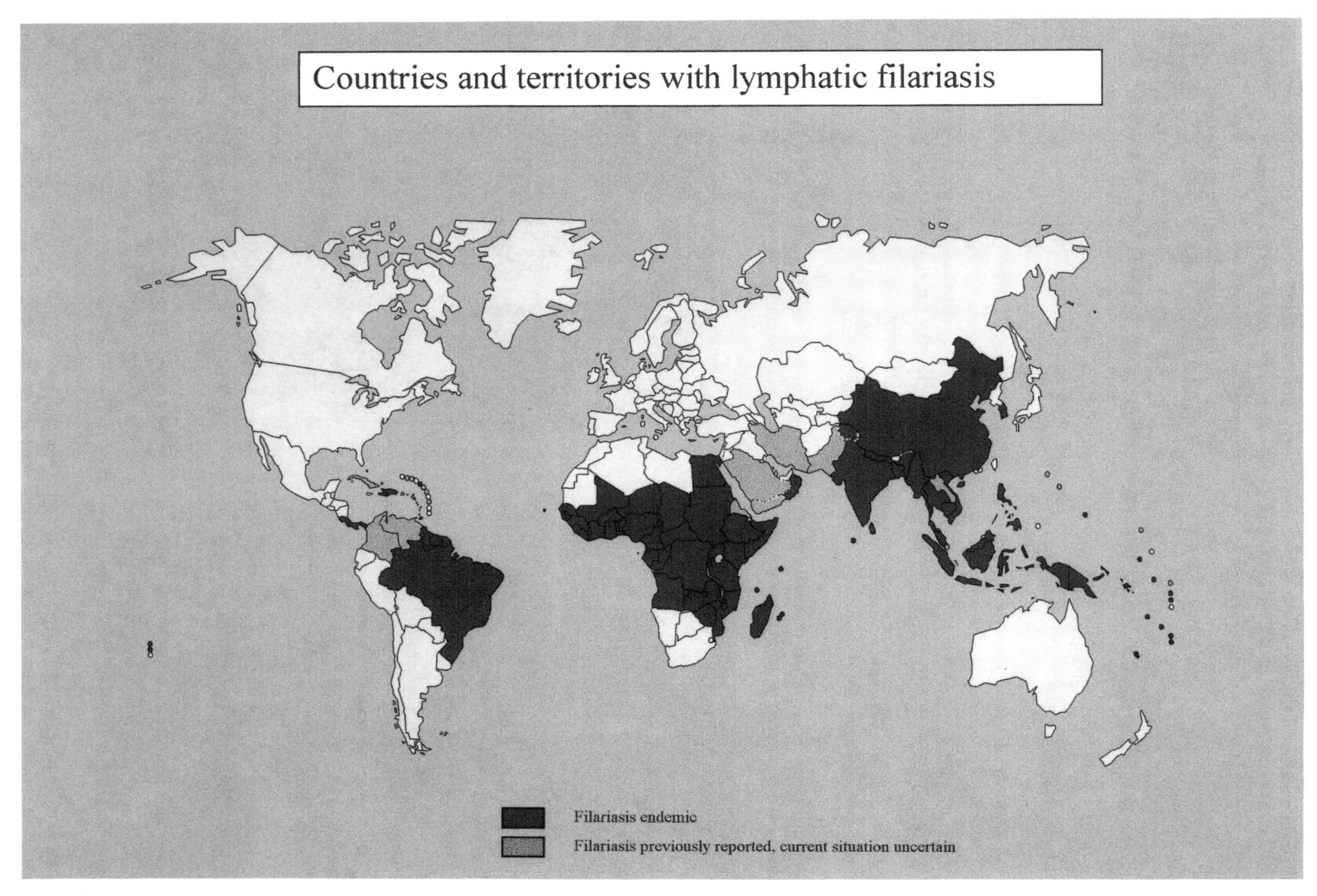

Figure 22.6 The distribution of filariasis.
(Source: World Health Organization, WHO/CTD/FIL, 1998)

bacterial infections, as well as the worms, cause a lot of the inflammation, scarring and block of the lymphatics.

Symptoms and signs

Lymphangitis caused by filaria causes attacks of acute inflammation of part of a limb or a joint or of a testis or of other areas. Acute lymphadenitis caused by filaria causes attacks of swelling and tenderness of the lymph nodes. Severe general symptoms and signs of infection can also occur. Usually you cannot tell if the inflammation is caused by filaria or bacteria. These conditions do not improve a lot with antibiotics if they are due to the worms; but they usually get better without treatment after some days or weeks.

Some attacks of 'tropical arthritis' may be due to filaria (see Chapter 29 page 394).

If there are repeated or heavy infestations with filarial worms for some years, especially if there are repeated bacterial infections also, these cause not only repeated attacks of acute lymphangitis and lymphadenitis but also two further things.

Lymphoedema of legs, scrotum, vulva, arms or breasts, etc. may develop. The nearby lymph nodes are usually large and hard.

After many years of lymphoedema severe chronic oedema of the part can develop, with thick folded skin often oozing lymph, called elephantiasis (see Figure 22.7). Note that the other causes of lymphoedema and elephantiasis include:

1. Chronic infective (bacterial) lymphadenitis including some STDs especially lymphogranuloma venereum.
2. Tuberculous lymphadenitis.
3. Chronic chemical lymphadenitis from silica absorbed from some soils in some countries through repeated cuts on the feet.
4. Cancer of the lymph nodes themselves (lymphoma) or more likely cancer spread from nearby skin or other organs to the lymph nodes, as well as Kaposi's sarcoma.

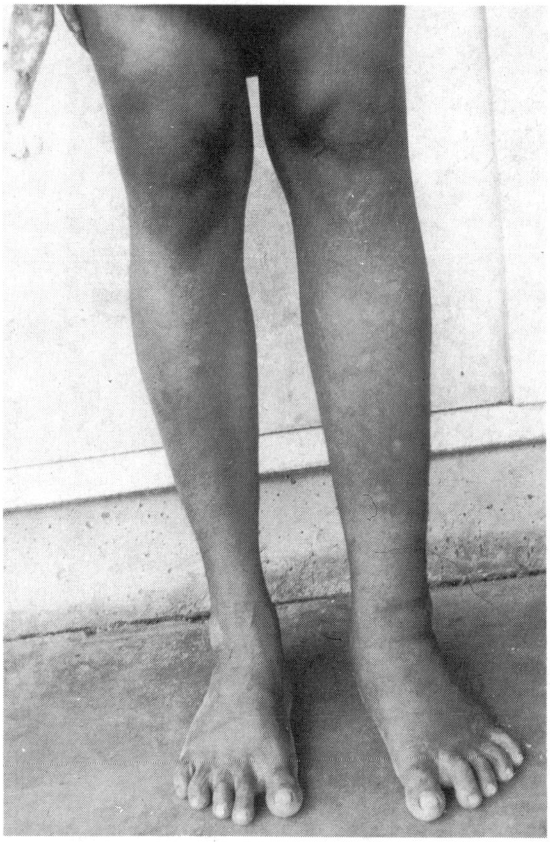

Figure 22.7A Lymphoedema left leg early in the course of the condition.

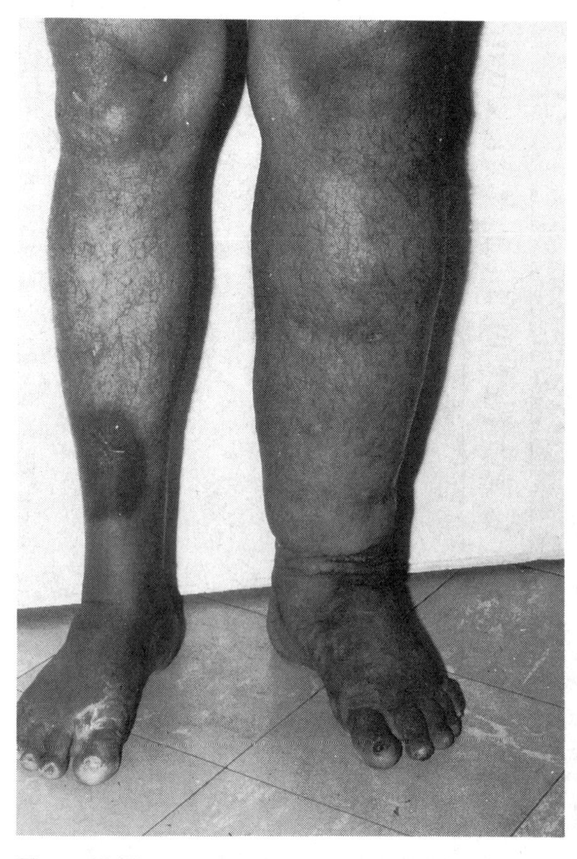

Figure 22.7B Lymphoedema both legs, 'Elephantiasis' left leg.

Test

The test for filarial worm infestation is to look for microfilaria in blood. Collect thick blood smears (as for malaria) between 10 p.m. and 2 a.m. on three nights or at midday in the Pacific (see Chapter 6 page 23.) Microfilaria are often not present when the patient has developed elephantiasis.

A much easier and more accurate blood test is now available in some places (e.g. ICT filariasis rapid immunochromatographic test for *Wuchereria bancrofti* antigen). This blood (serology) test, done on blood from just a finger prick collected at any time of the day, will show if the person is infected with filaria or not.

Showing that a patient is infected with filaria does not of course mean that the patient's symptoms and signs are necessarily due to this infection with filaria.

Do not, however, biopsy the lymph glands as this may make lymphoedema or elephantiasis worse. If the diagnosis is not certain, refer the patient to the next visiting Medical Officer for advice.

Treatment

Treatment depends on the stage and severity of the disease.

During attacks of acute lymphangitis or lymphadenitis

- Rest with the affected part elevated (keep as high as possible for as much of the day as possible).
- Dressings if any break in the skin and especially if any infection.
- Aspirin 600–900 mg (2–3 tablets) 4–6 hourly.
- Anthistamines, e.g. promethazine 25 mg (1 tab) 1–3 times daily.
- Antibiotics usually penicillin at first (see Chapter 11 page 46) as you cannot be sure the condition is not caused by bacterial infection and there is usually some bacterial infection present. Other antibiotics including doxycycline or tetracycline, or if staphylococci are causing infection, one of the cloxacillin group of drugs may be needed.
- Do not give diethylcarbamazine until the acute stage is over.

After the acute stage is over; and in the chronic stages

Give diethylcarbamazine 2 mg/kg three times a day for 3 weeks (usually 100 mg (2 tabs) three time a day). In some areas this dose causes severe allergic reactions by killing off many microfilaria quickly. In these areas therefore:

1. start with a low dose, e.g. 25 mg ($\frac{1}{2}$ tab) daily and double the dose daily until the usual dose (as above) is being given, and
2. give antihistamines, e.g. promethazine 25 mg (1 tab) 1–3 times a day as well for the first week.

Diethylcarbamazine kills the microfilaria easily but it does not kill the adult filaria worms as easily. You should therefore repeat the course after 6 weeks. After some months, you should examine slides for microfilaria. If microfilaria are present, treat with diethylcarbamazine again.

If there is onchocerciasis or *Loa loa* infection in your area, do not give diethylcarbamazine as severe reactions may occur when these organisms are killed by the drug. Ask advice from your local Medical Officer on how you should go about giving this drug or perhaps, more likely, use albendazole.

Lymphoedema

Give diethylcarbamazine tablets (see above).

Tell the patient to protect the limb from more damage by bacterial infection (e.g. wear shoes or sandals; get early antibiotic treatment and dressings if infection occurs, etc.).

Tell the patient to keep the affected part higher than the rest of the body when possible.

Treat any bacterial infection quickly and well.

Elephantiasis

Tell the patient to keep the affected part higher than the rest of the body when possible. He should not sit with the legs down for long periods.

Use compression dressings and bandages if possible.

Tell the patient to wear shoes or at least sandals.

Give antibiotics and use dressings for any infection that occurs.

Give diethylcarbamazine tablets (see above).

Discuss with a Medical Officer if surgery would help (surgery is not often helpful except for the scrotum).

Control and prevention

Control and prevention are at last possible. The programme is based on identifying populations affected (most easily by the serology test) and, if e.g. 5% or more of the population is affected, then treating the whole population with drugs to kill the adult worms, if possible. However it is more important, to stop the worms from producing microfilaria, as this will mean that mosquitoes can no longer get infected and spread the disease to other people. This is now possible as it has been found that a once-only dose of drugs, such as diethylcarbamazine and ivermectin and albendazole, given once each year works well.

Kill the parasite in the body of the original host and reservoir
Mass treatment of the whole population by diethylcarbamazine or albendazole as well as ivermectin is carried out. Ivermectin does not kill the adult worms although the other drugs do – although not all of them. This treatment will need repeating each year (6–18 months depending on what tests in your area show).

Ivermectin and the other drugs however do allow the body to destroy all the microfilaria and stop the adults producing more microfilaria. Then even if there are still adult worms present in the body, the infected person will not be able to pass the infection to mosquitoes by microfilaria. Ivermectin or diethylcarbamazine alone each control microfilaria for over a year and if both are given together, do it for over 18 months.

Treatment can be given by health workers or the community control distribution once each year (or as otherwise decided best). However everyone in the community needs to be treated so that no one keeps on infecting mosquitoes. The doses are ivermectin 400 micrograms/kg and diethylcarbamazine 6 mg/kg; but it has been found that standard doses such as diethylcarbamazine 300 mg for an adult and 150 mg for a child, are satisfactory and much easier to give out to the whole population.

Another effective way of getting drugs to the population is for all salt supplied to have 0.2–0.4 mg diethylcarbamazine/g of salt added. The diethylcarbamazine has no colour, smell or taste and is not hurt by cooking. It has reduced microfilaria by 97% from previous rates in some areas and has allowed eradication of filariasis in other areas when tests were done. However, all salt supplied has to have the diethylcarbamazine in it so that the whole population is treated. This, therefore, needs both company help and government legislation. In areas where there is onchocerciasis and *Loa loa* infection, drugs such as albendazole are given instead of diethylcarbamazine with ivermectin so that severe reactions do not occur.

Stop the means of spread
All the usual means of mosquito control are needed.

Personal protection from mosquito bites by clothing, repellents and mosquito nets at night time, especially if these are treated with permethrin, are helpful. New methods of controlling the *Culex* mosquito, which spreads the disease in urban areas, include the use of *Bacillus sphaericus*, a bacteriological agent, which kills the larva of the *Culex* mosquitoes which spread filariasis in towns and also the use of expanded polystyrene beads on the surface of non-flowing permanent water such as in pit latrines.

Raise the resistance of potential new hosts
This at present is not possible; but as some adults do develop some immunity to re-infection, it is possible that a vaccine will be able to be produced.

Prophylactic treatment
This is done in mass treatment with the diethylcarbamazine or albendazole.

Burkitt's lymphoma

Burkitt's lymphoma is a common cancer but occurs only where malaria is common. It is also related in some ways to previous infection with Epstein-Barr virus (EB virus causes infectious mononucleosis or glandular fever) and also to certain changes in the cell. It occurs mainly in children but also in some young adults.

Usually Burkitt's lymphoma causes tumours of the jaw. At first teeth near the tumour become loose. The tumour grows in the bone and becomes very large very quickly (e.g. in one month). The tumour often pushes the eye forward. It is soft and painless. The skin over the tumour is not ulcerated. The lymph nodes are not enlarged. There is no fever. Apart from the swelling, the patient seems well at first (see Figure 22.8). Dental abscesses can look similar; but an abscess has signs of inflammation and tenderness.

Abdominal tumours are almost as common as jaw tumours.

Paralysis or other nervous system changes also can occur from the tumour pressing on the brain or spinal cord.

Transfer suspected cases to a Medical Officer as soon as possible for diagnosis by biopsy and treatment with anti-cancer drugs as patients can get very much worse in a few days and good early treatment can cure some patients.

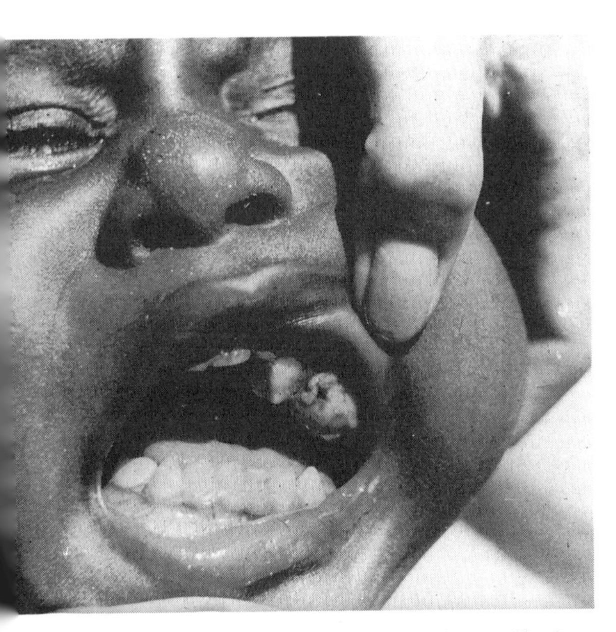

Figure 22.8 Photograph of Burkitt's lymphoma affecting the upper jaw. The teeth are loose in the swollen gum. If teeth look healthy (no holes in them) but you can very easily push the teeth back and forward in the gum with your finger, without hurting the patient, then it is likely the patient has a Burkitt's tumour.

Vaccines to prevent this tumour are being tried.

Cancer of the lymph nodes

There are two kinds of cancer that affect the lymph nodes.

The first kind is a primary cancer of the lymph nodes called a lymphoma. You will most often diagnose lymphoma when you biopsy a node to see if it is enlarged because of tuberculosis. Biopsy any lymph node that is enlarged and hard; (but not tender, red and hot); especially if there is no infection on the skin etc., or the gland has not much improved after treatment with antibiotics (see page 257). Sometimes the biopsy report will be that the lymph node shows no tuberculosis but does show Hodgkin's disease or non-Hodgkin's lymphoma. These are both primary cancers of the lymph glands. Sometimes they can be much improved by special treatment.

The other sort of cancer of lymph nodes you will diagnose is when cancer from the skin or an organ spreads to the lymph nodes, i.e. secondary cancer of the lymph glands. One particularly common site for a primary cancer which spreads to the lymph glands of the neck, is the back of the nose or throat (nasopharyngeal carcinoma). This tumour is also related to EB virus infection and perhaps diet. Often this cancer cannot be seen without special instruments or X-rays. Again this sort of cancer may be diagnosed when tuberculosis is expected. The lymph nodes in secondary cancer in most other cases are usually hard and stuck to each other or the muscles or the skin.

Refer or non-urgently transfer such patients to a Medical Officer. Do not biopsy lymph nodes unless they are very near the surface and you have been taught how to do it and you have actually done it under supervision (it is harder than it looks).

Enlargement of lymph nodes

Do a full history and examination (see Chapter 6). See which of the following your patient has:

1. Enlargement of a lymph node or some lymph nodes *and* tenderness of enlarged nodes *or* fever (see below).
2. Enlargement of a lymph node or some lymph nodes *but* no tenderness of enlarged nodes *and* no fever (see below).
3. Enlargement of *most* of the lymph nodes of the body *but* no tenderness of enlarged nodes *and* no fever (see below).

Enlargement of a lymph node or some lymph nodes and tenderness of enlarged nodes or fever

1. *Acute bacterial lymphadenitis*
   An infected lesion of some sort in the part of the body drained by the affected lymph nodes is usually present (the lesion may be very small).
   Treat with antibiotics (see page 257 and Chapter 11 pages 46–52).
2. *Acute filarial lymphadenitis*
   - The patient is from or in an area where filariasis occurs.
   - He has sometimes had previous attacks.
   - There are microfilaria in blood.

   Treat as for acute bacterial lymphadenitis and see page 261.
3. *Acute viral infections* such as rubella (German measles) or infectious mononucleosis.
   - Usually the patient is young.
   - Sometimes there is an epidemic.
   - Often the nodes affected are in the neck and not acutely inflamed.
   - Sometimes there are other symptoms and signs (especially a rash).

- Usually the patient is not very sick.

Give symptomatic treatment only and observe. (Do not give ampicillin or amoxycillin, which may cause a rash in these patients.)

4. *Bubonic plague*
   - The patient is in or has been in an area where plague occurs.
   - Sometimes there is an epidemic; but could be first case.
   - Usually there have been recent rat deaths.
   - The nodes usually severely inflamed and soon become large, fluctuant and discharge pus (bubo).
   - The patient is very sick, with fever, rigors etc.
   - Septicaemia often develops.
   - Pneumonia may develop.
   - The patient often dies within a week.

   If plague is a possible diagnosis, see Chapter 17 page 125 urgently for diagnosis and management.
5. *Some sexually transmitted diseases* especially:
   - Lymphogranuloma venereum.
   - Chancroid.
   - Donovanosis.
   - Herpes simplex,
   - lymph nodes in groin affected,
   - may be genital lesion.

   See Chapter 19 pages 170–8.

Enlargement of a lymph node or some lymph nodes but no tenderness of enlarged nodes and no fever

1. *Repeated acute or chronic bacterial infection*
   - Usually in the legs of a person who does not wear shoes.
   - Often there is a history of repeated injury or infection of feet, with swelling of lymph nodes in groin.
   - Chronic infection may still be present.
   - The nodes are hard and smooth.
   - Often there is lymphoedema.

   See page 261 for management.
2. *Filariasis*
   - The patient is in or from an area where filariasis occurs and usually other people near where he lives are affected.
   - There is often a history of repeated attacks of acute lymphangitis and lymphadenitis.
   - The nodes are hard and smooth.
   - Often there is lymphoedema.
   - Microfilaria may be present in the blood (but not necessarily).

   See page 261 for management.
3. *Tuberculosis*
   - The affected patient is often young (but not always).
   - The affected nodes are often in neck (but can be anywhere).
   - A node may be joined to other nodes under the skin.
   - Sometimes there is a sinus (hole) discharging pus over the node.
   - There is no infection or other cause for the node enlargement in the area of the body drained by the node.
   - Sometimes chronic cough or other symptoms or signs of tuberculosis are present.
   - Sometimes there is a family history of tuberculosis.
   - The tuberculin test is usually positive.
   - Treatment for 3 weeks with antibiotic does not cure the disease.

   Aspirate or biopsy all such glands (see page 258 and Chapter 14 pages 82–5).
4. *Some sexually transmitted diseases*

   See 'Enlargement of a lymph node and tenderness', No. 5 (above) as nodes are normally but not always tender.
5. *Chronic chemical lymphadenitis* of the groin nodes
   - Only in some countries where some soils have a lot of silica.
   - Patient has not worn shoes and has had numerous cuts on feet over many years.
   - Often lymphoedema.
   - No other cause.
6. *Cancer of the nodes*
   - As for tuberculosis (see 3 above) except no history suggesting tuberculosis and the tuberculin test is negative. *or*
   - The nodes are hard and lumpy and stuck to each other or the skin or the nearby muscles. *or*
   - There are other lesions which could be cancer in the area drained by the nodes.

   See page 263 for management.
7. *HIV infection*

   See 'Enlargement of most of the lymph nodes but no tenderness', No. 1 page 265.
8. *Trypanosomiasis*

   Often all the nodes are affected but sometimes it is mostly in the neck nodes.

   See Chapter 18 pages 144–7.

9. *Visceral leishmaniasis*
   Usually all nodes are affected but sometimes it is mostly in one part.
   See below and Chapter 18 pages 139–44.

Enlargement of most of the lymph nodes of the body but no tenderness of nodes and no fever

1. *HIV infection*
   - The patient is usually aged 15–50 years.
   - Unsafe sexual practices, blood transfusion, IV drug abuse etc. in last few years.
   - Nodes 1–3 cm in diameter not getting larger after 3 months.
   - No other cause obvious.
   - May have other symptoms and signs of HIV infection, although often none.
   - Blood test for HIV if available, is positive.

   See Chapter 19 page 178.
2. *Syphilis*
   - The patient has had sexual intercourse with a possibly affected person some weeks or months before.
   - There was a chancre (sore on genitalia) for 2–6 weeks about 6 weeks before.
   - Skin rashes are sometimes present.
   - Condylomata lata are sometimes present.
   - Mucous patches are sometimes present.
   - Malaise is sometimes present.
   - The serological test for syphilis is positive.

   See Chapter 19 page 172 for management
3. *Cancer of lymph glands (lymphoma)*
   - The spleen is often enlarged.
   - The liver may be enlarged.
   - Anaemia is often present.
   - Wasting is often present.

   See page 263 for management.
   Make certain that the patient does not have severe tuberculosis.
4. *Visceral leishmaniasis (kala azar)*
   - The patient is in or from an area where kala azar occurs.
   - There is fever at first and later.
   - The spleen is enlarged (often very enlarged).
   - The liver is enlarged, but not very enlarged.
   - Anaemia is present.
   - Repeated attacks of diarrhoea often occur.
   - Wasting is often present.
   - Lumps on skin are sometimes present.
   - There are leishmania organisms in blood or a biopsy.
   - The formaldehyde gel test is positive after a few months.

   See Chapter 18 pages 139–44 for management.
5. *Trypanosomiasis*
   - The patient is in or from an area where trypanosomiasis occurs.
   - There is a sore (in Africa) or a swelling (in America) at the place of the bite.
   - A fever may develop later.
   - The spleen is enlarged.
   - The liver is enlarged.
   - Anaemia is present.
   - The pulse is fast.
   - There may be meningitis or encephalitis or psychosis or unconsciousness (in Africa).
   - There are trypanosomiasis organisms in blood or aspirated from lymph gland.

   See Chapter 18 pages 143 and 148.

Swelling of one limb

Causes include:

1. injury,
2. infection,
3. chronic lymph vessel and lymph node disease with blocked lymph node channels (see this chapter).
4. clots in the main deep vein ('deep venous thrombosis' or DVT),
5. varicose veins, and
6. snakebite or allergic reaction to sting or toxin etc.

Swelling of both legs

See 'Generalised oedema' Chapter 36 page 485.

The spleen

Anatomy, physiology, pathology

The spleen (Figure 22.9) makes some of the white blood cells and also some antibodies. The spleen also takes 'worn out' red blood cells from the blood. It breaks them down and saves most of the parts for the bone marrow to make new red blood cells.

If the spleen collects and breaks down many more red blood cells than normal (e.g. in a patient with malaria which damages red blood cells), then the spleen enlarges. If the vein from the spleen (which goes through the liver) becomes blocked by disease

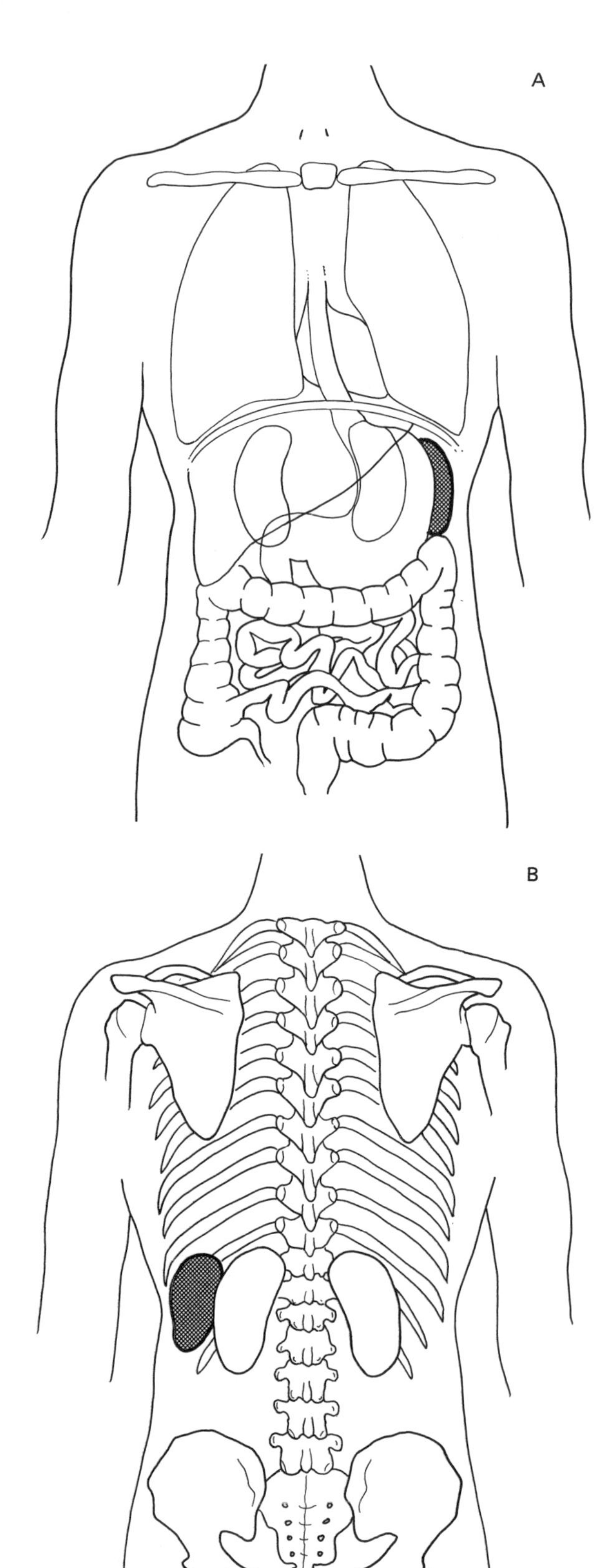

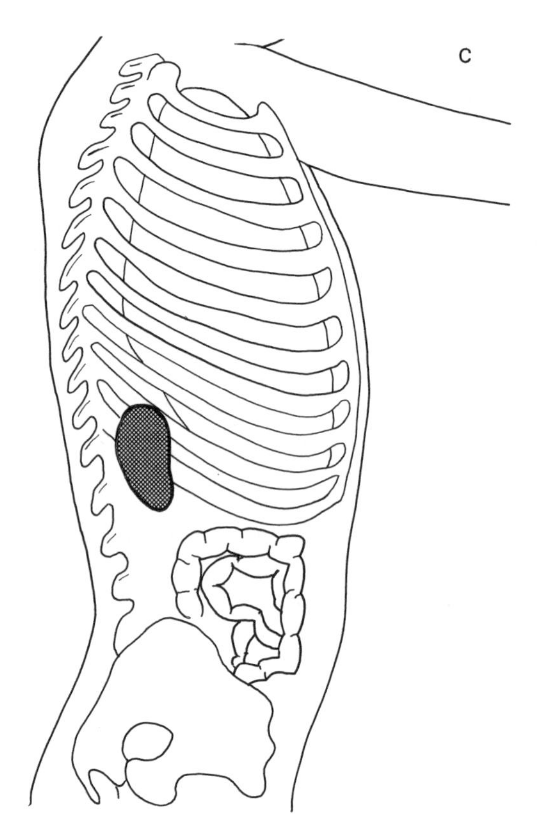

Figure 22.9 A, B and C. These diagrams show the normal position of the spleen (slightly enlarged). (A) Anterior or front view. (B) Posterior or back view. (C) Left lateral or side view. Note that the spleen is a posterior organ. Note that a normal spleen cannot be felt on examination of the abdomen. When a spleen enlarges it enlarges forwards, downwards and to the right. At first you can feel it right under the ribs on the left side, in the front. See Figure 22.10. Note also that the spleen is just under the ribs which protect it. If the left lower ribs are damaged (especially if they are fractured) the spleen is likely to be damaged too.

of the liver (e.g. cirrhosis or schistosomiasis), then the spleen becomes too full of blood and enlarges.

Anytime the spleen enlarges, it can start taking normal red blood cells, normal white blood cells, and normal platelets out of the blood. The body may then not have enough of some or all of these blood cells.

An enlarged spleen is more likely to rupture (break open) and bleed than a normal spleen.

Symptoms and signs

Disease of the spleen may cause these *symptoms*.

1. Pain in the left upper abdomen. This is usually caused by trauma or inflammation.

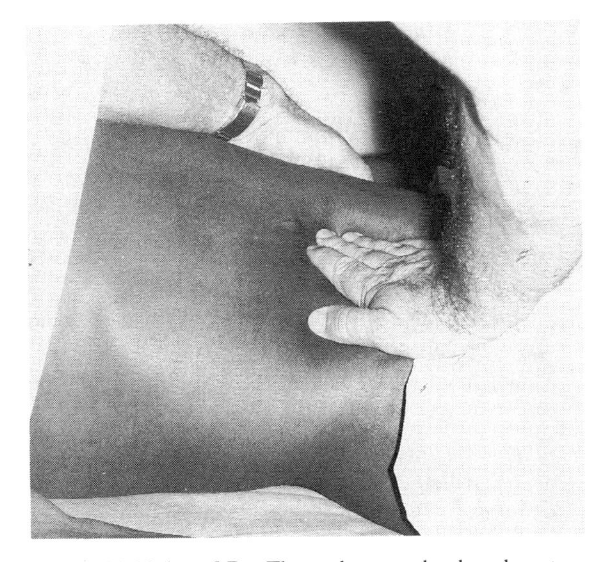

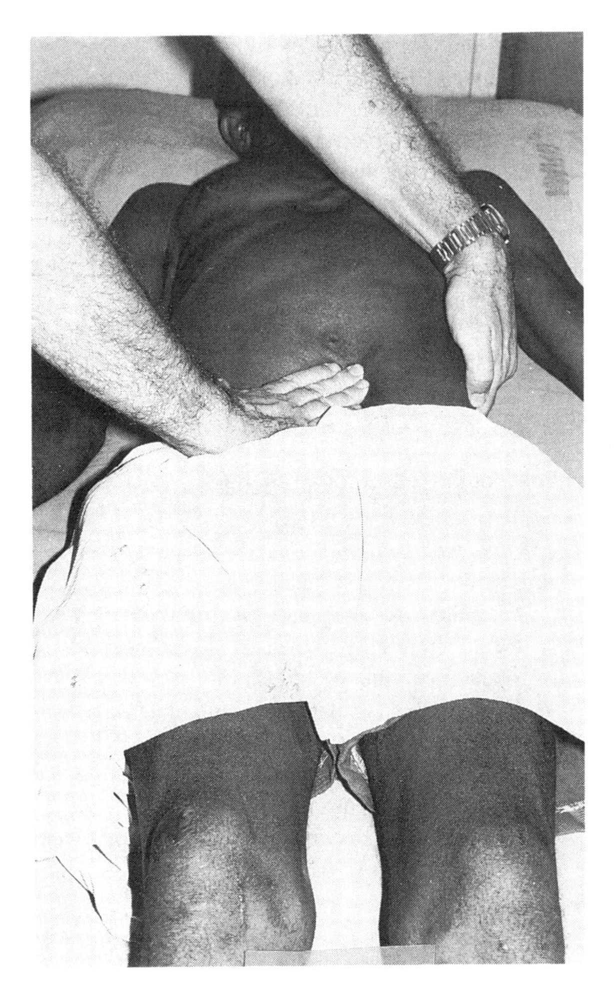

Figure 22.10 A and B These photographs show how to feel for a spleen. Place the left hand behind the left side of the patient's abdomen. Lift it upwards (forwards). Place the right hand with the palm flat on the patient's abdomen and the fingers pointing to the left upper abdomen. Start in the right lower abdomen (or you may not feel a very large spleen). Tell the patient to take slow deep breaths in and out. If the spleen is enlarged to where your fingers are you will feel it hit the tips of your fingers as the patient breathes in. If you do not feel the spleen, move the fingers towards the ribs and tell the patient to breathe deeply again. Keep moving the right hand up until the spleen is felt or you have felt along the edge of the ribs, and found no enlargement of the spleen.

2. Swelling of the left upper abdomen; or if the spleen is very enlarged, swelling of the whole abdomen.
3. Anaemia (and other blood disorders), if the spleen is enlarged and takes normal blood cells as well as 'worn out' red cells from the blood.
4. Shock and anaemia, if the spleen is ruptured and bleeds.

Disease of the spleen may cause these *signs*.

1. Tenderness in the left upper abdomen (see symptoms, 1).
2. Enlargement of the left upper abdomen or the whole abdomen (see symptoms, 2).
3. Anaemia (and other blood disorders) (see symptoms, 3).
4. Shock and anaemia (see symptoms, 4).

Common conditions affecting the spleen

Very large spleen

A very enlarged spleen may be caused by many conditions. In some areas, some of these causes do not occur. Do not worry about causes that do not occur in your area or areas where your patients may have been.

Your patient may have more than one cause for a very enlarged spleen. It is not always possible to know what causes a patient's enlarged spleen. But you must always try to find out.

If possible do these tests on your patient (do not test if the disease does not occur where your patient has been):

1. Blood slide for malaria parasites.
2. Thin blood film examination sickling test and laboratory blood tests for white blood cell diseases such as leukaemia, and red blood cell diseases such as thalassaemia and sickle cell anaemia.
3. Blood for whatever tests your laboratory can do for diagnosis of leishmaniasis.
4. Tests for trypanosomiasis on blood and fluid aspirated from lymph node.
5. Urine for schistosome eggs (or at least for miracidia).
6. Stool for schistosome eggs (or at least for miracidia).

Some of the causes for a very big spleen are:

1. *Chronic malaria*
   - The patient is in a malarial area; but he has not been there for long enough to have developed (semi-) immunity to malaria (which needs 4–10 years of continuous exposure).
   - He has repeated attacks of acute malaria.
   - Anaemia is present.
   - An enlarged liver is present.
   - Wasting is present.

   Treat acute attacks of malaria as soon as they start (see Chapter 13 page 61).

2. *Hyperreactive malarious splenomegaly* or *tropical splenomegaly syndrome*
   - The patient has lived in a malarial area for some years.
   - The spleen keeps on enlarging.
   - The liver is enlarged.
   - Anaemia is present.
   - Wasting is present.
   - There are episodes of haemolysis, when there is fever, jaundice, worsening of anaemia and the spleen becomes painful and tender.
   - The malaria smear is often negative.
   - Tests for schistosomiasis and visceral leishmaniasis are negative.

   Give prophylactic antimalarial drugs for at least 2 years, and probably for life (see Chapter 13 page 61 and Chapter 21 page 243).

   In an area where malaria occurs *always think of this condition* in any patient who has a chronically enlarged spleen as HMS is one of the few treatable causes of very enlarged spleen. But do not treat cases of chronic malaria as HMS (see Chapter 13 page 243).

3. *Visceral leishmaniasis (kala azar)*
   - The patient is in or from an area where kala azar occurs.
   - There is fever early in the disease.
   - The lymph nodes are enlarged
   - Anaemia is present.
   - Diarrhoea is present.
   - Wasting is present.
   - Sometimes skin rash is present.
   - Tests for leishmania in blood or formaldehyde gel test are positive.

   Management. See Chapter 18 pages 140–5.

4. *Trypanosomiasis*
   - The patient is in or from an infected area.
   - Sore or swelling at the site of the infecting bite.
   - Fever, fast pulse, swelling of lymph nodes and liver as well as spleen.
   - Lymph node aspirate or new special blood tests positive for trypanosomiasis.

   Management. See Chapter 18 pages 143 and 148.

5. *Schistosomiasis*
   - The patient is in or from an area where schistosomiasis occurs.
   - He has a past history of blood in the urine or dysentery.
   - There may still be urinary or intestinal symptoms and signs.
   - Late in the disease he may vomit blood or pass melaena (black tarry stools).
   - Late in the disease the abdomen may be full of fluid (ascites) and there may be some swelling of legs and back (oedema).

   Diagnose and treat as soon as possible. Once late stages are reached treatment is not likely to help as much. See Chapter 18 page 150.

6. *Chronic liver disease usually of an unknown cause (cirrhosis)*
   - No evidence of schistosomiasis is present.
   - A lot of ascites and some oedema are present with wasting of the muscles most noticeable around the shoulders.
   - Sometimes the patient may vomit blood or pass melaena (black tarry stools).
   - There may sometimes be a change in behaviour or level of consciousness; sometimes jaundice; sometimes bleeding, from anywhere. Diuretics help the ascites and oedema; but no treatment is much help. See Chapter 24 page 308.

7. *Blood diseases*
   - *Leukaemia* – The report of the blood film suggests this. Refer or non-urgently transfer to Medical Officer.
   - *Thalassaemia* – The report of the blood film and examination for abnormal haemoglobin confirms diagnosis.

   See Chapter 21 page 247.
   - *Sickle cell anaemia*:
     - The patient is usually an African.
     - Anaemia is present.
     - The patient has repeated infarction crises.
     - The spleen may become smaller.
     - The report of the blood film sickling test and examination for abnormal haemoglobin confirms diagnosis.

   See Chapter 21 page 244.

Painful or tender spleen

There are many causes of an enlarged, painful or tender spleen in tropical and developing countries. You can usually use other symptoms and signs to make the diagnosis. But never forget to check for the following conditions.

Traumatic rupture of the spleen

Small injuries can cause the spleen to rupture.

Be very suspicious if there has been a left-sided chest or abdominal injury.

Sometimes there is a haematoma (bruise) under the capsule (or covering) of the spleen for some hours or days after the injury before the capsule bursts and the spleen bleeds a lot.

The patient will become paler, the pulse rate faster and the blood pressure lower if the spleen is bleeding.

Generalised abdominal tenderness and later shifting dullness (see Chapter 36 pages 494 and 499) will develop.

Transfer urgently all suspicious cases to Medical Officer care after you have started an IV drip and any other necessary treatment (see Chapter 27 page 378).

Acute malaria

Always give antimalarial treatment (see Chapter 13 page 61) to any patient in a malarial area, unless you are certain he does not have malaria.

Septicaemia and typhoid fever

Always think of septicaemia in any patient who is very sick. Unless another cause for the illness can be found, treat for septicaemia (see Chapter 12 page 53).

Sickle cell anaemia

See above.

23

Disorders of the Gastrointestinal System

Anatomy, physiology and pathology

Food consists of proteins, carbohydrates, fats, salts, vitamins and water. Food is used as fuel for the muscles and other working parts of the body, and for growth and repair of the body.

Before body cells can use food, it must be crushed, digested (or broken down into simpler substances) and then absorbed (taken) into the body.

The parts of the gastrointestinal canal in which foods are crushed, digested and absorbed are the mouth, the oesophagus, the stomach, the small intestine and the large intestine.

First the food is crushed by the teeth, and mixed with saliva, which is a lubricant that also starts digestion of the food. The saliva is made by three sets of paired salivary glands. The parotid glands are on both sides of the jaw in front of the ears. The submandibular glands are on both sides under the jaw. The sublingual glands are under the tongue. (See Figure 23.1.)

Then the food is swallowed. The oesophagus has muscles in its wall which move the food into the stomach.

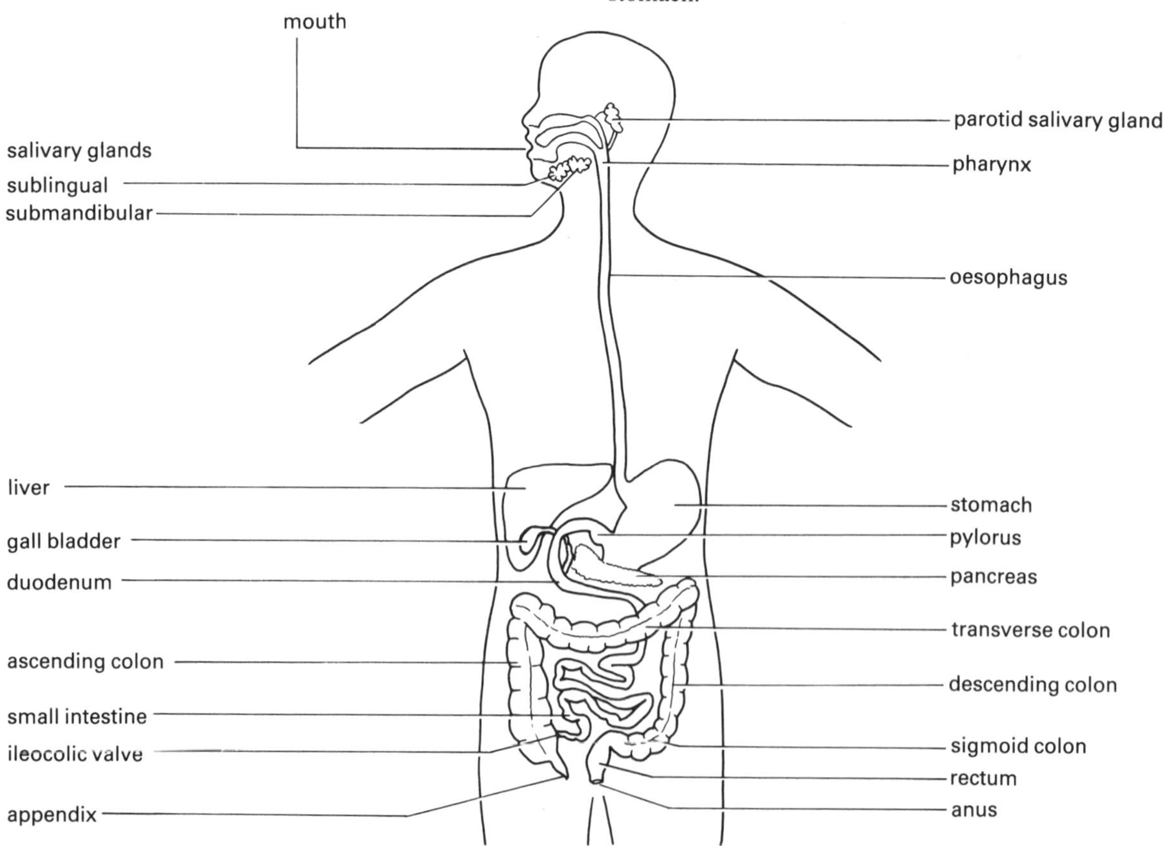

Figure 23.1 Diagram of the main parts of the gastrointestinal system.

The stomach is a storage bag. It lets small amounts of food into the intestine every few minutes until it is empty, which takes a few hours. In the stomach the food is mixed with two very powerful digestive juices – hydrochloric acid and pepsin. These are made in glands in the mucous membrane of the stomach.

When the food has been partly digested by the acid and pepsin, the ring of muscle at the outlet of the stomach (which is called the pylorus), opens a little. This allows the muscular contractions of the stomach (called peristalsis) to push a little food into the first part of the small intestine (called the duodenum).

In the duodenum the food is mixed with other digestive juices. Bile, made in the liver and stored in the gall bladder, is added and helps fats to be absorbed. Pancreatic juice from the pancreas is added and this contains an enzyme (trypsin), which breaks down proteins, and other enzymes, which break down carbohydrates and fats (see Figure 23.2).

The food is moved through the duodenum and the small intestine by contractions of the small intestine (also called peristalsis). The small intestine is about 6–7 metres long.

As the food travels along the small intestine, more digestive juices are added from glands in the mucous membrane of the intestinal wall. All these digestive juices break down (or digest) the food into simpler compounds.

These simpler compounds are then absorbed by the special mucous membrane of the intestinal wall. The digested and absorbed food is put into the blood, which goes to the liver through the portal vein (see Figure 24.3).

When the remains of the food reach the large intestine (also called colon), it is only the fibres and hard parts, which cannot be digested and absorbed by the small intestine, that are left. The remains of the food have been mixed with bilirubin (which is the remains of haemoglobin from worn out red cells which is excreted in the bile). This bilirubin gives the faeces their brown colour. The food remains are also mixed with many bacteria (both dead and alive) which normally live in the intestine. There is also a lot of water from food, drink and the digestive juices mixed with the food remains.

As all this material goes through the large intestine, most of the water is absorbed through the mucous membrane of the large intestine.

The lower part of the large intestine is called the rectum. The rectum is a storage bag for the remains of the food until they can be passed through the anus into the toilet.

The unabsorbed remains of the food and the other materials are called faeces or stool. If the faeces stay a long time in the rectum, they become hard and difficult to pass. This is called constipation. If the

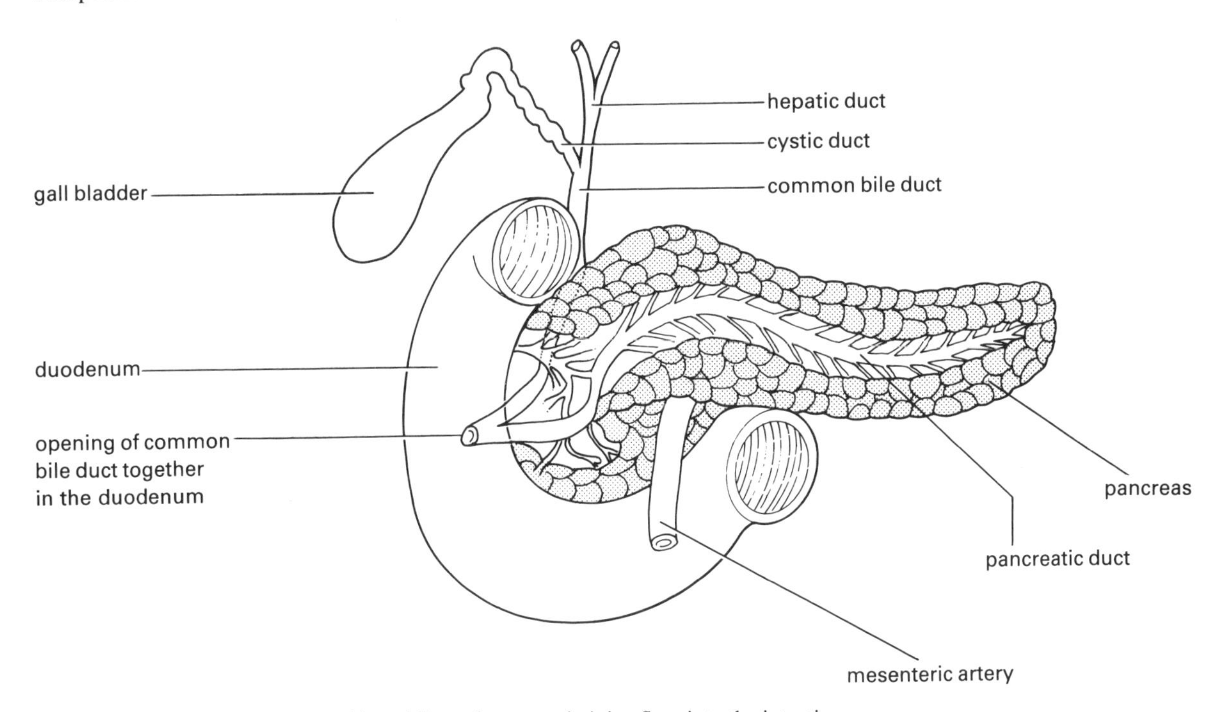

Figure 23.2 The duodenum and how bile and pancreatic juice flow into the intestine.

unabsorbed food goes through the large intestine very quickly there is not enough time for the water to be absorbed. The stools are then soft, watery, large in volume and frequent. This is called diarrhoea.

History and examination

These symptoms and signs can be caused by conditions of the gastrointestinal system. Always check for those marked* in a routine history and examination. See Figure 23.3.

Symptoms of gastrointestinal disease

1. Fever* – if there is infection.
2. Painful mouth or salivary glands.
3. Difficulty in swallowing (dysphagia).
4. Chest pain usually worse on swallowing or lying down (oesophageal disease).
5. Change in appetite.*
6. Vomiting*/haematemesis* (blood vomited).

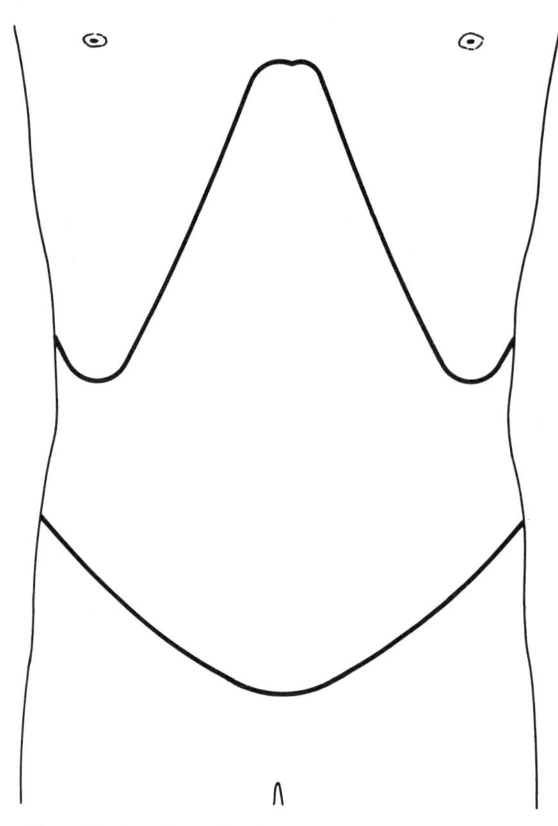

Figure 23.3 Use a simple diagram like this and mark the findings of your examination on it.

7. Diarrhoea*/dysentery (blood in loose stool)*.
8. Abdominal pain*
   (a) Epigastric (upper central abdomen) and if related to food (made worse or eased by food) – usually caused by stomach or duodenal disease.
   (b) Colic in epigastrium and around umbilicus – usually inflammation of or obstruction of the small intestine.
   (c) Colic in the side or lower part of the abdomen and around umbilicus – usually caused by inflammation of or obstruction of the large intestine.
   (d) Constant in any area – usually caused by inflammation or stretching of the peritoneum in that area.
9. Weight loss.*

Signs of gastrointestinal disease

1. Temperature raised* – if there is infection.
2. Dehydration and/or shock* – inelastic skin, fast pulse, low blood pressure, little or no urine passed, etc.
3. Wasting/malnutrition* – if not eating; or chronic vomiting; or not absorbing food (malabsorption); or chronic diarrhoea.
4. Pallor* – if gastrointestinal bleeding, acute or chronic; or poor absorption of iron, etc.
5. Inflammation of the mouth or salivary glands.
6. Enlarged lymph glands above the clavicles – some cancers in the abdomen.
7. Abdomen (details in Chapter 36 pages 449–501):
   (a) Inspection
   - size*
   - shape*
   - surface for scars*
   - movement when breathing*

   (b) Palpation
   - tenderness*
     – rebound tenderness
     – guarding
     – rigidity
   - enlarged organs*
   - lumps or masses*

   (c) Percussion (if necessary)
   - organs
   - masses
   - fluid (shifting dullness)

   (d) Ascultation (if necessary)
   - bowel sounds
     – increased

– absent
- splash

(e) Pelvic examination through the rectum ('PR') (if necessary) (see Figure 26.9 pages 352–3)
- tenderness
- enlarged organs
- masses
- faeces, blood or pus in rectum

(f) Pelvic examination through the vagina ('PV') (if necessary) (see Chapter 26 pages 352–3)
- tenderness
- enlarged organs
- masses
- blood or pus from vagina or uterus

Disorders of the gastrointestinal system

Parotitis

Parotitis is usually caused by mumps (see Chapter 16 page 119) in people who were healthy before.

Parotitis is often caused by acute bacterial infection (see below) in people who were already sick before. See Figure 23.4 for the position of the parotid glands.

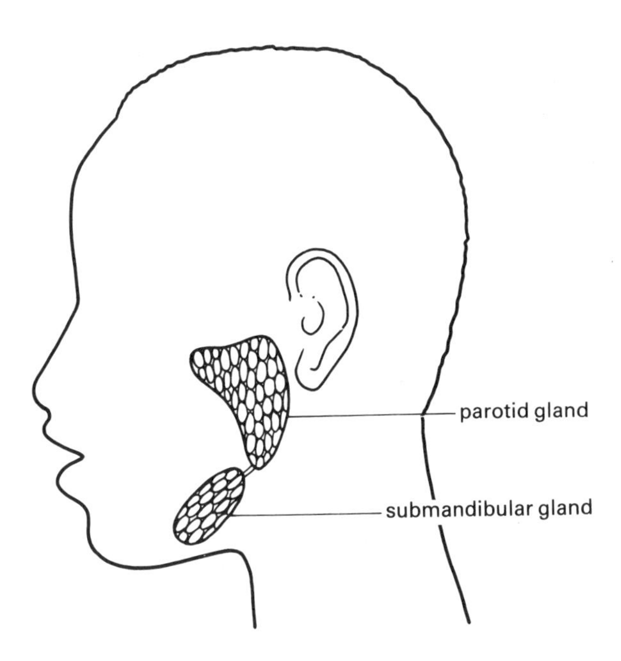

Figure 23.4 The anatomical position of the parotid and submandibular glands.

Acute bacterial parotitis

Acute bacterial parotitis usually occurs in sick people who are not eating, drinking or caring for their mouths properly.

Symptoms include pain in the side of the face (which is made worse by movement) and swelling of the parotid area.

Signs include:

- The parotid gland at the side of the face is swollen, hard, tender, often hot and sometimes red. It is difficult for the patient to open his mouth. The swelling is sometimes very large.
- The pulse is fast and the temperature is raised.

Differential diagnosis includes: parotid tumour (which is not acute); and mumps (see Chapter 16 page 119).

Treatment includes:

- antibiotics (start with penicillin),
- pain relief,
- mouth toilet, and
- proper hydration (intravenously, if necessary).

Prevention is by doing a mouth toilet and checking that sick patients have enough fluids.

Peritonitis

Peritonitis is an inflammation of the peritoneum (or lining or the peritonal cavity) in all parts of the abdomen. The inflammation is usually acute and is usually caused by bacterial infection. Blood in the peritonal cavity can cause similar symptoms and signs (see below). The inflammation is occasionally chronic, and is then usually caused by tuberculosis (see Chapter 14 page 80).

There may be a history or symptoms or signs of the condition which caused the peritonitis, e.g.

- inflammation of the bowel wall, e.g. appendicitis, enteritis necroticans (pigbel) or diverticulitis;
- a bowel obstruction, especially if strangulated;
- an abdominal wound, e.g. spear or knife;
- a peptic ulcer that has ruptured;
- a genital tract infection in the female, e.g. gonorrhoea or post-partum infection;
- ectopic pregnancy.

Symptoms and signs (See also Chapter 36 pages 489–502)

Symptoms may include:

- constant abdominal pain made worse by movement,
- vomiting, and
- constipation, usually.

Signs may include:

- temperature usually above normal,
- pulse usually fast,
- blood pressure low, late in the disease,
- the respiration rate may be fast late in the disease,
- dehydration may be present,
- the patient looks 'sick',
- the abdomen:
  - distension after some hours,
  - no movement on respiration,
  - tender all over with rebound tenderness, guarding and rigidity,
  - bowel sounds absent.

Tests

No tests are usually possible in a health centre.

If you do a white cell count, it is usually increased, with an increased percentage of neutrophils.

Treatment

Urgent (emergency) transfer to hospital is necessary if the patient agrees to surgery (to treat the cause; and to remove the pus, faeces or blood from the peritoneal cavity).

While waiting for transfer, treat like this:

1. IV fluids as necessary for dehydration or shock (see page 286 and Chapter 27 page 378) and then give maintenance fluids.
2. Nil orally. Insert an intragastric tube, and aspirate all the fluid every hour.
3. Antibiotics: chloramphenicol 1–2 g immediately and every 6 hours by IVI (or IMI).
4. Morphine 10 mg (1 ml) or pethidine 100 mg (2 ml) if necessary for pain while waiting for, and during, transfer.

Intestinal obstruction

Intestinal obstruction is present when the food and fluids in the intestine cannot go through a part of the intestine. The intestine above the part that is blocked contracts more than usual and secretes more fluids than usual, and then dilates (get bigger).

There may be a history or symptoms or signs of the disease which caused the obstruction, e.g.

- hernia,
- previous abdominal operation,
- enteritis necroticans ('pigbel'),
- cancer of the intestine,
- previous vomiting or passing of roundworms (*Ascaris*) which followed a dose of tetrachloroethylene (TCE),
- the swallowing of a large foreign body.

Symptoms and signs (See also Chapter 36 pages 489–502)

Symptoms include:

- abdominal pain, usually central, which lasts for about half a minute and which then goes away only to come back every few minutes, often with loud intestinal sounds,
- repeated vomiting and
- constipation (no faeces or gas passed).

Signs include:

1. Dehydration occurs if the condition has been present for more than a couple of hours (fast pulse, low blood pressure, inelastic skin, little or no urine passed, etc.).
2. General signs of peritonitis (see page 273) occur if the obstruction is strangulated, i.e. the blood supply to that part of the intestine is damaged. (The intestinal wall starts to die and is attacked by bacteria from inside the bowel which spread through the bowel wall into the peritoneal cavity.)
3. Abdomen
   Inspection:
   - distension of the whole abdomen,
   - the abdominal wall does not move well with respiration,
   - intestinal movements can sometimes be seen through the abdominal wall,
   - you must *always* look for hernias and scars.

   Palpitation:
   - Tenderness is not present. Tenderness is present only if the obstruction is strangulated. At first tenderness is only over the affected area. Later, when general peritonitis develops, the tenderness spreads to the whole abdomen.
   - You may feel a mass. It may be the affected length of intestine or a cancer or other mass which is causing the obstruction.

   Auscultation:
   - Intestinal sounds are increased (and pain occurs during the sounds).

- You can hear a loud splash if the abdomen is shaken while you listen with the stethoscope.

Treatment

Transfer to hospital urgently (emergency) is necessary for operation to remove the cause of the obstruction, if the patient will agree to surgery.

While waiting for transfer, treat like this:

1. Nil by mouth. Insert a tube into the stomach, and aspirate all the fluid every hour.
2. IV fluids (see: Fluid therapy – Dehydration and shock, page 286 and Chapter 27 page 378).
3. Treat for peritonitis if this is present (see page 274).

Gastro-oesophageal reflux (see page 302)

Peptic ulcer

A peptic ulcer is an acute or recurring acute or chronic ulcer of the wall of the stomach or duodenum caused by acid and pepsin and other factors.

Acid and pepsin are normally made by the stomach to digest food. But they do not normally digest the wall of the stomach or duodenum and so cause a peptic ulcer. A peptic ulcer can be caused by the acid and pepsin in some people at some times if other things are also present. The most common cause is infection with a special bacterium (*Helicobacter pylori*). Other causes include drinking alcohol, smoking tobacco, taking aspirin or NSAIDs or high dose adrenocorticosteroids, possibly worrying and unknown causes.

Peptic ulcer occurs everywhere; but it is common only in some areas.

Symptoms and signs

The main *symptoms* include.

1. Epigastric pain (i.e. in the upper central abdomen) related to food (i.e. pain made worse *or* better by food). At first the pain may occur for only a few days or weeks, and then get better. *Epigastric pain related to food is the main symptom.*
2. Later the pain may be there most of the time and may radiate (spread) to the back.
3. Sometimes there is vomiting after food (if food causes pain, the vomiting usually relieves the pain).
4. Weight loss (especially if food causes pain and there is vomiting).

The *signs* include:

1. 'The pointing sign'. When the patient is lying on a bed and you ask him to point with one finger to where the pain is, the patient points to one place, usually between the umbilicus and the lower end of the sternum. If the patient does this, there is usually a peptic ulcer. If the patient does not point to one place but instead rubs his hand in different parts of the abdomen, or if the pain is not between the umbilicus and the lower end of the sternum then there is usually not a peptic ulcer.
2. Epigastric tenderness. This is the main sign.
3. Weight loss (if there is pain and vomiting after food).
4. Anaemia (if the ulcer has bled).

Complications which the ulcer can cause include:

1. Penetration of the posterior (back) wall of the stomach or duodenum into the liver or back – this causes back pain which does not go away.
2. Perforation of the front wall of the stomach or duodenum – the food and acid inside the stomach or duodenum then go into the peritoneal cavity. This causes sudden severe abdominal pain and peritonitis.
3. Ulceration of a blood vessel – this causes bleeding into the stomach or duodenum with vomiting of blood (haematemesis); or digested black, tarry blood in the stool (melaena); also anaemia; and sometimes shock.
4. Obstruction of the stomach outlet so that food and later fluid cannot go from the stomach into the duodenum – this causes vomiting and wasting ('pyloric stenosis').

The *differential diagnosis* includes all other causes of upper abdominal pain (see Chapter 36 page 489). Sometimes an infection with many hookworms or a protozoal organism called *Giardia* in the duodenum may cause symptoms similar to a peptic ulcer.

Treatment

The treatment depends on how severe the attack is.

Mild attack:

- The epigastric pain is usually made better or worse by food.
- The epigastric tenderness is mild.
- There are no complications.

Severe attack:

- The epigastric pain may be present all the time.
- The epigastric tenderness is severe.
- There are no complications.

Mild attack
Treat as an outpatient.

1. Antacids.
   - Aluminium hydroxide compound tablet or liquid (or magnesium hydroxide or other antacid tablet or liquid). (Magnesium may cause diarrhoea; calcium may cause constipation.)
   - Give 2 tablets or 10–20 ml liquid 1 hour after every meal, and at night before sleeping, and at any other time if necessary for pain. Give this treatment regularly for 3 weeks.
   - If the patient gets better then give 2 tablets only if necessary for pain.
   - If no antacid tablets are available, give 1 cup of full cream milk (instead of 1–2 antacid tablets).
2. Tell the patient:
   - not to smoke,
   - not to drink alcohol,
   - not to drink strong coffee or tea or cola drinks,
   - not to take aspirin or codeine compound tablets or any other tablets for pain or arthritis except paracetamol, and
   - not to eat foods that he knows cause pain.
3. Tell the patient to eat at the same time every day (and, if possible, to eat 3–6 small meals every day rather than fewer larger meals).
4. Give no aspirin and as few other drugs as possible (many drugs can cause the symptoms of peptic ulcer). Give paracetamol if needed for other pain.
5. Give anti-hookworm drug (see Chapter 23 page 278).
6. Treat anaemia if present (see Chapter 21 page 238) but do not give oral iron while the pain is still present.

Severe attack:
Admit for inpatient treatment.

1. Rest in bed for 3 weeks. Give diazepam 5 mg (1 tab) three times a day if the patient will not rest.
2. Give treatment as for mild attack (see above).
3. If the patient does not improve:
   (a) Check that he does not have another disease (peritonitis, amoebic liver abscess, etc.).
   (b) Increase antacid dose. Use liquid if available. Give regularly every 3–4 hours or even every 1–2 hours if necessary.

Note that rest in bed in the health centre is the most important and effective part of this treatment. The reason for this is not known. However, it often stops the patient's symptoms and signs.

Note also that new drugs called histamine$_2$ (H_2) blockers and even more effective drugs called proton (acid) pump inhibitors can stop the stomach making acid and cause most peptic ulcers to heal. The ulcer, however, may come back when the drug is stopped. Also it may be more likely to get infections from organisms that are swallowed if there is no acid in the stomach to kill them. (H_2 blockers include famotidine 20 or 40 mg, ranitidine 150 or 300 mg, nizatidine 150 or 300 mg and cimetidine 200, 400 and 800 mg. These doses are given once or twice daily. Proton pump inhibitors include lansoprazole 30 mg, omeprazole 20 mg and pantoprazole 40 mg, and are given once daily). These drugs are expensive.

Note also that the best treatment, however, is to kill the *Helicobacter pylori* organisms. To do this the patient has to take proton pump inhibitors in twice the normal dose and also amoxycillin and metronidazole for 2 weeks (or even better more complicated and more expensive drugs). These are unlikely to be available for years in health centres.

Transfer

Transfer to Medical Officer care if:

1. Severe pain is not relieved by treatment for severe attack (non-urgent).
2. The pain comes back many times (non-urgent).
3. Perforation causing peritonitis occurs (urgent – emergency).
4. Haematemesis (vomiting blood) or melaena (black stool which looks and smells like tar) occurs, even if there is no shock or anaemia (urgent – emergency).
5. There is vomiting and weight loss caused by obstruction of stomach outlet (non-urgent).
6. There is constant pain in the back caused by penetration of the pancreas or back (non-urgent).

Prevention

Prevention is by not smoking, not drinking too much alcohol and not taking drugs (such as aspirin) when they are not needed (non-urgent).

Carcinoma (cancer) of the stomach

Usually old people are affected. Early symptoms and signs include:

- epigastric pain and/or

- a feeling of fullness after only a little food and/or
- anaemia.

Later symptoms and signs include:

- all of the above, and/or
- epigastric mass, and/or
- obstruction of the stomach outlet, and/or
- weight loss, and/or
- enlarged lymph glands above the clavicle.

If cancer of the stomach is suspected, treat as an inpatient for peptic ulcer for 3 weeks. If the patient is not cured after 3 weeks, transfer him to hospital for investigation. Surgery does not often cure the patient.

Roundworm (*Ascaris lumbricoides*)

Infestation (infection) with roundworms is very common everywhere.

The adult worms are about 15–25 cm long. They live inside the tube of the small intestine.

The female adult roundworm puts about 200,000 eggs into the patient's intestine everyday. These eggs are then passed in the patient's faeces. Inside fertilised eggs, infective larvae develop after about 2 weeks. The larvae will grow best when the patient passes faeces in those places where it is cool, shady and moist; but eggs can survive in other places for years. If an infective egg from dirt or in food is swallowed, the larva hatches and travels through the small intestinal wall, portal vein, liver, right heart, lungs, bronchi, trachea and then oesophagus and stomach into the small intestine, where it develops into an adult roundworm. (See Figure 23.5.)

Symptoms, signs and complications

Symptoms, signs and complications are all uncommon.

1. Usually there are no symptoms or signs. You can only make the diagnosis if an adult worm is seen in the stool or is vomited up or if eggs are seen when the stool is examined under the microscope.
2. If there are many worms, abdominal discomfort or mild colic and distension (swelling) sometimes occurs.
3. If there are many worms in children who eat a poor diet, malnutrition can occur.
4. If there are many worms, especially in children and especially if tetrachloroethylene is given (which irritates but does not kill the worms), a tangled mass of worms can cause intestinal obstruction (this is rare). (Obstruction of other organs such as bile ducts, pancreatic duct or appendix, etc. by a worm does occur but is rare.)
5. Pneumonia and asthma can be caused as the larvae travel through the lungs. (This may not be rare but the diagnosis is not often made.)

Treatment

Treat only if:

1. roundworms are vomited or passed in stool; or
2. you are giving tetrachloroethylene (TCE) to children (give roundworm treatment before giving the TCE); or
3. there is malnutrition; or
4. there is abdominal discomfort and you can find no other cause; or
5. the whole community is being treated as is sometimes done if 50% or more of the population has infection.

Treat as an outpatient.

Use whichever of the following drugs (see Table 23.1) is cheapest and is available.

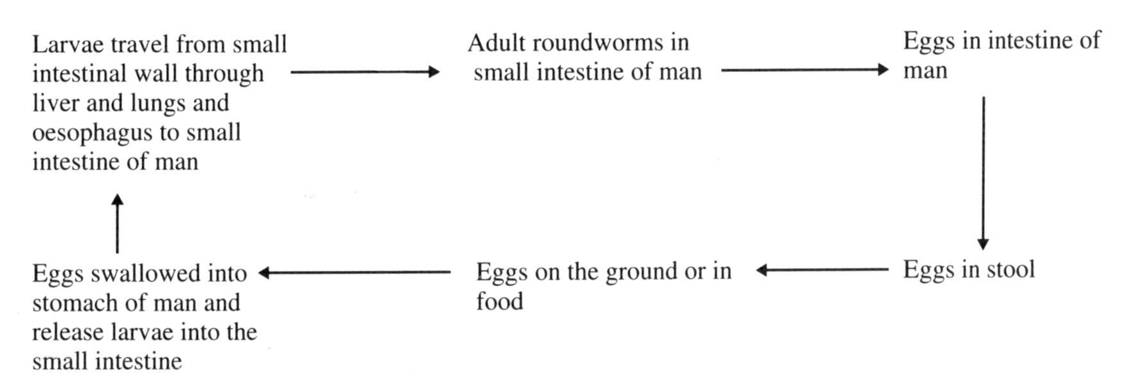

Figure 23.5 The life cycle of the roundworm.

Table 23.1 Effect of drugs on internal parasites

	Levamisole	*Pyrantel*	*Mebendazole*	*Albendazole*
Ascaris lumbricoides	+++	+++	+++	+++
Necator americanus	++	++	++	+++
Ancylostoma duodenale	+++	+++	+++	+++
Trichuris trichiura	++	++	+	++
Strongyloides stercoralis	+	+	+	++

+++ very effective ++ moderately effective + not very effective

- Pyrantel (pamoate or ambonate) (250 mg base tablets or 250 mg/5 ml of syrup).
  Give 10 mg/kg (maximum dose 1 g) once.
  This drug can be used during pregnancy after the first 3 months.
- Albendazole (200 mg and 400 mg tablets).
  For children 2–5 years 200 (possibly 400) mg once.
  For patients over 5 years 400 mg once.
  Do not give during pregnancy (or at least in the first 3 months) or 7 days after last normal menstrual period or in the first 2 years of life.
- Mebendazole (100 mg tablets).
  A single dose of 5 tablets once only is best. A dose of 100 mg twice daily for 1 day is usually adequate although some recommend 3 days. Do not give if pregnant (or at least in the first 3 months) or more than 7 days after the last normal menstrual period or in the first 2 years of life.
- Levamisole (40 mg, 50 mg and 150 mg tablets and 40 mg/5 ml syrup).
  A dose of 2.5–5 mg/kg (maximum dose 150 mg) once only. Do not give during the first 3 months of pregnancy.
- Piperazine (numerous strengths of tablets and mixtures).
  A dose of 75 mg/kg of the hydrate (maximum 4 g of the hydrate or maximum 5 g of the citrate or other salts) once daily between meals or half of this dose for 2 days. Note that piperazine is not effective against the other parasites and is now more expensive than the other drugs and often needs more than one dose and has more side effects.

Prevention

Tell the patient, family and village about the life cycle of the worm and that prevention is by the use of proper toilets by everyone (including children) always.

Hookworm (*Necator americanus* or *Ancylostoma duodenale*)

Infestation with hookworm is very common. The adult worms are about 1 cm in length. They live in the upper small intestine attached by their mouths to the intestine wall. They suck blood and protein from the intestine wall.

The female adult puts eggs into the patient's bowel. These eggs are then passed in the patient's faeces. In shady moist soil, fertilised eggs develop into larvae. After about 1 week the larvae can pass through the skin of a person who touches them. The larvae travel through the blood vessels, right heart, bronchi and trachea, and then the oesophagus and stomach into the small intestine where they develop into the adult worms (Figure 23.6).

Symptoms, signs and complications

1. Anaemia: with weakness, tiredness, dizziness, shortness of breath, pallor, etc. (see Chapter 21 page 238). This is caused by the loss of the blood that the hookworms suck from the intestine wall. (Some hookworms can suck 0.5–1 ml blood daily. Some patients have up to 1000 worms.) The body stores of iron are soon used up by the bone marrow making new blood. When this happens the bone marrow cannot make as much blood as before.
   Anaemia is the only common and important result of hookworm.
   Anaemia occurs only if there are a large number of hookworms in the patient and the patient also has a poor diet.
2. Heart failure (if the anaemia is severe).
3. Oedema (if the anaemia and heart failure and protein loss is severe).

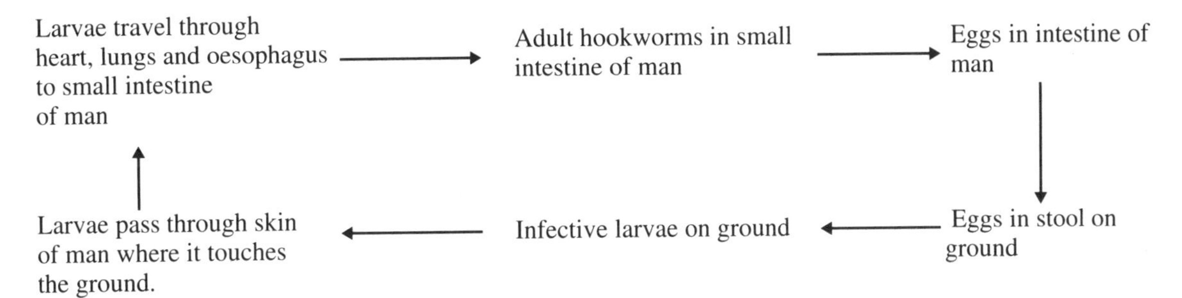

Figure 23.6 The life cycle of the hookworm.

4. Sometimes there is epigastric pain like the pain of a peptic ulcer. Sometimes there is just a little abdominal discomfort.
5. Sometimes a rash occurs (an itchy red rash which may be hard to see and lasts for only a few days) where larvae went through the skin (usually between the toes).
6. Sometimes a cough or wheeze (like bronchitis or asthma) can be caused by the worms travelling through the lungs.

You cannot be certain of the diagnosis of hookworm in the intestine at a health centre as you cannot normally examine the stool by microscope. But if you examine the stool under a microscope, you can see the eggs if the patient has hookworm.

Assume hookworm infestation is present in all patients who have anaemia.

Treatment

1. Give drugs to kill hookworms (Table 23.1). See page 278.
   Use whichever of the following drugs is the cheapest and available.
   - Albendazole (see page 278).
     A single dose of 400 mg will remove 80% of the worms and 400 mg daily for 3 days will remove almost all of the worms. Do not give if pregnant (or at least in the first 3 months of pregnancy) or more than 7 days after the last normal menstrual period or if less than 2 years old.
   - Mebendazole (see page 278).
     A dose of 100 mg twice daily for 3 days is very effective against both types of hookworm. A single dose of 500 mg is also effective. Do not give if pregnant (or at least in the first 3 months of pregnancy) or more than 7 days after the last normal menstrual period or if less than 2 years old.
   - Levamisole (see page 278).
     Give 2.5–5 mg/kg, maximum dose 150 mg. This drug is less effective against *N. americanus*. A second dose after 7 days may be needed. Do not give in the first 3 months of pregnancy.
   - Pyrantel (pamoate) (see page 278).
     Give 10 mg/kg, maximum dose 1 g. Do not give in the first 3 months of pregnancy.
     In heavy hookworm infestations, three further doses in the next 3 days may be needed.
   - Tetrachloroethylene (TCE) (not recommended)
     Treat for roundworm first (see page 277) as otherwise these roundworms are not killed but are irritated and may cause intestinal or other obstruction. The patient should not eat on the night before and on the morning of the treatment, although he can have water. Give TCE 0.1 ml/kg (one tenth of a ml/kg of body weight to a maximum dose of 6 ml). Do not give TCE to a patient whose haemoglobin is less than 5 g/dl or who is jaundiced or sick or who is in the first 3 months of pregnancy.
2. Give routine anaemia treatment.
   Give antimalarials usually chloroquine, iron, folic acid, good diet (containing iron, protein and vitamins) and advice on family planning if needed. (See Chapter 21 page 238.)

Prevention

Tell the patient, family and village about the life cycle of the worm and that prevention is by the use of proper toilets by everyone (including children) always. Wearing proper shoes to stop larvae going through the skin is important but for some populations, not practicable.

Threadworm (*Enterobius vermicularis*)

Threadworm infestation is very common, especially in children.

Adult worms are up to 1 cm in length. They live in the large intestine and cause no pathology.

The fertilised female comes through the anus at night, and lays eggs on the skin around the anus. This causes itching and scratching.

The eggs are taken by fingers or clothes from the skin around the anus to the mouth and are swallowed. Then they pass into the intestine where they hatch and grow into adults.

Management of the patient includes:

1. Treat the *whole family* with an anti-threadworm drug.
2. Cut the fingernails short and keep them short.
3. Wash the whole body every morning.
4. Wash clothes and bedclothes often.
5. Apply ammoniated mercury ointment to the anus every night (while taking the anti-threadworm drug).
6. Wash hands well after using the toilet.

Drugs for treatment: see page 278.

- albendazole 10–40 mg/kg to a maximum dose of 400 mg once only,
- mebendazole 100 mg once only, and
- pyrantel (pamoate) 10 mg/kg to a maximum dose of 1 g once only.

Note that albendazole and mebendazole should not be given to a pregnant woman or 7 days after the last normal menstrual period or to children less than 2 years of age, and pyrantel should not be given in the first 3 months of pregnancy. These drugs may have to be repeated in 6 weeks, as well as all the other treatment carried out, to get rid of the infection in the family.

Whipworm (*Trichuris trichiura*)

The whipworm is 2.5 cm long with a thin front half and lives in the mucosa of the large intestine of humans and pigs.

Whipworm may cause gastrointestinal symptoms and signs, but only if they are present in large numbers, and even then, usually only in children. These include diarrhoea with blood, prolapse of the rectum and anaemia.

Treatment is needed only if there are symptoms and signs and is carried out with mebendazole 100 mg twice daily for 3 days, although for adults 500 mg once is just as effective, or albendazole in a single dose of 400 mg. Do not give if the patient is pregnant or more than 7 days after the last normal menstrual period or the child is less than 2 years old. See page 278.

Strongyloides

Strongyloides is a very small worm which lives in the upper small intestine but can spread through the whole gastrointestinal tract, and also sometimes through it to other parts of the body.

Strongyloides has a life cycle similar to roundworm and hookworm; but as well can also reproduce inside the body (usually bowel and lung) and also in the soil without having to pass through man.

Symptoms are not usually caused but there may be abdominal discomfort, diarrhoea, failure to absorb food, allergic type skin rashes and another unusual rash with an inflamed line in the skin which disappears after a few hours.

However, if a patient has damage to their immune system caused by (1) drugs given for cancer or adrenocorticosteroid drugs (such as cortisone and prednisolone) or (2) severe malnutrition and now also (3) HIV infection, then worms may spread through the bowel through the whole body causing severe generalised symptoms, severe diarrhoea and bowel obstruction (paralytic ileus), pneumonia, empyema, meningitis, septicaemia, etc. These are caused by the spread and growth of both the worm and the bacteria (usually from the bowel) that are in the worm.

Treatment is not usually given unless there are some symptoms; but it is given if worms are in the bowel, before adrenocorticosteroid-like drugs or anti-cancer drugs are given. Albendazole 400 mg once daily (or thiabendazole if not pregnant 25 mg/kg up to 1.5 g twice daily) for 3 days – is the usual treatment. Ivermectin in a single dose of 200 micrograms/kg is very effective.

Prevention is by all people, including children, always using proper toilets and by washing hands after going to the toilet.

Tapeworm and cysticercosis

Two large tapeworms, the beef tapeworm (*Taenia saginata*) and the pork tapeworm (*Taenia solium*), and a number of very small tapeworms affect man.

The adult *Taenia* live in the gastrointestinal tract of man.

They can become metres long, but the adult worms do little harm. The patient usually diagnoses the condition when a part of the worm forces itself out of the anus or he sees part of the worm wriggling in the stool. You can see eggs if the stool is examined under the microscope.

If the eggs in the stool are not passed into a proper toilet, the eggs may be swallowed by beef cattle or pigs. The larvae travel all through the animal but most go into the muscles. When the animal is killed you can see the larvae as little white marks in the meat. If the meat is not properly cooked (and the larvae not killed) before it is eaten, then the larvae develop into an adult worm in the intestine. (See Figure 23.7.)

The big danger to man from tapeworms is from the pork tapeworm, if the pork tapeworm eggs get into the upper gastrointestinal tract. This occurs (1) if a person gets some of his own faeces on to his food or into his mouth, or (2) if a person gets some else's faeces containing the eggs on uncooked vegetables etc. or (3) during vomiting when the contents of the small intestine return to the stomach (Figure 23.8). If the eggs of a pork tapeworm get into the upper gastrointestinal tract of man, then the larvae develop and travel all through the body (just as they do in pigs). The larvae cause painful muscles, fever and later muscle lumps. More importantly the larvae can also go to the brain. If very many go to the brain, then a meningoencephalitis (see Chapter 25 page 327) develops, often with epilepsy. If only a few go to the brain, then there is often little trouble for some years. But, when the worm dies, the cyst it formed starts to swell. This causes symptoms and signs like a brain abscess or a brain tumour, with epilepsy or headaches or psychosis etc. (see Chapter 25 page 332). This condition, where pork tapeworms cause cysts in the muscle and brain, is called 'cysticercosis'.

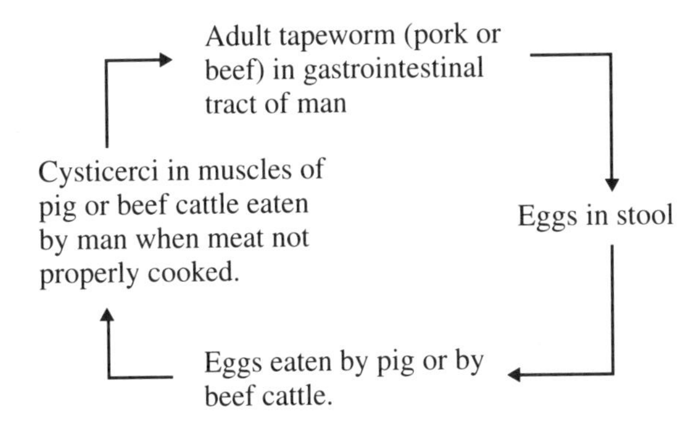

Figure 23.7 The normal life cycle of the pork and beef tapeworm.

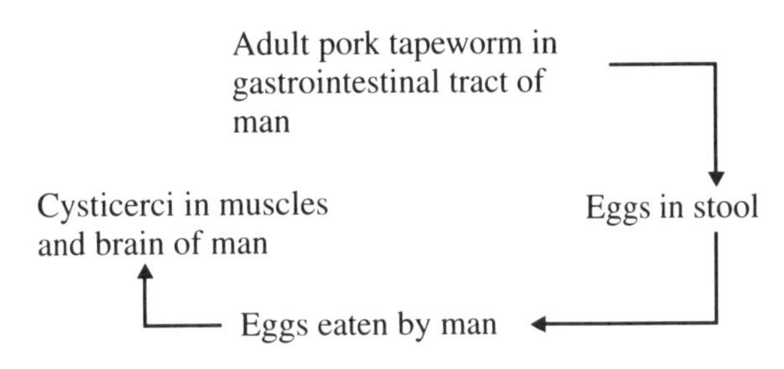

Figure 23.8 How the pork tapeworm causes cysticerci in man. The beef tapeworm cannot cause cysticerci in man.

You can diagnose the type of tapeworm infection a person has by examining the worm. But if the worm is a pig tapeworm, the worm and stools are dangerous to the patient and others. In the health centre *treat all cases immediately* as if the worm is a pork tapeworm, as follows.

Stop food and give clear fluids only until the worm is passed.

Give an anti-vomiting drug. e.g. chlorpromazine 25–50 mg or promethazine 25–50 mg.

After 2 hours, give niclosamide 1 g and 1 hour later another 1 g (or 2 g in a single dose) for an adult. One hour later give a laxative, e.g. 30 g of magnesium sulphate (Epsom salts) (30 ml in a measuring glass dissolved in warm water).

If the old treatment of mepacrine 1 g for an adult is used, this drug does not kill but only paralyses the worm. It is necessary then to collect all the stools and make sure the whole worm, *including the head*, which is as small as a pin head, has been passed. If the head is not passed, repeat the treatment.

Make sure no stools from the patient get on anyone at any time and all go into a safe toilet.

Check the stool test for ova 3 months later to see that the worm is not present.

Praziquantel or albendazole in one dose can be used instead of niclosamide for treatment of the worm. These drugs in repeated doses can also be used in the treatment of human cysticercosis. However they must not be given in a health centre as the dying cysticerci may swell and may make the patient worse at first, and special drugs and even surgery on the brain may be needed.

Prevention of tapeworm infection includes:

1. Kill the parasite in the original host. Treat all patients.
2. Stop the spread:
   (a) All people must use a proper toilet at all times.

(b) All meat must be properly inspected for cysticerci, and not sold if cysticerci are seen.
(c) All meat must be properly cooked. All the red colour of all the way through the meat must go before the meat is eaten.

Hydatid disease

Echinococcus granulosus is a very small tapeworm of dogs. When the dog passes faeces on to grass, these break down but the eggs are left on the grass and may be eaten by sheep or cattle. The eggs hatch in the animal's bowel and an infective organism gets carried in the portal vein to the liver but sometimes through the liver to the lung and occasionally to the brain, bone or other places. It grows in these places to a large fluid-filled cyst, sometimes many centimetres in diameter, with organisms infective to dogs on the inside of the cyst. If a dog eats these infective organisms with the rest of the organ, when the animal is killed for meat or dies, then these organisms form into the small tape worms in the dog's bowel.

Man can be infected instead of sheep or cattle if he gets eggs from dogs' faeces in his mouth. Cysts in the liver, lung, brain, bone or elsewhere can then develop in that person. Children who spend a lot of time with dogs and sheep and on grass are infected most.

The cysts can cause the following:

- painful enlargement of the liver, if in the liver;
- cough and shortness of breath, if in the lung;
- symptoms like a brain tumour, if in the brain;
- pain and fracture of bone, if in a bone;
- allergic reactions if fluid from the cyst gets into the circulation – these reactions can range from just urticaria to allergic type shock;
- sudden death if the cyst ruptures and a severe allergic reaction develops;
- typical X-ray changes, eosinophils in the blood and positive serology tests for circulating hydatid antigen if these tests are possible.

If you suspect the patient has a hydatid cyst because it occurs in your area and the patient has suspicious symptoms and signs, do not try to aspirate the cyst (as this may cause death from an allergic reaction or spread the infected material to other parts of the body where new cysts will form) but transfer the patient to a Medical Officer for investigations and if necessary treatment with albendazole and cutting out the cyst without letting it burst.

Prevention is by not allowing dogs to eat animal offal (liver, lung, etc.) from animals killed for meat or which die. If possible, dogs should be de-wormed regularly and all people should wash their hands after touching dogs.

Visceral larva migrans

Visceral larva migrans cannot be diagnosed in the health centre but you may hear of patients with it. This occurs when the eggs or ova of roundworms of dogs or cats (*Toxocara canis* or *T. cati*) are swallowed by people. The worms (larvae) are not able to develop into adults in the bowel as they are not in dogs or cats. The larvae wander (migrate) around in the organs (viscera) of the person. This causes fever, enlarged and tender organs such as the liver, more eosinophils and gamma globulin in the blood than normal, etc. Treatment is with thiabendazole.

Gastroenteritis (or acute diarrhoeal disease) (see Table 23.2 page 289)

Definition

Gastroenteritis is a very common and sometimes serious or fatal syndrome. (It is not a specific disease with only one cause; there are many causes.)

Gastroenteritis is diagnosed when there is:

1. diarrhoea, and
2. abdominal pain of bowel (intestinal) colic type (usually), and
3. vomiting (usually), and
4. other symptoms and signs such as fever (in some but not all).

Causes

Causes of gastroenteritis include:

1. '*Food poisoning*'
    - Poisonous foods, especially certain fish and certain plants.
    - Poisons or chemicals in food (including large volumes of alcohol).
    - Drugs including antibiotics given for infections.
    - Toxins in food made by organisms which have grown in the food but may be dead or cannot cause infections in the intestine (e.g. streptococci and staphylococci).
    - Organisms in food which can cause infections in the bowel (see below).

2. *Infections in the intestine*
   - Viruses (especially rota virus).
   - Unusual types of normal intestinal bacteria (e.g. *Escherichia coli*).
   - Special bacteria, such as:
   - *Shigella* (bacillary dysentery organisms).
   - Salmonellae which cause gastroenteritis.
   - Salmonellae which cause typhoid fever.
   - Clostridia which cause enteritis necroticans ('pigbel').
   - *Campylobacter* which cause dysentery.
   - Cholera organisms.
   - Amoebae (amoebic dysentery organisms).
   - *Giardia.*
   - *Schistosoma mansoni* and *Schistosoma japonicum.*
   - Sometimes other worms.
3. *'Medical causes'*
   - Any cause of fever, but especially malaria.
   - Any acute infections, but especially middle ear infections, pneumonia, and urinary tract infections.
   - Many chronic infections, especially visceral leishmaniasis.
   - Malnutrition.
   - Malabsorption, especially lactose intolerance and tropical sprue.
   - Change of diet.
   - Anxiety.
4. *'Surgical' causes*
   - Enteritis necroticans ('pigbel').
   - Intestine obstruction – early or incomplete.

Usually you cannot find the cause of gastroenteritis at a health centre, unless there is a medical or surgical cause. But you must always look for evidence of the cause. (Details of some of the causes are found above.)

You must also ask if other people are affected, because this is the only way to diagnose 'food poisoning' in a health centre. You may need to control an epidemic.

Epidemiology

The *spread* of gastrointestinal infections is usually:

- *From* the faeces (occasionally vomit) of an infected case or carrier.
- *To* the mouth of a susceptible person.
- *By* direct contact (personal contact) *or* vehicles (food or milk or water) into which organisms from faeces were introduced (put) by fingers or flies, or directly from improper or dirty toilets. See Figure 23.9.

Symptoms

Symptoms include:

1. Diarrhoea (frequent watery stool), dysentery (diarrhoea with blood and pus as well) if the intestine wall is ulcerated
2. Abdominal pain
   Pain due to gastroenteritis is bowel colic, i.e. it comes for some seconds and then goes away for some minutes. The pain is usually in the centre of the abdomen, but large intestinal colic can be at the side low down.
   Constant abdominal pain is NOT usually caused by gastroenteritis
   Cramps in the abdominal and limb muscles if the patient has severe diarrhoea suggest cholera.
3. Vomiting
   This is not always present; but it can be frequent.
   You must find out how often vomiting is occurring and how much fluid is being lost in the vomit each time.
   This helps you to know if dehydration will occur.
   Vomiting is dangerous, because it stops fluid from entering the body, and means dehydration will occur much more quickly and be more serious than if the patient can drink and absorb fluids.
4. Symptoms of infection in the gastrointestinal tract or elsewhere or of an underlying disease, may or may not be present.

History

Ask if the patient has eaten possibly poisonous food, 'bad' foods, pig meat or other high protein food when this is not usually in the diet, food that was cooked a long time before it was eaten; or if he has taken drugs, etc.

Family and contact history

Ask about contacts with similar disease.

> You can usually only diagnose 'food poisoning' at a health centre if a group of people develop gastroenteritis together.
> Always ask if other people are affected. You may need to control an epidemic. Think of cholera if there is an epidemic in which there are some cases of very rapid dehydration and death.

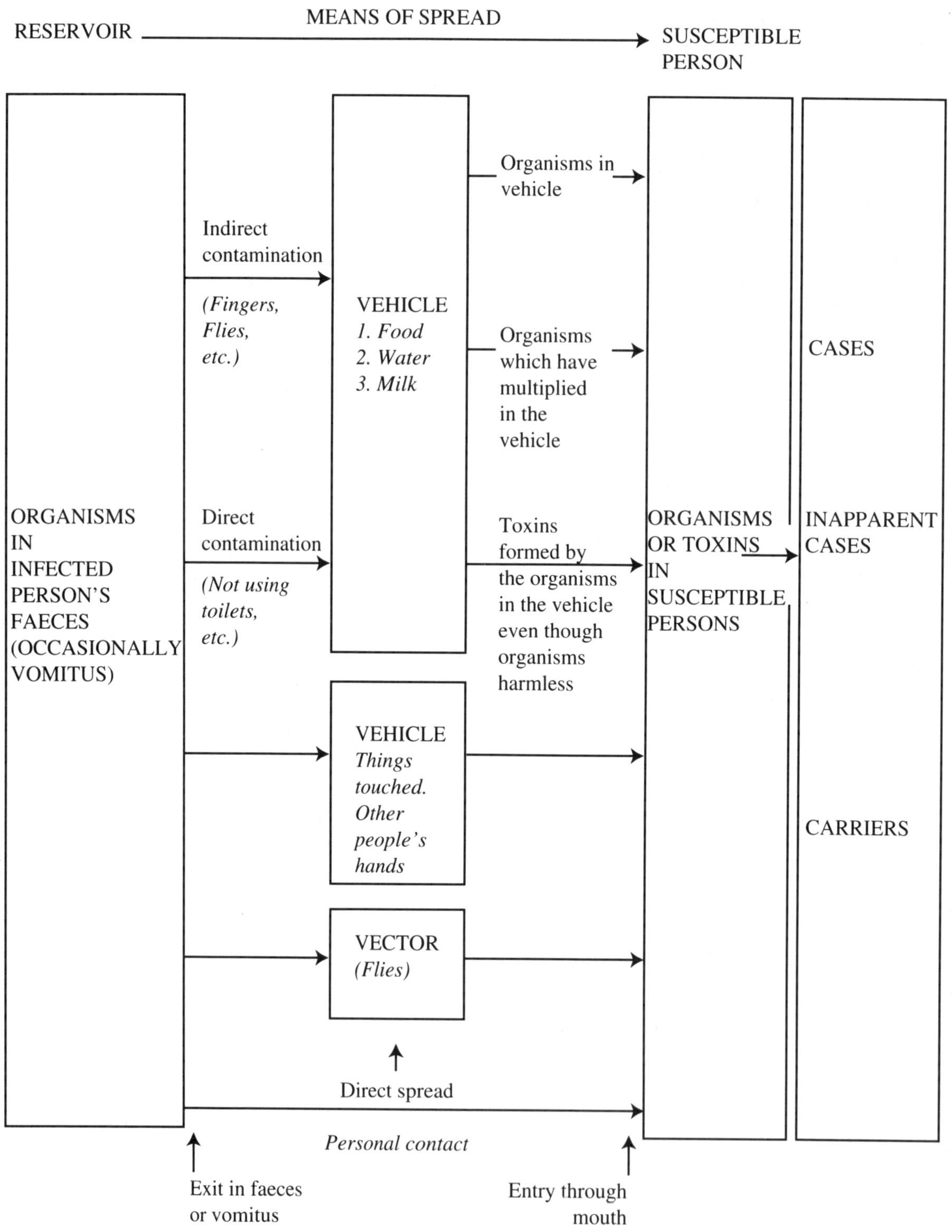

RESERVOIR — MEANS OF SPREAD → SUSCEPTIBLE PERSON

ORGANISMS IN INFECTED PERSON'S FAECES (OCCASIONALLY VOMITUS)

Indirect contamination →
(Fingers, Flies, etc.)

Direct contamination →
(Not using toilets, etc.)

VEHICLE
1. Food
2. Water
3. Milk

Organisms in vehicle →

Organisms which have multiplied in the vehicle →

Toxins formed by the organisms in the vehicle even though organisms harmless →

VEHICLE
Things touched. Other people's hands

VECTOR
(Flies)

Direct spread

Personal contact

Exit in faeces or vomitus

Entry through mouth

ORGANISMS OR TOXINS IN SUSCEPTIBLE PERSONS →

CASES

INAPPARENT CASES

CARRIERS

Figure 23.9 The epidemiology of most cases of gastroenteritis.

Signs

1. *Signs of dehydration* (these develop if a large volume of fluid is lost and not replaced quickly enough):
   - the number of times the patient has had vomiting and diarrhoea and the volume of the vomitus and stool – each time you check a patient ask about these during the last 6 and the last 24 hours,
   - urine volume small and urine of dark colour (concentrated urine),
   - rapid loss of weight,
   - loss of full consciousness,
   - decreased elasticity of skin, especially the skin of the neck (but do not mistake the inelastic skin of old age or of malnutrition or wasting for the inelastic skin of dehydration),
   - sunken fontanelle (children only),
   - sunken eyes,
   - dry mouth,
   - fast pulse,
   - low blood pressure,
   - cyanosis,
   - fever.

> PR, BP, skin elasticity and urine volume and colour are the best signs of dehydration in adults.

2. *Signs of gastroenteritis*:
   The abdomen
   - is normal in shape and moves normally on respiration;
   - has no marked tenderness and definitely no guarding or rigidity;
   - has increased intestinal sounds (which can be heard at the same time as the patient gets pain).
3. *Signs of cause of gastroenteritis*:
   You must look for all medical causes, especially malaria, other infections and malnutrition.
   You must look for all surgical causes, especially the signs of intestinal obstruction and peritonitis.

Complications

Look for these especially in the old, children, those with malnutrition, and certain virulent infections.

Complications include:

- dehydration which can cause shock and death – *dehydration is the usual cause of death*;
- dysentery, with the loss of large amount of blood, causing anaemia or shock;
- septicaemia which can cause infections in other organs or shock or death;
- paralytic ileus – because of loss of potassium the intestinal muscles become paralysed; this causes vomiting, abdominal distension, constipation but not colic;
- continuing diarrhoea, because of lactose intolerance caused by the gastroenteritis but milk with lactose in it is still in the diet;
- malnutrition;
- anaemia.

Diagnostic features

Diagnostic features are:

- diarrhoea or dysentery,
- colicky (not constant) pain, usually in the centre of the abdomen,
- vomiting (not always),
- no significant signs in the abdomen except increased intestinal sounds,
- sometimes an underlying cause not in the gastrointestinal tract,
- dehydration (if vomiting or if diarrhoea is often or is of large volumes or goes on for a long time).

See Table 23.2 about differential diagnosis; but these things do not need to be known to treat the patient correctly.

> Treatment includes four things:
> 1. Treat dehydration by oral fluids *or* by IV then oral fluids (page 286)
> 2. Treat any underlying surgical or medical disease **(page 286)**
>   Always give antimalarial drugs.
> 3. If necessary treat any infection in the intestine (page 287)
>   Most cases do NOT need chloramphenicol or metronidazole.
> 4. Treat symptoms; but only if necessary and only after you have done the other three things (page 287).

Treatment

In *all cases*, look carefully for dehydration:

- fast pulse (if severe),
- blood pressure low (if severe),

- inelastic skin,
- sunken eyes,
- dry mouth, and
- urine volume small and colour dark.

Mild case, with no or mild dehydration:

- treat as an outpatient;
- tell the patient to return if he does not improve and especially if vomiting is repeated.
  Severe case, with definite signs of dehydration:
- treat as an inpatient.

Treat dehydration
Oral rehydration. If

- there is no clinical dehydration, *or*
- only mild clinical dehydration, *or*
- moderate clinical dehydration but the vomiting is not repeated, *and*
- the abdomen is not distended (swollen),
  then give oral rehydration fluid (see page 287).

Give the patient 2–4 large cups (400–800 ml) of fluid to drink. Tell the patient to drink it immediately if he has no nausea or vomiting. Tell the patient to sip it slowly over the next hour if he has nausea or vomiting.

If the patient has moderate dehydration, he must continue to drink till the signs of dehydration are gone (100 ml/kg or 3–6 litres). The patient can do this as quickly as he can if he has no nausea or vomiting. He should do it slowly over 6 hours (i.e. sip 2–4 cups during each hour for 6 hours) if he has nausea or some vomiting.

When the patient has no (or only mild) clinical signs of dehydration and does not vomit (or only vomits a little), the patient can then go home. Tell the patient to drink at least 2–4 cups of fluid in every 3-hour period (i.e. 3–6 litres/day) until the diarrhoea and/or vomiting stops.

If most of the oral fluids are refused or vomited or they are not effective, or abdominal distension (swelling) develops or there is severe dehydration, *then* admit for IV fluids.

Intravenous rehydration. If

- there is shock, *or*
- severe dehydration, *or*
- repeated vomiting, *or*
- abdominal distension (swelling), *or*
- the patient does not improve after oral fluids, *or*
- oral fluids are vomited or refused,

then give IV rehydration. The method for IV rehydration is as follows:

1. *Give 0.9% sodium chloride solution*[1] 'fast'
   Give 40 ml/kg (2 litres) as fast as possible (e.g. in 1 hour).
2. *Review the hydration of the patient after (1).*
   - If he has improved, start (3).
   - If he is still shocked or very dehydrated, give another 40 ml/kg (2 litres) 0.9% sodium chloride solution[1] as fast as possible. Then review the hydration of the patient again.
   - If he still has shock, see Chapter 27 page 378.
   - If he has improved, start (3).
3. *Give 0.9% sodium chloride solution*[1] more slowly to complete rehydration in 6 hours.
   - Give 60 ml/kg (3 litres) over the next 4–5 hours.
   - When the signs of dehydration have gone, start (4).
4. *Give 0.18% sodium chloride in 4.3% dextrose solution.*
   Give 1 litre every 6 hours.
5. *Start oral rehydration solution.*
   When you have done (1) to (4) and the patient has stopped vomiting start oral rehydration fluids 400–800 ml every 3 hours.
6. *Stop IV fluids.* When the patient can take enough oral fluids (400–800 ml every 3 hours) to maintain hydration stop IV fluids.

> If the patient has cholera, if available use Hartmann's solution (see page 291 and a reference book for details).

Treat any underlying medical or surgical disease

- Antimalarial drugs must *always* be given, unless you are certain that the patient does not have malaria.
- Give at least the first dose by injection.
- See malaria (Chapter 13 page 61).

1 Hartmann's solution (lactated Ringer's solution) is better than 0.9% sodium chloride solution; but it is not usually available. But 0.9% sodium chloride solution is not good for cholera. If the patient has cholera you must try to get Hartmann's solution or another special IV fluid for cholera.

If necessary treat any infection of the intestine
If the patient has

- severe dehydration with shock, *or*
- severe toxaemia which continues after correction of dehydration and injection of antimalarials (i.e. after 6 hours), *or*
- fever of unknown cause for more than 2 days, *or*
- new red spots appearing on the skin of the trunk, *or*
- spleen getting larger, *or*
- more than mild abdominal tenderness, *or*
- severe dysentery (blood and/or pus in the stools which does not improve after a few days or returns),

then give chloramphenicol 25 mg/kg every 6 hours *either*

- 1 g (1 bottle) every 6 hours for 14 days by
  - IVI if there is shock *or* by
  - IVI or IMI if there is vomiting, or severe diarrhoea, or the patient is very sick, *or*
- 1 g (4 caps) every 6 hours orally if there is no shock, no vomiting and diarrhoea not severe and the patient is not very sick for 14 days.

Note that **most** cases do **not** need chloramphenicol

If:

- dysentery does not get better during the course of chloramphenicol, *or*
- dysentery returns after the course of chloramphenicol, *or*
- dysentery has occurred a number of times before the present attack, *or*
- dysentery has been present for 5–7 days already, *or*
- diarrhoea does not stop after 2 weeks,

then give metronidazole 800 mg t.i.d. for 5 days (possible amoebic or giardia infection).

If there is another infection or infestation especially schistosomiasis (see Chapter 18 page 154) shown by tests then give the necessary treatment.

Treat symptoms if necessary
Treat symptoms only after you have done rehydration, given antimalarial injection and excluded surgical conditions especially peritonitis and intestinal obstruction.

1. If there is severe colic, cease oral food and fluids, and give IV fluids only.
2. If there is severe abdominal colic or severe diarrhoea (and also vomiting), you can give morphine 10 mg (1 ml) and atropine 0.6 mg ($\frac{3}{5}$ mg) (1 ml) IMI once.
3. If there is abdominal colic or diarrhoea (but no vomiting), give codeine phosphate 30 mg (1 tab) every 4–6 hours if necessary.
4. If there is repeated vomiting, give chlorpromazine 0.5 mg/kg ($\frac{1}{2}$ mg/kg) but not more than 25 mg (1 ml) IMI every 6 hours if necessary. Do not give more than two doses. Look instead for the cause of the repeated vomiting.

Transfer these cases to Medical Officer care

1. If a surgical condition is possible – peritonitis, enteritis necroticans ('pigbel'), intestinal obstruction, etc. (urgent).
2. If vomiting continues for more than 2 days after you give IV fluids and IV or IM treatment and stop oral food, drugs and fluids (urgent).
3. If abdominal distension develops especially if there is also constipation and repeated vomiting (paralytic ileus) (urgent).
4. Diarrhoea which does not improve after the proper treatment (non-urgent).
5. Dysentery which does not stop after treatment with chloramphenicol and then metronidazole (non-urgent).

Oral rehydration solution

1. Oral Rehydration Salts (for a glucose/electrolyte solution): 1 packet dissolved in water (boiled, if possible) in the volume as directed on the pocket.
   Use a special bottle from the Medical Store, if available.
   Throw away any you have not used after 24 hours. Wash the bottle carefully, and if possible sterilise it, before using it again.

   or

2. 1 pinch of salt (only what you can hold between *one* finger and the thumb) and
   1 teaspoon sugar and

1 cup clean water (boiled, if possible) or tea
and
a little lemon juice (if possible)

or

3. Sodium chloride (common salt) 3.5 g
   Sodium bicarbonate 2.5 g
   Potassium chloride (each tablet of potassium chloride is 0.5 g) 1.5 g
   Glucose 20 g
   Clean water (boiled, if possible) 1 litre

or

4. Coconut water

Control and prevention

Control and prevention includes giving health education about hygiene, food handling, water supply and toilets to the patient, his family and his village.

It is important to recognise any epidemic of gastroenteritis. An epidemic is usually caused by a common source of the disease. This is usually food or water. You must discover the cause of any epidemic so that you can stop it.

You must think of cholera if there is an epidemic of very rapid dehydration and early deaths. Special treatment and control methods are necessary (see this page).

Methods of control and prevention of gastroenteritis caused by infections include:

1. Kill the organism in the body of the original host or reservoir (e.g. treat infected persons with antibiotics).
   You cannot usually do this. If you treat all cases and carriers with antibiotics, then soon many of the organisms become resistant to the antibiotics.
2. Stop the spread of the organism.
   Cases and carriers
   - do not allow them to handle food,
   - they must wash their hands after using the toilet.

   Proper disposal of faeces
   - proper toilets so that faeces do not contaminate water,
   - proper toilets so flies, etc. cannot walk on faeces and later walk on food.

   Provide a large supply of safe water.
   Cook food properly. Keep food covered and cool after cooking; but it is best to eat it immediately.
3. Raise the resistance of susceptible persons.
   Improve nutrition and health.
   - People with good nutrition usually have mild attacks.
   - People with malnutrition often have severe attacks.

   Immunisation against cholera and typhoid are available; but these immunisations are not very effective.
4. Prophylactic treatment.
   Do not give prophylaxis, except to special groups of people in a cholera epidemic.

For details of descriptions of special kinds of gastroenteritis, see pages 282–7 and a reference book.

Cholera

Definition and cause

Cholera is an acute illness caused by the cholera bacterium *Vibrio cholerae*. There are a number of different types of this bacterium, including the El Tor type. If the organism grows in the small intestine, it can cause severe diarrhoea and vomiting, with rapid dehydration and often shock and death.

Frequency

Cholera is endemic in India and Pakistan in the Ganges basin but has now spread to many other parts of the world where sanitation, water supplies and personal hygiene are poor, especially at the time of war or disaster.

Epidemiology

Man is the only host. The reservoir includes cases, inapparent cases and carriers. The cholera organism is passed from the gastrointestinal tract in the faeces or in the vomit. The organism then spreads to the mouths of other people. The usual way this happens is when the faeces or vomit contaminate drinking water. Contamination of food by contaminated water, hands and flies, can also occur. Direct spread from person to person can occur; but is not common.

All people are susceptible if there is an epidemic in a new area. But many infected people do not develop the clinical disease. And many people who do develop clinical disease have only mild disease. In endemic areas, most of the clinical cases are children.

A person can be a carrier for months.

Immunity after an attack only lasts for a short time.

The disease occurs mostly in countries where there is poor sanitation and the water supplies are not safe.

Table 23.2 The causes of gastroenteritis/diarrhoea/dysentery according to the length of time these symptoms present and whether blood is in the stools (dysentery) or not. However the cause of gastroenteritis does not need to be known for proper treatment to be carried out in the health centre (see text).

Diarrhoea/Dysentery/Gastroenteritis – acute (less than 2 weeks)				*Diarrhoea/dysentery – chronic (greater than 2 weeks)*
Fever & dysentery (often vomiting)	*Fever and no dysentery (often vomiting)*	*No fever Dysentery*	*No fever No dysentery (often vomiting)*	
Bacillary (*Shigella*) *Campylobacter* *Salmonella* *Escherichia coli* Visceral leishmaniasis	Malaria Any infection – especially upper respiratory tract infection; lower respiratory tract infection and urinary tract infection *Salmonella* *Shigella* *Campylobacter*	Amoebic (*Entamoeba histolytica*) *Balantidium coli* Schistosomiasis *Trichuris* and other GI worms Antibiotic caused (*Clostridium difficile*)	Poisonous foods Preformed toxins, e.g. Staphylococci *Clostridium perfringens* *Escherichia coli* Viral, e.g. rota virus Cholera Incomplete bowel obstruction	*Giardia lamblia* Amoebic (*Entamoeba histolytica*) GI roundworms Schistosomiasis Other systemic illnesses HIV infection Visceral leishmaniasis Diasaccharidase deficiency Post-infective malabsorption 'Tropical sprue' Bowel cancer

Pathology

There are no pathological changes in the structure of the gastrointestinal tract. The organism does not get into the blood or other parts of the body. The toxin from the cholera organism makes the gastrointestinal tract secrete very large volumes of salt and water. These are then lost by continuous vomiting and diarrhoea. This causes rapid dehydration (within hours), shock and death. If the lost salt and water is replaced quickly enough in the right quantity, the patient will get better.

Symptoms

If cholera comes to an area where it is not endemic, the first thing you will notice is a *group* of people with gastroenteritis. Some of the people will develop significant symptoms.

At first all of the normal faeces in the bowel are quickly passed. Then large amounts of watery stool are passed repeatedly, or almost continuously. Several litres may be passed in the first few hours. The stools often look like the water in which rice has been boiled; but sometimes they are different.

There is usually little abdominal pain or colic.

Vomiting usually occurs after the diarrhoea, but sometimes occurs first. There is little nausea. Large volumes of fluid are vomited.

Cramps in the muscles of the abdomen (and other areas) can cause severe pain.

Signs

When you see a patient with these symptoms, he is usually severely dehydrated, shocked and cyanosed and often unable to speak.

Signs may include:

1. The patient is conscious, but very weak.
2. The temperature is not raised; it may be lower than normal.
3. The pulse is very fast and weak; or you cannot feel it.

4. The BP is very low; or you cannot record it.
5. The respiration rate is fast.
6. The weight is decreased.
7. Severe signs of dehydration are present with wrinkled skin with no elasticity sunken eyes and cheeks, etc.
8. There is cyanosis.
9. The abdomen
   - is sunken,
   - is not tender, guarded or rigid,
   - has bowel sounds which are loud,
   - is usually soft; but sometimes there is spasm of all of the muscles of the body which may seem like guarding of the abdomen.
10. Spasm (tightening) of muscles, with cramps in the hands and feet and the calves of legs is quite common.
11. No urine is passed.

Course and complications

The disease has a course of 2–7 days.

Without treatment, over 50% of severely affected cases will die. Death can occur within a few hours.

With proper treatment, less than 1% will die.

After proper rehydration, vomiting usually stops.

Diarrhoea may not stop for 2–6 days. Usually 4–6 litres of fluid treatment over 1–2 days are needed (occasionally 60 litres over 6 days).

Miscarriage is common if the patient is pregnant.

Affected children may not be fully conscious, fits may occur and the temperature may be raised.

Without antibiotic treatment, many patients become carriers for some days or weeks or months.

Many mild cases and many unnoticed cases occur for every severe case.

Tests

There is no test for the disease that you can do at the health centre.

If you suspect cholera, you must take specimens to send to the laboratory urgently (stools, rectal swabs and vomitus), to confirm the diagnosis. If antibiotics are given before the laboratory tests are collected, the chance of a positive culture is less; so you must collect at least one specimen before you start the antibiotic treatment.

Collect faeces in a sterile pan which is free from disinfectant or antiseptic. Avoid contamination with urine if possible. Use a sterile wooden spatula or a spoon to put 10–15 ml of faeces (two or three spoonfuls), containing blood and mucus, if present, into a sterile screw-topped glass or plastic container and send this to the laboratory. Put the spoon into antiseptic. When the patient is incontinent, put a sterile, stiff-walled, 1.5-cm wide, 15-cm long, rubber or plastic tube, which is cut at an angle at the end and well lubricated, into the rectum (with the lubricated angled end in the rectum) and drain the faeces into a sterile container. If you take swabs, take them from the rectum, not only the anus.

Send the specimen to the laboratory *immediately*. If the laboratory is not close to the place of collection, send for a suitable transport medium such as alkaline peptone water. Put 1–3 grams of faeces ($\frac{1}{2}$ spoonful) into 10 ml of the medium in a screw topped bottle and mix it thoroughly.

Send a letter with the specimen which gives all the details of the specimen, full clinical notes, and a request for examination for cholera organisms. If you could not collect a specimen before you gave antibiotics, then the request form must give the name of the antibiotic, the dosage and how long the patient has been having it.

You must also make a request for a microscopic examination and culture of the specimen for all other organisms which could cause a similar disease.

Differential diagnosis

This is the same as for gastroenteritis (see page 282 and Table 23.2.).

Diagnostic features

Suspect cholera if:

1. A single patient who has returned from a cholera area within the last week develops gastroenteritis of *any* type; but especially if they have the typical signs and symptoms. *or*
2. There is an epidemic of gastroenteritis with some cases with the typical signs and symptoms especially if some die.

Treatment

Treatment includes three things:

1. Treat and prevent dehydration and shock.
   - Correct the dehydration and loss of salts.
   - Replace continuing loss of water and salts.
   - Give maintenance fluids.
2. Treat the infection in the intestine.
3. Treat symptoms if necessary, and give good nursing care.

Treat and prevent dehydration and shock
First you should correct the dehydration (loss of water and salts).

For severe dehydration use IV Hartmann's solution (also called lactated Ringer's solution).

For moderate or mild dehydration, use Oral Rehydration Solution (see page 287).

Table 23.3 Treatment of dehydration. For severe dehydration use IV Hartmann's solution. For moderate or mild dehydration use oral rehydration solution.

Dehydration	*Route*	*Adult*	*Child*
Severe	IV	40 ml/kg *very fast* Then 60 ml/kg *over 2 hours*	40 ml/kg *very fast* Then 60 ml/kg *over 4 hours*
Moderate	Oral	25 ml/kg/hour *for 4 hours*	25 ml/kg/hour *for 4 hours*
Mild	Oral	15 ml/kg/hour *for 4 hours*	15 ml/kg/hour *for 4 hours*

Note about children. Hartmann's solution does not contain enough potassium or sugar or water for children. As soon as they can drink at all, give children as much Oral Rehydration Solution (see page 287, but not just salt and glucose and water) as they can drink *and* the IV Hartmann's solution.

Note: If you have no Hartmann's solution – use WHO IV diarrhoea treatment solution or dextrose 2.5% in half strength Darrow's solution; or if you do not have these, use 0.9% sodium chloride. If you do not have Hartmann's solution start Oral Rehydration Solution (see page 287 but not just salt, glucose and water) as soon as possible, as the other IV fluids do not contain everything the patient needs. This is especially important if you give 0.9% sodium chloride.

The best signs to use to judge hydration are:

- pulse volume and rate,
- blood pressure,
- skin elasticity,
- normal fullness of neck and veins,
- loss of cramps, nausea and vomiting,
- weight increased,
- urine passed, and
- loss of thirst.

After 2–4 hours of intravenous hydration the patient will become alert and look well. Vomiting will stop and he will start to pass urine. But diarrhoea will continue for 1–3 days; but it should become less, and the stool less watery.

After correcting the dehydration you should *replace continuing loss of salt and water, and give maintenance fluids.*

Maintain the rehydrated state during the continuing diarrhoea by oral fluid.

Check the patient's hydration every 2 hours (see above). Keep a record of all the fluid you give (intravenous and oral). Also record the stool volume, appearance (clear, whitish, watery, yellow-watery, faecal) and frequency and how much urine is passed.

Give oral fluids every 4 hours. Give a volume of $1\frac{1}{2}$ times the stool volume passed over the previous 4 hours. Continue this until the diarrhoea stops. Give Oral Rehydration Solution (see page 287 but not just the salt and glucose and water), which is either drunk or else put down an intragastric tube. If the stool loss is not more than 500 ml per hour, further intravenous fluids are not necessary.

Only rarely will further IV fluid be necessary; but you may continue it at 10–20 ml/kg each hour for the 4 hours after rehydration if it is really necessary, while you start oral fluids.

If you do not have much intravenous fluid, you can use oral fluids immediately for most moderately or mildly dehydrated patients, and even in severely dehydrated patients immediately after they have been rehydrated intravenously. In most cases you can replace the continuing stool loss with an oral rehydration solution.

Treat the infection in the intestine with antibiotics
Give either tetracycline or chloramphenicol. Start the drug only when the patient has been rehydrated and is taking oral fluids, so that the antibiotic will not be vomited.

The dose of tetracycline for adults is 500 mg (2 caps) every 6 hours for 2 days.

Children under 10 kg are given chloramphenicol 125 mg ($\frac{1}{2}$ cap) (*do not use the suspension*) every 6 hours for 2 days.

Children weighing over 10 kg are given chloramphenicol 250 mg (1 cap) (*do not use the suspension*) every 6 hours for 2 days.

Antibiotics help to reduce the time and volume of diarrhoea, and the time the patient passes the bacteria.

Treat symptoms if necessary
This is not usually necessary. The above treatment will usually cure the symptoms.

- *Do not* give diuretics – rapid rehydration will make the patient pass urine.
- *Do not* give chlorpromazine for vomiting – rapid rehydration will stop the vomiting.
- *Do not* give morphine or analgesics for muscle cramps – rehydrate (and then if necessary give calcium gluconate 10% solution, 10 ml IV slowly).
- *Do not* use stimulants like adrenaline.
- *Do not* use adrenocorticosteroids.
- *Do not* use plasma volume expanders.
- *Do not* use oxygen to try to correct cyanosis.

These complications all improve with rapid IV rehydration.

Nurse patients on a bed with the mattress made of a waterproof sheet or mat with a 22 cm (or nine inch) hole in it. Place his buttocks over the hole, with a bucket under the hole. Measurement of stool volume is then easy.

The patient can start to eat when the vomiting stops.

1. In an epidemic, check that the patient has cholera and not another disease.
2. Repeated vomiting is usually caused by not enough of the right IV fluid.
3. Watch for overhydration and heart failure in children.

Control of epidemic

You must immediately find out how the disease started and how it has spread so that you can use the correct methods of control. The usual means of spread is water.

Kill the organism in the body of the original hosts and the reservoir.
Admit patients. Isolate patients. Start treatment with tetracycline (or chloramphenicol) when vomiting stops. This will make the patient non-infectious and stop him becoming a carrier.

Close contacts of patients (i.e. family and others who may have been infected by the same reservoir of infection (usually water)), may develop the disease or be mild cases or carriers. Treat them also with tetracycline (or chloramphenicol) for 2–3 days.

The usual reservoir is contaminated water. Chlorinate all water supplies and boil all water used for drinking, cooking, preparing food, washing dishes, etc.

Stop the means of spread.
Use all usual methods of stopping faecal-oral spread.

Disinfect the faeces and vomit and articles used by patients.

Staff must practise good hygiene, especially removing gowns before leaving the ward and washing hands after nursing patients and before eating or drinking. (No eating or drinking by staff is allowed in the ward.)

Check that everyone uses proper toilets.

Tell everyone to wash their hands after using the toilet.

Protect and chlorinate all water supplies.

Tell people to boil all water used for drinking or cooking or putting on food or washing dishes, etc.

Tell everyone about hygiene, cooking, handling, storing, serving and eating of food.

Try to reduce the number of flies, and keep flies away from all toilets and food.

Raise the resistance of susceptible persons
Do not try to immunise everyone with cholera vaccine, as mass immunisation is not usually helpful in an epidemic. It does not give good protection to most people and is slow acting. But, you may be told to give it. If so, give 0.5 ml ($\frac{1}{2}$ ml) of cholera vaccine immediately, and then 1 ml 7–28 days later by subcutaneous injection. New oral vaccines may soon be available and be effective.

Staff of health centres should be immunised because of their possible repeated exposure.

Prophylactic treatment
During an epidemic, staff at the health centre should take tetracycline 500 mg four times a day to kill any cholera organisms that enter their gastrointestinal tracts.

Prevention

Quarantine procedures are carried out at border posts, ports and airports to try to shop cholera entering a country.

Good sanitation and a plentiful supply of safe water and good general hygiene would stop any case which did enter a country causing an epidemic.

Immunisation may give some personal protection.

Notification

You should report all suspected cases of cholera *immediately* to the Health Officer, by telephone or radio or fast transport.

Cholera is one of the diseases subject to International Health Regulations. The Government will immediately report to the WHO and neighbouring countries if any case occurs.

Enteritis necroticans (pigbel)

Pigbel is common in the Highlands of Papua New Guinea if the diet is poor in protein and high in sweet potato, especially in children. Cases have also been reported from Uganda and Ghana and no doubt occur in other places.

The cause is a special type of special bacteria (*Clostridium*).

These organisms live in the intestines of animals or man or in the soil, and if they

1. contaminate food, and
2. are not all killed by proper cooking, and
3. are eaten,

then they

1. grow in any protein food in the intestine, and
2. produce a toxin in the intestine.

If the toxin (which is a protein) is not destroyed because there is

1. little of the digestive juice (trypsin) which digests protein (because of little protein normally in diet) and
2. sweet potato present in the intestine which stops what little protein digestive juice there is from working,

then the toxin attacks the bowel wall causing inflammation or even necrosis (death) of the bowel wall.

History

The history is of a person who:

- is usually a child from a known place for the disease, e.g. the Highlands of Papua New Guinea;
- usually does not have much protein in the diet;
- has eaten pig meat or other high protein food $\frac{1}{2}$–4 days before;
- then develops one of the four syndromes listed below.

Symptoms, signs, course and complications

1. As for gastroenteritis (see page 283) (diagnosis of pigbel is not made)

   or

2. • Severe upper abdominal pain which is constant, but there is also colic.
   - Vomiting; and vomitus soon becomes dark fluid (from blood) with flecks or spots in it (dead mucous membrane).
   - Blood in the stool sometimes with diarrhoea (this has often stopped by the time the patient has come to the Health Centre).
   - Raised temperature, fast pulse and dehydration.
   - Upper abdominal distension, with parts of the intestine visible.
   - Upper abdominal tenderness, often with guarding and rigidity.
   - You may feel intestinal masses.
   - Bowel sounds are decreased, though occasionally increased.
   - Death occurs in a few days if the patient does not get proper treatment.

   or

3. Soon after the start there is rapid development of severe general symptoms and signs of infection (septicaemia) and death.

   also

4. Patients who get better may have an incomplete intestinal obstruction or malnutrition, caused by a narrowing of the affected intestine.

Treatment

Treat as for acute gastroenteritis (see page 285) if there is no definite abdominal tenderness or distension.

Treat as for peritonitis if there are definite signs of 'pigbel' (nothing by mouth, IV fluids, IV penicillin (or chloramphenicol), IM pethidine) (see page 273).

Transfer

You should arrange transfer to *Medical Officer care* when:

1. The patient has a severe case: i.e. his abdomen is very swollen, and he has black flecked vomit and marked general symptoms and signs (urgent – emergency).
2. The patient has only a mild case (only some abdominal swelling, not toxic, no black flecked vomit), but does not improve after 2 days of treatment.

Control and prevention

1. Kill the organism in the reservoir.
   This is not possible.
2. Stop the means of transmission.
   Proper cooking of *all* foods to kill all organisms helps. It is difficult to make people do this.
3. Raise the resistance of susceptible persons.
   More protein in the diet and not eating sweet potato can increase the activity of the digestive juices from the pancreas. But it is also difficult to make people do this.
   People can be immunised against the disease. You should give immunisation if you work in a place where the disease is common, (e.g. in PNG in the Highlands). Give a dose of 0.5 ml of vaccine by IMI at the same time as each dose of DPT or triple antigen, (i.e. at 2 months of age, 2 months after the first dose and again 2 months after the second dose).

Amoebiasis

Amoebiasis is an infection with special amoebae (*Entamoeba histolytica*). These amoebae are protozoal organisms that usually live in the large intestine.

The amoebae in the large intestine make cysts, which are passed in the stool. These cysts are infective if swallowed. Direct faecal-oral spread can occur, but much more commonly, faeces with cysts contaminate food or water. When the food or water is swallowed, the cysts develop into amoebae in the intestine.

Most infected people have no symptoms or signs. The amoebae eat only bacteria and surface cells of the mucous membrane. But, these persons are infective to others.

Sometimes the amoebae eat into the intestinal wall and form ulcers. This is more common if the immunity is decreased, e.g. pregnancy or the patient is given adrenocorticosteroid drugs (e.g. prednisone or cortisone, for e.g. treatment of a leprosy reaction or asthma). Sometimes the ulceration is caused by other infections, e.g. bacteria or worms (e.g. *Schistosoma* or *Trichuris*). The invading amoebae can cause any or all of the following types of diarrhoea and dysentery.

1. Short periods of diarrhoea over many years; but examination shows nothing abnormal *or*
2. More severe attacks with malaise, fever, severe bowel colic and dysentery (frequent bloody stools). Examination shows general abdominal tenderness and an enlarged liver. Chloramphenicol does not cure the dysentery.
3. Sometimes very severe attacks with complications.

Chloramphenicol does not cure these conditions.

Sometimes large masses of chronic granulation tissue form in the intestinal wall. Symptoms and signs similar to cancer or obstruction of the intestine can occur. You can often feel the mass made by the amoebae in the abdomen, or on pelvic examination PR.

The amoebae can travel up the portal vein to the liver and cause liver abscess (see Chapter 24 page 311).

The amoebae can live on the skin and produce ulcers around the anus, or on the genitalia (see Chapter 19 page 174).

Treatment to kill amoebae in all parts of the body is metronidazole 750–800 mg three times a day for 5 days (400 mg three times a day for 10 days if nausea present). Tell the patient not to drink alcohol while taking metronidazole.

Albendazole in a large dose for 5 days, although not when possibly pregnant, is said to be as effective as metronidazole. You can also use chloroquine, tetracycline and emetine but only in certain circumstances (see Chapter 24 page 311 or a reference book for special doses of these).

If re-infection is not likely, then, and especially if previous attacks have occurred, it is best to ensure no amoebae are left alive in the bowel by following this treatment with diloxanide 0.5 g tablets one three times a day for 10 days.

Give treatment for gastroenteritis (see page 285) if present.

Control and prevention is the same as for all gastrointestinal infections. See page 288.

Bacillary dysentery (shigellosis)

Bacillary dysentery is an acute inflammation of the intestine caused by infection with *Shigella* – the dysentery bacteria. It causes diarrhoea or dysentery (frequent stools with blood and mucus), abdominal pain and fever. Sometimes mild cases with just diarrhoea occur and many infected persons have no symptoms. But, severe cases with complications can also occur.

The usual reservoir is man. Spread is from infected faeces to the mouth of another person. This spread is direct or in contaminated food or by flies.

In a health centre, there is no way that bacillary dysentery can be distinguished with certainty from other causes of acute diarrhoeal disease or gastroenteritis which have caused dysentery. However, if the dysentery does not need metronidazole to cure it (if metronidazole is needed it was probably due to amoebae) it is assumed that the cause was the bacillary dysentery organism

For symptoms and signs, course and complications, treatment, control and prevention, see page 282 or a reference book. Antibiotics should not be given unless the bacteria (1) invade deeply into the intestinal wall and cause severe disease with abdominal tenderness or (2) spread into the bloodstream and cause symptoms and signs of septicaemia. *Shigella* are often resistant to many antibiotics but fortunately most cases do not need antibiotics.

Salmonella causing typhoid

Typhoid is caused by only the very special *Salmonella typhi* organisms.

Infection with these organisms causes malaise, fever, abdominal pain and constipation with a slow pulse for the first week. During the second week the patient gets worse and diarrhoea, enlargement of the spleen and rash occur. In the third week intestinal haemorrhage or perforation and severe general symptoms and signs of infection may occur and the patient may die. (See Chapter 18 page 136 for details.)

You are not likely to mistake typhoid for one of the usual or undiagnosable forms of gastroenteritis.

Salmonella food poisoning

Salmonellae are bacteria that very often cause gastroenteritis. They can cause a mild or moderate or severe attack of acute diarrhoea and sometimes dysentery. The patient usually has a fever. There are no specific symptoms and signs which you can use to make the diagnosis in the health centre.

The reservoir of the salmonellae is the gastrointestinal tract of many animals and man. Spread can be direct, but it is usually by food or drink which is contaminated with the faeces of an infected man or animal. The organisms multiply in the food (especially milk, meat, eggs, fish, etc.), especially if it is stored for a time before eating. If there are enough organisms in the food when it is eaten, acute diarrhoeal disease with fever occurs, after an incubation period of 4–48 hours.

If group of people eat the infected food, there will be an epidemic of acute diarrhoeal disease with fever 4–48 hours later.

Treatment is as described for gastroenteritis (see page 285). Do not give antibiotics unless the conditions described on page 287 develop, especially spots on the skin of the trunk, increasing splenomegaly or fever for more than a few days.

However antibiotics are important if the patient has HIV infection and does not quickly improve, or if the patient has sickle cell anaemia (to stop salmonella causing osteomyelitis in the sickle cell patient).

Toxin type of food poisoning

If staphlococci or streptococci get into food or drink (especially milk), they grow in it and produce a toxin. The toxin is not destroyed by later boiling the food.

If the food or drink is swallowed, the bacteria do not cause disease; but the toxin causes acute gastroenteritis. There is usually the sudden onset of severe vomiting only. There is no fever. The other usual symptoms and signs of gastroenteritis can be present. The gastroenteritis usually gets better after a few hours, even without treatment.

The reservoir is the infected respiratory tract or skin of patients or carriers. These people contaminate food or drink with the organisms. Enough toxin can form to cause disease, especially if the food is milk, and especially if it is kept warm before eating. The incubation period is 1–6 hours. There is no infection of the patient by the organisms.

If a group of people eat the infected food there will be an epidemic of acute gastroenteritis without fever (probably just vomiting) 1–6 hours later.

Treatment is the same as for gastroenteritis (see page 285). Do not give antibiotics.

Giardiasis

Giardiasis is an infection of the small bowel with the protozoal organism, *Giardia lamblia*. It is a parasite of humans only. When the organism is carried into the lower bowel, it forms cysts which are able to survive outside the body for several weeks and are infective to other people as soon as they are swallowed. Infection is therefore common where sanitation is poor, water supplies are not protected from sanitation and personal cleanliness is not good.

The organism in the small bowel causes diarrhoea with pale, large, smelly stool or with a lot of flatus. There may be abdominal distension. There may be bowel sounds able to be heard by the patient and others; as well as burping bad tasting and smelling gas; as well as passing a lot of flatus. There may be loss of appetite and weight loss. Diarrhoea may continue for weeks or months. It is thought that eventually most adults start to lose their symptoms. However, if the patient has any abnormality of immunity, especially HIV infection, the giardia infection and its symptoms may become very severe.

The diagnosis may be made by finding the cysts on a microscopic examination of the stool. This is not usually possible in the health centre and the patient will be treated for gastroenteritis with metronidazole 800 mg three times a day for 5–10 days because he had diarrhoea which did not stop after 2 weeks of treatment. Metronidazole usually cures this condition.

See 'Gastroenteritis' page 285 and 'Post-infective malabsorption' this page.

Prevention is by good sanitation, safe water supply and good personal hygiene.

Schistosomiasis

See Chapter 18 page 150 for details if *Schistosoma mansoni* or *S. japonicum* affect people in your area.

Intestinal symptoms and signs start between 2 months and 2 years after infection.

There is often diarrhoea with blood and mucus in the stools and intestinal colic. All of these can be severe. These conditions can improve after some days or weeks; but they return some weeks later. On examination of the abdomen you can often feel the large intestine and it may be tender.

After some time, masses of infected tissue can form inside the intestine. You can often feel these masses on abdominal examination and they can prolapse (come out) through the anus.

It is difficult to tell the difference between amoebic infection and cancer of the large intestine and schistosomiasis, without tests.

Later, the eggs travel to the liver and damage the liver blood vessels causing portal hypertension with ascites and a large spleen (see Chapter 24 page 308).

If patients have only a few worms or if they do not have repeated infections, they may not have these symptoms and signs.

See Chapter 18 page 153 for diagnosis and treatment and control.

Hypolactasia (lactose intolerance), post infective malabsorption and tropical sprue

After some viral, bacterial, protozoal or worm infections of the gastrointestinal tract, patients may not be able to absorb the sugar called lactose which is in milk. This, then, becomes broken down in the bowel by organisms and causes chronic diarrhoea with a large amount of watery stool. If the patient has a milk product, he may get abdominal colic and swelling and pass a lot of flatus and watery stool. This can be diagnosed by testing the stool for sugar with a Benedict's test or tablet test for sugar. However, many of the stick tests for glucose do not work, as they do not show lactose (only glucose). Fortunately, most of these people get better without treatment if milk is kept out of their diet for a month or so and then only slowly put back into it. Fortunately many adults in developing countries do not drink milk and this condition is not a problem to them. The condition is called 'hypolactasia' or 'lactose intolerance'.

In the same sort of way, after many acute viral, bacterial, protozoal or parasitic infections of the bowel, other patients do not absorb fat, vitamins, electrolytes, protein, etc. properly. They develop chronic diarrhoea with large fatty stools which smell bad and pass a lot of flatus. They also lose weight as they do not absorb fat, and develop a sore mouth and anaemia as they do not absorb vitamins. This condition is called 'post-infective malabsorption'.

In some areas, a similar condition can occur suddenly and even in epidemics, and it is thought that this may be due to a bacterial infection. This condition is often called 'tropical sprue'. It is especially common in the Indian subcontinent and in the north part of South America as well as around the Mediterranean Sea.

It may well be that the 'post-infective malabsorption syndrome' and 'tropical sprue' are due to certain organisms being in the wrong parts of the bowel. A similar clinical state, however, may be caused by continuing infection with organisms such as *Giardia*, *Strongyloides*, HIV, tuberculosis, etc. The problem can also be due to lack of the enzymes in bile, pancreatic secretion and intestinal secretions (which help break down food so it can be absorbed) and can therefore occur in pancreatitis, liver disease, or if parts of the bowel have been surgically removed, etc.

Because of the difficulty of such cases, you need to refer them to the next visiting Medical Officer or transfer them non-urgently to the Medical Officer for investigation. Before doing this, however, you should test the stool for sugar and send stool tests for examination for ova, cysts and parasites and send blood for tests for HIV antibodies, full blood count, electrolytes, liver function tests and glucose. Ask the Medical Officer if you should try treating the patient with metronidazole for 10 days and then with tetracycline 250 mg four times a day for a month before sending the patient.

Appendicitis

Appendicitis is an acute inflammation of the appendix. The inflamed appendix may burst and cause a localised abscess or general peritonitis if it is not treated. (See a specialist surgery book for details.)

The patient usually complains of a central abdominal pain at first. After some hours the pain moves to the right iliac fossa and is constant. The patient loses his appetite from the start of the disease.

On examination there is usually:

1. mild fever,
2. pulse faster than normal,
3. abdomen:
   - not distended,
   - may not move well on respiration,
   - tenderness and rebound tenderness and guarding in the right iliac fossa, and tenderness on the right side on pelvic examination through the rectum.

Later, if it is not treated, an abscess with a tender mass in the right iliac fossa, or general peritonitis, develops.

Treatment is urgent transfer to Medical Officer care, if patient agrees to surgery, to remove the appendix.

Meanwhile give:

- nil by mouth;
- IVI fluids, 1 litre of 4% dextrose in 0.18% sodium chloride each 8 hours;
- IVI or IMI chloramphenicol 1 g (1 bottle) each 6 hours;
- pethidine 100 mg (2 ml) IMI before transfer.

Cancer (carcinoma) of the intestine

See a specialist surgery book for details.

Cancer of the intestine occurs more often in old people.

Cancer of the intestine may cause:

- anaemia from bleeding into the bowel;
- attacks of constipation and diarrhoea, often with blood in the stool;
- intestinal colic and later obstruction of the intestine;
- a palpable abdominal mass; and
- weight loss and malaise.

It may be difficult to distinguish cancer of the intestine from amoebic dysentery and amoeboma and schistosomiasis, which can have similar chronic histories and similar signs.

If cancer of the intestine is suspected, give the patient a full course of anti-amoebic treatment (metronidazole 400 mg three times a day for 10 days preferably with tetracycline (500 mg 6 hourly) and if the patient is in or from an area where schistosomiasis occurs, give praziquantel 30 mg/kg twice with 6 hours between doses.

If the disease does not improve rapidly and get completely better after some weeks, transfer the patient non-urgently to hospital.

Pain or difficulty swallowing (dysphagia)

Do a full history and examination (see Chapter 6).

Weigh the patient, test the urine and do the haemoglobin estimation.

Look for evidence of these conditions:

1. *Foreign body in throat or oesophagus*
   - often history of having swallowed bone or other object
   - sudden pain when swallowing
   - feeling of something stuck in the neck or chest
   - vomiting at first and if complete block cannot swallow saliva
   - no fever or other abnormal signs at first

   Urgently transfer to Medical Officer if you cannot see and remove the foreign body as severe, usually fatal, neck or chest infections can develop.

2. *Snake bite*
   - cannot swallow
   - cannot open eyes, talk or cough properly
   - history of snake bite
   - sometimes pain near the bite or abnormal bleeding from many places

   See Chapter 33 page 454 urgently and give anti-venom.
3. *Infection in the mouth or throat*
   - pain on swallowing
   - acute start
   - inflamed mucous membrane with patches of *Monilia* (thrush) or ulcers in the mouth or pus on the tonsils or tender swelling of abscess in throat or neck
   - sometimes fever
   - lymph nodes in neck often enlarged

   See Chapter 20 page 217.
4. *Diphtheria*
   - things swallowed come back through the nose
   - difficulty seeing
   - other paralysis at times
   - often no diphtheria immunisation
   - grey material stuck on to red inflamed throat (or sores on skin)

   See Chapter 20 page 216.
5. *HIV infection with oesophageal thrush*
   - age 20–50
   - other history or examination suggests possible HIV infection (Chapter 19 page 186)
6. *Rabies*
   - a history of dog (or bat) bite
   - symptoms and signs of encephalitis (Chapter 25 page 327) with episodes of over-activity or some paralysis
   - even the sight of water may cause spasms of throat muscles

   See Chapter 25 page 327.
7. *Tetanus*
   - starts over a few days
   - cannot open mouth widely
   - spasms of rest of body may be present
   - recent wound often
   - no tetanus immunisation

   See Chapter 25 page 330.
8. *Diseases of the oesophagus* including cancer, Chagas' disease, achalasia, stenosis etc.
   - slow start of difficulty in swallowing – at first only solid food; but later also soft food, then fluids
   - may vomit food and fluid eaten, but no bile in vomitus
   - weight loss

   Transfer all such cases to a Medical Officer at a hospital.
9. *Acting out*
   - the patient has a big problem
   - the patient has no abnormal signs on examination
   - the condition gets better if you discover his problem and solve it

   Discover and help solve the patient's problem.

Transfer

Transfer patients to Medical Officer care when there is:

1. a foreign body (urgent),
2. tetanus or diphtheria (urgent),
3. no improvement after treatment of the suspected cause (non-urgent), or
4. you cannot find the cause after observing the patient for a week (non-urgent).

Nausea or vomiting

Causes include:

1. Irritation of the gastrointestinal tract.
   (a) All causes of gastroenteritis (see page 282).
   (b) Alcohol. Some foods. Some drugs.
   (c) Peptic ulcer (see page 275).
2. Block or paralysis of the gastrointestinal tract.
   (a) Intestinal or 'pyloric' obstruction and gastro-oesophageal reflux (see pages 274, 275 and 302).
   (b) Paralytic ileus
   - after abdominal operation for 1–3 days,
   - water and salt problems after prolonged gastroenteritis,
   - pus or blood in the peritoneal cavity.

   (c) Peritonitis (see page 273).
   (d) Haemorrhage into peritoneum (e.g. ectopic pregnancy or ruptured spleen) (see page 273).
3. Irritation of vomiting centre in brain.
   (a) From disease of brain:
   - cerebral tumour or tuberculoma or abscess, etc. (see Chapter 25 page 337),
   - meningitis (see Chapter 25 page 322),
   - encephalitis (see Chapter 25 page 327).

   (b) From changes in blood going to the brain:
   - any fever (including malaria),

- any infection (especially middle ear inflammation),
- pregnancy (or other hormone changes),
- chemicals – drugs, poisons, toxins,
- kidney (renal) failure,
- hepatitis,
- diabetes.

(c) From 'higher' centre in the brain:
- fear,
- worry,
- severe pain of any cause.

Diagnosis

Do a full history and examination (see Chapter 6). Test the urine for protein, sugar, bile and pus. Diagnose the cause by the other symptoms and signs the patient has. Then treat the cause.

Which of these seven groups of symptoms and signs does your patient have?

1. Vomiting and
   - constipation *and*
   - abdominal pain, which is colic, *and*
   - abdominal swelling (distension).

   Then: intestinal obstruction. See page 274.
   If he *also* has constant abdominal pain or a tender area in the abdomen especially over a hernia.
   Then: strangulated obstruction. See page 274.
2. Vomiting and
   - constipation *and*
   - abdominal pain, which is constant, *and*
   - abdominal swelling (distension) *and*
   - abdominal tenderness all over.

   Then: paralysis of the intestine because of pus or blood in the peritoneal cavity (peritonitis or haemoperitoneum).
   See page 273.
3. Vomiting and
   - diarrhoea *and*
   - abdominal pain, which is colic, *but*
   - no abdominal tenderness.

   Then: gastroenteritis. See page 282.
4. Vomiting after food and
   - abdominal pain (in epigastrium, worse after food, relived by vomiting)
   - abdominal tenderness only in epigastrium.

   Then: peptic ulcer. See page 275.
5. Vomiting and
   - headache *or*
   - stiff neck *or*
   - confusion *or*
   - fitting *or*
   - paralysis *or*
   - unconsciousness.

   Then:
   - meningitis, *or*
   - cerebral malaria, *or*
   - encephalitis, *or*
   - head injury, *or*
   - brain tumour, etc.

   If the condition is acute and the patient is very 'sick' (but not if he has a head injury), do a malaria smear, give IMI quinine, do a lumbar puncture and see Chapter 25.
   If the condition is chronic and the patient is not acutely 'sick' or if he has a head injury and is not improving, transfer to the Medical Officer.
6. Vomiting and
   - conditions found that would affect blood going to brain.

   Then:
   - fever of any cause (especially malaria (see Chapter 13 page 61)), *or*
   - infection of any type (especially middle ear infection (see Chapter 20 page 212)), *or*
   - if menstrual period/s have been missed: pregnancy (see an obstetrics book), *or*
   - if jaundice: hepatitis, (see Chapter 24 page 307), *or*
   - if wasted, anaemic, BP high, protein in urine: kidney failure (see Chapter 26 page 359 and a medical reference book), or
   - if glucose in urine and blood glucose high: diabetes. (See Chapter 30 page 406.)
7. Vomiting and
   - pain *or*
   - fear *or*
   - worry *but*
   - no other abnormalities found on physical examination.

   Then:
   - pain (see Chapter 7 page 29), *or*
   - fear (see Chapter 35 pages 467 and 480), *or*
   - worry (see Chapter 35 pages 467 and 480).

Vomiting blood (haematemesis)

If a patient has recently vomited blood, then:

- Immediately start an IV drip (before doing the history and examination).

- Do a full history and examination and test the urine (see Chapter 6).
- Find out the answers to these four questions.

1. *Did the patient really VOMIT the blood?*
   Check that the patient vomited blood and did not:
   (a) cough up the blood, or
   (b) vomit up blood swallowed after coughing up blood (haemoptysis) or bleeding from the upper respiratory tract (e.g. bleeding nose).
   Look at the blood.
   (a) If it is brown it is from the stomach (the acid turns it brown).
   (b) If it is bright red it is more likely to be from haemoptysis or the upper respiratory tract; but if there is a lot of gastrointestinal bleeding the blood can be bright red.
   If the patient has blood in the gastrointestinal tract he will later pass melaena (black, smelly stools like tar).
2. *How much blood has been vomited up?*
   If more than 300 ml (1 cup), it is an emergency. Put in an IV drip *immediately*, in case the patient bleeds again and needs resuscitation.
3. *Is the patient shocked?*
   If he is shocked, start intravenous resuscitation immediately (see Chapter 27 page 378) and make arrangements for emergency transfer or blood transfusion.
4. *What is the cause of the bleeding?*
   (a) Stomach and duodenal diseases.
   - Peptic ulcer.
     - History of epigastric pain related to food.
     - Tenderness in the epigastrium.
   - Peptic ulcer caused by aspirin (or anti-arthritis tablet (NSAID)) or alcohol.
     - The recent taking of aspirin (even only a few) or alcohol (usually a lot).
   - Cancer of the stomach.
     - Older person.
     - Feeling of fullness soon after eating.
     - Weight loss.
     - Not cured by proper treatment for severe peptic ulcer.

   (b) Oesophageal diseases.
   - Cirrhosis of the liver with varicose veins in the oesophagus.
     - Ascites, often marked.
     - Some oedema.
     - Wasting and other signs of liver failure.
   - Schistosomiasis with liver disease and varicose veins in the oesophagus.
     - From area where schistosomiasis occurs, bowel symptoms, usually blood in the stool in the past.
     - Anaemia and ascites may not be present.
   - Tear in the oesophagus after vomiting from any cause.
     - Bleeding started AFTER vomiting.

   (c) Bleeding disease.
   - Snake bite.
     - History of being bitten by a snake.
   - Rare blood diseases.

If the patient:

- has vomited more than 1 cup of blood and/or
- has vomited blood more than once and/or
- has melaena too and/or
- is anaemic and/or
- is shocked;

then manage as follows:

1. Set up an IV drip. Give IV fluids/plasma volume expanders/blood as necessary (see Chapter 27 page 378).
2. Give sedation – diazepam 5–10 mg (1–2 ml) IMI; or if you are certain the patient does not have cirrhosis, morphine 10 mg (1 ml) IMI.
3. Insert an intragastric tube and aspirate till the stomach is empty; then aspirate hourly. When no blood comes back, give antacids every hour.
4. Transfer the patient to Medical Officer care in case he bleeds again and needs blood transfusion.
5. See index for other treatment of the diagnosed condition.

Diarrhoea or dysentery

Diarrhoea (frequent soft or watery stools) is a symptom – not a disease. You must try to find out the cause. Diarrhoea can cause dehydration and death.

Dysentery (diarrhoea with blood and often mucus) is a symptom – not a disease. You must try to find out the cause. Dysentery can cause: dehydration and death; but also anaemia and shock from blood loss; and also allow infection into blood (septicaemia).

Diarrhoea and dysentery usually occur with intestinal colic (often), vomiting (sometimes) and other symptoms and signs (sometimes), i.e. gastroenteritis.

Often you cannot find the cause in a health centre.

But it is always important to do the following three things:

1. Try to find the cause (see below).
   Treat any cause you find.
2. Look for dehydration of the patient (see page 285).
   Prevent or treat dehydration (see page 285).
3. Find out if others are also affected (i.e. an epidemic).
   Control and prevention may be necessary.

Do these things by doing a full history and examination (see Chapter 6) and see pages 282–288.

Causes to look for include:

1. 'Food poisoning'
   Often there is a history of others who ate the same food also being affected (i.e. an epidemic).
   Sometimes there is a history of eating food which may be poisonous (certain fish or plants); or food which did not look, smell and taste as it should; or food which was not eaten soon after it was cooked.
   Sometimes there is a history of taking drugs.
2. Infections in the intestine.
   These include viruses, bacteria (*Escherichia coli*, *Shigella*, *Campylobacter*, *Salmonella typhi*, other *Salmonella*, *Clostridium*, cholera), amoebae, *Giardia* and *Schistosoma*.
   Dysentery is caused by some of these infections.
   Fever is often caused by infections.
3. 'Medical' causes include:
   - any cause of fever, especially malaria,
   - any acute infection, especially middle ear infection,
   - any chronic infection, especially visceral leishmaniasis and HIV infection,
   - malnutrition,
   - lactose intolerance (if the patient has also drunk milk), or malabsorption including tropical sprue,
   - change in diet, and
   - anxiety.
4. 'Surgical' causes:
   - intestinal obstruction, early or incomplete,
   - enteritis necroticans.

   See also Table 23.2 page 289.

Management includes:

1. Prevent or treat dehydration (see page 286).
2. Treat any underlying cause you find (see above).
   Always give antimalarial drugs (see Chapter 13 page 61 unless you are certain that the patient does not have malaria).
3. Give chloramphenicol or metronidazole only if necessary (see page 287).
4. Transfer to Medical Officer care if necessary (see page 287).
5. Do any control and prevention that is necessary (see page 288).

Blood in stools

Always look at stools:

- to check there is blood in the stools, and
- to see what kind of blood there is, and
- to see where the blood is.

1. If fresh blood is on the outside of the stool, then it is probably due to:
   - haemorrhoids (see a surgery book), or
   - anal fissure (see a surgery book).
2. If blood is mixed with diarrhoeal stool, then it is:
   - dysentery, see gastroenteritis (page 282) for cause, (note especially – bacterial dysentery, amoebic dysentery, and schistosomiasis); or
   - cancer of the intestine (see page 297).
3. If blood is mixed with solid stool, then it is most likely to be:
   - cancer of lower large intestine (see page 287).
4. If black smelly stools (like tar), then it is:
   - upper gastrointestinal tract bleeding (see haematemesis, page 299).

Constipation

Constipation is present when the patient does not pass faeces for longer than is normal for that person.

Complete constipation:

- no faeces or gas passed,
- usually serious and important,
- causes – bowel obstruction (see page 274) or paralytic ileus (see page 285).

Incomplete constipation:

- less frequent bowel movements than normal,
- usually it is not serious,
- causes – not eating much, dehydration (see page 285), incomplete bowel obstruction (page 274), drugs, e.g. codeine or morphine.

Abdominal pain – tenderness – guarding – rigidity

See Chapter 36 page 489–502.

Abdominal swellings

See Chapter 36 page 495–502.

Loss of weight

See Chapter 36 page 488.

Gastro-oesophageal reflux (from page 274)

Gastro-oesophageal reflux (GOR) is said to happen when acid, pepsin and food from the stomach come back into the oesophagus. This happens if the 'one-way' valve into the stomach does not work properly (e.g. when there is a hiatus hernia and the stomach can partly slide through the bigger than normal hole in the diaphgram into the chest).

Acid and pepsin cause inflammation and even ulceration of the oesophagus; and of the lungs if they get up as far as the mouth and are then aspirated (breathed in) during sleep.

Symptoms and signs can include:

1. Pain in the front of the chest behind the sternum, called 'heartburn'. This is felt especially after meals or on bending or lying down and when acid reflux gets into the mouth and at other times too. It may be relieved by drinking or antacids.
2. Haematemesis and melaena if a peptic ulcer in the oesophagus forms, eats into an artery and bleeds.
3. Difficulty in swallowing if an ulcer causes scarring and then obstruction of the oesophagus.
4. Cough, sputum, haemoptysis, shortness of breath, etc. if acid etc. is aspirated into the lungs and causes asthma, bronchitis, pneumonia, etc.

Diagnosis can be made only by special tests (barium swallow, endoscopy, etc.) by a Medical Officer.

Treatment includes

1. Keep upright as much as possible (it is harder for the acid to flow upwards):
   - do not lie down soon after meals,
   - sleep with the head end of the bed higher than the foot end.
2. Have small meals and small volumes of fluid often rather than large meals and drinks less often.
3. Lose weight if overweight and do not use tight clothes around the abdomen (these, and pregnancy, push acid etc. up into oesophagus)
4. Drugs as for peptic ulcer. See page 275.

24

Disorders of the Liver and Bile Ducts

Anatomy

Figure 24.1 A and B (below) The normal position of the normal liver (A) on the front of the body and (B) on the right side of the body. Note that most of the normal liver is under the right ribs. In the mid-clavicular line at the right side the liver is almost as high as the nipple and is only about 1 cm below the edge of the ribs.

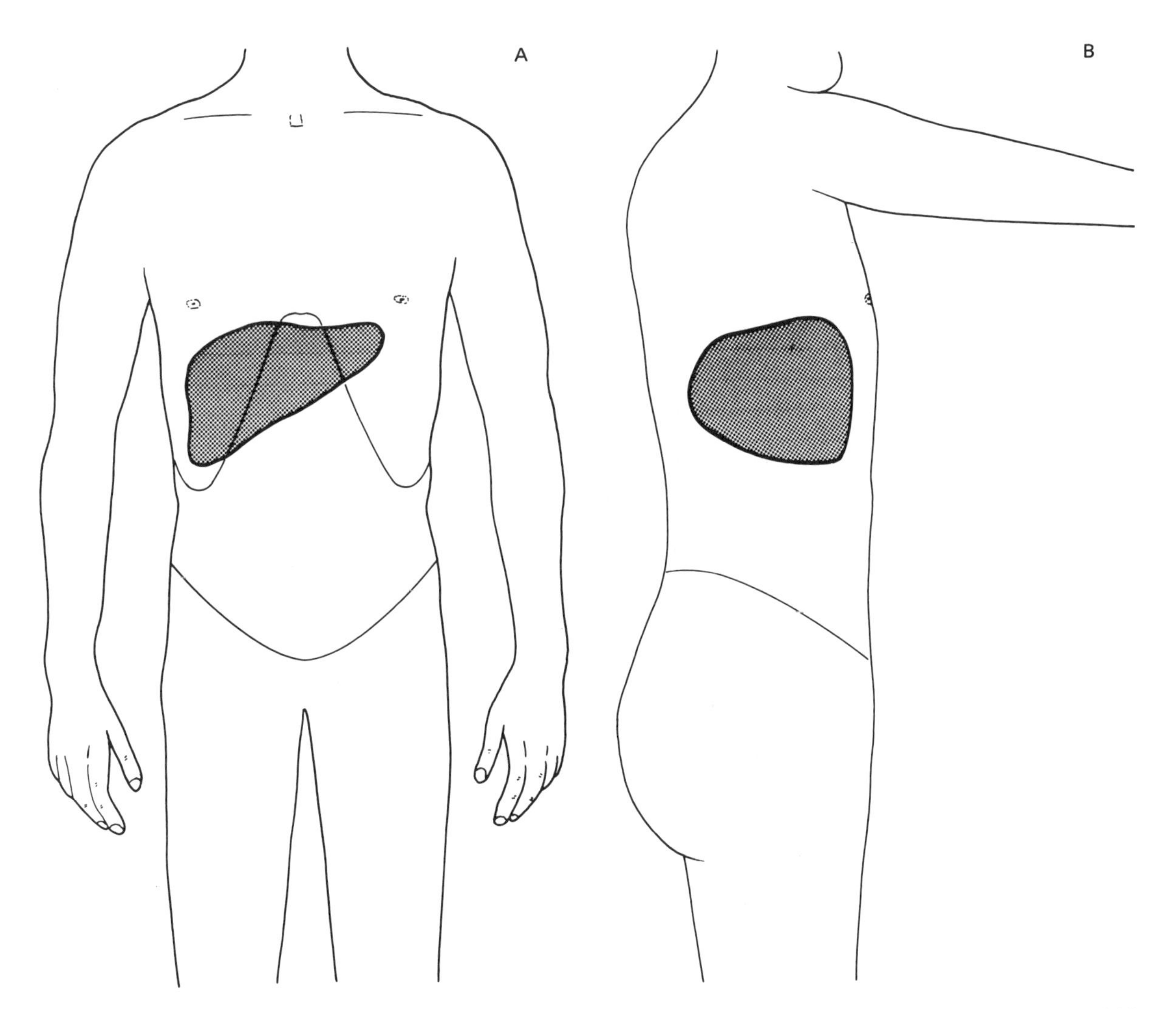

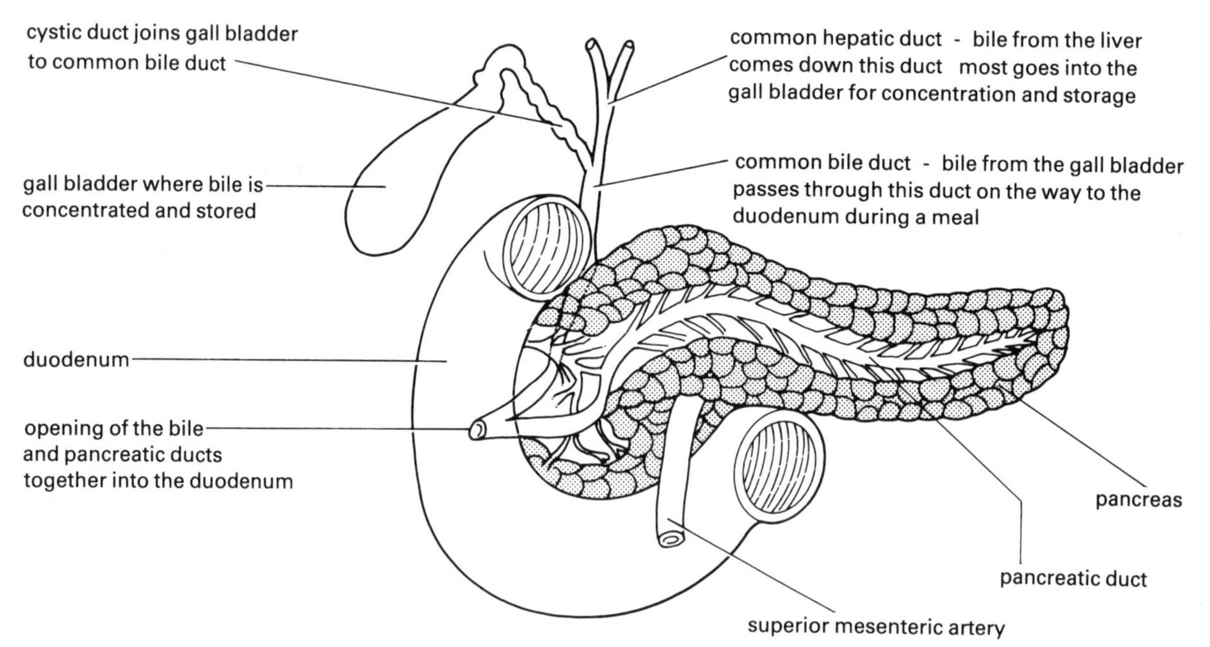

Figure 24.2 The anatomy of the bile ducts, pancreas and duodenum.

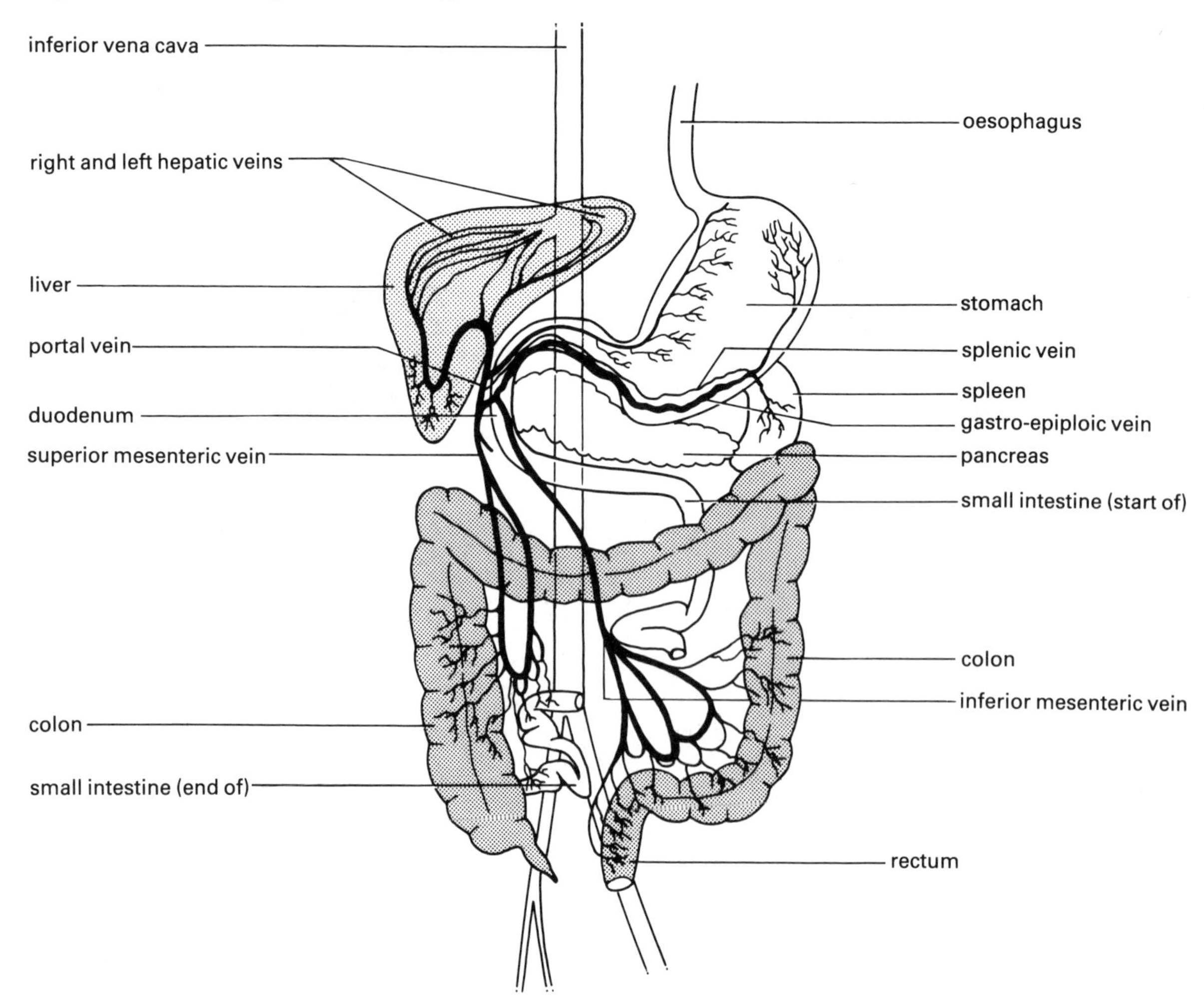

Figure 24.3 The anatomy of the liver portal venous system. Blood is carried from the stomach, intestines, spleen and pancreas into the liver by the portal vein. Hepatic veins then carry the blood from the liver to the inferior vena cava. The liver also has its own supply of arterial blood from the hepatic artery.

Physiology and pathology

The liver has many functions including:

1. manufacturing and storing bile;
2. storing sugar and controlling the amount of sugar in the blood;
3. manufacturing proteins and other substances; and
4. removing toxins, poisons, drugs and hormones, etc. from the blood.

Manufacturing and storing bile

The liver cells make bile. Small tubes or ducts take the bile from the liver cells. These join to form larger tubes, until they all join into one large tube called the common hepatic duct. The cystic duct goes from this to the gall bladder (see Figure 24.2) where the bile is concentrated and stored. When a person eats, the gall bladder squeezes the bile back through the cystic duct to the common bile duct which takes the bile into the duodenum. In the duodenum the bile mixes with the food.

Bile contains bile salts which help the fat in the food to be digested. Bile salts are re-absorbed further down the intestine so that they can be used again.

Bile also contains bilirubin. Bilirubin is a yellow waste product from worn out or damaged red blood cells. These red blood cells are usually destroyed in the spleen. The spleen then puts the bilirubin into the blood. This bilirubin is insoluble (not able to dissolve) and cannot get into the urine from the blood. So, the liver cells take it out of the blood, change it to make it soluble, and then put it into the bile. When the bilirubin in the bile reaches the intestine it becomes brown, and makes the faeces brown. If any of this changed bilirubin in the bile gets back into the blood, it is soluble and is taken out of the blood by the kidney and passed in the urine. The urine then looks brown or black (like tea or coffee without milk or like 'cola' drinks), though many patients say it looks 'red'. (Also the colour of the froth on the urine shaken in a test tube is yellow – normally urine froth is white, even if the urine is yellow.)

In haemolytic conditions, when many red cells are destroyed, much bilirubin goes into the blood. If the amount of bilirubin in the blood is more than the liver can take out, the amount of bilirubin in the blood rises. The patient therefore looks yellow; he is jaundiced. But the urine colour and the faeces colour remain normal (as the bilirubin cannot get into the urine and the faeces cannot be any more brown than they are).

In conditions which obstruct (or block) the bile ducts, the bile is reabsorbed into the blood. The bile salts cause itch. The bilirubin, which is the sort changed by the liver to be soluble, is taken from the blood by the kidney and put in the urine, which becomes dark. No bile reaches the intestine so the faeces become light or even white.

In hepatitis, the liver cells are damaged and cannot take all the bile out of the blood. The small bile ducts are also damaged, and bile with changed bilirubin goes back into the blood. The patient becomes jaundiced. The urine becomes dark. The faeces may become lighter; but they do not become white.

Storing sugar and controlling the amount of sugar in the blood

The blood which comes to the liver through the portal vein (see Figure 24.3) after eating is often full of sugar absorbed from the intestine. The concentration of sugar is often far more than the body needs. The liver cells receive messages from the pancreas (through a hormone called insulin) to remove much of the sugar and store it. When the concentration of sugar in the blood falls, the pancreas makes less insulin and the liver puts some of the sugar back into the blood. In that way the body does not have too much sugar after eating and not enough between meals.

Manufacturing proteins and other substances

The liver is the main place for building up the proteins the body needs. These proteins are built up from the substances which the intestine absorbs from the food, and which come to the liver in the portal vein (see Figure 24.3). Some of these proteins (albumin) stay in the blood to hold water inside the blood vessels, and stop it going out of the blood vessels and causing oedema and ascites. Other proteins made in the liver have other functions, including helping blood to clot.

If the liver does not work properly, the person may develop oedema and ascites, wasting of muscles and bleeding.

Removing toxins, poisons, drugs and hormones etc. from the blood

The liver also destroys many poisons, toxins, drugs and hormones etc. which enter the blood. If the liver is not working properly, ordinary doses of some drugs may be dangerous; hormones may stay in the blood and cause such things as enlargement of the breasts in men; and toxins from the intestines which come to the liver through the portal vein (see Figure 24.3) may damage the brain causing mental disturbance or unconsciousness.

History and examination

If you suspect liver disease or jaundice, try to find out if there is:

1. Liver structure abnormality
   - pain or tenderness of the liver
   - swelling of or lumps in the liver
2. Obstruction of the bile ducts
   - jaundice
   - dark urine
   - pale stools
3. Liver cell failure (failure of the liver cells to do their work)
   - jaundice
   - fluid in the body tissues – oedema and ascites
   - wasting of muscles
   - bleeding
   - loss of full consciousness or abnormal mental state
4. Haemolysis, if jaundice is present
   - anaemia
   - enlarged spleen, etc.
5. Infection in the liver or other parts of the body
   - fever, malaise, etc.
   - temperature raised
   - fast pulse

   } general symptoms and signs of infection
   - symptoms and signs of pneumonia, malaria or septicaemia
6. Signs of high pressure in the portal vein
   - ascites
   - gastrointestinal bleeding usually with vomiting of blood if one of these veins bursts

In the routine clinical examination of a patient, you may find these things in liver disease or jaundice:

- Loss of full consciousness
- Mental abnormally

} if there is liver (cell) failure.

- Temperature raised, if there is infection.
- Pulse fast, if there is infection; but sometimes the pulse is slow in deep jaundice.
- Wasting, if there is liver failure (usually chronic).
- Oedema, if there is liver failure (usually chronic).
- Pallor, if there is haemolysis.
- Jaundice if there is haemolysis or liver cell disease or obstruction of the bile ducts.
- Bleeding if there is liver failure (and especially gastrointestinal bleeding if there is high portal venous pressure).
- Ascites if there is liver failure (especially if there is high portal venous pressure).
- Liver enlargement (see page 313 for causes).
- Liver tenderness (see page 313 for causes).
- Splenomegaly if there is haemolysis or high portal venous pressure (but the spleen is often enlarged because of malaria or kala azar).
- Enlarged veins on the abdomen which suggest high pressure in or obstruction of the portal vein.
- Urine – dark (like tea) and bile present on testing, which suggests liver cell disease or obstruction of the bile ducts (urine is normal in haemolysis).
- Faeces – light or white if there is obstruction of the bile ducts.

Method of examination of the liver

Gently put the right hand with the fingers pointing to the patient's head flat on the right lateral abdomen. Place the hand outside the rectus muscle (the long strong muscle which runs down the middle third of the abdomen). Put the other hand either on top of the right hand or at the back of the patient to hold the liver forward. Ask the patient to take a deep breath. As the patient breathes in, gently press the hand inwards and upwards. (See Figure 24.4.)

Start low down in the abdomen (in the right iliac fossa). Move the hand up a little each time the patient breathes out until the fingers reach the edge of the liver, on the edge of the ribs. The edge of the liver hits the ends of the fingers as the patient breathes in.

Feel the surface of the liver for tenderness and lumps.

If you are not sure about the size of the liver, percuss in the mid-clavicular line from high up in the chest down to the dullness of the liver. (Just below the right nipple.) Check how far down the dullness of the liver goes.

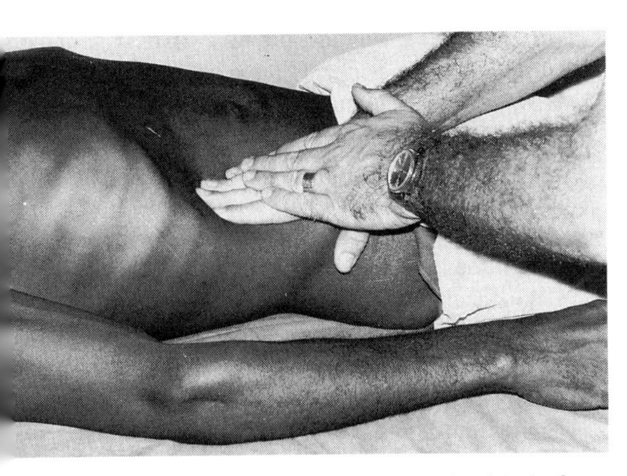

Figure 24.4 Method of palpating for the edge (size) of the liver. See text for description of the method.

Disorders of the liver and bile ducts

Acute viral hepatitis

Viral hepatitis is a viral infection of the whole body, but it causes mainly inflammation of the liver.

The *cause* is one of several viruses. Hepatitis A virus (HAV) (previously called infectious hepatitis virus) spreads by faecal–oral means. In many developing countries most adults have had HAV infection during childhood and are immune. As health standards improve, fewer adults will be immune and epidemics will occur. Hepatitis B virus (HBV) (previously called serum hepatitis virus) spreads mainly from blood, semen, vaginal secretions or saliva at the time of birth or during childhood (when there is close skin contact, sores, scratches, etc.); during sexual intercourse; when blood is transfused; from unsterilised needles and syringes at health centres; or among IV drug addicts. Hepatitis C, D, E and G viruses (apart from HEV), spread like HBV. In many developing countries most adults have had HBV or HCV as an infant or in childhood and most are immune to HBV infection. However, up to 15–30% may still in fact carry the virus in their blood as up to 90% of infected infants and up to 10% of infected older children and adults, become carriers.

Other viruses (especially arbor viruses, e.g. yellow fever virus) cause hepatitis but often a much more acute disease (see Chapter 17 page 129 and 131).

The incubation period for HAV is long (2–6 weeks) and for HBV very long (6 weeks to 6 months).

Symptoms and signs

For the first week the patient complains of:

- mild fever (a high fever is not common),
- malaise,
- loss of appetite, nausea, vomiting, etc.,
- mild right upper abdominal pain (over the liver).

After the first week

- dark urine (like tea – test for bilirubin positive),
- jaundice (yellow skin and sclera),
- liver smooth enlarged and tender (but not very enlarged or very tender).

The patient feels much better soon after the jaundice appears; but he may not feel completely well for months.

The jaundice usually gets worse for about 2 weeks and then slowly (sometimes very slowly) gets better.

Hepatitis B or C is a more serious disease. The patient may die from severe acute hepatitis with liver failure. After months or years some patients develop chronic liver disease (see page 308). After some years, some patients develop hepatoma or primary cancer of the liver (see page 312).

Some patients with hepatitis B or C infection cannot destroy all the virus in their body even when they become well. The virus stays in their blood. They are then 'carriers' of hepatitis B or C.

Differential diagnosis

See jaundice page 314, tender liver page 313, or fever with jaundice Chapter 17 page 134 if the patient is very sick or has bleeding.

The condition you are most likely to confuse with viral hepatitis is hepatitis caused by drugs, especially drugs for leprosy, tuberculosis, schistosomiasis, or chlorpromazine given for vomiting. If a patient becomes jaundiced or develops hepatitis, stop all drugs, discuss the problem with a Medical Officer and transfer tuberculosis and leprosy cases.

Treatment

There is no cure.

Admission is not normally necessary.

If he is 'sick', the patient must rest in bed.

If he has repeated vomiting, give IV fluids for dehydration and maintenance fluids (see gastroenteritis Chapter 23 page 285).

Encourage the patient to drink as much sugary fluid and eat as much good food as possible. Tell him not to drink beer or alcohol.

Give antimalarial drugs as indicated, usually chloroquine 450–600 mg (3–4 tabs) daily for 3 days and 300 mg (2 tabs) weekly until he is well.

Do not give drugs which could affect the liver, especially chlorpromazine or TCE (tetrachloroethylene). Stop all drugs the patient is taking, including oral contraceptives. If the patient is taking tuberculosis or leprosy drugs, stop these drugs and transfer the patient to a Medical Officer urgently. (Do *not* just stop tuberculosis or leprosy drugs and take no other action.)

Control and prevention

1. Kill the organism in the body of the original host and reservoir. This is not possible (even with the people who are carriers of HBV or HCV).
2. Stop the means of spread.
   (a) Stop faecal–oral spread
   See Chapter 23 page 288.
   Check toilets, water supply, hand washing and personal hygiene if an epidemic occurs.
   (b) Stop spread by sexual intercourse.
   See Chapter 19 page 194.
   See also about immunisation.
   (c) Stop spread by blood in the health centres (see Chapter 19 page 195). If an epidemic occurs, check that your staff are doing proper sterilisation.
   (d) Stop spread by transfusion of infected blood. Do not transfuse blood unless the test for HBV has been done and is negative. See Chapter 19 page 195.
   (e) Stop the spread by IV drug addicts.
   See Chapter 19 page 195.
   (f) Stop the spread in the home.
   See Chapter 19 page 195.
   (g) Isolation of the patient does not help. The patient with HAV is infectious before the jaundice appears but for less than 1 week after it appears. Carriers of HBV and HVC are infectious for life.
3. Raise the resistance of susceptible people.
   (a) Normal human immunoglobulin (gamma globulin) contains antibodies against HAV. A killed HAV vaccine exists and live HAV vaccines are being tested. Immunisation is helpful in areas where contacts of patients are not likely to be immune. HAV vaccine is likely to be helpful if a non-immune person is going to an area where there is much HAV infection. These situations are uncommon in many developing countries at present.
   (b) Hepatitis B immunoglobulin (HBIG) is made from the serum of people previously infected with HBV and now immune and not carriers of HBV. Killed HBV vaccines are effective.
   HBIG should be given to HBV non-immune people who are exposed to HBV infection (e.g. health worker with needle stick injury and newborn children if the mother is HBV patient or carrier).
   HBV vaccine should be given to:
   - all newborns but see Chapter 10 pages 39 and 41 (as well as HBIG if the mother is a carrier of HBV),
   - all health workers (together with HBIG if exposed to infection),
   - all persons in institutions or where HBV infection commonly occurs,
   - all sexual and household contacts of HBV-positive patients,
   - all patients with decreased immunity,
   - persons in high risk groups (e.g. IV drug addicts, prostitutes, prisoners, etc.).

   However, apart from the newborn, many of the above reasons for giving HBV vaccine do not apply in many developing countries as many people have already been infected.

What should be done in your area will depend on the prevalence of infection, the availability of blood testing for infection or to detect carriers, and the availability of immunoglobulin and vaccines. The WHO recommends that all infants receive vaccination for HBV at birth and later or as in Chapter 10 pages 39 and 41. Find out what the policy of your health department is, and write it in the book here.

Cirrhosis of the liver (chronic liver disease)

Cirrhosis of the liver is a disease which slowly destroys liver cells in all parts of the liver. Fibrous scar tissues and some, but not enough, new liver cells grow. All this slowly destroys the structure and function of the liver.

Cirrhosis is a common disease. It usually affects middle-aged adults; but it can also affect the young and the old.

Pathology and clinical features:

When a patient has cirrhosis, liver cells die. After a long time there are not enough liver cells for the liver to function properly (see pages 305–6).

The following very important effects of liver failure occur:

1. If the liver does not make enough of the serum proteins (albumin) which hold fluid inside the blood vessels; fluid goes out of the blood vessels causing oedema and ascites.
2. If the liver does not metabolise hormones, hormone levels get too high and this causes changes in the sexual characteristics of the patient.
3. The liver does not metabolise drugs; the effects of some drugs last a very long time.
4. The liver does not metabolise toxins from the intestines; and these toxins may stop the brain working properly.

The new fibrous scar tissue presses on the portal veins (see Figure 24.3). The pressure in the portal vein is more than normal and the vein becomes overfilled and stretched. Fluid from the vein goes into the peritoneum causing ascites. Sometimes the vein bursts and the blood goes into the gastrointestinal tract causing vomiting of blood (haematemesis) or passing of faeces which are made of digested blood and so are black tarry and smelly (melaena).

You cannot find out the cause of cirrhosis in a health centre. Previous infection with hepatitis B virus is the most common and important cause in a health centre. Drinking a lot of alcohol every day for a long time can cause cirrhosis. Toxins which form in badly stored grains or groundnuts can cause cirrhosis. In parts of the world where schistosomiasis occurs, schistosomiasis is the common cause of liver damage; but the damage is mostly to the portal vein not the liver cells.

Symptoms usually include:

1. swelling of the abdomen (usually the first symptom),
2. swelling of the legs,
3. malaise, weakness, etc.
4. haematemesis (vomiting blood) or melaena (black tarry smelly bowel motions made of digested blood).

Signs (Figure 24.5) usually include:

1. Wasting. This is not marked at first; but later it is very severe. You can see it most in the arms and shoulders (as the legs are swollen with oedema). (This is caused by liver cell failure.)
2. Oedema of the legs and back. (This is caused by low protein in the blood from liver cell failure.)

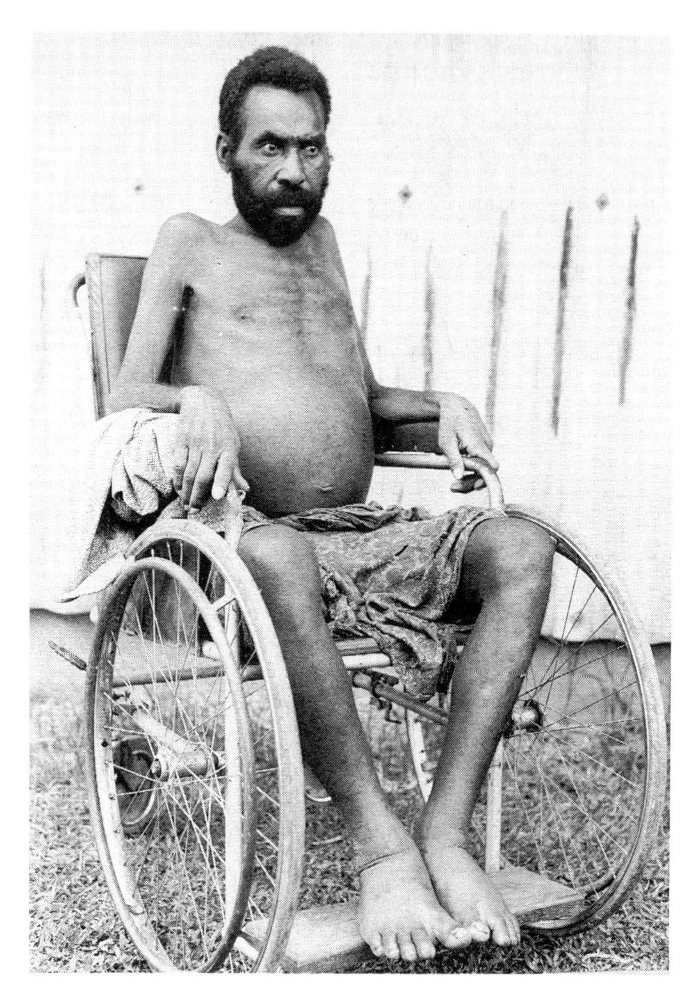

Figure 24.5 A typical patient with cirrhosis: an adult, very swollen abdomen (ascites), some swelling of the legs (muscle wasting but hidden by oedema), very thin arms and shoulders (muscle wasting).

3. Very swollen abdomen caused by ascites. (This is caused by both low protein in the blood from liver cell failure and high portal vein pressure.)
4. The spleen is enlarged. (This is caused by high portal vein pressure; but there are often other causes for an enlarged spleen as well.)

Note two things.

1. The liver is often not enlarged.
2. Jaundice is not common until late in the disease.

Check the patient does not have one of the other common causes of these symptoms or signs.

- Oedema see Chapter 36 page 485.
- Wasting see Chapter 36 page 488.

- Splenomegaly see Chapter 22 pages 265–9.
- Ascites see Chapter 36 page 499.

Check the patient does not have abdominal tuberculosis which causes ascites *but*:

- little or no oedema,
- abdominal pain or tenderness (sometimes),
- abdominal masses (sometimes), and
- no help from diuretic treatment.

Test the stools and the urine for schistosomiasis to see if this is the cause (see Chapter 18 page 153).

Complications may develop:

1. Gastrointestinal bleeding
   This comes from burst varicose veins in the oesophagus or stomach caused by high portal pressure. Haematemesis, melaena, anaemia or shock may develop. In most places there is nothing a Medical Officer can do to help, so do not transfer the patient. Find out what you should do in your area in case injection of the oesophageal veins through an endoscope (sclerotherapy) or even an operation is available, as these can help especially if the cause is schistosomiasis. Treatment at the health centre is with IV fluids. See Chapter 27 page 378 but do not give morphine. Treat also for peptic ulcer in case the patient has bled from an ulcer. See Chapter 23 page 275. Be ready to treat for brain disturbance (see 2 below).
2. Brain function disturbance
   If there is high protein food or blood in the gastrointestinal tract, toxins from this may go past the liver (as there are not enough liver cells left to take the toxins out of the blood) and these toxins can stop the brain working properly. The patient may become psychotic or unconscious. If this happens, give proper nursing care, give neomycin, or if not available streptomycin powder for injection *orally* or down an intragastric tube (not by injection), 1 g every 6 hours until the patient improves. Give enough magnesium sulphate (e.g. 10–15 mg or ml in water) as often as needed to make the patient pass faeces 2–3 times every day.

Treatment

Cure is not possible.

If the cause is schistosomiasis, give praziquantel. Do not give the previous drugs used for treatment for schistosomiasis as these are dangerous if the patient has liver disease. See Chapter 18 page 154.

Manage complications as described above.

Routine treatment is for the ascites and oedema to make the patient feel better for the rest of his life.

1. Diuretics – hydrochlorothiazide 25–100 mg (1–4 tabs) should be given every morning.
   - You can also give frusemide (furosemide) 40–160 mg (1–4 tabs) every morning if hydrochlorothiazide alone is not effective.
   - You can give frusemide 20–60 mg (2–6 ml) by IVI every morning for some days if the tablets are not effective.
   - Sometimes other diuretics which act in another way and can be more effective (e.g. spironolactone or amiloride or triamterene) could be given instead of, or as well as, the hydrochlorothiazide and frusemide.
   - Always give a small dose of each drug first. If the drug is not effective after 3–4 days, increase the dose.
2. If the patient is not eating a tuber diet (i.e. sweet potato, yam, taro, etc.) or if you have given him frusemide, then add potassium chloride 1200 mg (2 tabs) three times a day. Do not give potassium if giving the spironolactone, amiloride or triamterene group of diuretics.
3. The patient must eat food with high protein but no added salt. He should not eat tinned meat or fish as these contain a lot of salt. He should eat fresh foods if possible.
4. Usually you should *not* drain the ascitic fluid through a needle. See a medical reference book.

Check the effect of the treatment every time you see the patient by measuring his:

1. weight,
2. amount of oedema of legs and back, and also,
3. the abdominal circumference, at the level of the umbilicus.

After some months or years, even increased doses of diuretics will not help the oedema, and the patient will die.

Note that if you give large doses of diuretics quickly this may damage the brain function and cause death.

If the patient only has ascites, or if intravenous diuretics do not cure the ascites, refer or transfer (non-urgently) the patient to a Medical Officer to check if he or she has another disease (e.g. tuberculosis of the abdomen or ovarian cyst).

Spirit glass with 30 ml drink
Sherry glass with 60 ml drink
Wine glass with 100 ml drink
1/2 pint (285 ml) glass of heavy beer
3/4 pint (425 ml) glass of light beer

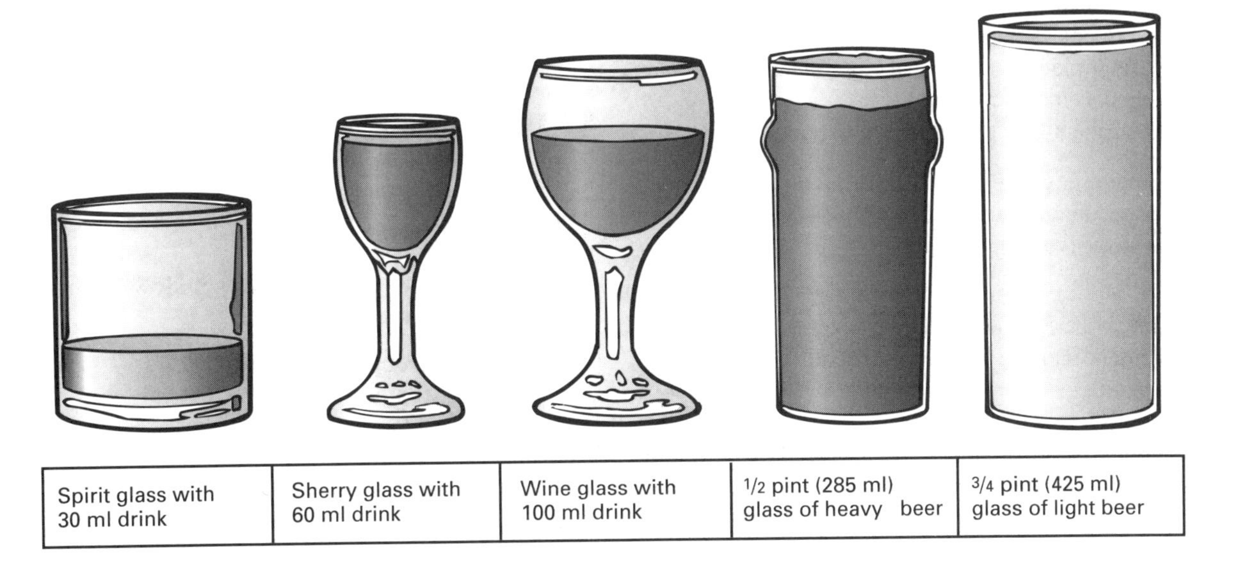

Figure 24.6 Standard drinks. From left: One standard drink, 30 ml of spirits or liquers, 60 ml of fortified wine, 100 ml of wine, 285 ml of heavy beer or 425 ml of light beer.

Prevention of the main cause of chronic liver disease, i.e. hepatitis B infection, is now possible with immunisation. See Chapter 24 page 308. Prevention of schistosomiasis is also possible (see Chapter 18 page 154). Dry storage of grains and groundnuts (so that toxins do not form in them) may help.

Educate people not to drink more than two standard alcoholic drinks per day if a woman, or three if a man (Figure 24.6).

Liver abscess

Liver abscess is an acute (but sometimes chronic) infective inflammation of the liver. It is usually caused by amoebae. Acute abscesses are occasionally caused by bacteria. The infecting organism causes inflammation, then pus and then an abscess forms in the liver.

A liver abscess is not very common; but it is important. If it is treated, it is cured. If it is not treated, the patient dies.

The amoebae spread to the liver from the intestine through the portal vein. The patient often does not have symptoms or signs of amoebic infection in the intestine (or a history of these).

Symptoms include:

1. Pain and swelling of the abdomen, especially the right upper part.
2. The general symptoms of infection – malaise, weight loss, fever, etc.

Signs include:

1. The liver is tender and enlarged. Sometimes you can feel a soft area. Percussion of the right lower ribs causes pain (see Figure 24.7).

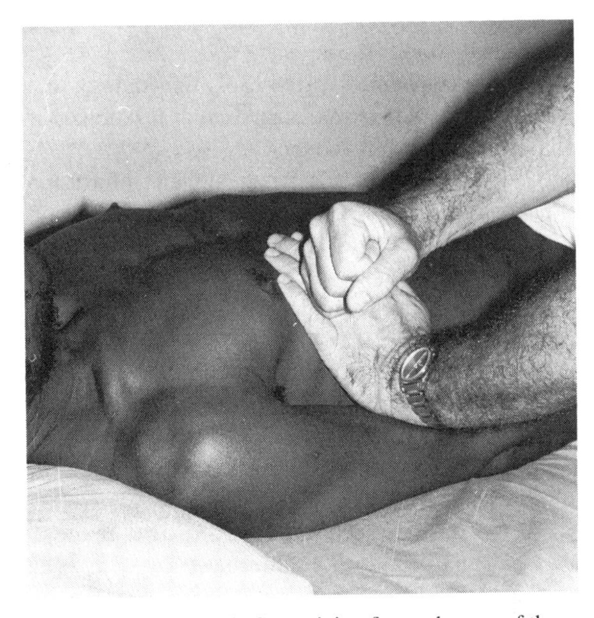

Figure 24.7 Method of examining for tenderness of the liver (which is under the ribs) by percussing over the ribs. It is usual for the liver to be tender if a liver abscess is present. Sometimes you can find the tender area in the liver caused by an abscess by palpating with the fingers between the patient's right ribs, low down at the side or the back.

2. Fever, fast pulse, anaemia, weight loss, etc. may be present. Jaundice is not common.
3. A right pleural effusion of right sided pneumonia may develop.

   The patient gets progressively worse and dies.

Hepatoma causes a similar clinical appearance. Occasionally tuberculosis in the liver can cause similar symptoms and signs.

Management includes:

1. Check there is not another cause for the enlarged, tender liver, (e.g. malaria, acute heart failure, hepatitis).
2. Admit for inpatient treatment.
3. Take 10 ml of venous blood and send the serum to the hospital laboratory with a request for examination for alpha-fetoprotein (AFP). (AFP is positive if it is hepatoma.)
4. Give treatment for abscess while waiting for the result of the AFP. Note the effect of the treatment.

   (a) Metronidazole 800 mg three times a day for 10 days. If this dose causes nausea, reduce the dose to 400 mg three times a day. Advise the patient not to drink alcohol until the treatment is finished.

   (b) Chloroquine 600 mg daily for 2 days until cured, transferred, diagnosed as hepatoma, or finished 3 weeks' treatment.

   (c) Chloramphenicol 1 g (4 caps) four times a day until cured, transferred, diagnosed as hepatoma, or finished 2 weeks' treatment.
5. If AFP is positive, stop this treatment. Inform the patient's relatives of the diagnosis (hepatoma) and prognosis. (See below.) Allow the patient to go home if he wants to. Give analgesics (see Chapter 7) as necessary at home, or in the hospital, or health centre.
6. Transfer these cases to Medical Officer care:

   (a) High fever, toxicity, etc. (i.e. general symptoms and signs of severe infection) which do not improve after 2 days or are not cured after 5 days (?pyogenic liver abscess). (Urgent.)

   (b) If signs develop suggesting the abscess is about to burst, i.e. fluctuant area in liver (urgent).

   (c) Not cured by treatment and AFP is negative. This is especially important in the first 4 months of pregnancy. In other cases a liver biopsy will probably be necessary. (Non-urgent.)

Hepatoma

Hepatoma is a primary cancer of the liver cells themselves. It is common in many tropical countries. It affects young people and older adults.

The usual cause is now known to be infection with the hepatitis B virus, usually many years before. Some cases may be caused by toxins in badly stored groundnuts or grains.

Symptoms usually appear and get slowly worse over weeks or months and include:

1. pain in the right upper abdomen,
2. abdominal swelling, and
3. weight loss and weakness and malaise.

Signs include:

1. wasting, and
2. an enlarged hard lumpy liver, which is usually very tender.

Late in the disease liver failure with oedema, ascites and jaundice may occur.

The alpha-fetoprotein (AFP) test is positive. Send the serum from 10 ml of clotted blood to the hospital laboratory for this test immediately if you suspect hepatoma.

The patient usually gets quickly worse and dies in a few months.

Check the patient does not have amoebic abscess.

1. Send blood for AFP.
2. Meanwhile treat for amoebic abscess.
3. If AFP comes back positive, stop anti-amoebic treatment.
4. If AFP comes back negative and the anti-amoebic drugs have not cured the patient, transfer him to hospital for liver aspiration or biopsy.

See page 311 for details of the above.

No cure is possible. But, aspirin, codeine co., pethidine or morphine can be given for pain as necessary (but only if the diagnosis is confirmed by AFP). (See Chapter 7 page 29.) Arrange for care and analgesics with the relatives at home; or, if the patient prefers, in the health centre.

Biliary colic, acute cholecystitis and obstructive jaundice

If something suddenly blocks the bile duct (which goes from the liver to the duodenum) or the cystic duct (which goes to and from the gall bladder), the patient feels severe pain called *biliary colic*. If the obstruction remains, infection may occur behind the obstruction. *Obstructive jaundice* may also occur. The patient will become yellow, the stools will become pale and the urine will become dark. These conditions are uncommon. They can be caused by gall stones or sometimes by a liver fluke or a roundworm going from the duodenum into the bile ducts.

The patient feels *biliary colic* as a sudden upper central abdominal pain that gradually increases in waves and usually moves to the right upper abdomen. He may feel it in the back, the right side and the right shoulder. The pain is extremely severe and may cause vomiting. The pain usually lasts several hours and then suddenly stops, leaving a feeling of soreness in the right upper part of the abdomen. During the attack, there is some muscle spasm and guarding in the right upper part of the abdomen, but no fever.

Give an injection of pethidine 100 mg (2 ml) and atropine 0.6 mg (1 ml) for biliary colic. If the pain stops, the patient needs non-urgent transfer to a hospital for investigation. If the pain does not stop after one or two injections, you must refer the patient to the Medical Officer urgently.

If obstruction and infection of the gall bladder occurs it is called *acute cholecystitis*. In acute cholecystitis following an attack of biliary colic, some pain remains. The patient develops both the general symptoms and signs of infection and the localised symptoms and signs of infection over the gall bladder in the right upper part of the abdomen. There is fever and a fast pulse. There is tenderness and guarding over the gall bladder.

Transfer a patient with acute cholecystitis urgently to hospital. Meanwhile manage like a case of peritonitis – nil by mouth, intravenous fluids, pethidine and chloramphenicol if necessary. (See Chapter 23 page 373.)

Slow obstruction of the bile duct which finally becomes complete occurs when a cancer presses on the main bile duct. This does not usually cause pain or infection. It causes *painless obstructive jaundice* with marked jaundice with itching, very dark urine and pale or almost white faeces. The liver may be enlarged. If the obstruction is in the common bile duct past the gall bladder (see Figure 24.3), the gall bladder may be enlarged: you can feel it as a soft lump underneath the front of the liver.

You should transfer the patient non-urgently to hospital to confirm the diagnosis, and for surgery if necessary, as also some cases are due to gallstones.

Liver flukes

Liver flukes with the names *Clonorchis* and *Opisthorchis* are small worms about 10–25 mm long which live in the bile ducts of dogs, cats and other animals. Eggs are passed through the bile ducts and bowel. If they reach fresh water, they develop in certain snails and then attack certain fish and crayfish and live in their muscles. Dogs and cats then eat these fish and the larvae hatch in the bowel and eventually become worms in the liver.

Humans are affected when they eat uncooked freshwater fish or crayfish.

Symptoms include a feeling of something moving about in the liver and episodes of fever, enlargement and tenderness of the liver and jaundice. If a worm completely blocks a large duct, obstructive jaundice can occur.

The *diagnosis* is made by finding the ova or eggs in the stool.

Treatment is with praziquantel 30 mg/kg twice daily for 3 days or 25 mg/kg three times a day for 2 days.

Prevention is not eating uncooked fish or crayfish, even if they are pickled.

Diagnosis of liver symptoms and signs

Enlargement of the liver

The normal liver is not more than 1 cm below the ribs of the right side of the chest.

Causes of enlarged liver include:

1. Malaria. Where malaria is common 70% of the normal population has an enlarged smooth non-tender liver. The liver functions normally. No treatment is needed for this liver enlargement.
2. Unknown. Up to 20% of normal people in tropical developing countries have an enlarged smooth non-tender liver even in areas where malaria is not common. The liver functions normally. The cause is not known. No treatment is possible or needed.

3. Other diseases.
   - viral hepatitis
   - amoebic hepatitis or bacterial liver abscess
   - tuberculosis of liver
   - hepatoma
   - secondary cancer
   - hydatid cyst
   - heart failure
   - kala azar – visceral leishmaniasis
   - trypanosomiasis
   - brucellosis
   - schistosomiasis
   - sickle cell disease
   - rare blood diseases
   - others – see a specialist reference book.

Tenderness of liver

The liver may be tender for any of these reasons:

1. Enlargement which happened quickly, e.g. acute heart failure.
2. Acute inflammation, e.g. amoebic abscess, viral hepatitis, infarction in sickle cell anaemia.
3. Hepatoma (tenderness is unusual if it is a secondary cancer).
4. Others – see a specialist reference book.

Jaundice

There are three types of jaundice (see page 305). There may be more than one type at the same time in a patient (see below, four groups).

Do a full history and examination (see Chapter 6).

Test the urine for protein and bile (Chapter 26 page 355).

Look at the colour of the stools.

Diagnose and treat the cause.

Find out which of the four groups of symptoms and signs your patient has.

1. *Acute severe infections with red blood cell and liver cell damage* (i.e. acute haemolysis and acute hepatitis in varying degrees)
   The *symptoms* and *signs* are:
   - fever, often high,
   - 'sick',
   - sometimes diagnostic symptoms and signs,
   - sometimes diagnostic tests if available,
   - jaundice,
   - dark urine with bile,
   - stools not white.

   Causes include:
   - malaria, } the most common
   - pneumonia, } the most common
   - relapsing fever,
   - yellow fever,
   - septicaemia, etc.

   See Chapter 17 page 133.
   Treat with antimalarials and antibiotics if diagnosis is not possible (see Chapter 12 page 53 and Chapter 17 page 134).
2. *Hepatitis caused by a virus or a drug*
   The *symptoms* and *signs* are:
   - feels sick with nausea or vomiting,
   - right upper abdominal pain,
   - dark urine,
   - stools not pale,
   - fever (not high),
   - tender enlarged liver (not severe),
   - bile in urine.

   Treat like this:
   (a) If he feels 'sick', the patient must rest in bed.
   (b) If he has repeated vomiting, give IV fluids for dehydration and maintenance fluids (see Chapter 23 page 285).
   (c) Encourage him to drink as much sweet fluid and to eat as much good food as possible.
   (d) Give an antimalarial drug as indicated (see Chapter 13 page 61).
   (e) Stop all drugs including oral contraceptives.
   If the patient is on tuberculosis or leprosy treatment, stop all drugs and urgently transfer the patient to Medical Officer care.
   Give no drugs which could affect the liver, especially not chlorpromazine or TCE (tetrachloroethylene).
   (f) Check the patient's home and village sanitation and water supply.
   Check sterilisation procedures of the patient's health workers if the disease could be hepatitis B. Give health education about these things if required.
   (g) If a case of viral hepatitis occurs in a closed community (e.g. college) consult with the Medical Officer about using immunisation or immunoglobulin to prevent an epidemic.
3. *Obstructive jaundice*
   The *symptoms* and *signs* are:
   - jaundice,
   - urine dark and test for bile positive,
   - stool light colour or white,
   - often an itch.

Causes include:

- cancer, } pressing on and
- enlarged lymph nodes } blocking the bile duct,
- gall stone or liver fluke or roundworm in the bile ducts, and some drugs including chlorpromazine.

Treat like this:

(a) Stop all drugs except antimalarials.

(b) Transfer to Medical Officer care – urgent if the patient has a fever or is sick, non-urgent if he has no fever and is not sick.

4. *Haemolytic jaundice*

The *symptoms* and *signs* are:

- jaundice,
- stools normal colour,
- urine normal colour and test for bile negative.

Causes include chronic haemolytic anaemias including:

- hyperreactive malarious splenomegaly
- sickle cell anaemia and
- thalassaemia.

Causes also include acute haemolysis in hyperreactive malarious splenomegaly or sickle cell anaemia as well as drugs, snakebite, etc.

Find and *treat* the cause if possible.

Transfer to Medical Officer if a blood transfusion is necessary.

25

Disorders of the Nervous System

Anatomy and physiology

The nervous system consists of three parts:

1. the brain and spinal cord – the central nervous system;
2. the peripheral nervous system; and
3. the special sense organs (organs of sight, hearing, smell, taste).

The nervous system is made of nerve cells and some other cells which support and help the nerve cells. The nerve cells have a body, and some have very long extensions (like tails) called axons (see Figure 25.2). These axons conduct (or carry) messages from one part of the nervous system to other parts of the nervous system, or to other systems (in a way similar to the wires which carry electrical messages in a telephone system).

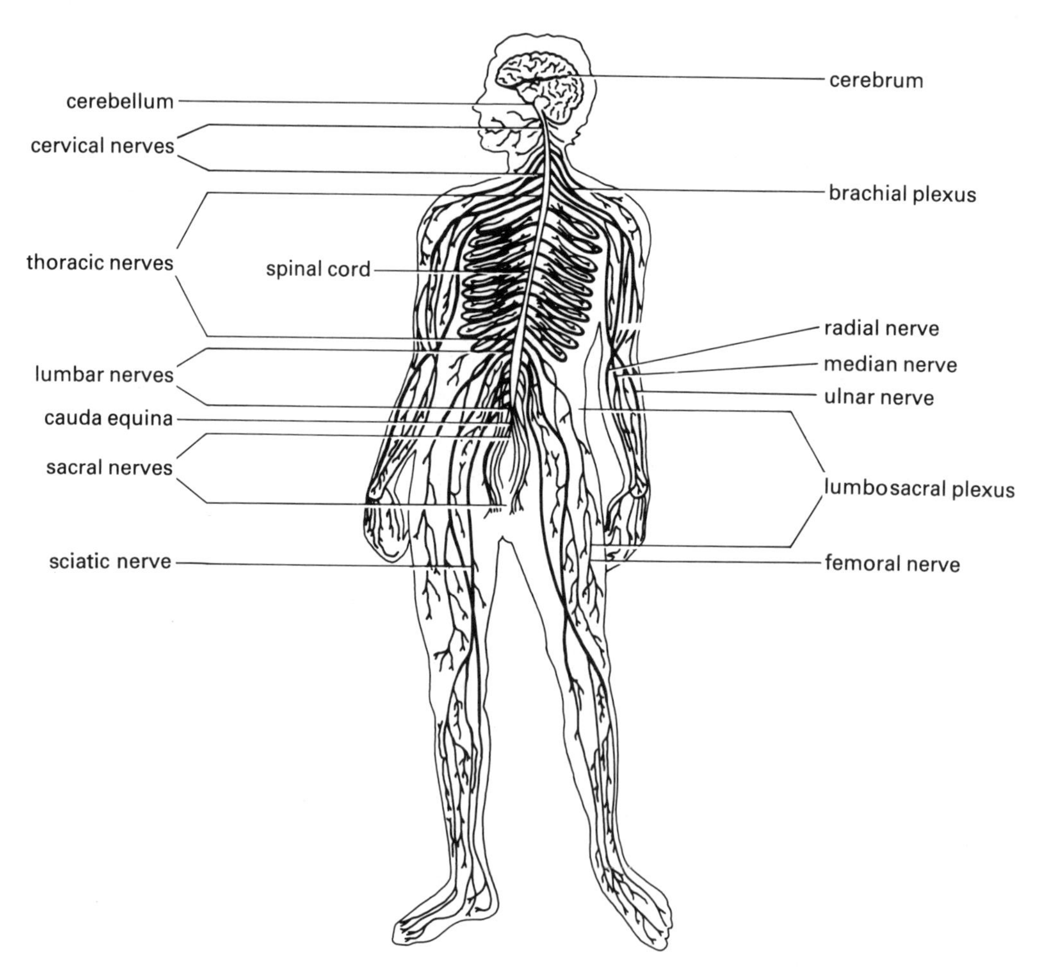

Figure 25.1 Two parts of the nervous system. 1. The central nervous system, i.e. brain (cerebrum and cerebellum etc.) and the spinal cord. 2. The peripheral nervous system, i.e. the peripheral and cutaneous nerves.

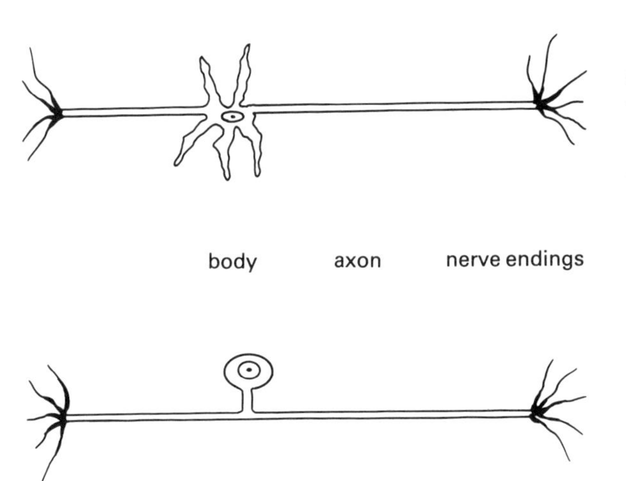

Figure 25.2 The microscopic structure of two types of nerve cell.

The nerve cells in the nervous system that have the same function are grouped together in one or more areas.

In the brain the bodies of the nerve cells which deal with speech or movement or sensation etc. are grouped together in special areas on the surface (or cortex) of the brain, and these areas are called the speech area, motor (movement) area, sensory area, etc. (see Figure 25.3).

In the *spinal cord* the bodies of nerve cells which deal with movement are in the front of the cord, and those which deal with sensation are in special extensions of the spinal cord, called 'dorsal root ganglia', attached to the back of the cord (see Figures 25.4, 25.5 and 25.10).

The *axons* of nerve cells which run from one part of the nervous system to another are also grouped together (like the wires of a telephone system, which run in a cable). These groups of axons are called '*tracts*' if they are in the central nervous system. They are called '*nerves*' if they are in the peripheral nervous system (see Figure 25.4, 25.5 and 25.6).

The central nervous system

The central nervous system consists of the brain and spinal cord.

The central nervous system is like a telephone exchange. Messages about sensation travel from many parts of the body through nerves (called 'sensory nerves') to the central nervous system. These messages are then sent to other parts of the central nervous system and/or to the nerves which go from the central nervous system to other parts of the body. The nerves that go from the central nervous system

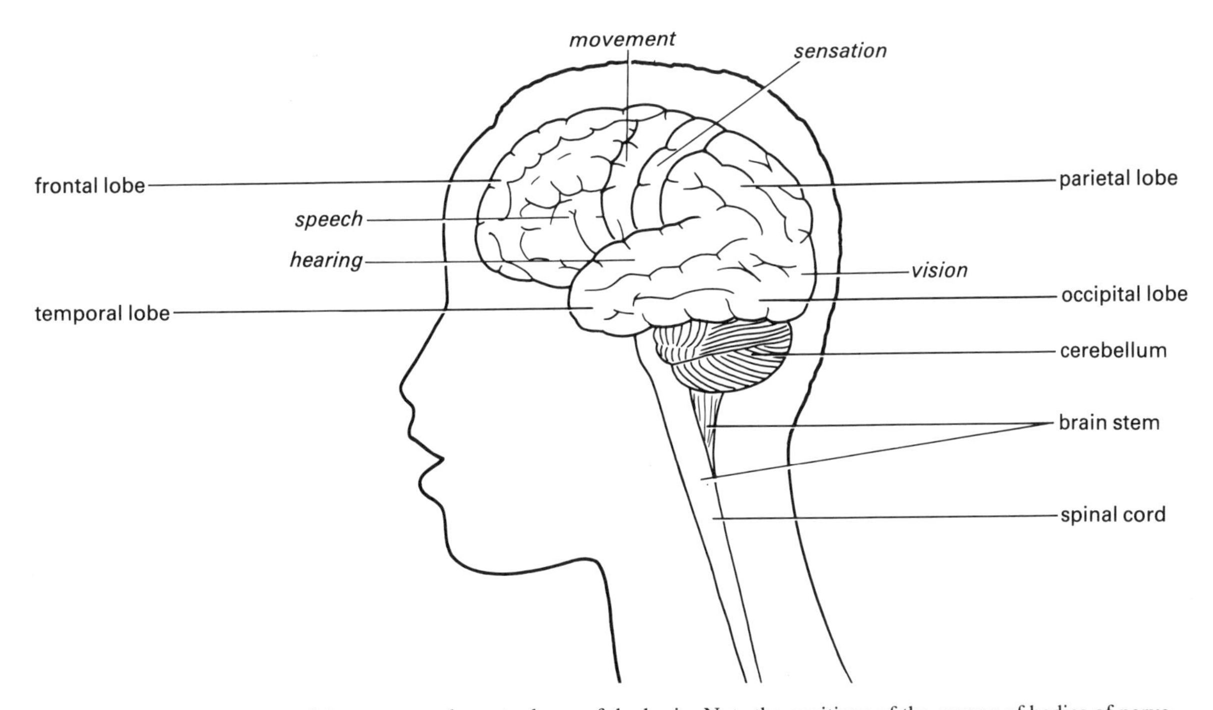

Figure 25.3 The anatomy of the cortex or the outer layer of the brain. Note the positions of the groups of bodies of nerve cells that have the same special function (e.g. hearing).

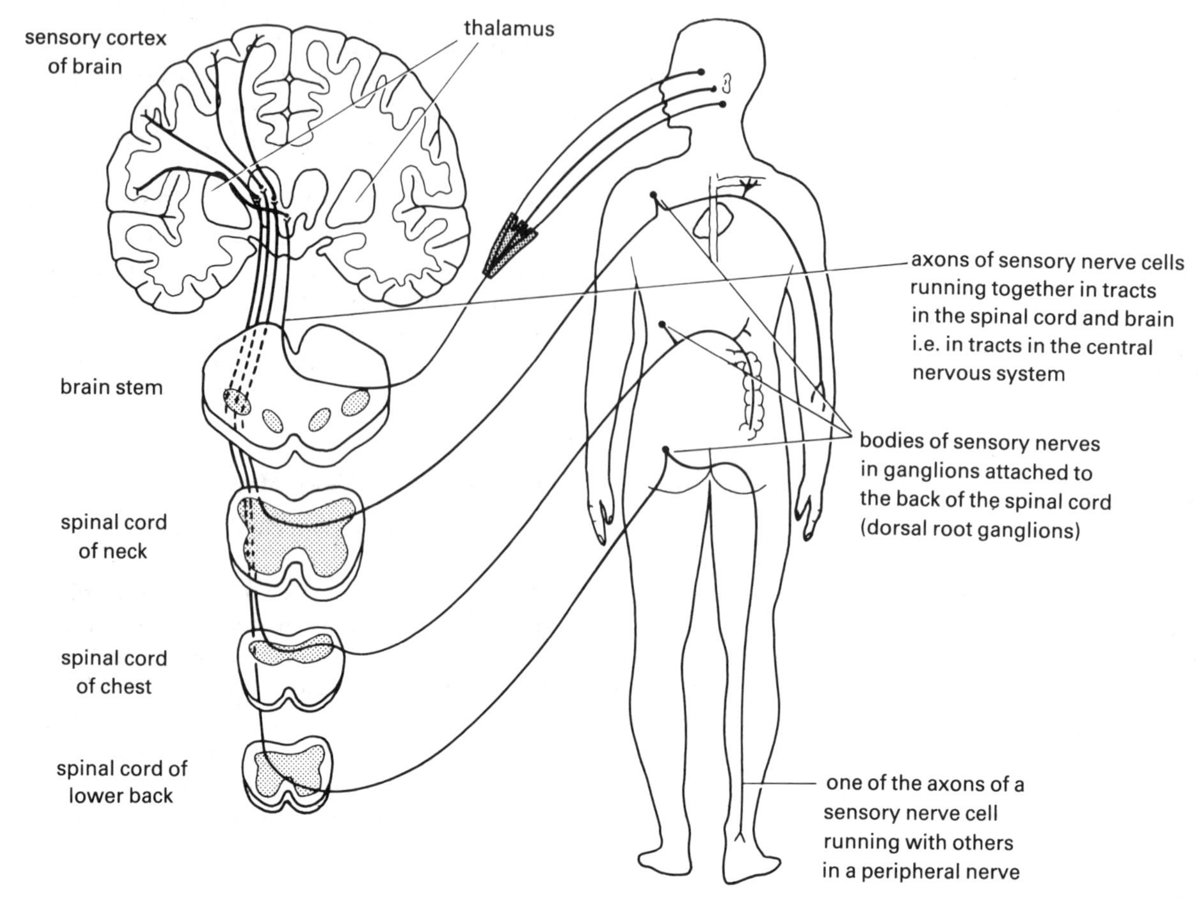

Figure 25.4 This diagram shows how one of the sensations of the body (pain) is taken from the skin to the cerebral cortex of the brain where the person can feel it. Pain nerve cell axons are all grouped together in one tract after they enter the central nervous system. Other sensations have other tracts. Note that tracts also go to the cerebellum (not shown).

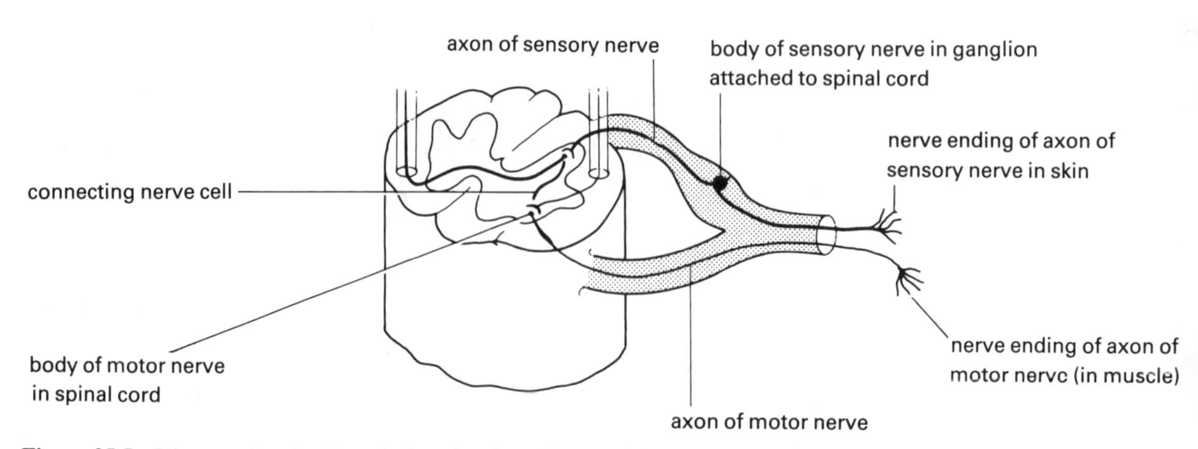

Figure 25.5 Diagram showing the spinal cord and a reflex arc. Pain sensation from sensory nerve endings in the skin goes along the axon of the sensory nerve and into a connecting nerve cell. The message then goes into the motor nerve cell. The motor nerve cell then sends a message to the muscle to move that part of the body away from what is causing the pain. The sensation of pain is also sent up to the cerebral cortex of the brain (see Figure 25.4) and the cerebellum.

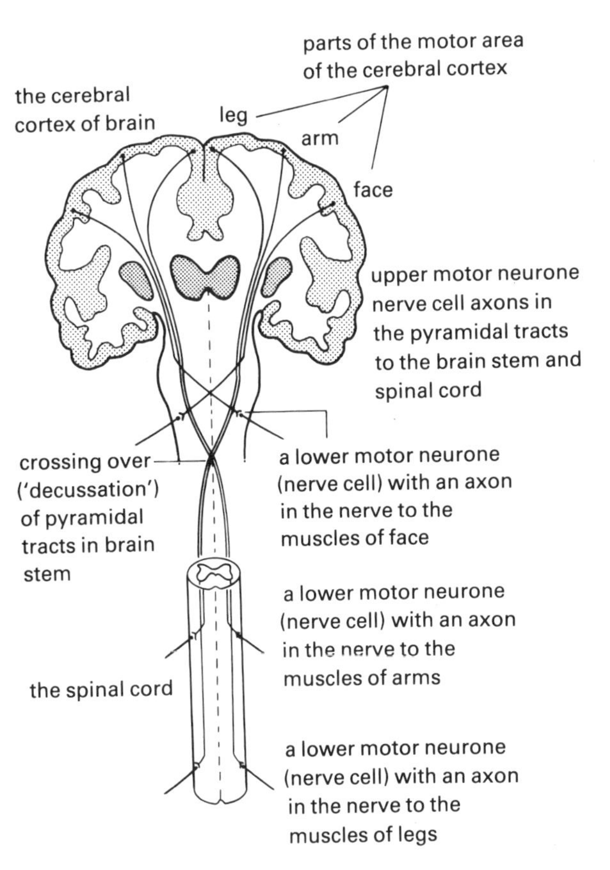

Figure 25.6 Diagram to show the axons of the nerves in the motor area of the cerebral cortex which go in tracts to the brain stem and spinal cord. Note that the motor tracts cross to the other side of the body in the brain stem.

are called 'motor nerves' because they carry messages to make parts of the body move.

The sensory system

Sensory messages coming into the central nervous system can go to three different places.

1. Sensory messages can go up the spinal cord to the cerebral cortex of the brain. The person then knows what is happening and can decide to do something or not.
2. Sensory messages from joints and muscles, about the position of limbs, can go to the cerebellum. The cerebellum then sends messages back to the muscles to help the person stand or move properly (the way he has decided in the cerebral cortex).
3. Sensory messages coming into the spinal cord do not all go up the spinal cord (to the cerebral cortex or cerebellum). Some go to other nerves in the spinal cord and may cause reflex action. For example, if a sensory message comes into the cord that says the hand is being burned by fire, the message immediately goes to the correct nerve in the spinal cord to pull the hand away from the fire. This reflex action pulls the hand away without the person thinking.

Usually, when a sensory message comes into the central nervous system, it causes all these things as necessary:

- reflex action,
- control of movement by the cerebellum, and
- decision about action by the cerebral cortex.

The motor system

The cerebral cortex controls movement through motor nerve cells whose fibres go from the cortex through the brain to the spinal cord. In the spinal cord, they join other motor nerves which go to muscles. Motor messages travel in tracts and nerves to the muscles in the same way that sensory nerve cells take sensation to the brain from the body.

Note that *movement and sensation of one side of the body are controlled by the opposite side of the brain*. This is because the nerve axons cross over to the other side of the body where the cerebellum and spinal cord meet (at the brain stem) or in the spinal cord. See Figures 25.4 and 25.6.

Note also that the *control of the body in the brain is upside down*, i.e. the sensation and movement of feet are at the top of the brain, and the face at the lower part. See Figures 25.7 and 25.8.

Note also that there are large areas of the brain connected to the parts of the body that have many sensations and many complicated movements (e.g. face and hands). See Figures 25.7 and 25.8.

Damage to the special motor or sensory parts of the cerebral cortex will cause loss of sensation or movement on *the opposite* side of the body. Damage to the spinal cord will cause loss of movement and loss of joint and touch sensation on *the same* side of the body, but pain sensation on *the opposite* side of the body, below the lesion. Damage to the brain stem (where the cross-over of nerve fibres occurs) may cause a mixture of motor and sensory losses on different sides of the body and face.

The meninges

The *meninges* surround the whole of the central nervous system. The meninges are three layers of membranes (see Figures 25.9 and 25.10). In the middle layer, there is a mesh-work of fibres in which circu-

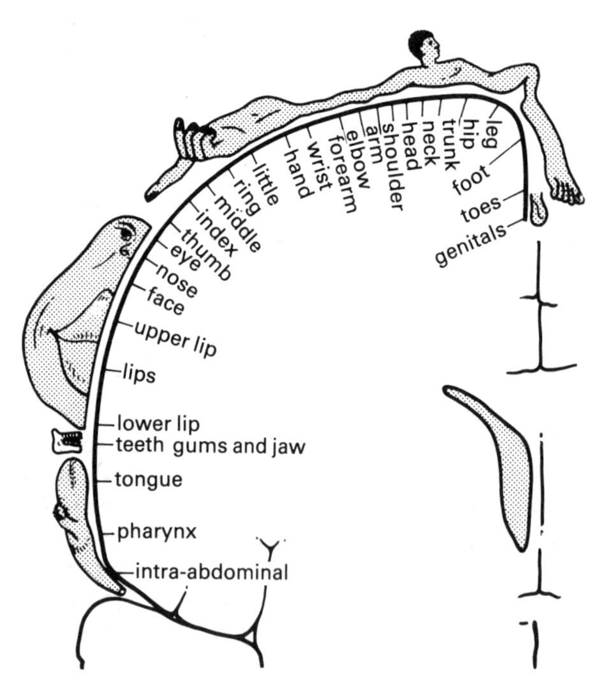

Figure 25.7 A diagram of a section cut through one half of the brain at the level of the sensory cortex (see Figure 25.3). This diagram shows which parts of the sensory cortex make the person aware of sensation in various parts of the body.

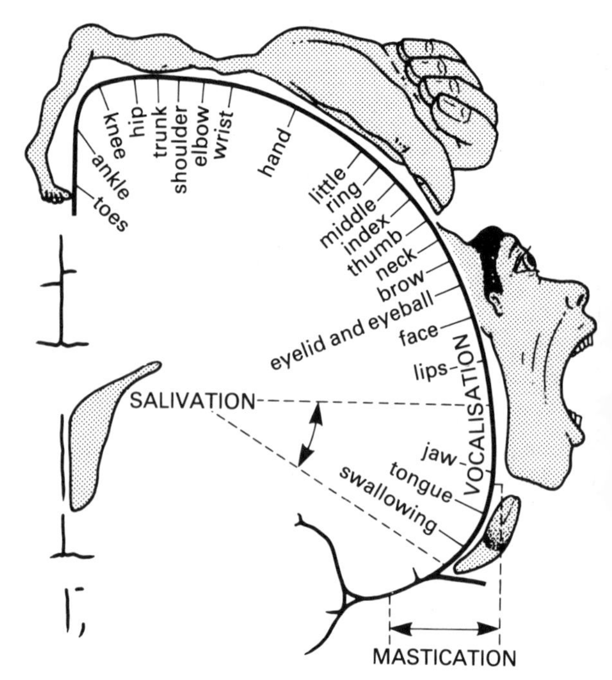

Figure 25.8 A diagram of a section cut through one half of the brain at the level of the motor cortex (see Figure 25.3). This diagram shows which parts of the motor cortex move the various parts of the body.

lates a fluid called the cerebrospinal fluid (CSF). The meninges and CSF protect and give food to the central nervous system.

The peripheral nervous system

Nerves are the white cords which take messages between parts of the body and the central nervous

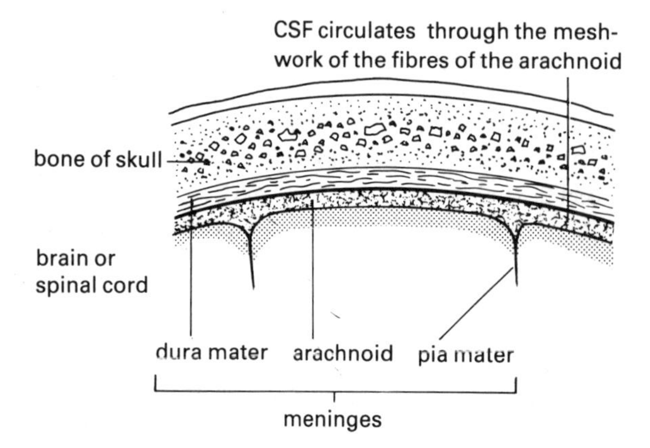

Figure 25.9 Diagram showing the structure of the meninges around the brain.

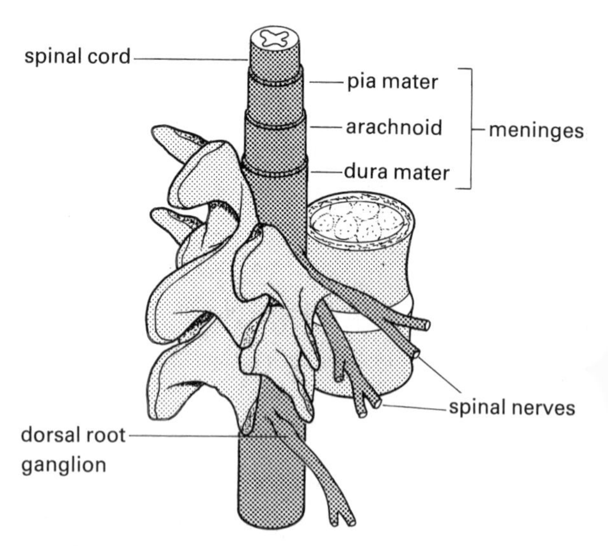

Figure 25.10 Diagram showing the three layers of the meninges surrounding the spinal cord in the vertebral canal. The structure of the meninges which surround the cord is the same as the structure of the meninges which surround the brain (see Figure 25.9).

system. They go to and from the spinal cord and brain through gaps between the vertebrae of the spine or holes in the skull. They consist of very many axons (thin fibres which are the tails of nerve cells which are in the spinal cord or in ganglia). (Ganglia are special groups of nerves cells attached to the spinal cord.)

Most nerves contain both sensory and motor fibres. Most nerves therefore both take sensation to the central nervous system and take motor messages back to parts of the body. The small nerves in the skin are called *cutaneous nerves* and contain only sensory nerve fibres.

Symptoms and signs of disease of the nervous system

Note that you will find only those symptoms and signs marked with an asterisk (*) in a routine history and examination. If you have a special reason to suspect nervous system disease, then check for the other symptoms and signs too.

Symptoms

- Headache
- Fits or convulsions
- Change or loss of sight, hearing, smell or taste
- Weakness or paralysis of arm/s and/or leg/s
- Weakness of the bladder
  - retention of urine (the patient cannot pass urine)
  - incontinence of urine (the patient cannot stop the passing of urine)
- Change or loss of sensation
- Clumsiness
- Fever and general symptoms* (if there is infection)

Signs

- Change in level of consciousness*.
- Confusion*. Poor memory. Disorientation. Not thinking properly, sometimes with mixed up thoughts, hallucinations or delusions (organic psychosis).
- Meningeal irritation* (stiff neck, stiff back, positive Kernig's sign, bulging fontanelle but only in infants.)
- Fitting*.
- Change or loss of sight, hearing, smell or taste.
- Change or loss of speech.
- Stiffness or weakness or paralysis of eye/s and/or face, and/or arm/s, and/or leg/s.
- Paralysis of the bladder, with retention or incontinence of urine.
- Change or loss of sensation of the face, and/or arm/s, and/or trunk and/or leg/s.
- Shaking or clumsiness.
- Reflexes
  - plantar – if abnormal, the big toe goes up if you scratch the outside of underneath the foot
  - tendon – decreased or increased; – right side not equal to left side; – arm not equal to leg on same side } if abnormal
- Fever*, fast pulse, etc., if there is infection.

Pathology tests in diseases of the nervous system

You can get CSF for naked eye and laboratory examination by doing a lumbar puncture (LP). (For the proper method of doing a lumbar puncture and for the laboratory examination of CSF, see Appendix 1, at the end of this chapter.)

Naked eye examination of the CSF

Normal CSF should look clear like clean water.

If CSF does not look clear, assume that it contains pus, and treat for bacterial meningitis. In viral meningitis and encephalitis the CSF usually looks clear (because there are not enough mononuclear cells for you to see with the naked eye). The same is true for some early cases of tuberculous meningitis.

Sometimes a few red cells can make the CSF look cloudy and you may treat some patients for meningitis who do not have it. But this is better than not treating some patients with meningitis.

Sometimes the CSF is red and obviously has red blood cells in it. Find out if this is caused by a 'traumatic tap' or if there is blood in all the CSF (see page 344).

Sometimes the CSF is clear but yellow. This is called 'xanthochromia'. Xanthochromia is caused by red blood cells that are destroyed and release their haemoglobin and other pigments into the CSF, i.e. there has been a haemorrhage into the CSF. Xanthochromia appears 4 hours after the haemorrhage. There are also other causes of yellow CSF including tuberculous meningitis, cerebral tumours, etc. So, unless the patient has clinical evidence of a haemorrhage, transfer him for tests to find the cause of the 'xanthochromia'.

If you leave the CSF for a day in a cool area, a clot (sometimes like a spider's web) may form. This is not normal. There are various causes for this, including tuberculous meningitis.

Common conditions affecting the nervous system

Acute bacterial ('purulent') meningitis

Acute bacterial meningitis is an acute bacterial infection of the meninges (the coverings) of the brain and spinal cord. This infection causes:

1. acute inflammation with pus in the meninges, and
2. damage to the brain, and
3. toxaemia or septicaemia.

It is a common disease and often causes death. The *cause* is one of many bacteria including *Neisseria meningitidis* (the meningococcus – the most common cause), *Streptococcus pneumoniae* (the pneumococcus), *Haemophilus influenzae* (both cause pneumonia) and others.

Many healthy people (up to 10%) may carry these organisms in their throats. For no reason that is clear, these organisms in some people can then infect the blood and the meninges. Of course if there is a compound fraction of the skull, the organisms can go directly from the nasal cavity onto the meninges or directly through the cuts on the scalp to the meninges.

Meningitis is usually a disease of children; but anyone can be infected by droplets spread from patients or carriers; and any of these infected people can then develop meningitis although most do not. However, young adults recently crowded together (e.g. army recruits or children in boarding schools) are commonly affected. Regular epidemics occur in Africa and Asia.

Symptoms and signs

Symptoms may include:

- Headache
- Fever
- Photophobia (pain in the eyes and head, if the eyes are open in the light)
- Pains in the back, neck and other parts of the body
- Nausea and vomiting

(In children there may be few symptoms.)

Signs (see Figure 25.11) include any of these:

1. Signs of damage to the brain.
   - Any loss of full consciousness, e.g. sleepiness, drowsiness, unconscious, etc.
   - Any irritation of the brain, e.g. restlessness, irritability, confusion, delirium, psychotic behaviour, muscle twitching, fitting, etc.
2. Signs of inflammation of the meninges.
   - Full or bulging fontanelle (infants only)
   - Stiff neck
   - Stiff back
   - Positive Kernig's sign

   (In children these signs may not be present.)
3. General signs of infection are usually present, e.g. fever, fast pulse, fast respiration, dehydration. Signs of septicaemia may be present, e.g. haemorrhagic rash, shock, etc.

Tests

You must do a lumbar puncture on *every* person who has symptoms or signs which could be caused by meningitis.

Do a lumbar puncture for anyone who:

1. is not fully conscious or is unconscious, or
2. has fitted (and is not known to be epileptic), or
3. who is not mentally normal (and is not known to suffer from a mental disease), or
4. who has signs of meningeal irritation (neck stiffness, back stiffness, etc.), or
5. who has a severe illness with a fever which you cannot diagnose.

If the CSF is cloudy or like pus, treat as bacterial meningitis.

If the CSF is blood-stained, treat as bacterial meningitis.

If you do not get any CSF (lumbar puncture failed), treat as bacterial meningitis.

If the CSF is clear but the patient has the clinical signs of meningitis, he must have:

- cerebral malaria, or
- viral meningitis, or
- encephalitis, or
- tuberculosis meningitis, or
- very early bacterial meningitis (before much pus has formed).

} Sometimes the CSF may look clear (applies to the last two items)

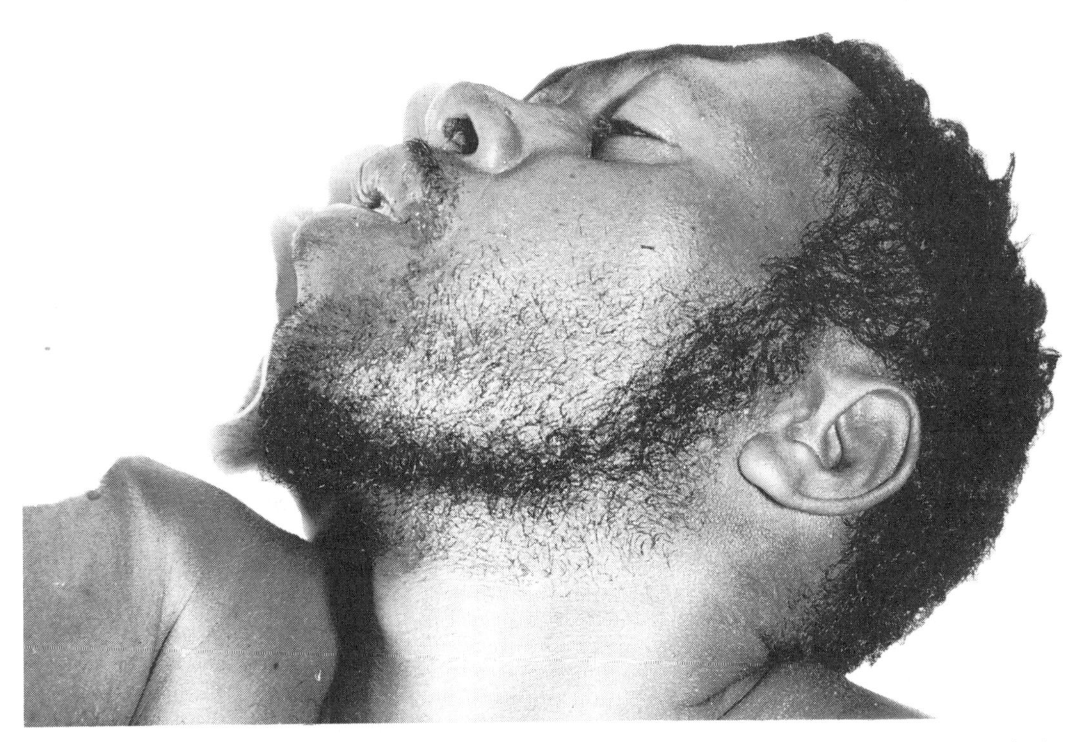

Figure 25.11 This patient has meningitis. Not only does he have a stiff neck but he also lies with his neck bent backwards (sometimes called 'neck retraction'). This is a sign of severe meningeal irritation.

If it is possible keep the CSF cool and send it to the hospital laboratory for examination for cells, bacteria, protein, sugar and culture with sensitivity testing (see Table 25.1 page 346).

If you strongly suspect acute bacterial meningitis in a very sick patient, give an extra dose of chloramphenicol or penicillin by IMI immediately (while you are doing the lumbar puncture and starting the IV drip).

Management

Treat for meningitis if:

- CSF is not clear (cloudy),
- CSF is bloody,
- you cannot get CSF (LP failed).

Treat all cases of meningitis also for cerebral malaria with quinine (or chloroquine) (see Chapter 13 page 64) unless you are sure that the patient does not have malaria.

If the CSF is clear, treat only for cerebral malaria with quinine. But, if there is no improvement after 24 hours, repeat the lumbar puncture.

Treatment includes five things:
1. An antibiotic, preferably chloramphenicol, in a large dose, for at least 2 weeks (see below)
2. IV fluids; but only if necessary (see below)
3. Anti-convulsants if necessary (see below)
4. Antimalarial drugs, usually quinine (see below)
5. Care of unconscious patient if necessary (see below)

1. *Antibiotics*

Give chloramphenicol *or* penicillin.

(a) Chloramphenicol – (25 mg/kg each 6 hours) For an adult of average weight give 2 g immediately then 1 g every 6 hours.

Give it by IVI *if*:

- there is shock (essential), or
- an IV drip is needed for another reason and is running.

Give by IMI to *all other cases* until they can take oral doses.

Give orally (4 caps) *only if* the patient:

- is not shocked, and
- is not very sick or after he improves (when oral drugs are reliable enough), and
- can swallow, and
- has no vomiting or severe diarrhoea.

(b) Benzyl (crystalline) penicillin
You can give penicillin *instead of* chloramphenicol. Chloramphenicol is better as penicillin resistant organisms can sometimes cause meningitis.
Give 1.2 g or 2,000,000 units by IVI immediately.
Give 1.2 g or 2,000,000 units by IVI every 3 hours after the first dose.
Give by IMI if a drip is not running. However IVI is essential if the patient is in shock.
If you cannot give injections every 3 hours then give 2.4 g or 4,000,000 units *slowly* (at 1 ml/minute) by IVI or by IMI every 6 hours instead.

(c) Continue the antibiotic for at least 2 weeks or for 1 week after the fever stops – whichever is longer.
Do *not* reduce the dose of chloramphenicol unless the patient appears to be cured very quickly (see Chapter 12).
You can reduce the dose of penicillin to 1.2 g or 2,000,000 units every 6 hours when the patient appears to be cured.

2. *IV fluids* if necessary
   Do not give more IV fluids than necessary. Too much IV fluid can cause cerebral oedema with convulsions and death.
   If shock is present, see Chapter 27 page 378. If dehydration is present, see Chapter 23 page 285.
   If only maintenance is needed, or if there is a drip to allow repeated IV instead of IM injections, give 0.18% sodium chloride in 4.3% dextrose solution – 1 litre each 8–12 hours.
3. *Anticonvulsant drug* if necessary for fitting or restlessness
   Give paraldehyde 0.2 ml/kg ($\frac{1}{5}$ ml/kg) (5–10 ml) IMI immediately. Repeat after 10 minutes if necessary; if further fits occur, repeat every 6–12 hours until the patient improves (usually 2–3 days).
   Give diazepam by slow IVI if paraldehyde (every 6 hours) is not effective. But also continue the regular paraldehyde.
   See Convulsions (page 334).
   Do not use phenobarbitone if you are giving the patient chloramphenicol (because it may reduce the concentration of chloramphenicol in the body).
4. *Antimalarial drug* as for cerebral malaria.
   Give IMI quinine 10 mg/kg. If you cannot weigh the patient, give 600 mg for a large adult (> 50 kg) or 450 mg for a small adult (< 50 kg). (See Malaria Chapter 13 page 64).
5. *Routine care of unconscious patient* if necessary
   See page 332.

Transfer

Transfer the patient to Medical Officer care if:

1. He is still inconscious after 24 hours of full treatment (urgent).
2. He is not improving after 2 days of full treatment (urgent).
3. He still has a fever after 1 week of full treatment (urgent – but not emergency).
4. He is not cured after 2 weeks of full treatment (urgent – but not emergency).
5. Any complications develop which you cannot manage in the health centre (urgent).

Prevention

1. *Kill the organism* in the body of the original host or reservoir.
   It is not possible to kill the organisms in the reservoir as most carriers are completely healthy and do not know they have the infection; and after passing it to others probably get rid of the organism themselves.
2. *Stop the means of spread.*
   Carry out all the usual means of stopping droplet spread of respiratory infections.
   In an epidemic in an institution avoid overcrowding and separate people in eating, and especially sleeping, quarters as much as possible and ventilate the rooms as well as possible.
3. *Raise the resistance* of possible new hosts.
   Routine immunisation against meningococcal infection is not at present recommended as the vaccines are not very effective for the (B serotype) meningococcus usually responsible for endemic meningococcal infections.
   If, however, 15 cases of meningococcal meningitis or septicaemia occur in 2 weeks for each 100,000 of the population then immunisation with the correct (A or C serotype) meningococcal vaccine will

be very effective in controlling the epidemic. If therefore you have an outbreak of meningitis, always notify your Medical Officer and ask about immunisation.

Haemophilus influenzae type b (Hib) vaccine and a conjugate (combined) DPT-Hib are effective against *Haemophilus influenzae* infections in infants. Trials are being done to see if it is effective enough in stopping enough infections in developing countries, to make it worthwhile being added to the routine immunisations.

Pneumococcal vaccines are also being developed but at present the meningitis problem in adults due to pneumococci does not warrant their use (though in some populations pneumococcal vaccines are indicated to try to prevent pneumonia).

4. *Give prophylactic antibiotics* (e.g. procaine penicillin or tetracycline or doxycycline) for 5 days to other members of the family who live in the same house as the patient, or who live in a closed community with them (e.g. boarding school).
   Also give prophylactic antibiotics to staff who have close personal contact with an untreated patient (e.g. who do mouth-to-mouth ventilation).
   Check close contacts daily. Educate all contacts and the public to come for examination and if needed treatment at the first sign of meningitis or septicaemia.

Cerebral malaria

Cerebral malaria is the acute damage of the brain (encephalitis) and meninges caused by falciparum malaria parasites and their toxins in the blood vessels of the brain.

Cerebral malaria is clinically similar to acute bacterial meningitis (see page 322) but there are some differences.

The *history* is similar *but* the history may also suggest malaria, e.g.

- the patient is a non-immune person recently in a malarial area,
- he has had recent attacks of fever.

The signs of brain damage are similar, i.e.

- loss of full consciousness,
  e.g. the patient may be sleepy, drowsy, unconscious, etc.
- irritation of the brain,
  e.g. the patient may be restless, irritable, confused, delirious, psychotic, twitching, fitting, etc.

The *signs of inflammation of the meninges* are similar, e.g. stiff neck, stiff back, etc.

The *general signs of infection* are similar, e.g. fast pulse, fast respiration, dehydration, etc. *but* there are no signs of septicaemia.

There may be other signs of acute or chronic malaria, e.g. anaemia and/or jaundice, enlarged tender spleen, or enlarged liver.

But you cannot tell the difference between acute bacterial meningitis and cerebral malaria without a lumbar puncture.

Always do a lumbar puncture if you suspect cerebral malaria *or* meningitis.

In cerebral malaria the CSF will be normal and look clear. The CSF will also look clear in:

- viral meningitis,
- encephalitis,
- tuberculous meningitis (sometimes), and
- a very early acute bacterial meningitis (rarely).

Treatment

Treatment includes five things:

1. Antimalarial drugs by injection (see Malaria, Chapter 13 page 61)
   Give quinine 10 mg/kg by *slow* IV drip or by IMI
   - immediately, *and*
   - 6–8 hours later, *and*
   - 24 hours after first dose, *and*
   - then repeat every 8–12 hours until the patient can take oral antimalarial drugs.

   Quinine should be given by slow IV drip. But if you are not successful in having the drip running in 15 minutes or you are not certain that the staff can care for the drip, give IMI quinine instead of IVI quinine.
   Give choroquine by IMI if you cannot get quinine.
   Quinine takes effect faster than chloroquine, and quinine is essential if there is any chance of the patient having chloroquine resistant malaria.
   If the above treatment is not possible, artesunate suppositories (Artesunate Rectocaps) if available would be the best treatment to be given immediately.

If none of the above are possible, put down a nasogastric tube and give quinine and other antimalarial drugs through this tube into the stomach.
(See Chapter 13 page 65 for details of giving these drugs.

As both malaria and quinine can cause low blood glucose, do a test for blood glucose. If it is low or if you cannot do the test, give glucose 50 ml or 50% solution glucose stat and use 5% or 4.3% dextrose in the drip for the quinine.

2. Anticonvulsants if there is fitting.
   Give paraldehyde 0.2 ml/kg ($\frac{1}{5}$ ml/kg) (10 ml usually) by IMI immediately. Repeat in 10 minutes if necessary. If further fits occur repeat every 6–12 hours until the patient improves (usually 1–2 days).
   Give diazepam by IVI slowly for fitting that is not controlled by paraldehyde.
   See Convulsions page 335 for details of giving these drugs.
3. If the patient is unconscious, give routine care for unconsciousness.
   See page 332 for details. Patients may be unconscious for some days and still make a complete recovery.
4. Reduce temperature if 40°C or above.
   See Chapter 13 page 65 for details.
5. IV fluids if necessary.
   Do not give more fluid than necessary. Too much fluid can cause cerebral oedema and death. See meningitis page 326. Use 5% or 4% glucose.

Transfer patients to Medical Officer care:

1. if they are unconscious for more than 1 day;
2. if they are not greatly improved after 2 days; or
3. if they are not cured in 2 weeks.

Tuberculous meningitis

See also Chapter 14 page 79.

Tuberculous meningitis is a sub-acute or chronic infection of the meninges with tuberculosis organisms.

Tuberculous meningitis is clinically similar to acute bacterial meningitis (see page 322).

Symptoms and *signs* include:

- headache, and other symptoms and signs of brain damage;
- signs of meningeal irritation, with stiff neck, stiff back etc;
- general symptoms and signs of infection;
- abnormal CSF (but sometimes you cannot see this without a microscope).

But there are differences from acute bacterial meningitis:

- The history is often longer (days or weeks, not hours or days).
- The patient is often not as 'sick' at first.
- Evidence of tuberculous infection is sometimes present in other parts of the body.
- The CSF may only be yellow; or, when left standing for some hours, form a spider's web type clot; or be almost clear.
- Proper antibacterial meningitis treatment causes no improvement in 2 days, no loss of fever in 1 week and no cure in 2 weeks.

The tuberculin test is often negative.

Suspect tuberculous meningitis if any of these things occur and *transfer* all suspected cases urgently to a Medical Officer for diagnosis and treatment with special drugs.

In areas where African trypanosomiasis (sleeping sickness) occurs, this may cause similar signs and symptoms. This patient needs urgent transfer to a Medical Officer for diagnosis and treatment. A lumbar puncture would not be done until after diagnosis and the start of treatment.

Whenever you see meningitis that does not respond to treatment or is chronic, ask yourself if there is any history or signs that would suggest tuberculosis infection.

Virus meningitis

Virus meningitis is an inflammation of the meninges caused by infection with one of many viruses.

It is clinically similar to acute bacterial or tuberculous meningitis (see above) *but*

1. The CSF looks clear.
2. Most cases get better with no treatment. Antibiotics do not help.

You will diagnose most cases in a health centre (where laboratory tests are not available) incorrectly as cerebral malaria. This does not matter as the management is as for cerebral malaria.

Treat as for cerebral malaria (see page 325).

Transfer to Medical Officer care if the patient is unconscious for more than one day, *or* not improving after 2 days, *or* not cured after 2 weeks.

Encephalitis

Encephalitis is inflammation of the brain itself, usually caused by one of many viruses. Often the meninges are also inflamed (i.e. it is meningo-encephalitis).

It is similar to acute bacterial or tuberculous meningitis (see pages 322 and 326), *but*:

1. The CSF looks clear.
2. Many cases get better with no treatment. Some cases may have permanent brain damage. A few cases (and any case due to rabies) die. Antibiotics do not help.

You will diagnose most cases incorrectly as cerebral malaria; but this does not matter because management is as for cerebral malaria (see page 325). If you could be certain that the patient did not have malaria, you would not give the antimalarial drugs.

Arborviruses (see Chapter 17 page 133) are a common cause especially if there is an epidemic.

However, always think of rabies (see below) if you are in an area where rabies occurs.

Cases may be caused by African trypanosomiasis (see below) or cysticercosis. See Chapter 23 page 280.

Transfer to Medical Officer care if the patient is: unconscious for more than one day, *or* not improving after 2 days, *or* not cured after 2 weeks.

African trypanosomiasis (sleeping sickness)

See Chapter 18 page 144 for details.

The patient is in (or from) an area where African trypanosomiasis occurs.

Early *signs* may be:

1. fast pulse, and perhaps heart failure,
2. anaemia,
3. enlarged lymph glands,
4. enlarged spleen, and
5. proteinurea.

Chronic meningoencephalitis follows and causes:

1. headache;
2. tiredness, sleepiness and no interest in anything (the patient may not even eat);
3. sleeping in the day, but sometimes not at night;
4. changes in personality, confusion, and development of organic psychosis (see Chapter 35 page 470–1) (these may be the first signs);
5. shaking, weakness, pains, difficulty in walking;
6. coma and death.

Transfer all such cases for diagnosis and treatment by a Medical Officer.

Rabies

Rabies is an acute viral disease of the brain (encephalitis) and the salivary glands of animals, which sometimes affects man.

It is spread from one animal to another animal by infected secretions (usually saliva). The means of spread is usually a bite by an infected animal. All warmblooded animals can be infected with rabies.

Rabies occurs in most countries. Find out if it occurs in your area.

Symptoms and *signs* of rabies in man include:

1. There is a history of an animal bite, usually from a dog which was behaving abnormally.
2. The disease has a long incubation period (1 week to more than 1 year), before the first signs appear.
3. The patient becomes 'sick' for a few days with fever, headache, etc.
4. The patient then has a period of encephalitis. This produces over-activity or paralysis or a mixture of both. Some patients become very anxious. Sudden noises and lights, etc. cause strange behaviour. There are episodes of wild behaviour and muscle spasms and fear. The patient cannot swallow because of the spasms of the throat muscles. Even the sight of water causes these spasms. The spasms can cause 'foaming at the mouth'. Other patients become very depressed and quiet, and become paralysed. But even they can get spasms of the throat and cannot swallow.
5. The patient dies, usually within 10 days (but it can be shorter or longer).
6. Cases that are not typical may be common. Suspect rabies in any unusual disease of the nervous system in an area where rabies occurs.

Signs of rabies in the dog or other animals are similar to those in man.

Confirmation of the *diagnosis* is by special tests.

If you strongly suspect rabies in a patient or an animal, notify the nearest Medical and Veterinary Officer urgently.

No *treatment* can cure rabies once it has developed. Give morphine, chlorpromazine and diazepam in large regular doses each 4–6 hours to relieve the stress and pain.

Prevention of rabies includes:

1. Kill the organism in the body of the original hosts (reservoir).
   In areas where rabies occurs:
   (a) All dogs without owners should be killed.
   (b) All dogs with owners should be immunised against rabies.
   (c) If wild animals in the area carry the disease they can be immunised by spreading live virus vaccines on baits.
2. Stop the means of spread.
   Control dogs.
   Do not get bitten by dogs, cats or bats or go into bat caves.
   When nursing patients with rabies, use strict barrier nursing including use of gloves and goggles as the saliva is infectious if it gets into the eyes or mouth as well as through the skin – and the patients sometimes spit.
3. Raise the resistance of persons who are bitten.
   Treat local wounds.
   Give passive immunisation with anti-rabies hyperimmune serum, preferably from human, but if not available, from animals. However it is probably needed only if there has been a large dose of virus from a large bite or many bites or if the bite was in a central part of the body.
   Give active immunisation with whatever is available. Brain tissue vaccine is effective but quite a number of patients develop encephalitis from the vaccine. Purified duck embryo vaccine is safer. The best, however, are tissue culture vaccines, e.g. HDVC, PCECV and PVCU but they are very expensive although only 0.1 ml given intradermally immediately and on days 3, 7 and 14 gives good protection.
   Find out what is available in your area and what you should do.
   If a person is bitten by an animal, manage as follows:

1. *Give proper treatment for the bite*
   - Wash the wound with a lot of soap and water.
   - Rinse with a lot of water.
   - Then apply iodine in spirit.
   - Then do the necessary surgical toilet.
   - Do not stitch the wound.
   - Dress the wound and apply a compression bandage to stop bleeding.
   - Give tetanus prophylaxis (see page 331).
2. *Try to find out if the animal has rabies and transfer the patient for immunisation if necessary.*
   (a) If the animal looks healthy, lock it up for 10 days. If it is still alive and well after 10 days, the animal did not have rabies and no immunisation of the patient is necessary. If the animal shows any sign of sickness before the 10 days are finished, start immunisation or transfer the patient immediately for immunisation.
   (b) If the animal has disappeared, start immunisation or transfer the patient for immunisation.
   (c) If the animal has been caught and looks sick, lock up the animal carefully (make sure that it does not bite anyone) and inform the local Veterinary Officer. Transfer the patient for immunisation.
   (d) If the animal has been killed leave the body for the Veterinary Officer. If the Veterinary Officer cannot come and you do not have special ways of removing animal brains, or cutting off the head and keeping it in ice without infecting yourself, bury the animal carefully. Start immunisation or immediately transfer the patient for immunisation.

Poliomyelitis

Polymyelitis is an acute inflammation of parts of the brain and spinal cord caused by one of the polio viruses. Polio viruses are spread by the faecal–oral route or, less often, by respiratory secretions.

Infection can cause one or more of the following:

1. An asymptomatic infection.
2. A non-specific viral gastroenteritis or febrile illness.
3. In only a very few of the above clinical virus meningitis (see Chapter 25 page 326).
4. In only a very few of the above an infection of the brain and spinal cord (encephalitis and myelitis). This can cause sudden paralysis of groups of muscles in one or two days. Other groups may then be paralysed in the next week or so. Often a number

of limbs are partly paralysed. This is different from a stroke or injury where usually the whole of one limb or the whole of one side of the body is paralysed. There is often severe pain and aching in the affected muscles. There is no loss of sensation. If the muscles used for breathing are affected, the patient will die because he cannot breathe. If the muscles which are used to swallow are affected the patient may die because saliva, food, etc. will be breathed into the lungs and cause pneumonia.

No treatment to kill the infection or cure the encephalitis and myelitis is possible. However if the patient can be kept alive, considerable improvement may later occur with physiotherapy, exercises, etc.

If you have a patient who could have poliomyelitis contact the Medical Officer urgently about *care* and *transfer* of the patient as breathing may later become affected and there will be the need for vaccination of contacts.

Killing the parasite in the body of the original host or reservoir is not possible. Stopping the means of spread by reducing faecal–oral spread and respiratory secretion spread will help. However, the main way of control is by raising the resistance of all people to polio. If everyone is made resistant to polio, the disease will have to die out. Sabin trivalent live attenuated oral polio vaccine (OPV) could be given at birth and then at 6, 10 and 14 weeks of age with the DPT or triple antigen and the polio vaccine again at 5 years of age and then each 10 years. All unimmunised adults should be given three doses of the vaccine. In an epidemic all contacts should be given a dose of the vaccine. If the contacts were not previously immunised, the vaccination course should be completed. In polio eradication programmes, extra doses will be given even if the person has been immunised before.

Polio is a 'disease under surveillance' by WHO and it is hoped to eradicate it by the year 2000. All cases must be notified immediately to your Medical Officer so that the government can control the disease and notify the WHO.

Polio can cripple people so that they cannot care for themselves (see Figure 25.12). Many people who have suffered from polio become beggars. You can make cheap surgical aids to help these people care for themselves again (See Huckstep, R.L, 'Orthopaedic appliances for developing countries' *Tropical Doctor* 1971; **1**: 64–7.)

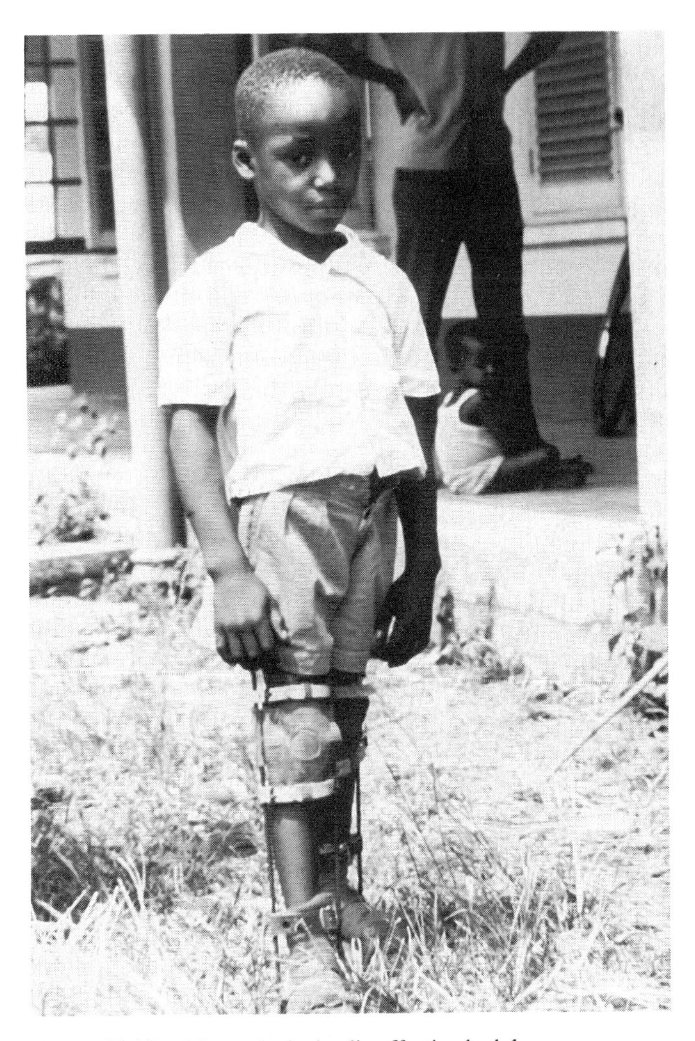

Figure 25.12 A boy who had polio affecting both legs and could not walk – he could only crawl. Calipers were made for him in a health centre at a cost of about US$1. He can now walk without help.

Cerebrovascular disease (stroke)

A stroke is a sudden paralysis or loss of one of the other functions of the body controlled by the brain. This is caused by disease of the blood vessels that bring blood to the brain.

When people get old, their blood vessels get narrower; and the blood in them may clot. If a person has high blood pressure, it can damage the blood vessels; one of these damaged blood vessels may burst or the blood in one of them clot. Some people are born with weakness in part of a blood vessel (called an aneurysm); the weak blood vessel can burst. Diseases, especially meningitis and syphilis, can damage blood vessels; and then the blood in these blood vessels can clot. A clot of blood from a diseased heart can break off and suddenly block a normal blood vessel. All of these blood vessel conditions can stop the flow of the blood to a part of the brain which then does not work and then dies, i.e. they can cause strokes.

The *symptoms* and *signs* depend on which blood vessel disease is the cause and what part of the brain is affected.

If a haemorrhage occurs the stroke usually starts suddenly. If the blood goes into the subarachnoid space, it will cause symptoms and signs of meningeal irritation like meningitis (see page 322), i.e. a severe headache, stiff neck, etc. A lumbar puncture will show blood in the CSF which does not decrease in each bottle of CSF.

If a blood vessel clots then the stroke will start slowly over a few hours; and there will be no signs of meningeal irritation.

If the part of the brain which controls movement is affected, then the patient will have paralysis. The patient will have loss of sensation, blindness, loss of speech, etc., if other parts of the brain are involved.

Do a lumbar puncture to check that the patient does not have meningitis. If the patient is young, do a serology test for syphilis (see Chapter 19 page 170) to check that the patient does not have syphilis.

The patient often dies in the first 2 days. If the patient lives for the first 2 days, he will often greatly improve for the next 6 months or more (sometimes even up to 24 months).

Treatment includes:

1. Nursing care as necessary. If the patient is unconscious, see page 332.
2. Physiotherapy. All limb joints must be moved 10–20 times each, twice daily. If the patient cannot do this, the nurse or orderly must do it.
3. Early mobilisation. The patient must get out of bed as soon as possible after the first 2 days. Help the patient to walk as well as he can even if it takes two strong people to hold him up while he tries. The patient must not stay in bed all the time. If he does, many complications will develop, and he will not get better.
4. If the patient improves, but his blood pressure stays high (more than 160/100), then see Chapter 27 page 380 or refer the case to a Medical Officer for treatment of the high blood pressure.

Tetanus

Tetanus is an acute disease of the nervous system caused by tetanus toxin. Tetanus toxin is made if tetanus bacteria grow in the body.

Tetanus bacteria (*Clostridium tetani*) normally live in the intestines of animals and in dirt. They can get into a person's body when dirt gets into the body, e.g. through wounds or burns, the female genital tract at delivery, and the cut end of a baby's umbilical cord at birth. Usually the tetanus bacteria grow and make the toxin in special types of wounds: puncture wounds, wounds or burns that get dirt in them and wounds infected by other bacteria.

The first *symptoms* are usually pain and stiffness of the jaw, difficulty in opening the mouth wide and difficulty in swallowing. The pain and stiffness then spread to the whole body. Several days later, spasms of the whole body usually occur (Figure 25.13). The spasms last from a few to several seconds. Movement of the patient's body or a sudden noise can sometimes start the spasms. During the spasms the patient is conscious and in great pain (this is different from 'fits').

There are *no tests* to make the diagnosis. If you have real doubt about meningitis or cerebral malaria, do a lumbar puncture and a blood slide, and start treatment as on page 323. Spasms can sometimes be caused by drugs such as chlorpromazine. If you suspect this, see Chapter 35 page 479. You can only diagnose tetanus from the history of the wound, the symptoms of jaw stiffness and the signs – the mouth will not open wide, general body stiffness and later spasms.

Treatment at a health centre is not usually possible. If you make the diagnosis, immediately arrange urgent transfer of the patient to hospital. Management before transfer includes:

1. Give IMI chlorpromazine 100 mg (4 ml) immediately.
2. Give IMI phenobarbitone 100–200 mg ($\frac{1}{2}$–1 ml) *or* IMI paraldehyde 10 ml immediately.
3. Set up an intravenous drip.
4. Also give IVI diazepam 10 mg (2 ml) slowly when necessary to control the spasms.
5. Give IMI human tetanus immunoglobulin 500 units (2 of the 250 international units vials) immediately. (In hospital a 3000 unit dose will be added.)
6. Give benzyl penicillin 2,000,000 units (1.2 g) immediately by IVI and continue 6th hourly.

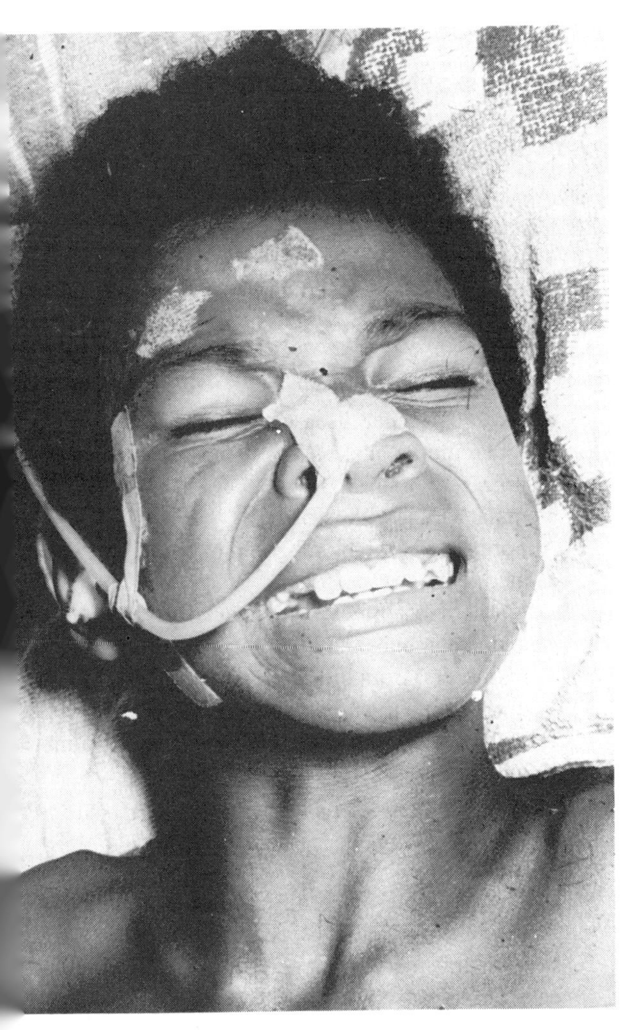

Figure 25.13 Tetanus. Note the muscles of the body are all in spasm, the head is bent backwards and the lips are pulled back (as in a smile). The patient is in great pain.

7. Nurse the patient on his side with the head lower than the feet. Gently suck out the patient's airway if it is blocked, or he is breathing noisily. Do not disturb the patient if possible.
8. Give nothing to eat or drink by mouth.
9. Clean and dress any wound.
10. A good health worker must go with the patient to the hospital. This person will care for the patient's airway, suck out the airway if necessary and give more of the above drugs for spasms if necessary.

Prevention includes:

1. Immunise all children with DPT or triple antigen and all adults with DT or tetanus toxoid three times (See Chapter 10 pages 39 and 42) and then give tetanus toxoid each 10 years.
2. Treat wounds and burns properly. Clean them all well, and remove all dead tissue from wounds.
3. If the wound is:
   (a) a deep wound, a puncture wound or a compound fracture;
   (b) a wound which has a lot of dead tissue in it;
   (c) a wound which has foreign bodies especially wood, dirt or manure (animal faeces) in it;
   (d) many hours old before you treat it, or is already clinically, infected:
   then
   - give antibiotics,
   - give tetanus toxoid 0.5 ml IMI and complete the course, if not immunised,
   - give human tetanus immunoglobulin, if not immunised, 250–500 IU (1–2 ml) in different limb from toxoid.

Peripheral neuritis or peripheral neuropathy

These are the names for the condition when the nerves (page 320) that run to the edges of the body do not work properly.

Usually (but not always) the longest nerves in the body are the most affected and therefore the legs and the arms are usually the most affected parts.

If the nerves do not work properly, sensation from the part of the body to the brain may not be normal.

1. The patient may complain of numbness or not being able to feel things in the affected area.
2. The patient may get injuries or burns without feeling them and therefore they let the cause continue until large injuries or burns or ulcers form. Even then they do not cause the pain that would be expected.
3. On the other hand, if the nerves are not completely stopped from working, the patient may feel pains or a burning sensation or a 'pins and needles' sensation or a 'crawling' sensation in the areas supplied by the nerves.
4. On examination there will be loss of some touch and pain and other sensations in the area (see Chapter 15 page 99) for ways of testing sensation.

The muscles that are supplied by the affected nerve may become weak and wasted and eventually paralysed unless the cause is stopped.

See Chapter 13 pages 99–102 for ways of testing for some of the muscles.

Causes of peripheral neuropathy are many but include the following:

- Traumatic injury including just pressure on them when lying still during drunkenness or general anaesthesia and also if the nerve is trapped by normal structures at the wrist, elbow, neck or knee.
- Infections especially: leprosy, HIV, diphtheria, typhoid.
- Post-infectious (after infections) immunological reactions (Guillain–Barré syndrome) which causes both legs to start to get weak about 3 weeks after a viral type infection and the weakness slowly goes up the legs and into the trunk and can cause death if it reaches the breathing muscles and this is not treated.
- Non-infectious immunological inflammatory conditions, especially leprosy reactions.
- Autoimmune diseases, especially rheumatoid arthritis.
- Drugs especially isoniazid if given without pyridoxine.
- Vascular causes, especially diabetes mellitus.
- Vitamin deficiencies, especially some of the vitamin B group deficiencies (e.g. pellagra, beri beri), folic acid and vitamin B_{12} deficiency.
- Poisons especially alcohol excess.
- Effects of cancers elsewhere in the body.
- Many others known.
- Many others not known (up to 50% of cases have no cause found).

If a patient has a peripheral neuropathy:

1. Treat any cause you can, especially:
   - give pyridoxine 100 mg daily if on isoniazid;
   - give vitamin B group vitamins and improve diet if any suggestion of malnutrition or alcoholism;
   - advise patient to stop any excess alcohol intake;
   - treat any leprosy reaction quickly and transfer if you are not successful;
   - control any diabetes better;
   - treat any diphtheria and transfer for anti-toxin if needed.
2. Discuss the case with your Medical Officer to see if there are any special tests you should do or special treatment you should give or if the patient should be transferred for further investigation.

Brain tumour/Intracranial mass (see page 338)

Diagnosis and management of common symptoms and signs

Unconsciousness (coma)

Causes of unconsciousness include:

1. Disease of the brain and meninges.
   - head injury
   - meningitis – bacterial, viral, tuberculous
   - cerebral malaria
   - encephalitis/African trypanosomiasis (sleeping sickness)
   - cerebrovascular disease
   - tuberculoma, abscess, cysticercosis, schistosomiasis, tumour
   - malnutrition with beriberi
2. Abnormality of the blood going to brain.
   - alcohol, drugs, poisons
   - toxins from infections, especially septicaemia and pneumonia and typhoid
   - toxins, etc. from the body – chronic kidney failure, chronic liver disease
   - low oxygen from anaemia, shock, heart failure, lung diseases
   - high sugar from diabetes; low sugar from too much insulin
   - eclampsia
   - small volume of blood circulation because of severe dehydration, especially cholera
3. Non-organic mental illness.
   - acting out

Management of the unconscious patient

Management of unconsciousness includes:

1. Give routine nursing care to the unconscious patient.
2. Record the level of consciousness hourly.
3. Diagnose and treat the cause.
   Take a full history from the patient's relatives or friends.
   Do a full physical examination.
   Make a malaria smear and give quinine and glucose.
   Do a LP. Treat for meningitis if necessary.
   Test the urine.
4. Transfer to Medical Officer care if the level of consciousness gets worse, if complications develop or if the patient is still unconscious after 24 hours.

1. *Routine nursing care of the unconscious patient*
   Maintain the airway (check that the patient can breathe):
   - lay patient on his side (never on his back) (see Figure 25.14),
   - bend his head back,
   - pull his jaw forward,
   - suck out his pharynx every hour or when there is noisy or blocked breathing (noisy breathing or snorting means blocked breathing),
   - raise the foot of the bed to let secretions run out of his mouth,
   - insert 'airway' if necessary, and
   - give artificial ventilation if the patient stops breathing because of something you can treat (e.g. snake-bite, poisoning by drugs, etc.).

   Care of pressure areas – turn every 2 hours.
   Give intravenous fluids if necessary. If you give intragastric fluids nurse the patient with his head down and on the side, and maintain his airway carefully.
   Use an indwelling catheter if the bladder becomes distended and cannot be emptied by gentle pressure every 2–4 hours (bladder distension is one of the common causes of restlessness in an unconscious patient).

2. *Record the level of consciousness*
   You should also record the size of the pupils of the eyes. Repeat these observations every hour to see if the patient is improving or getting worse. Observations will show if the patient:
   - is fully conscious, or
   - answers only simple questions, or
   - obeys only simple commands, or
   - responds (moves) only if hurt,
   - does not respond (move) if hurt, or
   - is dead.

3. *Diagnose and treat the cause*
   (a) Always take a full *medical history* from the patient's relatives or friends (see Chapter 6). Ask about the possibility of drug overdose or poisons (including alcohol) or if he has had recent treatment for an illness (including insulin) or a head injury.
   (b) Always do a full, careful *physical examination* of the patient. (See Chapter 6.)
   - Smell the breath for alcohol, diabetes and kidney failure.
   - Look carefully for a head injury.
   - Check the BP (especially if pregnant (eclampsia)).
   - Check for shock, especially from bleeding or severe dehyrdration (cholera), and treat if present (see Chapter 27 page 378).
   - Check for severe infection (e.g. septicaemia), and treat if present (see Chapter 12 page 53).
   - Check for chronic conditions (e.g. cirrhosis, kidney failure, African trypanosomiasis).

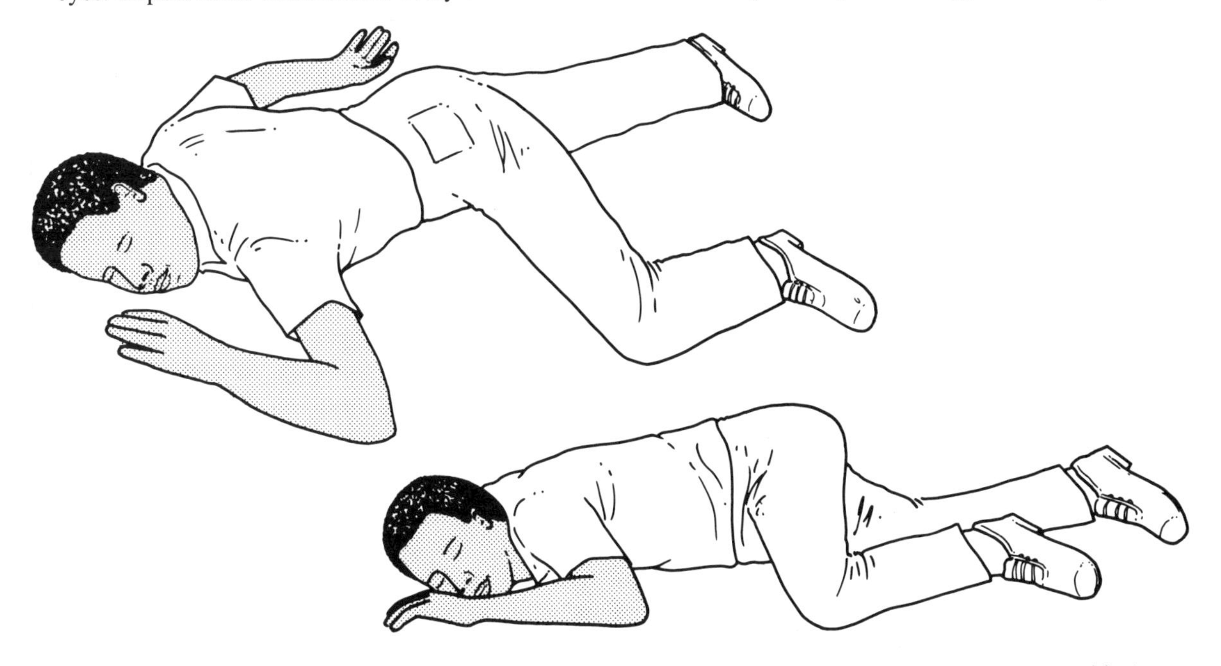

Figure 25.14 Diagram showing the position in which you should nurse an unconscious patient (the recovery position).

(c) Always do a malaria smear and *give antimalarials* for cerebral malaria (see page 325). Unless you are certain that the patient does not have malaria give quinine 10 mg/kg by IMI immediately or by SLOW IV drip (if you cannot weigh the patient, give 600 mg for large adult and 450 mg for small adult).

(d) Always do a *lumbar puncture*. Treat for meningitis if:

- the CSF is cloudy, or
- the CSF is blood stained, or
- the CSF is not obtained (failed LP).

(e) Always *test urine* for sugar, protein and bile (diabetes, eclampsia and chronic kidney failure).

(f) Always do a *blood glucose test*. If glucose low or you cannot do the test, give 50 ml of 50% glucose IV.

(g) Try to find out if patient has a psychiatric condition ('acting out') (see Chapter 35 page 476). But do not diagnose this until the patient is fully conscious again.

4. *Transfer*

   Transfer to Medical Officer care:

   (a) if the level of consciousness gets worse every hour for 4 hours (urgent – emergency) (especially important if the cause can be treated); or

   (b) if the size of one pupil does not stay the same as the size of the other pupil (urgent); or

   (c) if another complication develops which you cannot treat at the health centre (e.g. the patient is not breathing enough) (urgent); or

   (d) if the patient is still unconscious after 24 hours and not obviously improving (urgent).

   Do not transfer if the cause cannot be treated.

Simple faint (syncope)

In a faint (or attack of syncope), the patient feels light headed, is not able to see properly, has muscle weakness, cannot stand, and loses full consciousness.

If you lay the patient down, he will recover quickly – in 1–3 minutes.

Check that the patient does not have another condition, especially a fit.

Look for and treat the cause:

1. diseases of the brain,
2. abnormality of the blood going to the brain, or
3. mental disturbances.

See 'Unconsciousness' page 332 for list of causes.

Most cases are caused by:

1. standing still for a long time (blood stays in the legs and not enough goes back to the heart to go to the brain);
2. anaemia (not enough oxygen in blood going to the brain); and
3. fear, worry, disgust and pain.

Dizziness (vertigo)

This is a feeling of movement (e.g. things going around) often with faintness and nausea or vomiting.

Causes include:

1. diseases of brain (see 'Unconsciousness' page 332 for list);
2. abnormalities of blood going to brain (see 'Unconsciousness' page 332 for list);
3. some eye conditions; and
4. some ear conditions.

Treat the cause, as symptomatic treatment cannot cure the condition. Symptomatic treatment would be something such as prochlorperazine 5–12.5 mg, chlorpromazine 10–12.5 mg or promethazine 10–25 mg, as long as the blood pressure was not already low, each 4–6 hours if needed.

Convulsions (fits) and epilepsy

Convulsion (fit)

In a convulsion or a fit, the patient suddenly loses consciousness, and falls. All the muscles of his body suddenly contract and stay contracted. The face and the limbs become stiff. The patient cannot breathe and so goes blue. He may pass urine and faeces. Usually after about 30 seconds, the muscles relax. Then the muscles start to contract and then relax again and again quickly. This makes the patient's limbs jerk, and his mouth and eyes open and close. Often the patient bites his tongue. Breathing starts again but it may be very noisy. This period can last a very short or very long time; but it usually stops without treatment. Then the patient usually sleeps deeply for about half an hour. When the patient wakes, he cannot remember anything about the convulsion. Sometimes he is confused and has a headache. This is a general convulsion (grand mal).

These symptoms and signs are caused by the patient losing control of all of his brain. Without control the brain makes the body act abnormally. You can easily see the loss of control and the abnormal working of the area of the brain which makes the muscles move. All the other parts of the brain are also without control and also working abnormally during a general convulsion (or fit).

Some convulsions (fits) are different from these general convulsions. The patient may have a feeling which tells him that the fit is about to start. If only one part of the area of the brain which controls muscles is affected, only one part of the body may jerk (e.g. the face or one limb or one side of the body), and the patient may stay conscious. If only one part of the area of the brain which controls sensations is affected, the patient may only have abnormal sensation in one part of his body. If only another part of the brain is affected, the patient may have only abnormal (often violent) behaviour.

But any of these other types of fit may develop into a general convulsion if the abnormal working of part of the brain spreads to all of the brain, including all the areas that control the muscles.

Sometimes convulsions do not stop but continue for hours or longer. This is a very dangerous condition that often results in death. This is called 'status epilepticus'.

The *causes* of convulsions or fits are the same as the causes for unconsciousness (see page 332).

A convulsion (or a fit) is not a disease and is never the only diagnosis. A convulsion is caused by something which upsets the normal working of the brain. There is a disorder of the brain or the blood coming to the brain. The cause of the convulsion must always be diagnosed too and treated.

Epilepsy

Epilepsy is diagnosed if there are *repeated convulsions* over weeks, months or years. The *causes of epilepsy* are the same as the cause of a single fit. See page 332. Often it is not possible to find the cause of epilepsy. But this does not mean that there is no cause.

Epilepsy is not a disease and is never the only diagnosis. Epilepsy is caused by something which affects the normal working of the brain. You must diagnose the cause of the epilepsy if possible. Epilepsy is not infectious.

Management of a patient with convulsions (fits) or epilepsy

Management include six things:

1. When the patient is fitting, check that he does not hurt himself.
2. When the patient is unconscious, give the nursing care for an unconscious patient.
3. Stop the fit with anticonvulsant drugs: give IMI paraldehyde; if not successful give IVI diazepam.
4. Find and treat the cause.
   Take a full history from the patient's relatives or friends.
   Do a full clinical examination.
   Always check the BP, especially if pregnant.
   Make a malaria smear and give quinine.
   Do an LP. Treat for meningitis if necessary.
   Do blood glucose and give IV glucose if needed.
   Test the urine.
5. Give phenobarbitone or phenytoin when the patient can swallow, until you cure the cause of the fits (if possible).
6. Transfer if you cannot stop the fits or if you cannot find or treat the cause of the fits in the health centre.

1. *When the patient is fitting*
   Check that he does not hurt himself, e.g. fall off a bed, fall into a fire, etc. Do not try to stop the movements as this is not possible and you may injure the patient. When the mouth is opening and closing, put something between the teeth so that the patient does not bite his tongue.

2. *If the patient is unconscious*
   Give nursing care (see page 333). Check that the airway is clear (i.e. the patient can breathe) – keep on his side, keep his neck bent back, keep his jaw forward, clear his airway and suck out his throat if necessary.

3. *Give anticonvulsant drugs*
   Paraldehyde 0.2 ml/kg ($\frac{1}{5}$ ml/kg) or 10 ml for the average adult, immediately, by IMI. Repeat in 5 minutes if the patient is still fitting. After this give it once every 4–6 hours if necessary.
   If paraldehyde does not stop the fitting, give diazepam when necessary; but continue paraldehyde regularly every 6 hours.
   Diazepam by slow IVI (less than 5 mg/minute). Stop the injection as soon as the fitting stops or if

the patient is not breathing enough. Maximum dose is 15 mg. Give artificial ventilation if breathing stops. Repeat the dose after 20 minutes if the patient has not stopped fitting or starts again.
Diazepam IMI is very slow acting.
Diazepam rectally is effective if IVI not possible.

4. *Find and treat the cause* (if the patient is not a known epileptic). (See page 333.)
   (a) Always take a full medical *history* from the patient's relatives or friends (see Chapter 6). Ask about the possibility of drug overdose or poisons (including alcohol) or if he has had recent treatment for any illness (including insulin).
   (b) Always do a full careful *physical examination* (see Chapter 6):
   - smell the breath for alcohol.
   - look for head injury;
   - check the BP, especially if pregnant;
   - check for shock and treat if present;
   - check for severe infection (e.g. septicaemia) and treat if present;
   - check for chronic conditions (e.g. cirrhosis, kidney failure, African trypanosomiasis).

   (c) Always do a *lumbar puncture*. Treat for meningitis if:
   - the CSF is cloudy, or
   - the CSF is blood stained, or
   - the CSF is not obtained (failed LP).

   (d) Always do a *malaria smear* and give *antimalarials* for cerebral malaria unless you are certain that the patient does not have malaria. (See page 325.) Give the patient quinine 10 mg/kg by IMI immediately or by SLOW IV drip. If it is not possible to weigh the patient give 600 mg for large adult and 450 mg for small adult.
   (e) Always *test the urine* for protein, sugar and bile.
   (f) Always check the *blood glucose* and give 50 ml 50% glucose if blood glucose low or cannot be done.
   (g) Always *check that the patient did have a fit* and does not have another condition, e.g. tetanus, rigor, rabies, or psychiatric condition ('acting out').

5. *Give phenobarbitone or phenytoin*
   Give phenobarbitone 90 mg (3 of the 30 mg tabs) twice daily *or* 180 mg (6 of the 30 mg tabs) daily when the patient can swallow (and then stop paraldehyde) until the cause of the fits is found, treated and cured (if possible). But do not give phenobarbitone if the patient is taking chloramphenicol; use paraldehyde instead. Other drugs such as phenytoin can be added if there is still fitting. The dose is about 300 mg daily – more if the fits are not controlled or less if there are side effects, especially dizziness, unsteadiness on the feet, swelling of the gums, anaemia, rashes, enlarged lymph nodes or encephalitis.

6. *Transfer*
   Transfer to Medical Officer care:
   (a) if you cannot stop the fitting by treatment in the health centre (urgent);
   (b) if the patient has his first fit or has only recently become epileptic and you cannot find the cause (non-urgent);
   (c) if patient has another abnormal sign in the nervous system which has recently developed or is getting worse (non-urgent);
   (d) if phenobarbitone alone will not control the fits (first check that the patient is taking the phenobarbitone) (non-urgent).

Paralysis

Paralysis is when the patient cannot make a muscle or group of muscles work.

The cause is not usually in the muscle although check that the patient does not have a *muscle* injury or infection (pyomyositis) or a *bone* injury (fracture) or infection (osteomyelitis) which makes it too painful to move the muscle. The cause is usually a disease of the *nerves* which normally make the muscle move. Common diseases which cause paralysis include:

In the limbs:
- leprosy, HIV, diphtheria, etc.,
- trauma, when a nerve is cut or pressed on,
- nerve damage from drugs, especially isoniazid without pyridoxine; or diabetes; or lack of vitamin B.

In the spinal cord:
- poliomyelitis,
- fracture of the spine,
- tuberculosis or bacterial infection of the spine,
- encephalitis, schistosomiasis, African trypanosomiasis.

In the brain:
- cerebrovascular disease (stroke),
- trauma,
- encephalitis or African trypanosomiasis,
- brain abscess or tuberculosis or tumour, etc.

Mental disturbance:

- acting out.

There are other causes in all of these places. See a specialist medical reference book if it is not one of the above.

Paraplegia and quadriplegia

Paraplegia is paralysis of both legs.

Quadriplegia is paralysis of both legs and both arms.

The usual *causes* are:

- injury to spinal bones, or
- tuberculosis of spinal bones pressing on the spinal cord.

Transfer all cases for Medical Officer investigation and treatment.

If the paralysis started recently take great care not to make it worse. Do not bend or twist the patient's spine in any direction (especially the neck). Transfer the patient lying flat with sandbags or pillows packed around him so that he cannot bend or move the spine.

Headache

Headache is common. It occurs with many different kinds of illness.

Unless headache is the only symptom, use another symptom for *diagnosis*, e.g. headache and cough – find out and treat the cause of the cough, and the headache will probably go away.

If headache is the only symptom, think of all the structures in the head and neck. Take a history and do the examinations and tests to find if there is disease of one of them. Start with the structures on the inside of the head and neck, and work out towards the skin (see below).

If there is no evidence of disease, remember that anxiety is the most common cause of headache.

But do not miss the common curable causes – meningitis (especially the chronic meningitis of tuberculosis) and cerebral malaria.

Causes include diseases in the following structures:

1 *Brain* (*acute* diseases)
   - cerebral malaria
   - encephalitis

   Do a lumbar puncture if necessary. Take a malaria slide and give quinine if necessary.
2. *Brain* (*chronic* infections/tumours)
   - African trypanosomiasis (sleeping sickness)
   - tuberculoma (a 'lump' of tuberculosis); abscess
   - cysticercosis, schistosomiasis
   - brain tumour (cancer)

   Ask about epilepsy and other nervous symptoms.
   Look for weakness or change in reflexes or other nervous system signs. Are these getting worse?
   Look for other symptoms and signs of the above.
   Do these occur where patient is/was?
   Do not do a lumbar puncture.
   Transfer to a Medical Officer.
3. *Meninges*
   - meningitis – bacterial and tuberculous
   - cerebral haemorrhage

   Do lumbar puncture if necessary
   See pages 322, 326 and 329.
4. *Skull*
   - trauma

   History of trauma
   Haematoma or tenderness under scalp.
5. *Muscles*
   - tension from work, worry or habit

   Feel for tenderness of muscles.
   Move neck in all directions for stiffness and painful movements of muscles.
6. *Ears*
   - infection

   Examine ears with auriscope.
7. *Nose*
   - sinusitis

   Press over the sinuses for tenderness.
   Look for pus in nose.
8. *Mouth*
   - tooth decay and dental abscess

   Tap each tooth gently for tenderness.
9. *Eyes*
   - doing close work if long sighted

   Test eyesight with small print.
   - iritis or glaucoma

   Pupil too large or small and irregular (see Chapter 31 pages 420 and 421)
10. *Blood vessels*
    - hypertension
    - pre-eclamptic toxaemia

    Take BP.
    Look for oedema.
    Test urine for protein.
    - migraine

    Pain on only one side of the head.
    History of changes in sight and/or nausea and vomiting usually before headache.
    Treat attack with aspirin and metoclopramide
    Ask Medical Officer about treatment with ergotamine if above treatment not enough and

prevention with propranolol or amitriptyline etc. if numerous attacks.

11. *Blood coming to head*
    - other diseases especially those causing fever

    Take temperature.
    Do examination of the rest of the body.

Neck stiffness

There are four common causes of neck stiffness:

1. *Real 'neck stiffness'*, i.e. meningeal irritation. The patient cannot move his head forwards and the head is often held backwards (See Figure 25.11 page 323). If you try to bend the neck forward, this causes pain and the patient will stop you.
   Other signs of meningeal irritation may be present and are helpful if you are not certain if the neck is stiff or not (e.g. full fontanelle but only in infants, back stiffness, positive Kernig's sign).
   Very import causes include:
   - acute bacterial (purulent) meningitis,
   - cerebral malaria,
   - tuberculous meningitis, and
   - subarachnoid haemorrhage.

2. '*Meningism*' or '*meningismus*'
   No organic disease of the meninges is present and the CSF is normal.
   This sometimes occurs with other infections, especially middle ear inflammation and pneumonia.
   You must always do a lumbar puncture and find clear CSF *before* you make this diagnosis.

3. *Tetanus*
   See page 330.

4. *Torticollis and diseases of the muscles and bones of the neck*
   The patient also cannot move his head from side to side. Causes include:
   - muscle spasm,
   - arthritis of the spine, and
   - infections in the neck.

   If you have any doubt about the diagnosis always do a lumbar puncture before you make this diagnosis.

Brain tumour/Intracranial mass (from page 332)

Brain tumours or intracranial masses are lumps of tissue within the skull which progressively become larger. This diagnosis is suggested by:

1. slowly increasing loss of some part of the brain's function, e.g. slowly increasing paralysis starting in the thumb and then slowly involving more of the hand, arm, etc. and/or
2. onset of epilepsy in someone previously not epileptic and/or
3. generalised abnormality of brain function e.g.
   - headache especially on coughing, sneezing, straining, etc. or lying down; the attacks of headache gradually getting longer and at times being accompanied by vomiting,
   - change of personality,
   - development of dementia.

The diagnosis can be made only by special X-rays or scans in a hospital. If this condition is strongly suspected and there is not a strong suspicion of some type of meningitis, a lumbar puncture should not be done in a health centre as this could make the condition quickly worse. Instead the patient should be transferred to the hospital.

If the condition is due to a primary cancer of the brain cells or to secondary cancer spread from elsewhere in the body to the brain, no curative treatment is possible.

If, however, the mass is due to:

1. a tuberculoma – a mass of tuberculous inflammation tissue,
2. schistosomiasis – a mass of inflammation around eggs,
3. cysticercosis,
4. a bacterial abscess from the nose or ear or blood stream or head injury,
5. syphilis,
6. other more rare infection including *Nocardia* and *Toxoplasma*,
7. or others;

then, treatment with:

1. anti-tuberculosis drugs,
2. praziquantel,
3. praziquantel or albendazole,
4. chloramphenicol or penicillin probably with metronidazole
5. penicillin or chloramphenicol,
6. sulfadoxine 500 mg and pyrimethamine 25 mg two tablets twice daily for 6 weeks,
7. or other drugs

may help.

Similar conditions may affect the spinal cord.

Discuss such patients with your Medical Officer or transfer.

Appendix 1 The proper method of doing a lumbar puncture

First you must understand the anatomy of the spine and the spinal canal. Look at Figure 25.15.

The front of the vertebra is a strong short cylinder of bone which is called 'the body' of the vertebra. It is joined to similar bodies above and below it by 'intervertebral discs' (see Figure 25.16). This column of bone and discs is called the spine. It supports the weight of the body and allows the body to bend. (See Figure 25.17.)

Behind the body of a vertebra are thinner plates of bone which have several functions.

1. They form a hole surrounded by bone. The hole in each vertebra is lined with strong ligaments. These ligaments also go inside the hole in the next vertebrae, above and below. This makes a long cylindrical space surrounded by bone and strong ligaments, behind the vertebral bodies. This space is called the spinal *canal*. The spinal *cord* goes out of a hole at the bottom of the skull and down the spinal canal to the level of the 1st lumbar vertebra.
2. They have joints with the vertebrae above and below which make the spine stronger.
3. They have pieces of bone on each side and at the back called 'spinous processes'. These spinous processes are joined by strong ligaments and muscles to the spinous processes of vertebrae above and below them. These ligaments and muscles make the spine stronger and also move (bend and straighten etc.) the spine.
4. They fit together with the vertebrae above and below leaving holes at the sides. Nerves pass through these holes from the spinal cord to the body. (See Figure 25.16.)

A

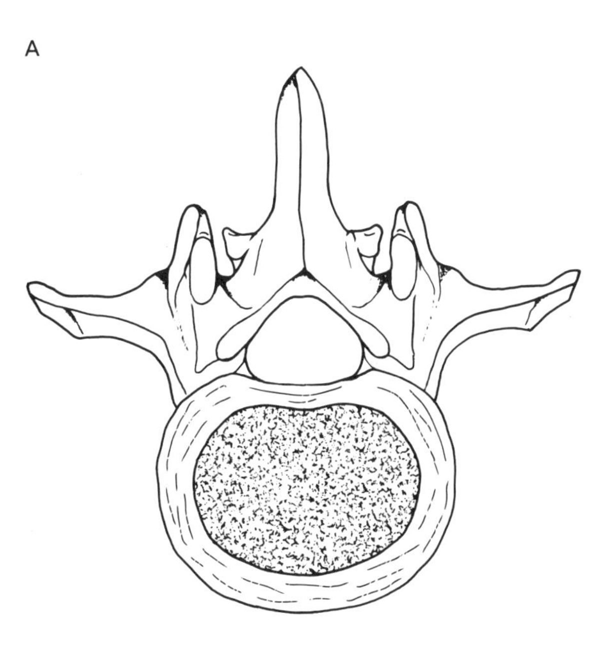

B

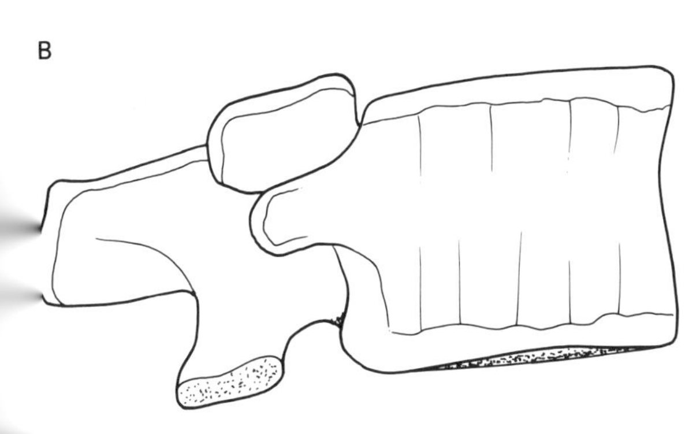

Figure 25.15 Diagram to show a single lumbar vertebra (A) from above and (B) from the side.

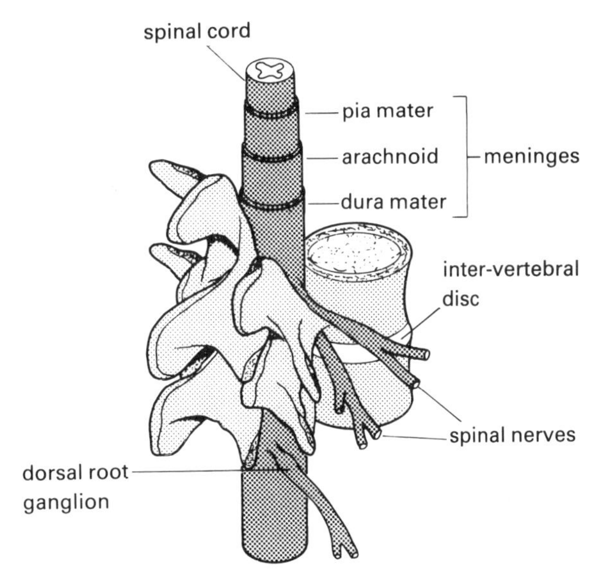

Figure 25.16 Diagram to show how vertebrae fit together and form the spine and spinal canal. The spinal cord goes through the canal, and nerves come through the holes in the spine.

In the lumbar puncture you push a needle through the skin and ligaments between the posterior spinous process of the fourth and fifth (or the fourth and third) lumbar vertebrae, and then into the spinal canal (see Figures 25.18, 25.19 and 25.20). The needle will then go through the outer layer of the meninges (dura mater) and CSF will flow back through the needle. As the spinal cord ends at about the first lumbar

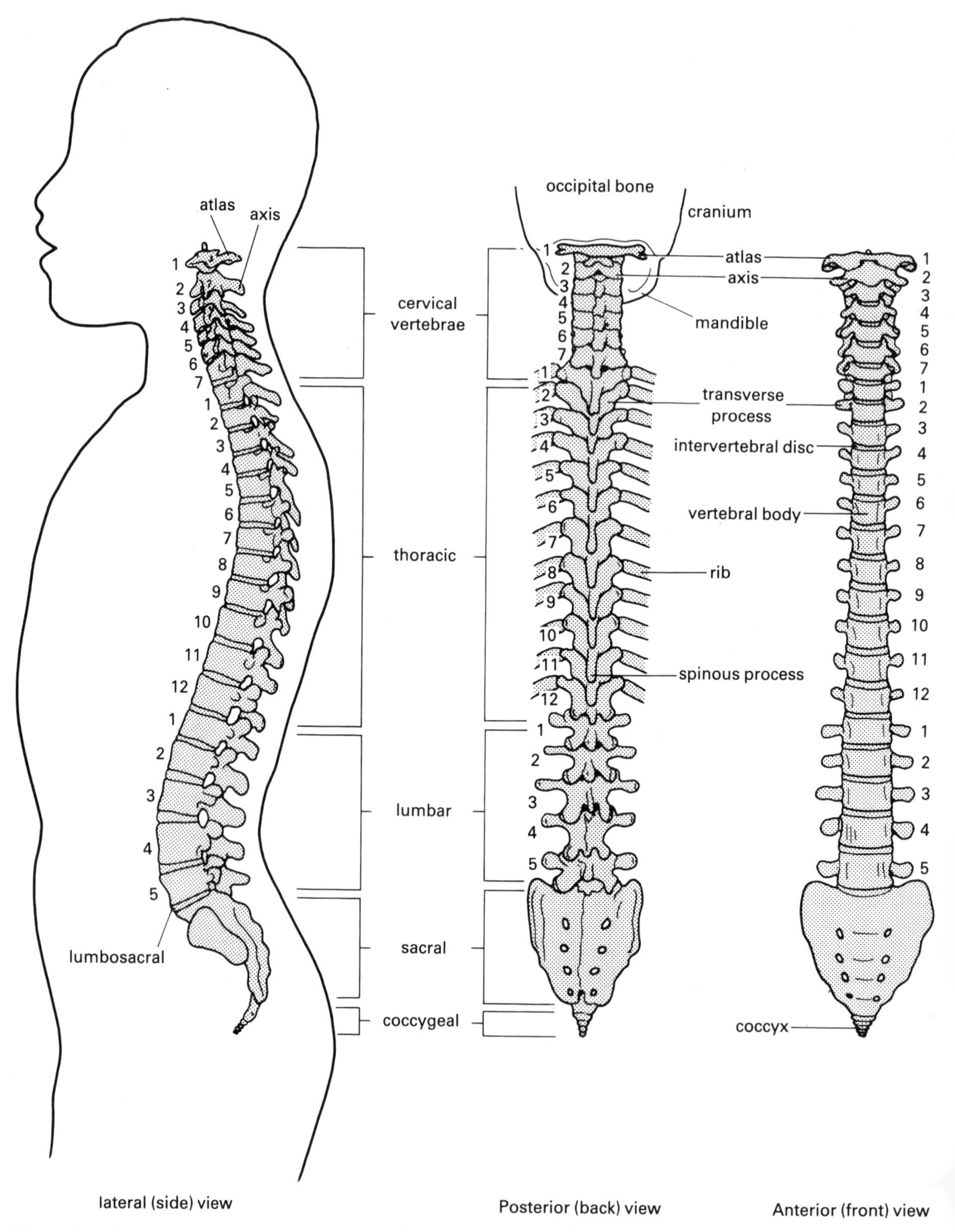

Figure 25.17 Diagram to show the vertebrae (or the spinal bones). The spinal cord goes from the brain through the spinal canal and ends at about L1. Lumbar puncture is done at L3–4. Note how flexion (bending forward) of the spine will open up the space the lumbar puncture needle must go through into the spinal canal.

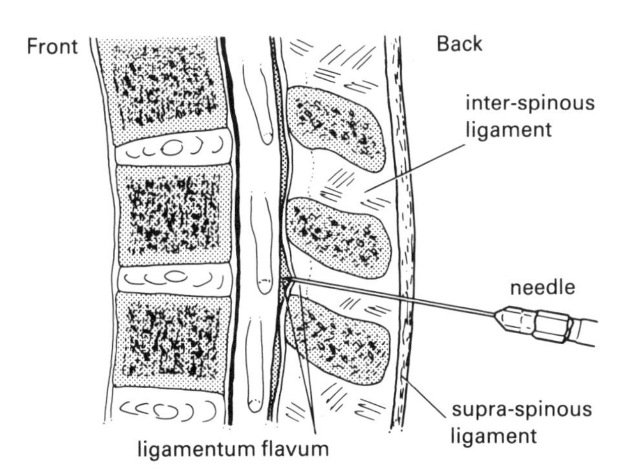

Figure 25.18 Diagram to show the ligaments through which you must push the lumbar puncture needle to get into the spinal canal. The ligaments join the bones of the spine. The diagram shows the 2nd, 3rd and 4th lumbar vertebrae in section from the front to the back.

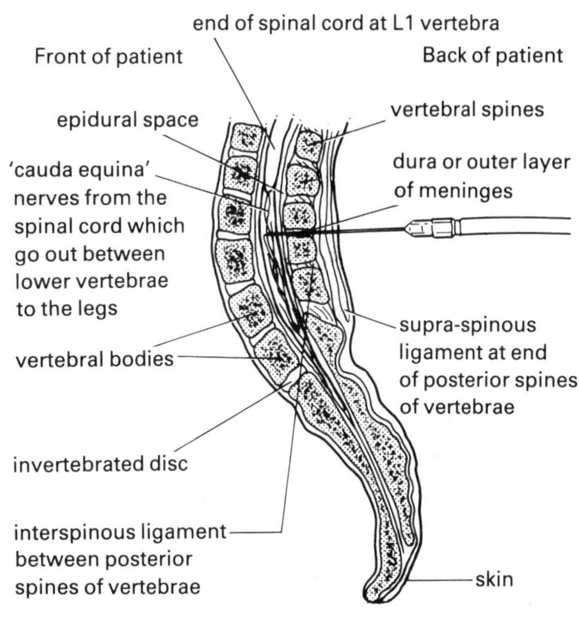

Figure 25.19 This diagram shows the lumbar and sacral spine in section from the front to the back. Note the anatomy of the spine and spinal cord. Note the structures through which the lumbar puncture needle goes to get into the spinal canal between the 3rd and 4th lumbar vertebrae. If the needle is directed too high or too low it will hit bone and not enter the spinal canal. Note that flexing (bending forward) the lumbar spine will open up the spaces between the lumbar vertebral posterior spinous processes and leave more space for the needle.

vertebra (a little lower in infants) there are only some nerves in this area. You cannot damage the spinal cord here. You should not damage nerves; but if they are damaged, they will probably recover.

To do a lumbar puncture successfully, you must put the patient in the proper position and put the needle into the patient in the proper place and in the proper direction. This is the proper method:

1. Before you start, sedate the patient with paraldehyde 0.1–0.2 ml/kg ($\frac{1}{10}$–$\frac{1}{5}$ ml/kg) (5–10 ml) by IMI if he is likely to be unhelpful.
2. Train an assistant to hold the patient properly. Good assistants often hold a patient well by

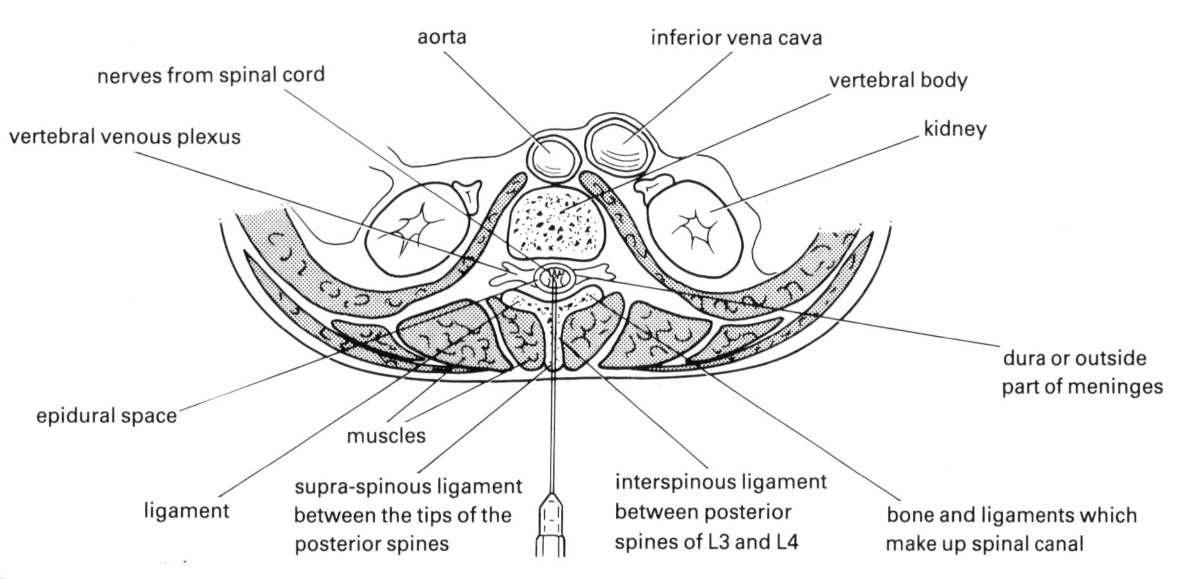

Figure 25.20 This diagram shows the third lumbar intervertebral disc (in section from side to side). Note that a lumbar puncture needle must go straight in to reach the spinal canal. If it goes to one side it will miss the spinal canal.

putting one arm at the back of the patient's bent neck and the other arm behind the patient's bent knees, and then holding his own hands together.

3. Use a flat, hard surface such as a wooden bed, table or bench (a sagging bed is not good).
4. Put the patient with his head to your left.
5. The vertebral column (backbone) must be close to the edge of the bed.
6. The lumbar vertebral column must be parallel with the edge of the bed.
7. The head must be bent forward, with the chin on the chest.
8. The knees and hips must be completely bent and the knees pushed up onto the chest.

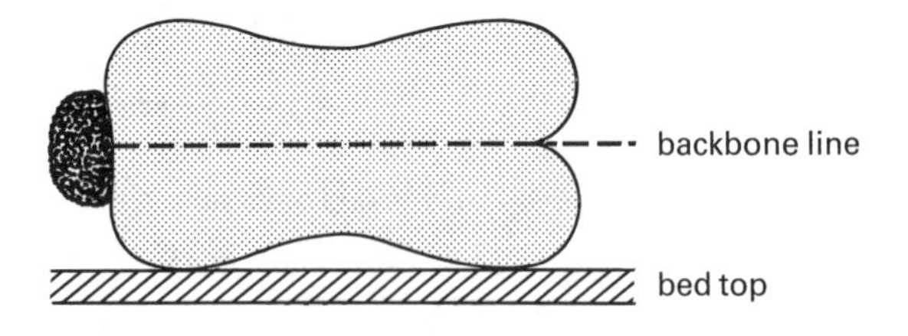

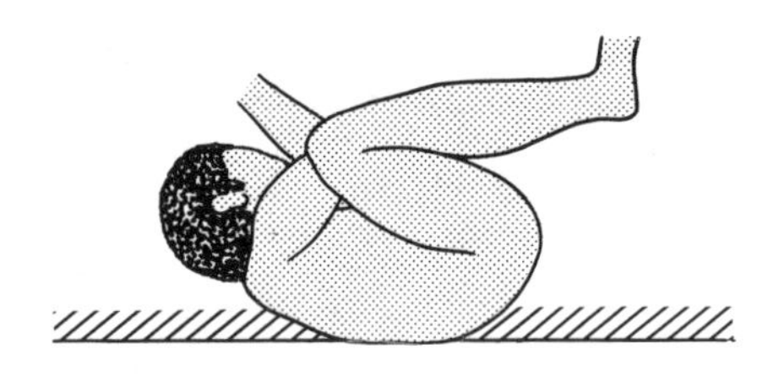

9. Check that the vertebral column is bent in a half circle.
10. Put a support (e.g. sandbag, folded towel) between the bed and the patient's waist, as the hips and shoulders are wider than the waist. (This is not necessary in children or very fat patients).
    If you do not do this, the vertebral column will be twisted.

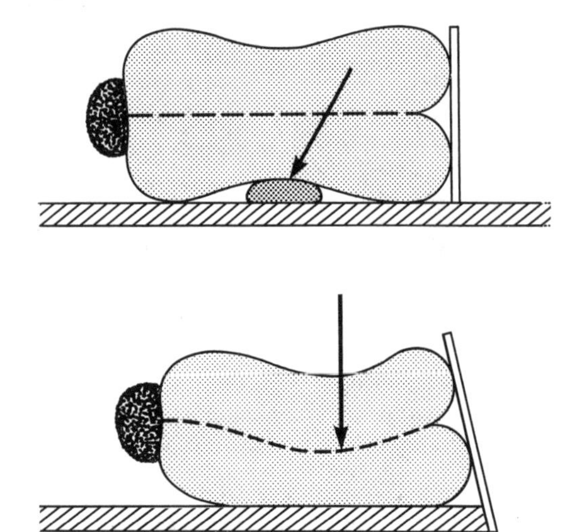

11. When looking from above the patient, check that the right shoulder is exactly above the left shoulder.
12. When looking from above the patient, the right iliac crest (hip) must also be exactly above the left one. Put the right knee on top of the left knee, with a pillow between them.

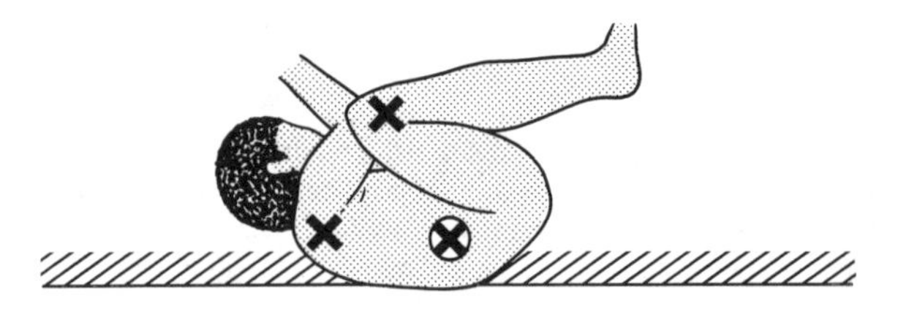

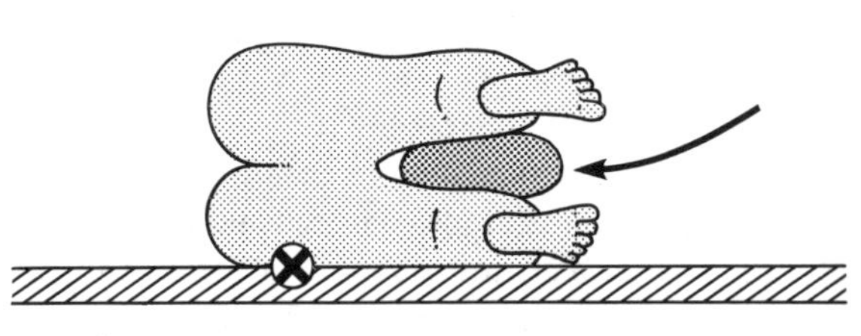

If you do all this properly the patient is now in the proper position for you to do the lumbar puncture. Do not attempt a lumbar puncture until the patient is in the proper position; or you will not get any CSF.

13. Wash your hands well. Then clean the patient's back with iodine in alcohol (or other antiseptic).
14. Put a drape on top of the right iliac crest and waist.

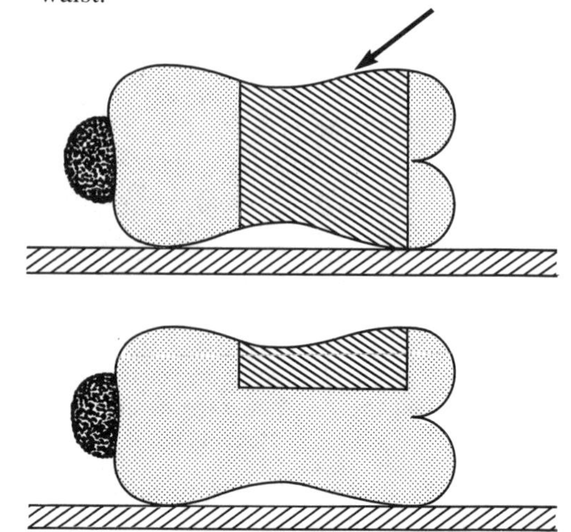

15. With your right hand, move a finger from the top of the right iliac crest straight down to the backbone. This will show you the position of the vertebral spine (bony lump) of the fourth lumbar vertebra.

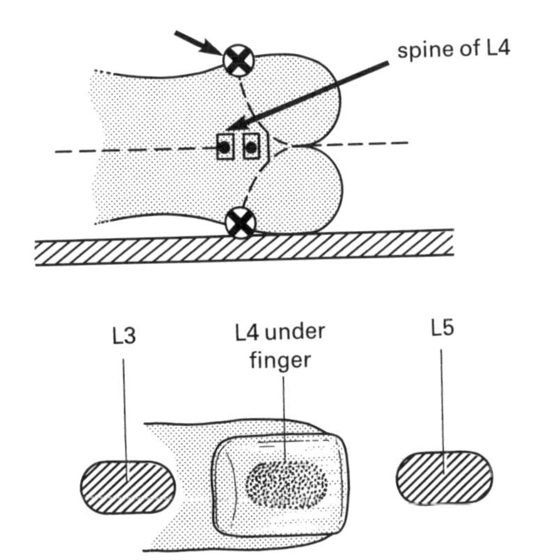

16. Move the finger which is on the spine of L4, straight down towards the patient's buttocks to find the space between L4 and L5 – this is where you will put the spinal needle in. Mark the skin vertically in the centre of this space by pressing firmly with your thumb-nail for half a minute.
17. Now you must find the centre line of the spine from the head to the buttocks. It is the line which joins the centre (highest parts) of the bony spines. It almost always is *not* the same place as the hollow of the skin along the spine. You must feel the bony spines to find it. Mark this horizontally with your thumb-nail on the skin.

    There will now be a cross on the skin between the vertebral spines and in the centre line of the spine. This is where you will put the lumbar puncture needle in.

    Gently clean the area again with iodine (or other antiseptic).
18. In an older child or adult, give 2–5 ml of 1% lignocaine using a 26G needle. Put the needle through the skin exactly in the centre of the cross. First raise up a swelling *in* the skin (i.e. give an intradermal injection). Then inject deeper between the spines of L4 and L5. So that you do not lose the place after injecting the local anaesthetic, disconnect the syringe but leave the needle in the skin until you are ready to put the LP needle in. Wait 3 minutes for the local anesthetic to work.
19. Put the lumbar puncture needle in the gap between L4 and L5 where the needle for the local anaesthetic was, exactly in the centre of the cross. Check that the LP needle is in the proper position. *It must be at a right angle (90°) to the patient's back* at the L4 level *in both directions.* Check that this is so by looking *both* from above the patient and from the end of the patient along his spine. Then push the needle in, always checking that it is at right angles to the patient in both directions.

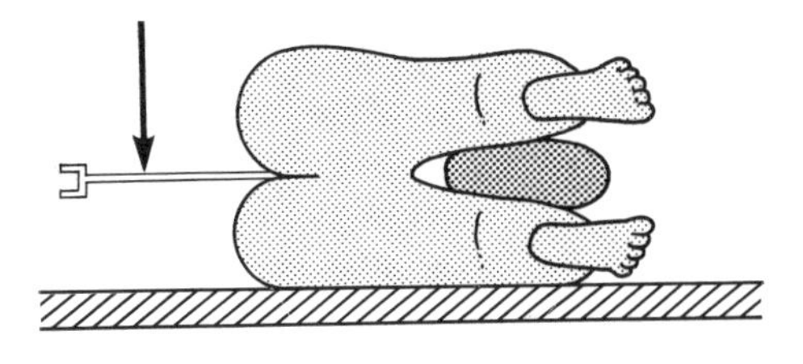

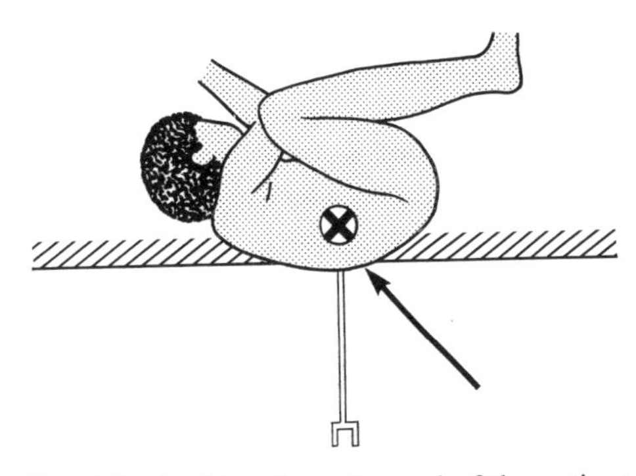

Check by looking from the end of the patient and from above the patient to see if the needle is straight.

20. In children you can use a needle from an IV drip set or a disposable needle.

    In adults, use a size 20 or 18 spinal needle with the proper fitting inner part (stilette or trochar) (as the disposable and drip set needles are often not long enough for adults).
21. The layers you push the needle through are in order

    (a) the skin
    (b) subcutaneous fat
    (c) spinal ligament
    (d) meninges (dura mater) – this is the last layer and you often feel the needle suddenly go through into the space where the CSF is.

    Push the needle in *very* slowly. Stop several times and remove the stilette and look to see if

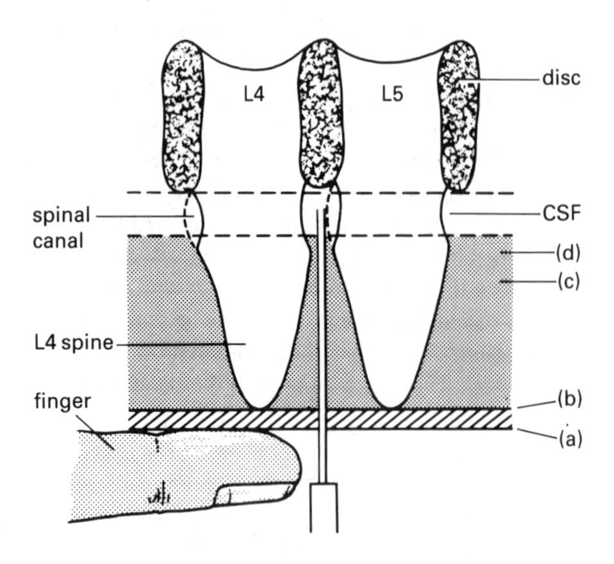

CSF comes out especially after you feel the needle has gone through something. Turn the needle round if you think the needle is in the proper position but no CSF comes out when you remove the stilette.

25. If you do not get CSF when you cannot push the needle in any further check that the needle:
(a) is exactly in between two vertebral spines; and that it
(b) is in the centre of the spine lengthways (and not in the centre of the skin fold in the back which often does not lie over the the centre of the spine); and that it
(c) has gone in the right direction (at right angles to the patient at L4 in both directions).
If all these are so, remove the stilette, continue to turn the needle around slowly, and slowly pull it out looking to see if CSF comes as you start to pull the needle out.
If you get no CSF put the needle in again in a slightly different direction – usually more towards the patient's head. Pull the needle right out to the surface of the skin before trying again.
If you still get no CSF after several changes of position (including pushing the needle towards the feet), take the needle right out.
26. Check that the needle was in fact in the centre line of the spine and in the middle of the space. Then try the LP again.
27. If you still do not get CSF repeat the whole process one space further up, towards the patient's head.
28. Collect the CSF in two sterile bottles, about 30 drops (2 ml) in each bottle.
29. If the CSF is blood stained, do not remove the lumbar puncture needle. Allow the bloodstained CSF to continue to come out. Collect 2 or 3 ml in three or four bottles. Note if the CSF becomes clearer in each bottle or if the amount of blood stays the same in each bottle.
30. Carefully remove the spinal needle, put on a small square of sterile gauze over the hole and lay the patient flat on his abdomen for 2–3 hours.
31. The whole procedure must be sterile. Wash or scrub the hands well, as for an operation. If possible, wear sterile gloves. Clean the patient well with an alcoholic solution of antiseptic. Only use a sterilised LP needle. *Never* touch the part of the needle which goes into the patient (especially the needle tip) with the fingers even after scrubbing up and putting on sterile gloves (i.e. use a 'no touch' technique).

Appendix 2 Examination of the CSF

Naked eye examination of the CSF

See page 321.

Laboratory examination of the CSF

Always send the CSF for laboratory examination if possible. Ask for the first five of these tests on all CSF samples. Ask for a Medical Officer to send you a report on what the tests mean. (See Table 25.1 page 346.)

Tests on CSF samples:

1. Cells, total count. Normally fewer than 5/cubic mm are present.
2. Cells, differential count. Normally all are mononuclears (usually lymphocytes). (No red blood cells.).
3. Protein. Normally 15–45 mg% or 150–450 mg/l.
4. Sugar or glucose. Normally 45–100 mg% or 2.5–4 mmol/l (varies with blood glucose and is about two-thirds of blood glucose).
5. Gram stain for organisms. Normally negative (or no organisms seen).
6. Ziehl–Neelsen (ZN) stain for AFB. Normally negative (or no AFB seen).
7. Culture/sensitivity for bacteria. Normally negative (or no growth).
8. Culture for tuberculosis organisms. Naturally negative (or no growth).
9. Other tests if necessary.

Table 25.1 Typical CSF test results in the common conditions for which CSF tests are necessary.

	Cells		*Gram stain*	*Protein*	*Sugar*	*ZN stain*	*Bacterial culture*	*TB culture*
	Total	*Differential*						
Normal	0–5	All lymphocytes	No organisms	15–45 mg%	40–100 mg%	No AFB	No growth	No growth
Acute bacterial meningitis	Increased (up to thousands)	N > L	Often bacteria	Increased	< 40; usually none	No AFB	Often growth	No growth
Cerebral malaria	Normal	L > N	No organisms	Normal or increased	Normal	No AFB	No growth	No growth
Viral meningitis	Increased (tens or hundreds)	L > N	No organisms	Increased	Normal	No AFB	No growth	No growth
Encephalitis	Normal or increased (tens or hundreds)	L > N	No organisms	Increased or normal	Normal	No AFB	No growth	No growth
Tuberculous meningitis	Increased (up to hundreds)	L > N usually; N > L early	No organisms	Increased	Decreased or none	Sometimes AFB	No growth	Often growth
Cerebral haemorrhage early	Many RBCs	Normal	No organisms	Increased	Normal	No AFB	No growth	No growth
Cerebral haemorrhage late	Normal or increased	L > N	No organisms	Increased	Normal	No AFB	No growth	No growth
Traumatic tap	Many RBCs	Normal	No organisms	Increased	Normal	No AFB	No growth	No growth
Cerebral tumour or tuberculoma or abscess	Normal or increased	Varies	No organisms	Increased or normal	Normal	No AFB	No growth	No growth

26

Disorders of the Urinary System

Anatomy and physiology

When the cells of the body do their work, they make several waste products, including urea, uric acid and carbon dioxide. The blood removes these waste products from the cells.

The carbon dioxide passes from the blood into the air in the lungs.

Each time the heart contracts (pumps), about one-fifth of the blood it pumps out goes through the kidneys. The kidneys remove most of the waste products from the blood which goes through them.

The kidneys remove the waste products from the blood so efficiently that when this one-fifth of the blood mixes with the other four-fifths of the blood, which did not go through the kidneys (and still has waste products in it), the concentration (or amount) of waste products in the mixed blood is never high.

The waste products removed from the blood by the kidneys are dissolved in water, and this is called urine. The urine goes down a tube, called a ureter, from each kidney, to the bladder. The bladder is a muscular storage bag in the pelvis. The bladder can hold about $\frac{1}{2}$ litre of urine before it must be emptied. The body passes the urine from the bladder out through the urethra. (See Figures 26.1, 26.2, 26.3.)

The urine also contains any salt or water which the body does not need. There is normally no protein and no sugar in the urine.

The body needs to pass about 800 ml of water in the urine everyday, in order to remove the normal amount of waste products made each day.

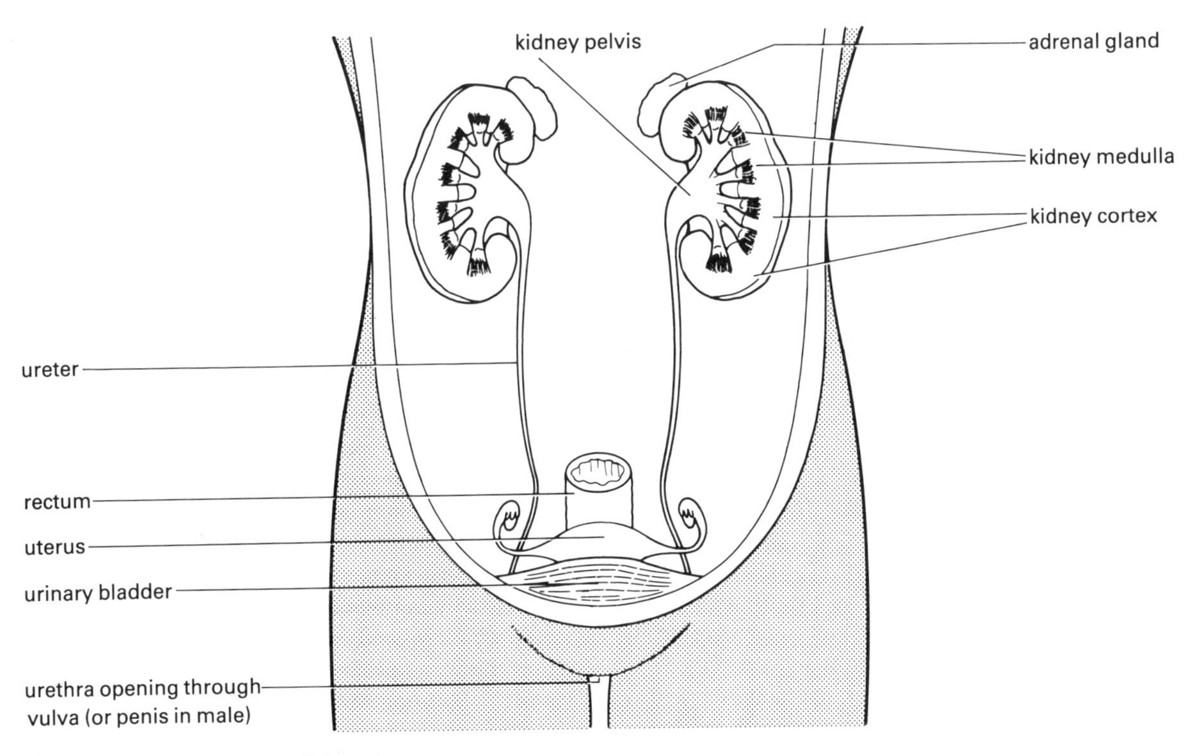

Figure 26.1 The anatomy of the urinary system.

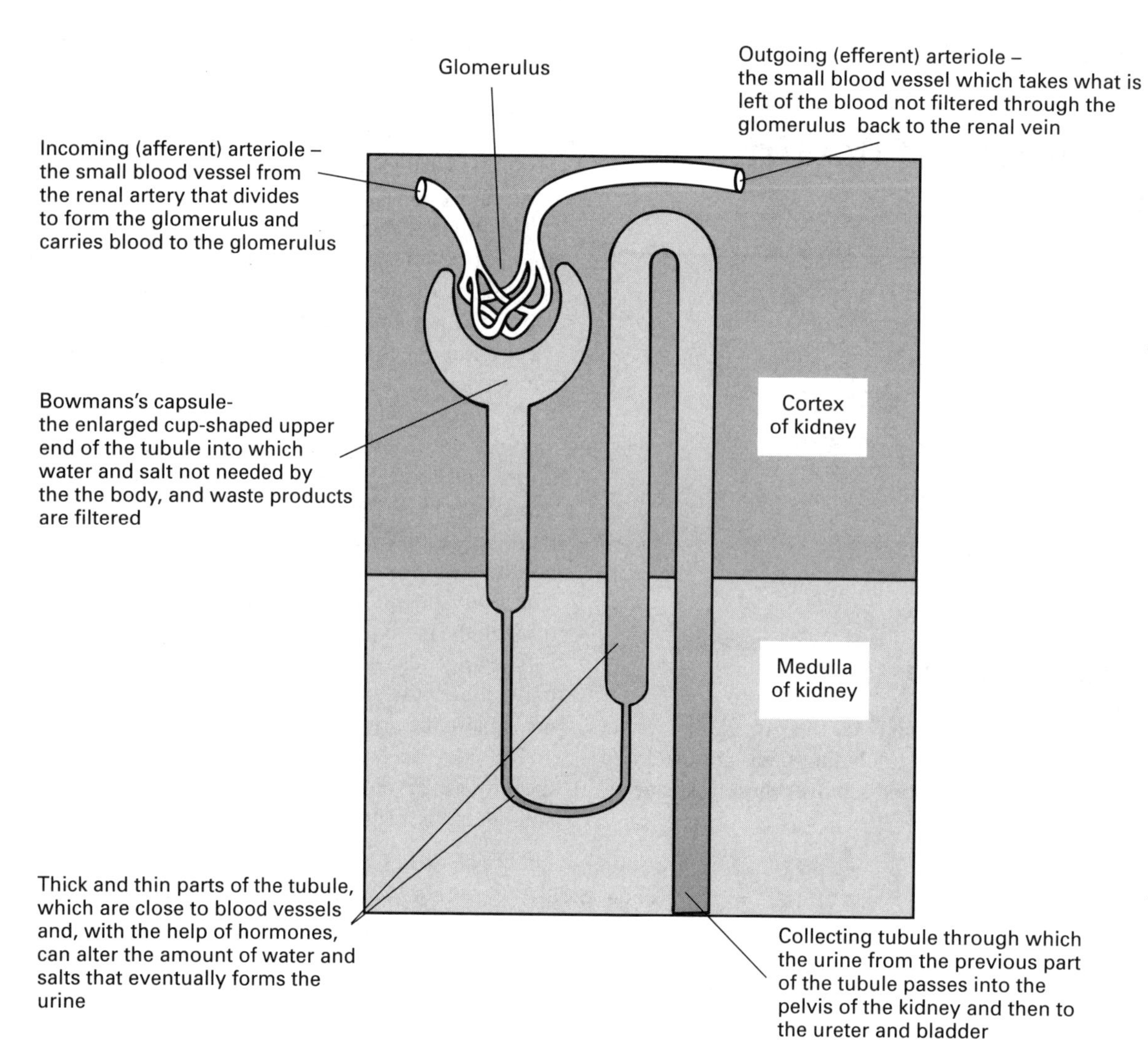

Figure 26.2 A diagram of one of the one million units in each kidney which take waste products and unwanted water and salt from the blood and put them into the urine.

Each kidney is made up of about one million separate little filters which do its work. The blood comes to the kidney in the renal artery which branches into more and more smaller vessels until it eventually ends up in little tufts (bunches or collections) of capillaries called 'glomeruli'. Water, salt and waste products are filtered out through these glomerular capillaries and red blood cells and protein are not allowed through. These tufts of capillaries are surrounded by the enlarged end of the tubules (little tubes) which collect the water, salt and waste products filtered through the glomeruli and carry them to the ureter and bladder. However, the tubules can also get back some of the water or the salt if the body needs it. (See Figure 26.2.)

Pathology

If the body is dehydrated, there is not enough water to make 800 ml of urine each day. So all the waste products in the urine are dissolved in only a little water. The urine is concentrated. The common causes of acute dehydration are gastroenteritis (when much fluid is lost from the body in vomiting or diarrhoea) and when the patient is too sick to drink enough. Chronic dehydration can occur in hot dry places in people who drink only a little water. In some of these people the waste products are not all dissolved in the water of the urine. The waste products then make small (or even large) stones in the kidneys or bladder. Infections in the urinary tract can make stones in the

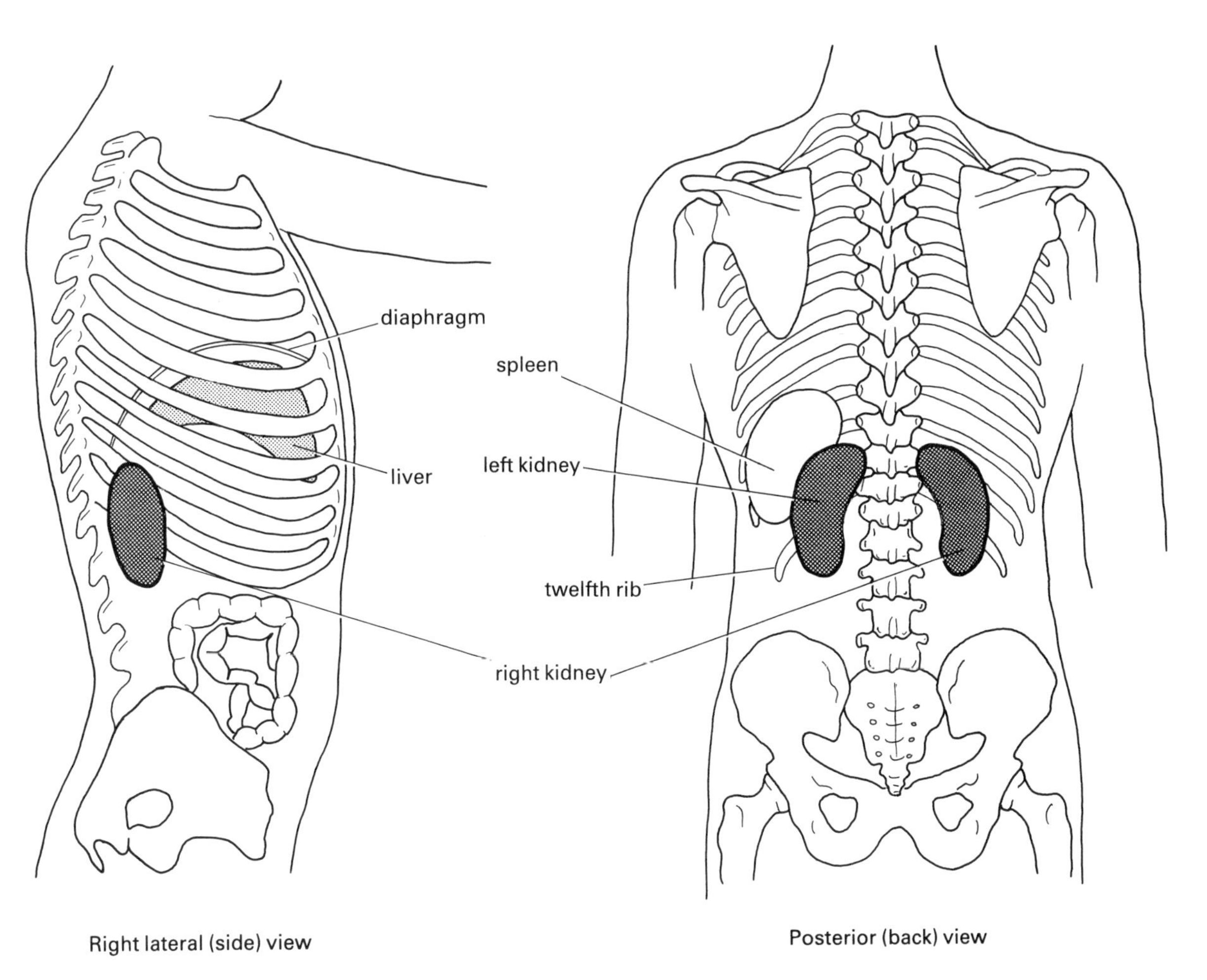

Figure 26.3 The position of the kidneys. Note that the kidneys are both posterior (at the back) and are also high in the abdomen, partly under the ribs.

kidneys or bladder even when there is no dehydration.

If the body is very dehydrated, it will make very little urine. Then the body cannot remove the waste products and salt, and the concentration of the waste products and salt rises in the blood. This is called 'kidney failure'. If this happens quickly, it is called acute kidney failure or 'renal failure'.

Some acute conditions can damage the kidney very severely – and stop the kidney working. The kidney cannot make urine, so the waste products and salt remain in the body and cause death in a few days. This is called acute kidney failure.

Some conditions damage the kidney so that it can still work; but it cannot work properly. It cannot dissolve all the waste products in only 800 ml of water. It needs much more water to remove all the waste products. And still more waste products than normal remain in the blood. This is called 'chronic kidney failure' or 'chronic renal failure'. If a person with chronic kidney failure does not get enough fluid, then the concentration of waste products in his blood quickly rises, and he also gets acute kidney failure.

Infection is the most common pathological condition of the urinary tract. Infection in one part of the kidney tract easily spreads to another part (or all parts) of the urinary tract.

In the kidney itself the glomeruli are the parts most often damaged by disease. Other parts can, and are at times, damaged and you may hear such words as 'tubular necrosis', 'vasculitis', etc. Damage to the glomeruli, however, is called 'glomerulonephritis'. If the glomeruli (which you remember are made up of tufts of little capillaries through which water, salt and waste products are filtered but red cells and protein are not allowed through) are damaged, any of all of the following can occur:

1. Protein can leak through the glomeruli and cause protein in the urine (proteinuria) (see page 365).
2. A lot of protein can leak through the glomeruli and cause nephrotic syndrome (see page 356).
3. Red blood cells can leak through the glomeruli and cause blood in the urine or haematuria.
4. Acute inflammation of the glomeruli can occur and cause acute nephritic syndrome (see page 358).
5. Acute kidney failure (see page 363) can occur if enough glomeruli are suddenly damaged and do not work.
6. Chronic renal failure (see page 359) can occur if more and more glomeruli are slowly damaged.

Conditions that cause glomerulonephritis are many, but in tropical countries most of them are due to abnormal reactions to infections including:

- hepatitis B virus and HIV infections;
- tuberculosis, leprosy and syphilis bacterial infections;
- malaria, especially *Plasmodium malariae*
- schistosomiasis, onchocerciasis, *Loa loa* and filariasis.

Note that these infections do not infect the kidney but there is an abnormal immunological or body reaction to them. The appearance of the glomeruli under the microscope also can be quite different from one condition to another, although glomerulonephritis can produce only the above six conditions.

Urea is the main waste product of the body and you can easily measure it in a laboratory. In the blood of a normal healthy person, there is less than 40 mg urea/100 ml of blood or less than 6.6 mmol urea/l (litre) of blood. If the blood urea is more than 100 mg/100 ml or more than 16 mmol/l, then the patient has kidney failure and may die unless you give him treatment. Creatinine gives an even better guide to kidney function but is a more difficult waste product to measure in the laboratory. The normal range is 15–35 mg/100 ml or 0.4–1.2 mmol/l.

Symptoms and signs of disease of urinary tract

Symptoms of urinary tract disease

1. *Urinary symptoms*
    - urethral discharge of pus, or white fluid, or watery fluid
    - dysuria
    - urinary frequency
    - change in colour or urine
    - blood in urine
    - pain in
        - urethra (felt in the penis)
        - prostate (felt in the perineum in front of the anus)
        - bladder (felt in the lower central abdomen)
        - kidneys (felt in the loin (or back where the lower ribs join the spine))
        - ureter (felt anywhere from one loin to the iliac fossa or genitalia or inner upper leg on the same side)
2. *Symptoms of infection*
    - fever
    - rigors
    - malaise etc.
3. *Symptoms of kidney failure*
    - see page 359.
4. *Symptoms of oedema*
    - swelling of ankles, back, face, etc.

> *Always ask all patients about these urinary symptoms:*
> 1. pain or a burning feeling when passing urine (called dysuria).
> 2. passing urine more often than normal (called urinary frequency) and more than once at night (called nocturia),
> 3. abnormal colour of the urine, including blood in the urine.

Signs of urinary tract disease

1. *Urinary tract signs*
    (a) kidney
    - tenderness (see Figures 26.3 and 26.4)
    - enlargement (see Figure 26.4)

    (b) bladder
    - tenderness
    - enlargement

    (c) urethra
    - discharge (see Chapter 19 pages 155 and 160)
    - tenderness

    (d) abnormalities of the external genitalia

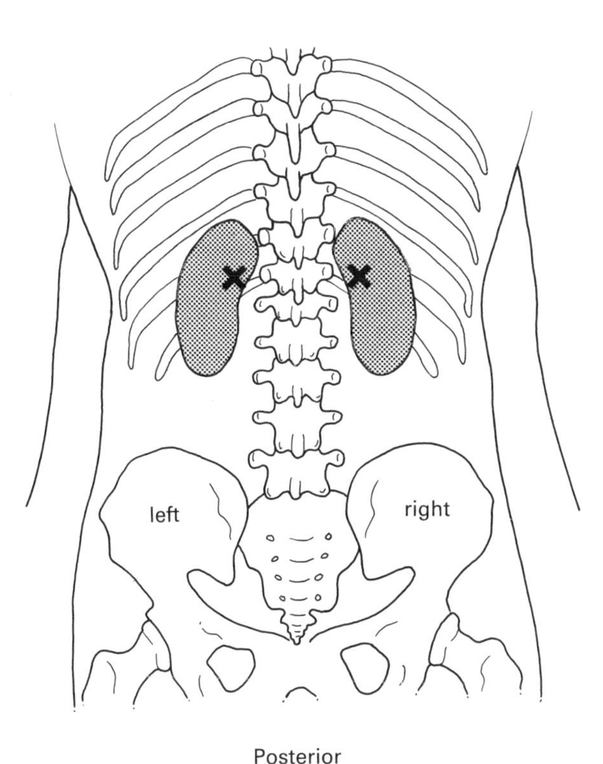

Figure 26.4 Diagram showing where (marked with a cross) you *gently* hit the patient with the side of your fist, to find out if the kidneys are tender.

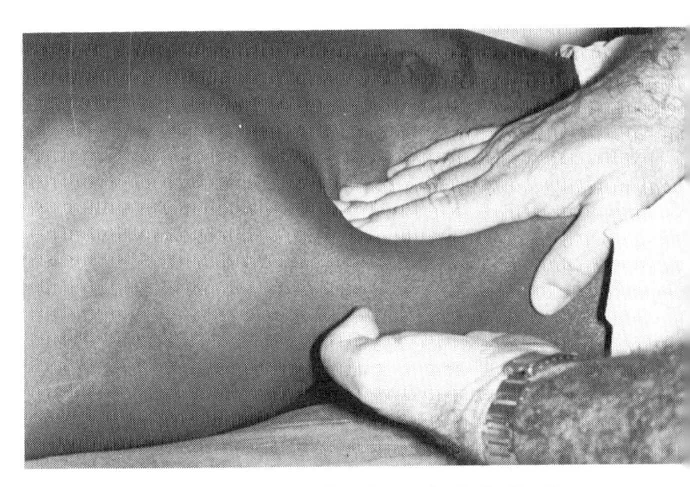

Figure 26.5 Photograph showing the method of palpation of the kidneys. Use both hands. Put one hand flat on the abdomen beside the long central abdominal muscle and below the edge of the ribs. Put the other hand in the angle between the ribs and the spine and gently lift the kidney upwards. Ask the patient to take a deep breath. When the patient has nearly finished breathing in, press the front hand gently down and quickly bend the fingers of the back hand upwards. If the kidney is enlarged you will feel the kidney hit the top hand. Then feel the kidney slide back between the hands as the patient breathes out. In thin people you can often feel the lower part of a normal right kidney.

(e) prostate or uterine { enlargement / lumpiness / tenderness } on pelvic examination through the rectum ('PR')

(See Figures 26.6, 26.7, 26.8 and 26.9.)

(f) vaginal, urethral, bladder or uterine abnormalities on pelvic examination through the vagina ('PV')

(See Figure 26.8 and an obstetrics and gynaecology textbook.)

2. *Signs of infection*
   - raised temperature
   - fast pulse rate
3. *Signs of kidney failure*
   See page 359.
4. *Signs of oedema*
   Swelling of the ankles, back, face etc. If you press gently with a finger you will make a hollow in the skin and underlying tissues which only returns to normal slowly.
   See Chapter 36 page 485.
5. *High blood pressure*
   See Chapter 27 page 380.

Always look for these urinary tract signs on all patients during a general medical examination.

1. Kidney tenderness, during abdominal examination.
   (See Figures 26.3 and 26.4.)
2. Bladder tenderness / bladder enlargement } during abdominal examination
3. Abnormalities of external genitalia, during abdominal examination.
   (See Chapter 19 page 158 and Figures 26.6, 26.7 and 26.8.)

Tests

Urethral and cervical (if female) smear

Take smears if you suspect urethritis – see Chapter 19 page 158.

Urine test

Test urine for:

- protein,

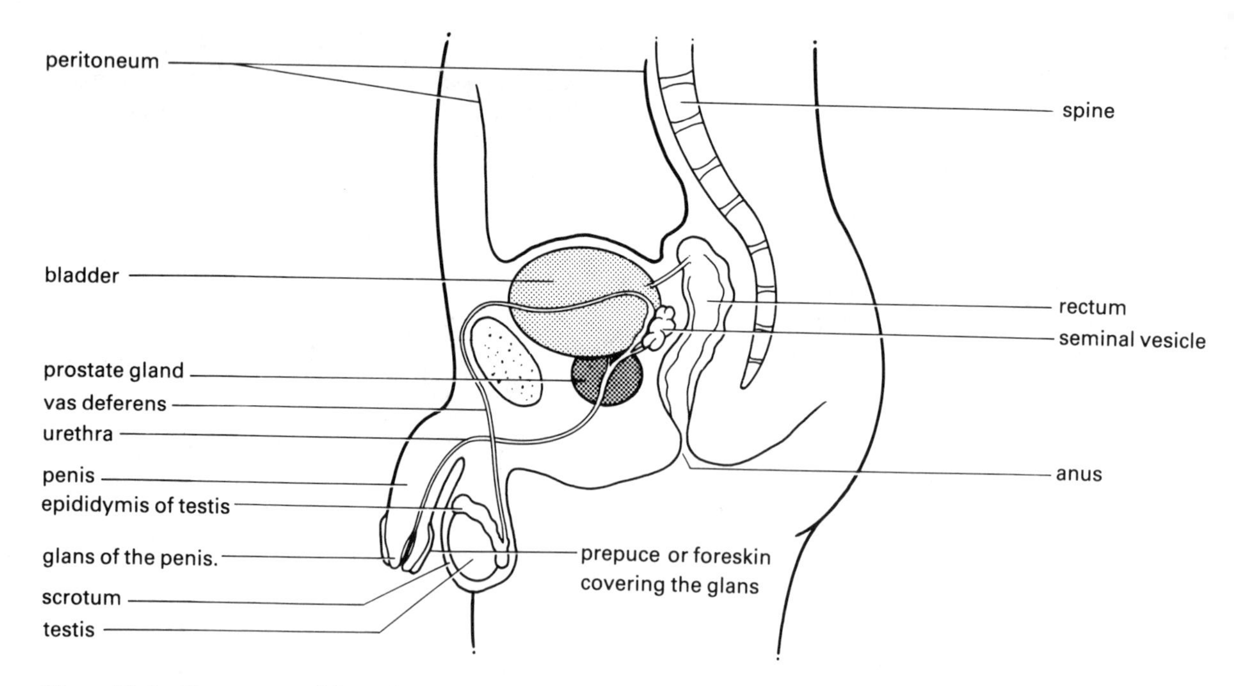

Figure 26.6 The anatomy of the male pelvis. The pelvis is shown in section from front to back. Note the structures which you can feel anteriorly (in the front) on pelvic examination through the rectum (per rectum or 'PR') – anal sphincter (muscle), prostate, seminal vesicles and bladder.

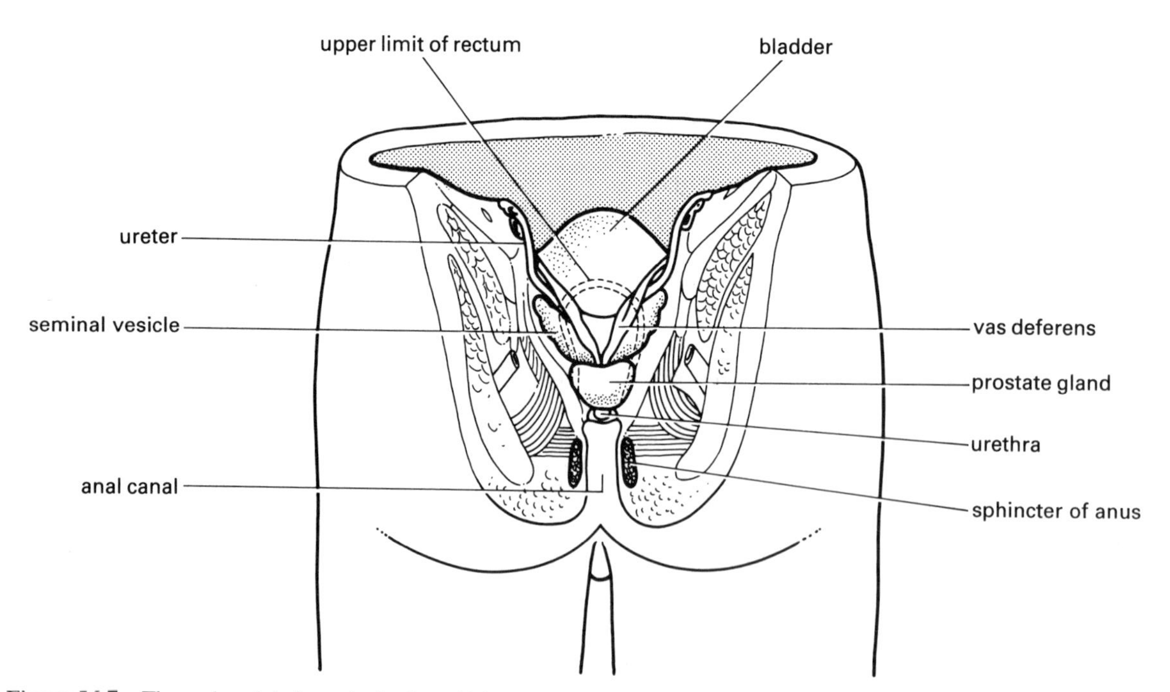

Figure 26.7 The male pelvis from the back, as if the buttocks and bones and rectum at the back had been cut away. Note again the structures which you can feel on rectal examination 'PR' – anal sphincter, prostate, seminal vesicles and bladder.

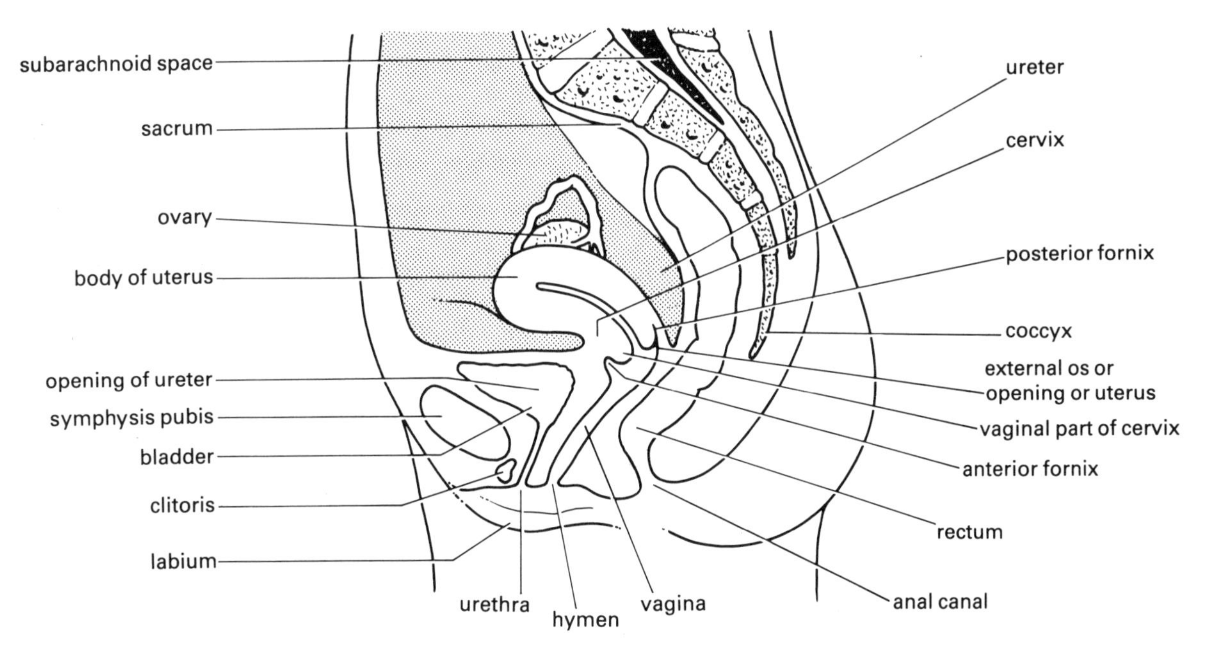

Figure 26.8 The anatomy of the female pelvis. The pelvis is shown in section from front to back. Note the structures which you can feel anteriorly (in the front). Through the rectum (per rectum or 'PR') you can feel the vagina and the cervix of the uterus. Through the vagina (per vaginum or 'PV') you can feel the urethra, bladder, cervix and uterus. For method of examination 'PV' see a specialist gynaecology/obstetrics book.

- sugar,
- blood,
- pus, and
- bile.

If you have no laboratory and no microscope, Figure 26.10 shows how you can still examine the urine and also what you may find.

Urine microscopy (examination of centrifuged urine under the microscope) normally shows fewer than 5 white cells (sometimes called pus cells) in each high power field (HPF) and fewer than 5 red blood cells (usually none) in each high power field (HPF). If you see more than 5 white cells/HPF this suggests inflammation of the urinary tract, which is most often caused by bacterial infection (see this page). If you see more than 5 red cells/HPF, this is called 'haematuria'. Haematuria usually means a serious disease (see page 364).

Proteinuria is present if there is more than a trace of protein in the urine (see page 365).

There should be no sugar in the urine. If sugar is present, see page 364.

Blood urea and serum creatinine

See page 350.

Diseases of the urinary tract

Urinary tract infection

Definition

Urinary tract infection (UTI) is present if there is an acute or chronic inflammation of one or more parts of the urinary tract. It can have these special names:

1. Urethritis – urethra only inflamed.
2. Prostatitis – prostate only inflamed.
3. Cystitis – bladder only inflamed.
4. Pyelonephritis – kidney or kidneys inflamed (but all the other parts of the urinary tract are also affected as the infected urine runs through them.
5. Urinary tract infection – it is not known which parts of the urinary tract are inflamed, or all of the urinary tract is inflamed.

If one part of the urinary tract is infected, you should treat the patient as if all the urinary tract were infected.

Causes

These organisms can cause infection:

1. Ordinary bacteria – these cause infections which are usually acute but can also be chronic.

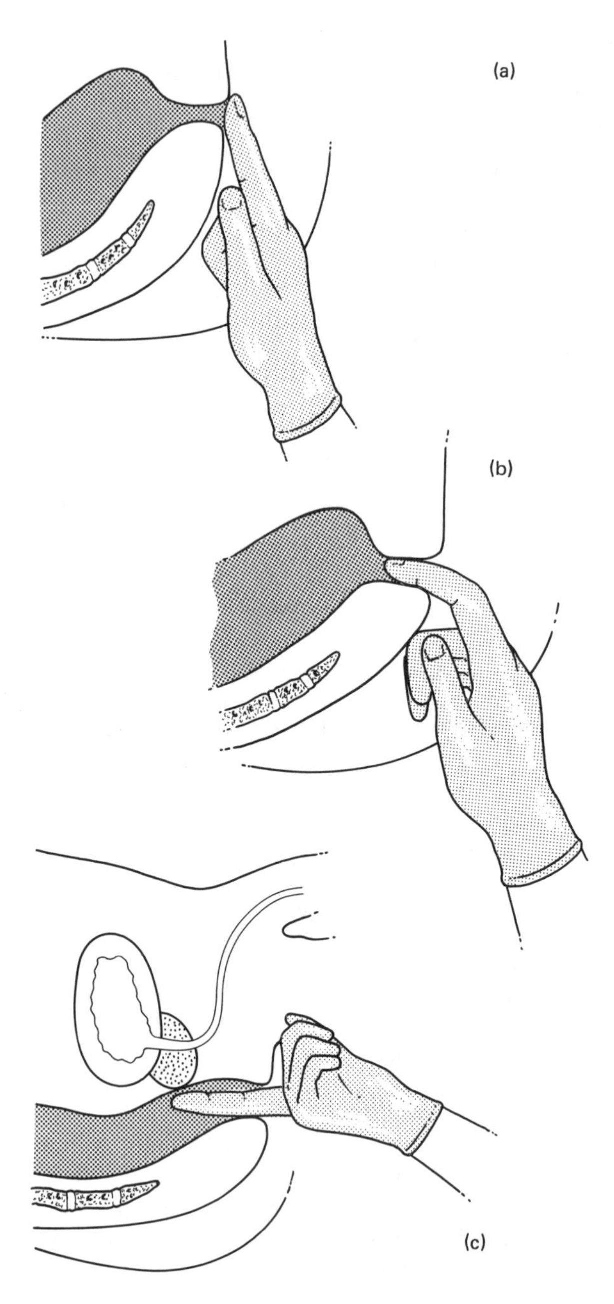

Figure 26.9 Method of examination through the rectum ('PR'). Explain to the patient what you will do. Lay the patient on his left side with his back and hips bent forward. Wear a glove and put a lubricant on the index finger. First put the finger flat on the anus as shown (A). Then press gently backwards. The finger will then gently go into the rectum (B). Do not try to push the finger straight into the rectum. Then turn the finger round to the front of the patient (C). Gently examine the structures shown in Figures 26.7, 26.8 and 26.9 for tenderness, lumpiness or enlargement. At the end of the examination gently clean any lubricant remaining outside the anus.

2. Tuberculosis bacteria – these usually cause chronic infections.
3. Schistosomiasis worms – there is usually chronic infestation. This only occurs in some countries. (See Chapter 18 page 150.)

Causes of bacterial urinary tract infection include:

1. Gonorrhoea or non-gonococcal urethritis (usually *Chlamydia*):
   Always ask about the possibility of these sexually transmitted diseases.
   Always suspect these, even if the patient says he could not have a sexually transmitted infection.
2. Use of an urethral catheter, even if done correctly. Try not to use an urethral catheter.
3. Intercourse or pregnancy or no special cause in some normal females.
   If the infection does not get better or if the infection returns often, look for an abnormality in the urinary tract.
4. Common abnormalities in the urinary tract include:
   - enlarged prostate gland,
   - stone in the bladder or kidney,
   - tuberculosis,
   - schistosomiasis (only in some countries), and
   - cancer.

Normal males do not get ordinary bacterial urinary tract infections, but normal females sometimes do. If a male gets urinary tract infection, always look for 1, 2 and 4 above.

Symptoms

Symptoms include:

1. Dysuria (pain or a burning feeling when passing urine).
2. Urinary frequency including at night.
3. Pain in the;
   - back (loin) if the kidney is affected,
   - lower central abdomen if the bladder is affected.
   - rectal area and perineum if the prostate is affected.
   - penis if the urethra is infected.
4. Toxaemia (general symptoms of infection including fever, rigors, malaise, etc.) if the kidney is infected. (Toxaemia is not usually present if the infection does not involve the kidney.)

Signs

Signs include:

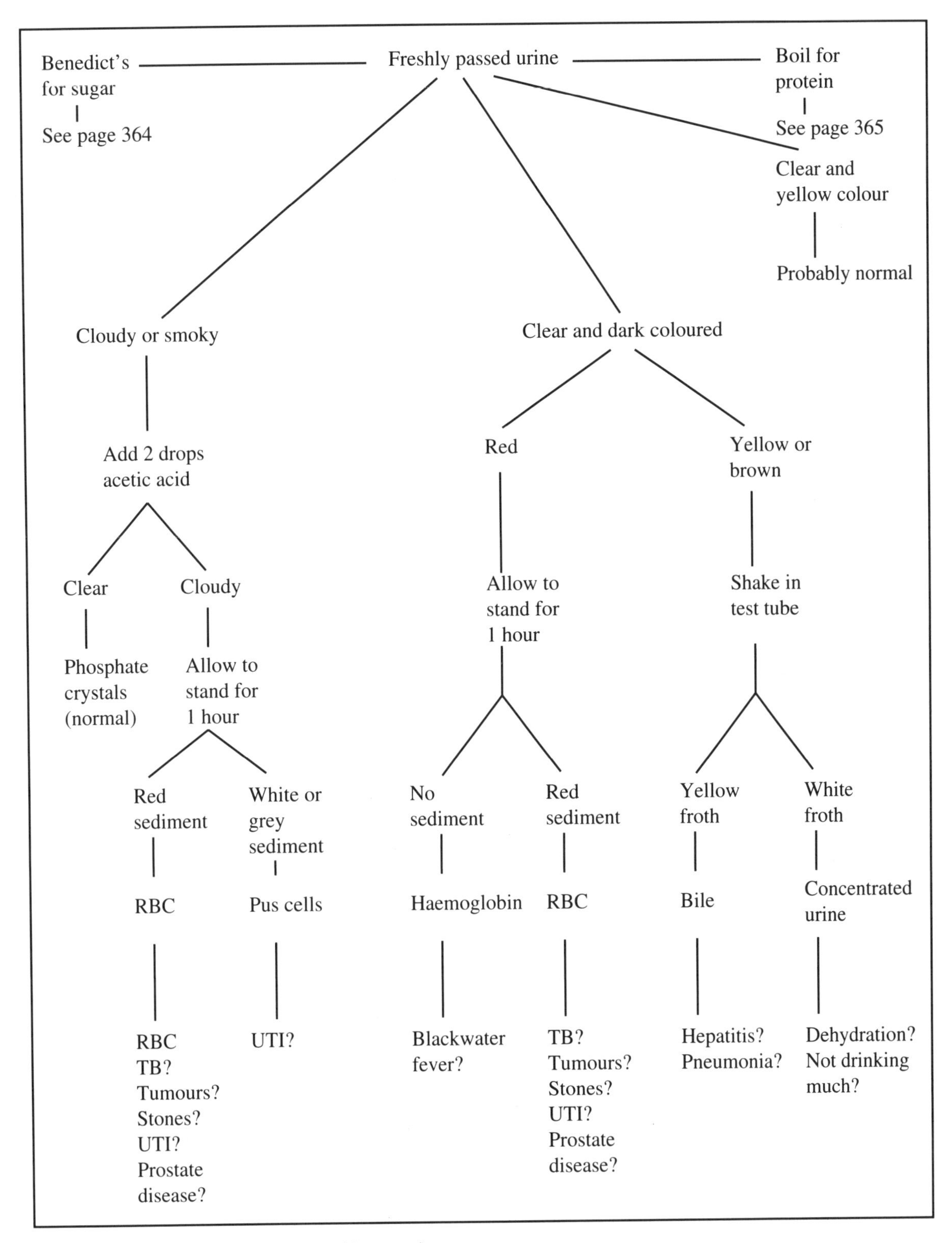

Figure 26.10 Examination of the urine without a microscope.
RBC, red blood cells; TB, tuberculosis, UTI, urinary tract infection

1. Tenderness over the affected area of the urinary tract (see above).
2. Toxaemia (fever, fast pulse, etc.) if the kidney is infected. (Toxaemia is not usually present if the kidney is not affected.)

Tests

Tests that you must do include:

1. Examination of a mid-stream specimen of urine for protein, sugar, pus cells and red blood cells. If a laboratory available send for culture and sensitivity test also (see also pages 353 and 355).
2. Take a urethral smear for gonococci and send it to the laboratory (if possible to do; and if urethritis is a possibility).
3. Test urine for schistosomiasis if patient from or in an area where this occurs. Send sample for ova or eggs to be looked for under the microscope. Otherwise look for miracidia (see Chapter 18 page 153).

Details of management

Examine a mid-stream specimen of urine for pus, blood, protein and sugar (if there is infection, pus and usually protein (trace to $\frac{1}{4}$) are present).

Ask if urethral or vaginal discharge is present and if a sexually transmitted disease is possible. Take a urethral and (in females) cervical smear for gonococci and treat for urethritis if the history or examination suggests it is possible (see Chapter 19 page 160).

Do an abdominal and pelvic examination (PV in women and PR in men) to check for genital tract disease (especially important if the infection is not quickly cured or it returns after treatment).

Check that the patient does not only have urinary frequency from normal pregnancy.

Treat as an outpatient. Admit for inpatient treatment only if sick.

1. *If* there is any possibility of urethritis:
   Give drugs to treat urethritis (See Chapter 19 page 160).
   Give treatment otherwise as follows.
2. Sulphamethoxazole 800 mg/trimethoprim 160 mg (co-trimoxazole) twice daily or trimethoprim 300 mg once daily or 200 mg twice daily or sulphadimidine 1 g (2 tabs) 4 four times a day for 10 days.
3. If the patient does not improve after 2–4 days or is not cured after 10 days give tetracycline or doxycycline (if not pregnant) or amoxycillin or ampicillin (if pregnant) 250–500 mg three or four times a day for 10 days.
4. If the patient does not improve after 2–4 days or is not cured after 10 days of tetracycline or ampicillin, give chloramphenicol 750 mg (3 caps) four times a day for 10 days.
5. Give antimalarial drugs as indicated, if there is any fever (see Chapter 13 page 161).
6. Tell the patient to drink plenty of fluid.
7. If tests show ova or eggs or miracidia of schistosome, treat with praziquantel. See Chapter 18 page 154.

Examine a mid-stream specimen of urine (for pus and protein) after the treatment is finished to check that the infection has gone.

Transfer or *refer* to Medical Officer care:

1. if the patient is not clinically cured and the urine tests are not clear after this treatment (non-urgent);
2. if a male has more than one attack (non-urgent);
3. if a female has an infection that returns often (e.g. three or more infections in less than one year) (non-urgent); or
4. if there is blood in the urine at any time which is not caused by schistosomiasis (see Chapter 18 page 150) (non-urgent).

Glomerulonephritis

See page 349.

Nephrotic syndrome

Definition

Nephrotic syndrome is a condition in which a patient has glomerular damage and enough protein leaks out of the capillaries in the glomeruli into the kidney tubules and then into the urine to cause the following.

1. There is much protein in the urine (more than $\frac{1}{8}$ or 1+ on boiling the urine or more than 3 grams per 24 hour output of urine).
2. There is oedema of the whole body (swelling because of an abnormal amount of fluid in the whole body) because not enough protein (albumin) is left in the blood to hold the water and salt part of the blood inside the blood vessels.
3. You can find no other cause for the oedema (such as malnutrition, severe anaemia, heart failure, chronic liver disease, toxaemia of pregnancy, acute nephritic syndrome, filariasis, etc.)

Causes

Many conditions damage the glomeruli in the kidney and lead to nephrotic syndrome including the following:

- diabetes mellitus,
- autoimmune diseases,
- the end result of some cases of acute nephritic syndrome,
- a reaction to certain infections such as *Plasmodium malariae*.
- damage to the kidney and other parts of the body by chronic infections and chronic inflammations which have lasted for a long time such as lepromatous leprosy and severe bronchiectasis,
- some drugs,
- and many others.

In many cases it is not possible to find out what condition has led to nephrotic syndrome but this does not affect your management of the disease. However, check to see that your patient does not have a cause you can stop.

Symptoms

Usually swelling caused by oedema is the only symptom (see Figure 26.11). Malaise may be present.

Signs

Usually oedema is the only sign.

Tests

The urine has much protein in it (more than $\frac{1}{8}$ or +). You must test the urine in all patients who have oedema.

Differential diagnosis

See Chapter 36 page 485 for causes of oedema of the whole body. Very important causes include:

1. kidney diseases, including nephrotic syndrome,
2. malnutrition,
3. heart failure,
4. severe anaemia, especially if caused by hookworm, and
5. chronic liver disease (cirrhosis).

Details of management

Do not diagnose nephrotic syndrome unless there is generalised oedema and much protein in the urine (more than + or $\frac{1}{8}$th).

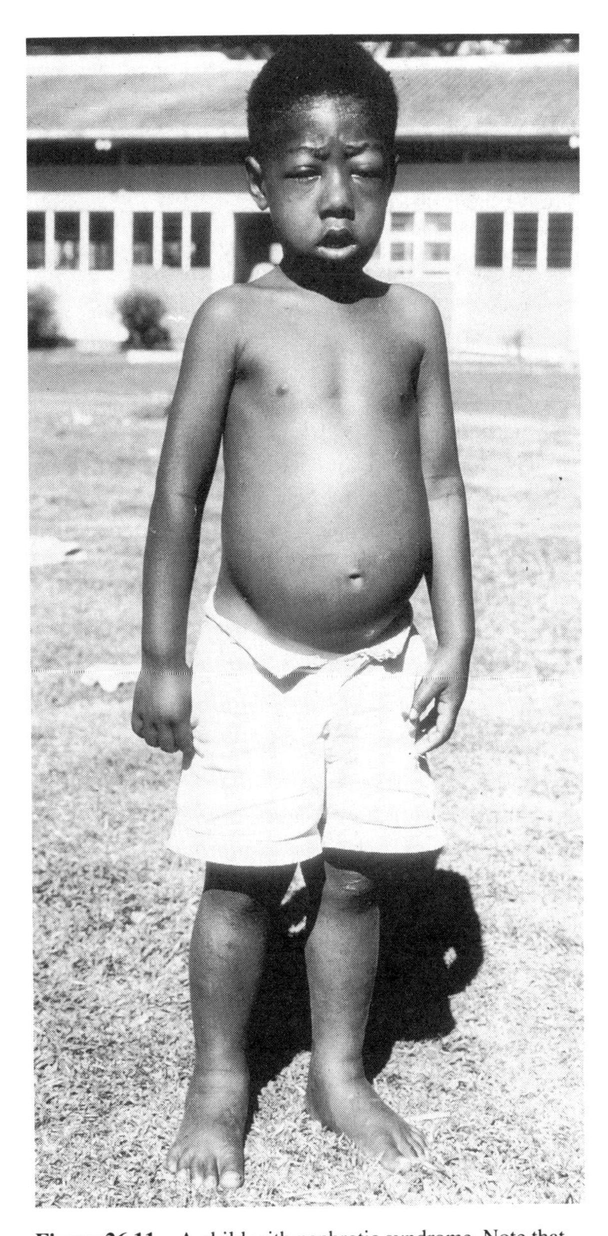

Figure 26.11 A child with nephrotic syndrome. Note that he has swelling of *all* of his body including his face. Swelling of the face suggests (but does not prove) a kidney cause for oedema of the whole body. General oedema (though often with a different distribution can be caused by: (1) kidney disease (especially nephrotic syndrome), (2) malnutrition, (3) chronic liver disease (cirrhosis), (4) severe anaemia, (5) heart failure, (6) filariasis (usually only the limbs affected), (7) other conditions (see text). Swelling of the face alone may be caused by an allergic reaction and needs urgent treatment with adrenaline and antihistamine, if the allergic swelling starts to block breathing.

Check that the patient does not have another cause for generalised oedema (other kidney disease, heart failure, malnutrition, severe anaemia, chronic liver disease filariasis, etc).

Admit for inpatient treatment to check the effect of treatment and the progress of the disease (but you can treat as an outpatient if necessary).

Give the following *treatment*:

1. No salt in the diet, i.e. no salty food, no salt added when cooking food and no salt added after food is cooked.
2. Routine diuretics.
   Hydrochlorothiazide 50–100 mg (1–2 tabs) each morning.
3. Normal protein diet with no added salt. High protein diet does not help as this gives more protein for the kidney to lose. (Tinned fish and meat are not satisfactory as they contain much salt. Give fresh foods if possible.)
4. Antimalarial drugs as indicated, usually chloroquine 450–600 mg 3–4 tabs) daily for 3 days then 300 mg (2 tabs) weekly.
5. Treatment for intestinal worms.
   See Chapter 23 page 278 (to stop any protein loss for worms in bowel).
6. Test the urine for protein every day and weigh the patient to check if he is improving.
7. Give powerful diuretics if the patient is not improving. Start with a small dose.
   Frusemide (furosemide) 40–160 mg (1–4 tabs) daily. If this is not successful give frusemide 20–60 mg (2–6 ml) IVI daily for a few days.
8. Special diuretics such as spironolactone or amiloride or triamterene would be helpful if ordinary diuretics and frusemide are not enough to control the oedema.
9. Potassium chloride 1200 mg (2 tabs) three times a day if you give frusemide and/or the patient is not on a tuber diet, but do not give potassium chloride if the patient is also taking spironolactone or amiloride or triamterene.
10. Look carefully for acute bacterial infections and malaria. Give proper treatment quickly if they occur.

Transfer the patient to Medical Officer care, but only after discussion with the Medical Officer:

1. if you cannot remove the oedema after 3–6 weeks; or
2. if the proteinuria has not gone after 3–6 weeks; or
3. if a micro-urine examination shows more than the normal number of red blood cells or white blood (pus) cells;

as special tests may show a cause that can be treated and as other drugs (e.g. prednisolone) can sometimes help special cases.

Schistosomiasis

Schistosomiasis is a very important cause of disease of the urinary tract.

Schistosomiasis only occurs in parts of Africa, the Middle East, India, South-East Asia including the Philippines, and South America. (See Figure 18.13 page 151.)

Find out if you are in an area where schistosomiasis occurs. If so, see Chapter 18 page 150 for details of schistosomiasis.

Acute nephritic syndrome

Definition

Acute nephritic syndrome is an acute inflammation of the glomeruli. It is not caused by infecting organisms in the kidney. It is caused by an abnormal reaction of the body's immune system. This abnormal reaction is often to a certain type of infection, which the patient had about 2–3 weeks before, but also to numerous other causes.

Clinical features

A respiratory or skin infection (usually caused by a *Streptococcus)* occurs 2–3 weeks before the start of the illness in many, but not all, cases. Then there is suddenly:

- malaise,
- swelling (oedema) of the face and legs,
- only a small volume of urine, which looks like black tea and has positive tests for red blood cells and protein, and
- high blood pressure (developing over a day or two).

See a specialist book for details of diagnosis and management.

Transfer such cases to a Medical Officer for exact diagnosis and treatment unless the patient starts to get better within a couple of days, as the treatment could be difficult, especially if very high blood pressure and especially if acute renal failure develops.

Treatment would include:

1. Penicillin in case any infection of skin or respiratory tract is still present.
2. Rest in bed.
3. Treatment of high blood pressure if above 160/100.
4. Treatment of acute kidney failure.

Chronic kidney (renal) failure

Chronic kidney failure is present when the kidneys are permanently damaged and cannot excrete (put) all the waste products made by the body into the urine. The amount of waste products in the body increases and damages many functions of the body. There are many causes of chronic kidney failure. You can treat very few of these causes successfully in the health centre. (See Figure 26.12.)

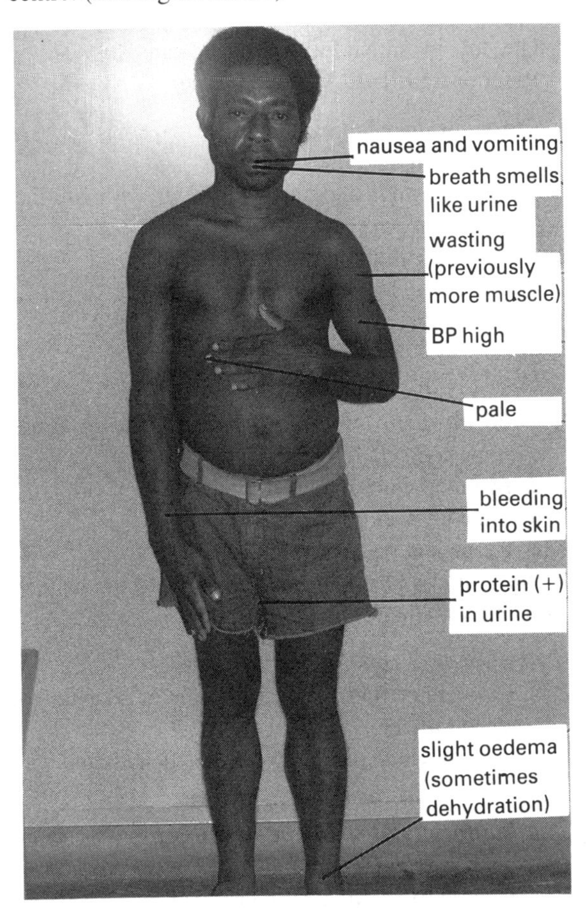

Figure 26.12 A patient with chronic kidney failure. The patient came to the health centre because he had the symptoms of anaemia. Routine treatment of the anaemia did not make him any better. The signs of kidney failure were then looked for and found. The diagnosis was confirmed by a blood urea test.

Think of chronic kidney failure in any patient who has:

- anaemia (especially if it does not improve with treatment),
- high blood pressure than 160/100),
- loss of appetite, nausea, and often vomiting (for no obvious reason),
- wasting of muscles (for no obvious reason),
- breath that smells like urine smells,
- deep breaths, even though the patient does not feel short of breath (usually late in the disease), or
- bleeding into the skin (usually only late in the disease).

A history of previous kidney disease makes the diagnosis more likely.

Test the urine for protein. Protein in the urine makes the diagnosis very likely if the other signs are present.

Send blood to the laboratory to confirm the diagnosis; ask for a blood urea and creatinine test (and electrolytes). (See page 353.)

Causes of chronic renal failure that can be treated need to be looked for in all patients. These causes include high blood pressure, urinary tract infection, including with tuberculosis and schistosomiasis, urinary tract obstruction including from an enlarged prostate and schistosomiasis, dehydration, infections, drugs or chemicals which cause kidney damage, etc.

Some things may help the patient's symptoms and slow the rate at which the kidney failure gets worse. These include the following:

- Drugs to keep the blood pressure down to about 140/90. See Chapter 27 page 380.
- Good diet with plenty of carbohydrate and fat but just a normal (and not increased) amount of protein.
- A large fluid intake of about 3 litres a day.
- Control of salt intake according to blood and urine tests, although it is more likely a large amount of salt is needed, but this may need to be reduced if the blood pressure becomes too high.
- Early treatment of any nausea and vomiting with anti-nausea drugs and if needed intravenous fluid; as mild dehydration can cause worsening of kidney failure.
- Blood test to see if the patient would be helped by calcium carbonate or aluminium hydroxide or sodium bicarbonate

In view of these things, *refer* the patient to the next visiting Medical Officer or discuss with him about non-urgent transfer about the above.

Acute kidney (renal) failure

See page 363.

Ureteric (renal) colic

Ureteric colic is a pain caused by something (usually a stone formed in the kidney) going down the ureter from the kidney to the bladder.

Ureteric colic is a very severe pain. It usually begins in the loin (one side of the back, where the lowest ribs join the spine) and then spreads to the iliac fossa (lower outer front of the abdomen), labia or penis or testes or inner leg on the same side. It is a constant pain which may slowly get much worse. It is not a true colic.

The attack may continue for only a few minutes; but sometimes it continues for hours. Passing urine is often painful. Blood is often passed in the urine. Tests show protein and blood in the urine.

Stones never dissolve themselves. But if they are small, they may be passed in the urine. If stones remain in the urinary tract for a long time, infection often occurs.

Treatment includes the following:

1. Treat any ureteric colic with IMI pethidine 100 mg (2 ml) and atropine 0.6 mg (1 ml) every 4 hours or more often if necessary.
2. Treat any urinary infection present. Do not use sulphadimidine. Use some other drug. See page 356.
3. Keep any stone that is passed. Give it to the Medical Officer for analysis in the laboratory.
4. Give 3–4 litres of fluid daily (to make a large urine volume).

Transfer the patient to a Medical Officer within 2 days to check if there is an obstruction of the ureter. This is especially important if there is continuous pain and tenderness over one kidney. The Medical Officer will do special tests and X-rays.

Some common diagnostic problems and their management

Urinary frequency (Passing urine more often than normal)

Do a full history and examination (see Chapter 6 and pages 350–53).

Do a pelvic examination PR and PV (see page 352–3).

Test the urine (see pages 353 and 355). If needed test the urine for schistosomiasis

Find out if the patient is passing large volumes (amounts) of urine often or if he is passing only small amounts of urine often.

Large amounts of urine passed often

Look for:

1. *Diabetes mellitus*
   - sugar (glucose) in the urine
   - drinking a lot
   - eating a lot
   - losing weight if young; or overweight if old

   See Chapter 30 page 406

   Treat dehydration if present (see Chapter 23 page 285).

   Diet low in animal fat and refined sugars.

   Refer or transfer to Medical Officer.
2. *Chronic kidney failure*
   - protein in the urine
   - anaemia that does not get better with routine treatment
   - blood pressure higher than normal
   - wasting

   See page 359.
3. *Taking of diuretic drugs*
4. *Neurotic disorder – acting out (drinking more than is necessary)*
   - no other abnormalities found on examination
   - urine tests all normal
   - the patient has a mental problem

   If you find and solve the problem, and the patient drinks less, the frequency stops.
5. *Rare medical conditions*

   If you cannot find the cause, refer or transfer to Medical Officer.

   Do not allow the patient to become dehydrated.

Small amounts of urine passed often

1. *Urinary tract infection*
   - dysuria (pain on passing urine) also
   - urethral discharge if there is urethritis
   - fever if the kidney is infected
   - tenderness over urethra, prostate, bladder or kidney/s if these are infected

   See page 353.

2. *Schistosomiasis*
   - patient in or from an area where schistosomiasis occurs
   - blood in urine, especially at the end of passing urine – worse after exercise
   - eggs or miracidia in urine on examination

   See Chapter 18 page 150.

3. *Obstruction of the urethra by an enlarged prostate gland or a urethral stricture*
   - older man if there is an enlarged prostate; or middle-aged man who has a history of gonorrhoea if there is a stricture
   - for months or years it has been difficult to pass urine – difficult to start, then a thin stream and difficult to pass all the urine
   - sometimes you can feel an enlarged or lumpy prostate on pelvic examination PR
   - no pus or protein in the urine unless there is also a urinary tract infection

   If there is pus and protein in the urine, treat for urinary tract infection (see page 353).
   If patient is not cured, refer or transfer non-urgently to a Medical Officer (probably for an operation).

4. *Normal pregnancy* pressing on the bladder
   - the patient is well, but is in either early pregnancy (1 or 2 periods missed) or late pregnancy
   - the urine tests are normal

   No treatment is necessary.

5. *Pelvic disease* such as pelvic inflammatory disease or schistosomiasis, or amoebiasis or cancer of the female genital tract pressing on the bladder.
   - vaginal discharge or bleeding
   - abnormal tenderness or enlargement of organs or lumps on pelvic examination PR and PV

   Treat pelvic inflammatory disease (see Chapter 19 page 166) and amoebic infections (see Chapter 23 page 294 and schistosomiasis see above).
   Refer or transfer most cases non-urgently to a Medical Officer.

6. *Blood in the urine* when schistosomiasis is not present (no eggs or miracidia in the urine), and you cannot find other disease.
   Refer or transfer to a Medical Officer all patients who have blood in the urine with no obvious cause. It may be disease which can be cured if treated early, but may cause death if not treated until late.

7. *Chronic disease of the bladder* such as a stone or late schistosomiasis or tuberculosis or cancer.
   - long history of urinary symptoms
   - urinary symptoms getting worse
   - blood or protein or pus in the urine

   Refer to transfer non-urgently to a Medical Officer.

Dysuria (pain on passing urine)

Do a full history and examination (See Chapter 6 and pages 350–3).

Test the urine (see pages 353 and 355).

Do a pelvic examination PR and PV (see Chapter 6 page 20 and pages 352–3).

Pull back the foreskin of the penis and look under it and on the glans of the penis.

Look for:

1. *Sores on, or inflammation of, the penis, vulva or vagina*
   - Urinary frequency may not be present.
   - The urine tests are usually normal.

   If sore, see Chapter 19 page 165.
   If discharge, see Chapter 19 page 165.

2. *Urethral infection*
   - Urine frequency is present.
   - Ask if there is urethral or vaginal discharge or pus or of white or watery material.
   - Ask about the possibility of a sexually transmitted disease.
   - Still suspect a sexually transmitted disease, even if the patient says it is not possible.
   - Look for urethral discharge.
   - The urine tests may not have much pus or protein in a mid-stream specimen.

   If urethritis is likely, see Chapter 19 page 160.

3. *Prostatitis*
   - Urinary frequency is usually present.
   - Ask about the possibility of a sexually transmitted disease in younger men.
   - Ask about symptoms of an enlarged prostate (increasing difficulty in passing urine, etc.) in older men.
   - Examine for tenderness of the prostate, on pelvic examination PR.
   - The urine test may not have much pus or protein in a mid-stream specimen.

   Treat as for urethritis and urinary tract infection. See page 356.

4. *Cystitis due to bacteria*
   - Urinary frequency is present.
   - Tenderness over the bladder may be present.
   - Symptoms and signs of pyelonephritis may be present.
   - Urine tests show pus and protein.

   Treat for urinary tract infection (see page 356).

5. *Cystitis due to schistosomiasis*
   - Patient from or in an area where schistosomiasis occurs.
   - Blood in the urine, especially at the end of passing urine and after exercise.
   - Severe pain if clots of blood are passed.

   Treatment – see Chapter 18 page 154.

6. *Pelvic disease* irritating the bladder, especially pelvic inflammatory disease.
   - Vaginal discharge or bleeding.
   - Abnormal tenderness, lumps, or enlarged organs on pelvic examination PR or PV.
   - Urine tests normal, unless urine has vaginal secretions in it.

   Treat for pelvic inflammatory disease (see Chapter 19 page 166) and amoebic infections (see Chapter 23 page 294).

7. *Pyelonephritis*
   - Urinary frequency.
   - Fever, fast pulse, toxaemia.
   - Tenderness in the loin/s.
   - Urine tests show pus and protein.

   Treatment – see page 356.

8. *Note* that people often complain of dysuria when they have pain all over or a fever, and pass concentrated urine. The dysuria improves as the person gets better. There is no disease of the urinary tract.

Incontinence of urine (the patient cannot control when urine is passed)

Do a full history and examination (See Chapter 6 page 17).
Examine the urine (see pages 353 and 355).

Do a pelvic examination PR and PV (see Chapter 6 page 20 and pages 352 and 353).

Look for:

1. *No proper control of the body and bladder by the brain*
   - Children
   - Old people with senile dementia – do not diagnose this until you have done all the examinations below with normal results *and* you fi[nd] that the patient has a chronic organic psycho[sis] (see Chapter 35 page 471).
   - During fitting (convulsions).
   - Unconsciousness from any cause.
   - Some psychoses.

   Treat the cause if possible.

2. *Damage to parts of the spinal cord which contr[ol] the bladder*
   - Injury to the back; or pain in the back, oft[en] with a lump in the spine.
   - Difficulty in walking or paralysis or the legs.
   - Loss of sensation with the legs.
   - Anus not closed or tight when pelvic examin[a]tion PR done.

   Transfer the patient urgently to Medical Offic[er] care, unless the condition has been present f[or] many months or for years.

3. *Vesicovaginal fistula or damage to the bladd[er] during labour*
   - Present soon after difficult childbirth.

   Transfer non-urgently to a Medical Officer.

4. *Infection in the bladder*
   - Dysuria and frequency.
   - Pus and protein in the urine.

   Treatment – see page 356.

5. *Obstruction of the urethra* causing the bladder t[o] be too full. A little urine goes through the narro[w] urethra constantly.
   - Older man if there is an enlarged prostate; o[r] middle aged man who has a history of gonor rhoea if there is a stricture.
   - For months or years it has been difficult to pas[s] urine – difficult to start, then a thin stream an[d] difficult to pass all the urine.
   - Sometimes you can feel an enlarged or lump[y] prostate on pelvic examination PR.

   If there is pus and protein in the urine, treat fo[r] urinary tract infection (see page 356).
   If the incontinence is not cured refer or transfe[r] the patient non-urgently to a Medical Officer (probably for an operation).

Anuria and Oliguria (the patient does not pass urine or passes little urine)

There is usually one of these causes of anuria.
Look for:

1. *The urine is made by the kidneys but the bladder cannot empty* ('acute retention of urine')
   - You can feel or percuss the bladder in the lower abdomen (see Chapter 36 pages 495–8).
   - The bladder is tender as well as enlarged.

   Find out why the bladder cannot empty.
   - There is a history and signs of an enlarged prostate gland or a urethral stricture (see page 362), *or*
   - There are signs and a history of damage to the spinal cord, usually trauma or tuberculosis. (See Chapter 29 page 397), *or*
   - There are signs of loss of control of the bladder by the brain, such as unconsciousness (see Chapter 25 page 332).

   Empty the bladder by *gentle*, continuous pressure over the bladder with your hand.
   If this is not possible, insert a urethral catheter with all the special care necessary to avoid infection of the bladder.
2. *The kidneys do not make urine* ('acute kidney failure')
   - You cannot feel or percuss the bladder because it is not enlarged (it is usually empty).
   - The patient is usually very sick with the condition that caused the acute kidney failure.

   Look for the cause of the acute kidney failure
   - Any condition that caused shock that continued for more than a short time before controlled: external or internal bleeding, and especially antepartum or postpartum haemorrhage; severe dehydration; septicaemia; malaria, etc.
   - Acute haemolysis (See Chapter 21 page 239) and especially blood which was wrongly cross-matched or malaria with 'blackwater fever' or some snake bites or certain drugs.
   - Some drug overdoses, e.g. streptomycin.
   - Many other causes (see a specialist book).

   Immediately treat the condition that caused the acute kidney failure, especially if it is shock (see Chapter 27 page 378).

   Insert an urethral catheter into the bladder if still no urine passed to make sure there is not a full bladder which cannot be felt.

   Arrange urgent (emergency) transfer to Medical Officer care.
3. *The patient is not telling the truth*
   - The bladder is not enlarged or tender.
   - The patient has no serious symptoms or signs, and looks well.
   - The patient usually has a big mental problem.

   Admit and observe the patient for 24 hours to see if he is telling the truth or not.

Abnormal colour of the urine

Normally the colour of the urine shows how much waste product is in the urine.

If the person is dehydrated or has no extra water to pass, the concentration of waste product in the urine is high. The urine is 'concentrated'. The colour of the urine is yellow (although the patient may say it is red).

If the person has much water to pass the concentration of waste product in the urine is low. The urine is 'dilute'. The urine colour is clear or like water.

If a person says his urine is an abnormal colour, always look at the urine yourself to see what colour it is and if it is abnormal. Do all the tests for urine (see pages 352 and 355).

Yellow urine
Look for causes of:

1. normally concentrated urine (see above);
2. abnormally concentrated urine, from dehydration (see Chapter 23 page 385);
3. bile in the urine – but this usually makes the urine dark (see Chapter 24 page 305).

Clear urine (like water)
Look for causes of:

1. normally dilute urine (see above);
2. dilute urine because the patient has kidney failure and cannot concentrate the urine (see page 359).

Cloudy urine
Look for causes of:

1. pus from a urinary tract infection (see page 351);
2. phosphate crystals – these do not mean any disease at all and they dissolve if acid is added to the urine; the urine then becomes clear.

Red urine
Look for causes of:

1. red blood cells in the urine ('haematuria') (see this page);

2. haemoglobin in the urine (although then the urine is usually brown or black, not red) (no red blood cells are in the urine) – causes for this include malaria with 'blackwater fever', some snake bites, and wrongly-crossmatched blood; the patient is very sick;
3. bile in the urine (the urine is really brown or black, not red) (see Chapter 24 page 305);
4. food, e.g. beetroot, or sweets (lollies) with red colour in them;
5. normally concentrated urine (the urine is really a yellow colour, not red).

Black urine (like tea or coffee without milk)
Look for causes of:

1. bile in the urine (see Chapter 24 page 305), or
2. haemoglobin in the urine (see above).

See page 355 for ways to test urine for pus, blood, bile, haemoglobin, etc. without laboratory help. If a laboratory is available, you can examine the urine for pus cells and red blood cells under the microscope, and for bile, blood, protein, sugar and haemoglobin with test tablets or paper strips.

Blood in the urine (haematuria)

Check that the patient does have blood from the urinary tract and not either:

1. menstrual blood in the urine, *or*
2. red urine not caused by red blood cells (see above).

If there is blood in the urine, look for:

1. *Trauma to the urinary tract*
   - History and signs of trauma are present.

   Transfer all cases to Medical Officer care urgently.
2. *Urinary tract infection*
   - Dysuria and urinary frequency.
   - Pus and protein with the blood in the urine.
   - Treatment removes the blood from the urine and it does not appear in the urine again.

   Treatment – see page 351.
3. *Schistosomiasis*
   - Patient is from or in an area where schistosomiasis occurs and usually a boy.
   - There is more blood at the end when passing urine, and more after exercise.
   - Eggs or miracidia are in the urine, on examination see Chapter 18 page 153.

   Management – see Chapter 18 page 154.
4. *Acute nephritic syndrome/glomerulonephritis*
   - Throat or skin infection 1–3 weeks before, but not always.
   - Oedema (puffy face, etc.)
   - Blood pressure high.
   - Urine has protein and blood in it and the volume is small.

   See page 358 and refer to Medical Officer.
5. *Stone in the urinary tract*
   - Ureteric colic (see page 360).
   - Persistent urinary tract infection. See page 353.
6. *Causes that you cannot diagnose at the health centre but must be diagnosed* (because some conditions, such as early cancer and tuberculosis, can be cured, but kill if not diagnosed and treated). Refer or transfer all patients who have blood in the urine for which you cannot find the cause.

Pus in the urine (pyuria)

Look for:

1. urinary tract infection (see page 353); or
2. acute nephritic syndrome (see page 358).

If these conditions are not present, or if treatment is not effective, refer or transfer the patient to Medical Officer care.

There may be other conditions, such as tuberculosis or stone, which must be diagnosed and treated.

Sugar in the urine

You can diagnose sugar in the urine with a positive Benedict's test. There are only two common conditions which cause sugar in the urine:

1. Diabetes mellitus – glucose in the urine
   - Benedict's test and Clinitest tablet test positive.
   - Stick tests, e.g. Clinistix test also positive.

   See Chapter 30 page 406 for management.
2. Pregnancy and lactation – lactose from breast milk in the blood and urine.
   - Benedict's and Clinitest tests positive.
   - Stick tests, e.g. Clinistix test *negative*

   No treatment necessary.

Protein in the urine (proteinuria or albuminuria)

If you find more than a very little protein in the urine, there is usually a serious disease of the kidneys. Look for the causes:

1. urinary tract infection (see page 353),
2. haematuria (see page 364),
3. pre-eclamptic toxaemia of pregnancy and eclampsia (see an obstetrics book),
4. nephrotic syndrome (see page 356),
5. acute nephritic syndrome (see page 358) or
6. chronic kidney failure (see page 359).

You may find small amounts of protein in the urine of people who have other conditions that do not affect the kidneys directly:

1. heart failure,
2. fever of any cause,
3. operation.

Bile in the urine

See Chapter 24 page 305.

27

Disorders of the Heart and Blood Vessels

Anatomy and physiology

The body is made of many cells. All these cells need food from the intestine and liver and oxygen from the lungs. Waste products and carbon dioxide must also be removed from the cells. The blood takes all things to and from the cells. Many other important things also go from one part of the body to another in the blood (See Chapter 21 page 236). The body, therefore, moves the blood in a big circle through the parts of the body in a special order. The blood moves round this circle in the blood vessels – arteries, capillaries and veins. The heart pumps the blood through the blood vessels. This is called the 'circulation' of the blood (see Figure 27.1). The system of the heart and blood vessels is called the 'cardiovascular' system. (See Figures 27.2, 27.3, 27.4, 27.5 and 27.6.)

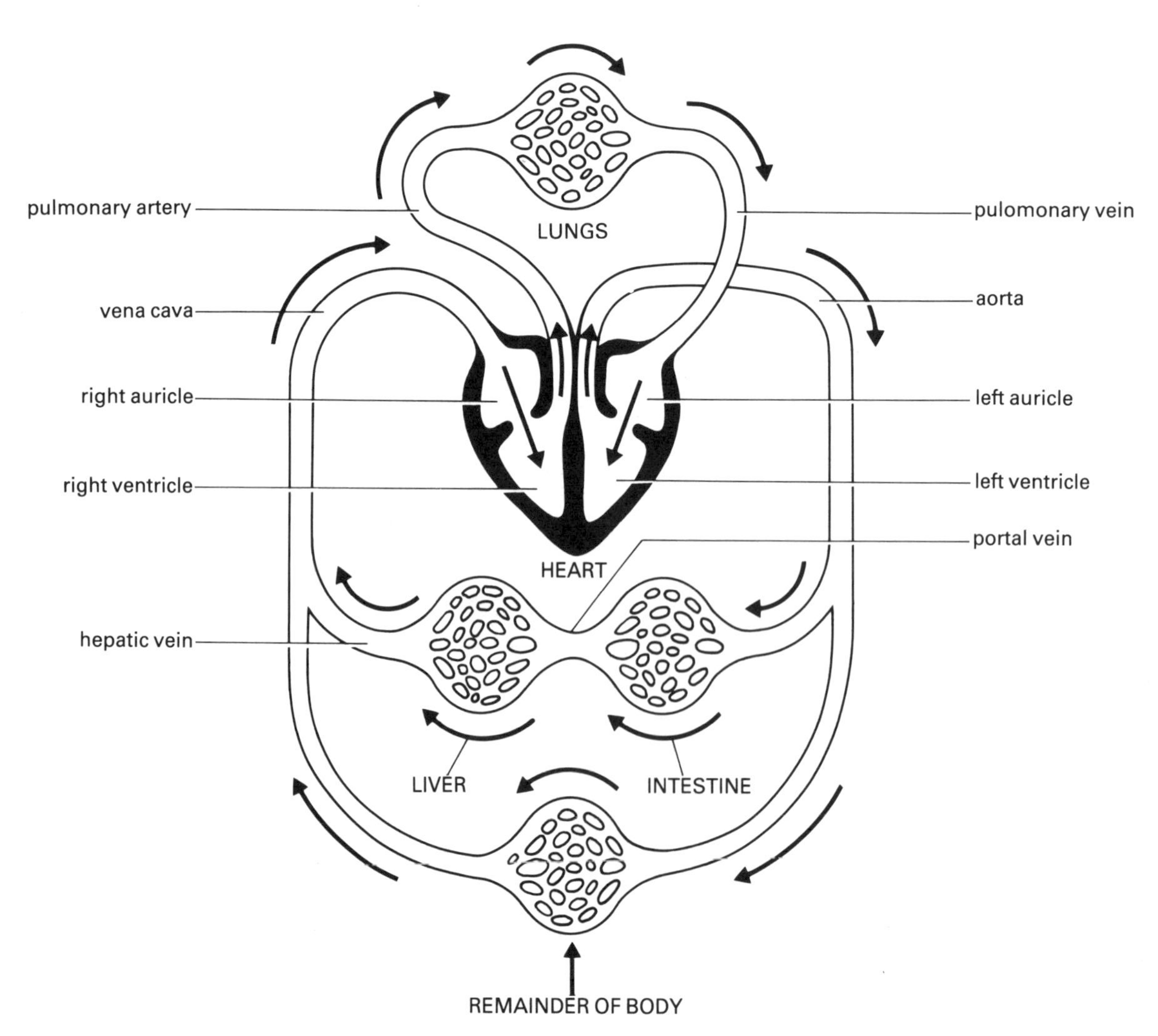

Figure 27.1 (on page 366) Diagram showing circulation of the blood. The blood goes from the lungs to the left side of the heart. This blood contains much oxygen and little carbon dioxide. The left side of the heart pumps the blood through the arteries to the capillaries in the body, and the intestine. Through the walls of these capillaries the blood gives food and oxygen to the cells and removes carbon dioxide and waste products. The blood then goes from the capillaries into veins. The blood in the capillaries of the intestine also takes food from the intestine and it then goes through the portal vein to the liver. In the liver the blood goes into capillaries which put most of the food from the intestine into the liver for storage. The blood from the liver, which contains enough food for the rest of the body, then goes into veins again and travels to the right side of the heart. The blood from the capillaries in the rest of the body travels in veins straight to the right side of the heart. The right side of the heart pumps the blood to the lungs through the pulmonary artery and then into capillaries again. The lungs remove carbon dioxide from the blood and put in oxygen. The capillaries in the lung then join to form the vein which goes to the left side of the heart. The circulation of the blood then starts again.

The heart normally pumps about 70 ml of blood into the blood vessels of the lungs and of the body with every contraction or beat. The heart normally contracts about 70 times every minute.

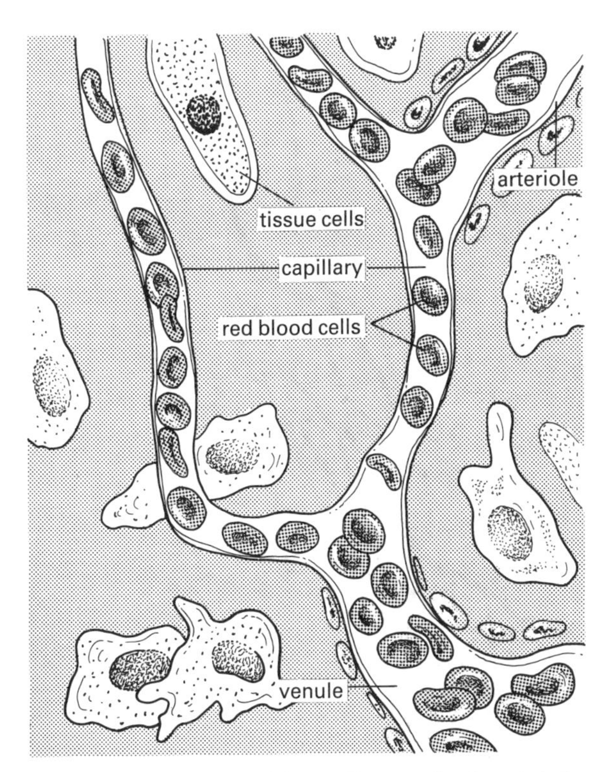

Figure 27.2 Diagram of the smallest arteries (arterioles) and the smallest veins (venules) of the capillaries as seen through the microscope.

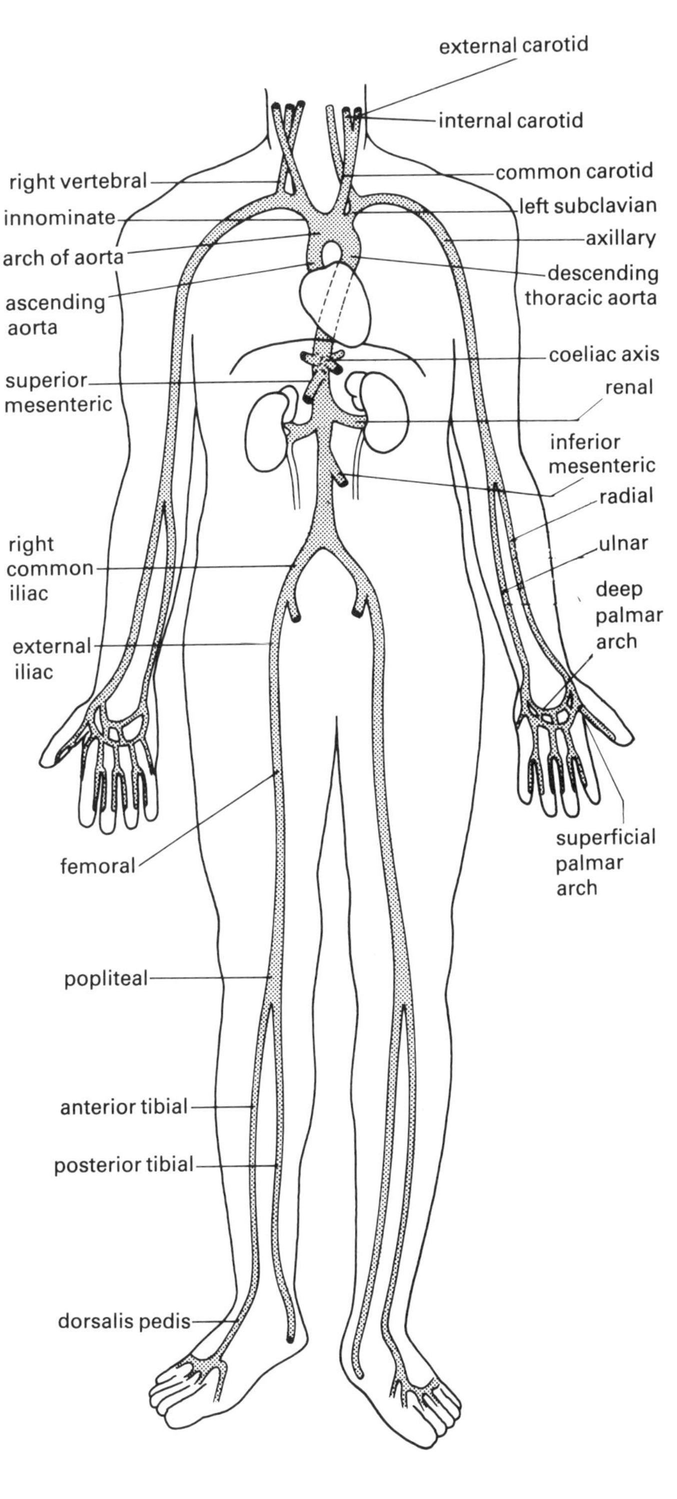

Figure 27.3 Diagram showing the main arteries of the body. The names of the arteries are not important.

The blood cannot go backwards into the heart because of the one-way valves (aortic and pulmonary) where the heart is joined to the blood vessels.

The small arteries (arterioles) let the blood go into the capillaries slowly. When the heart beats, the big arteries stretch to let all the blood into them. These stretched big arteries then slowly push the blood through the small arteries and arterioles into the capillaries before the next heart beat. Some blood remains in the arteries before the heart beats again, so there is always pressure in the arteries. When the heart pumps more blood into the arteries the pressure is highest – called the 'systolic blood pressure'. The systolic pressure is normally between 100 and 120 mm mercury when measured with a sphygmomanometer. The pressure in the arteries is lowest just before the heart pumps more blood into the arteries – called the 'diastolic blood pressure'. The diastolic pressure is

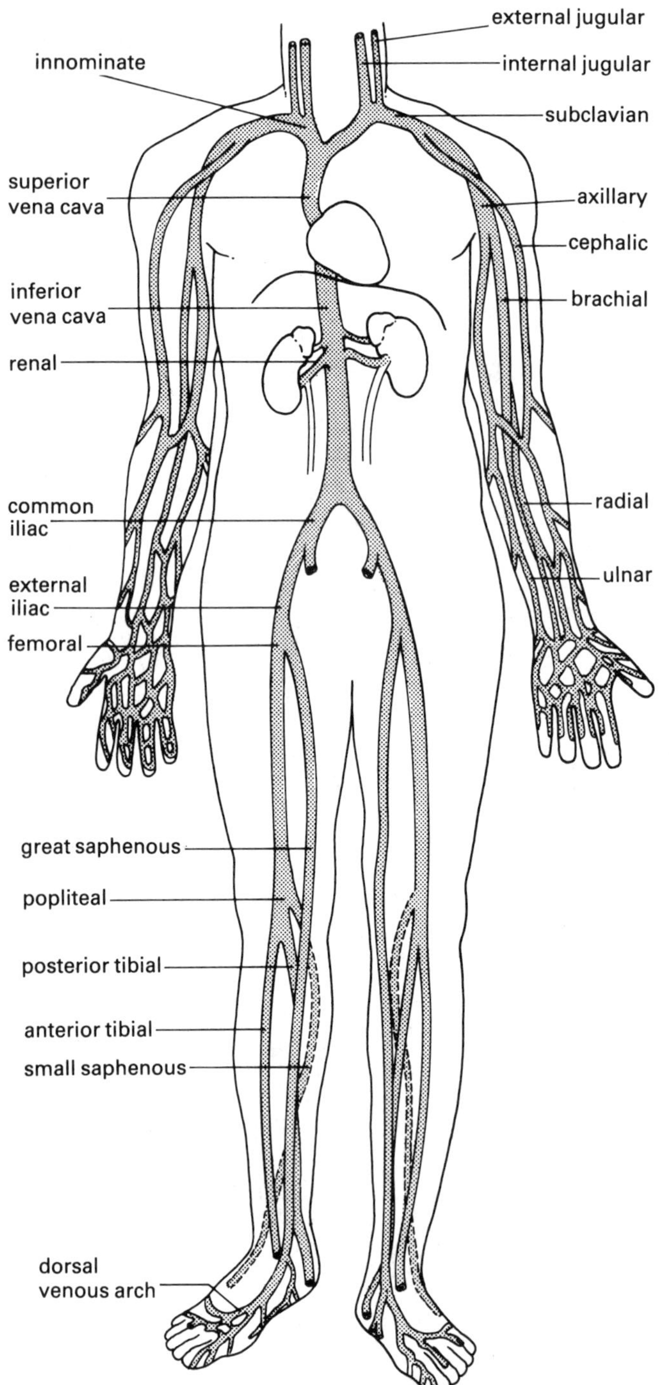

Figure 27.4 Diagram showing the main veins of the body. The names of the veins are not important.

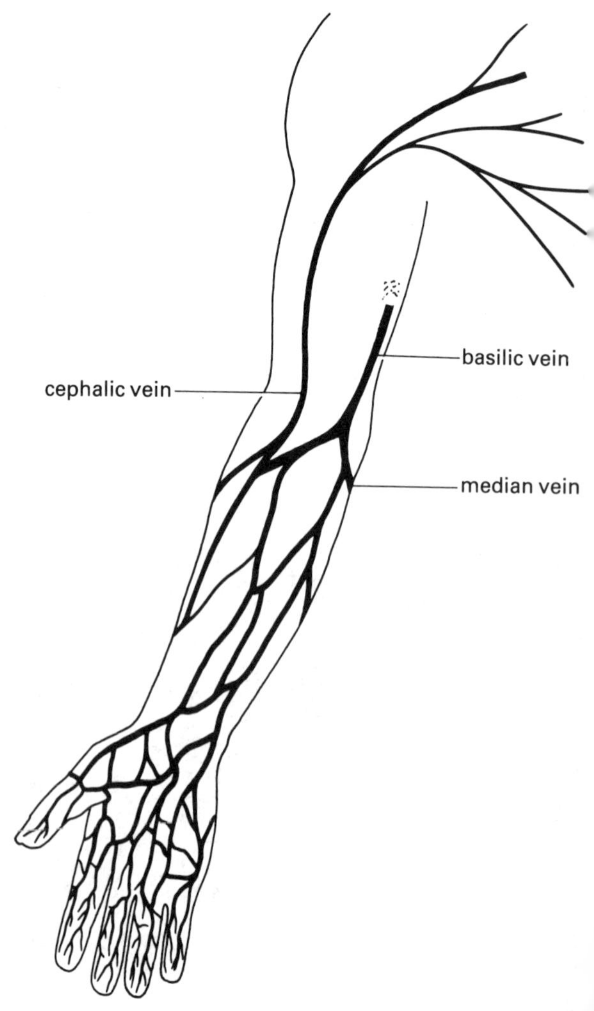

Figure 27.5 Diagram showing the veins of the arm.

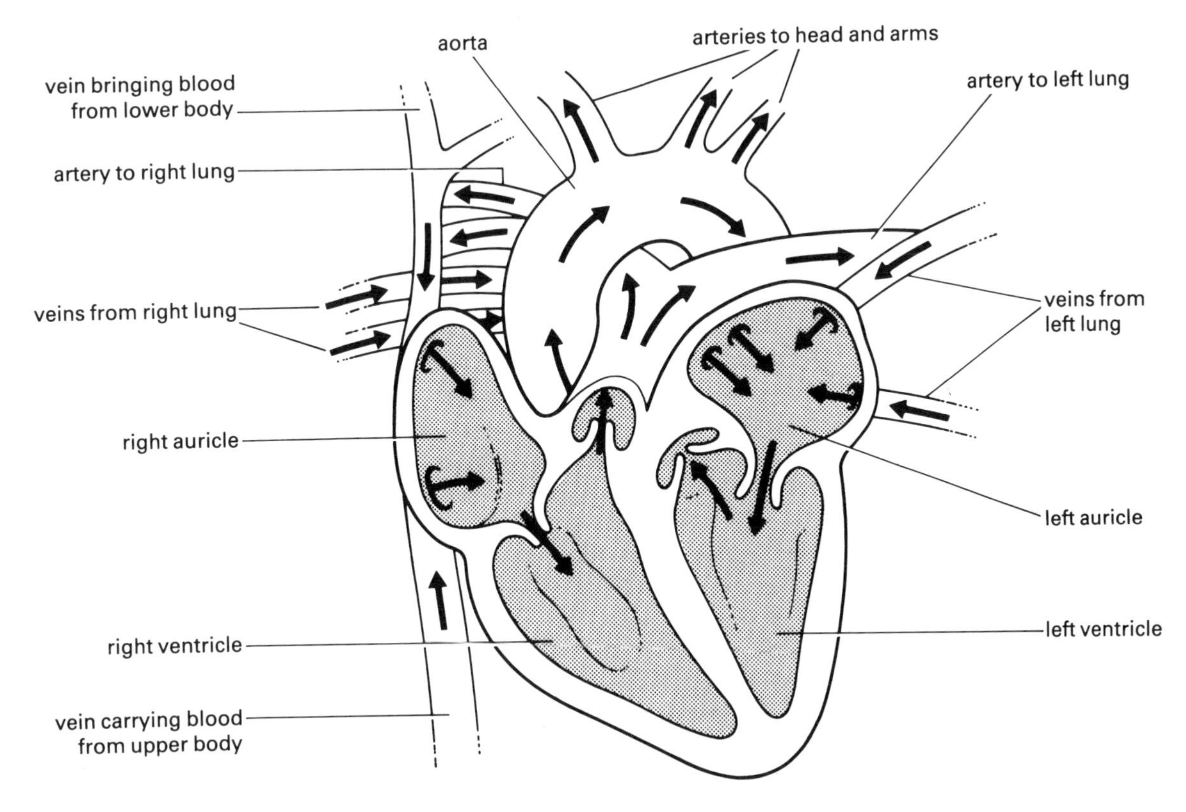

Figure 27.6 Diagram showing the internal anatomy of the heart. The arrows show the direction the blood goes. Note the 'one way' valves which make the blood go in one direction only when the heart muscle contracts (gets smaller) and squeezes the blood out of the heart.

normally between 70 and 80 mm mercury. The blood pressure (BP) is written with the systolic pressure (e.g. 120) first and the diastolic pressure (e.g. 80) second, like this: BP 120/80.

One special set of arteries is the coronary arteries. These are two small arteries which come out of the large blood vessel into which the left ventricle pumps all the blood (the aorta), just above the heart. These arteries then run back to supply the muscle of the heart from the outside. (The muscle of the heart wall is too thick for oxygen and food to spread into it from the blood inside the heart, and needs it own blood vessels.) See Figure 27.7.

Pathology

If the blood does not circulate (go round the body), then the body cells cannot work properly. If the circulation of the blood stops, the body cells start to die. If the circulation of the blood to the brain stops for more than 2 or 3 minutes, many of the brain cells die or can never work properly again – even if the circulation starts again.

The blood does not circulate properly if either of the following things happen.

1. Heart failure. If the heart cannot pump enough blood round the body quickly enough, then heart failure is present.
   For details of heart failure see page 371.
2. Shock. If there is not enough blood in the blood vessels for the heart to pump around the body, then shock is present.
   For details of shock see page 376.

If the blood pressure remains much higher than the normal blood pressure, this condition is called hypertension (high blood pressure). Hypertension can damage the arteries and the organs they go to. For details about hypertension see page 380.

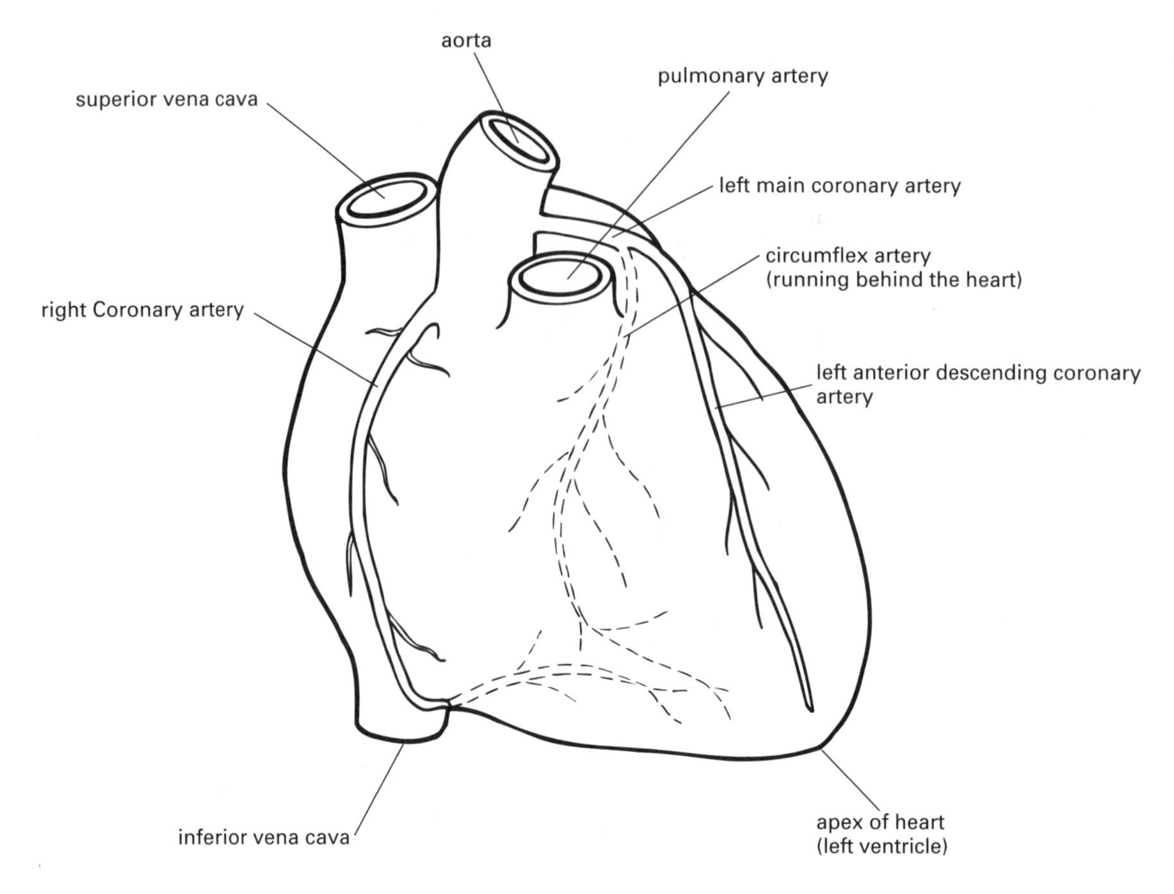

Figure 27.7 Diagram showing the coronary arteries of the heart from the front.

Symptoms and signs of cardiovascular disease

Symptoms of cardiovascular disease

Abnormal shortness of breath (dyspnoea)

With mild disease, shortness of breath occurs only after exercise (i.e. walking fast, carrying heavy things, working hard etc.).

With worse disease, shortness of breath also occurs when the patient is walking slowly and later just sitting.

With severe disease, lying down makes the shortness of breath even worse and sitting up makes it a little better.

There are many causes of shortness of breath other than heart disease. (See Chapter 20 page 232.)

Oedema

Oedema (swelling caused by fluid) of the ankles occurs if the patient usually walks around. Oedema of the back occurs if the patient spends most of the time lying down.

There are many causes of oedema other than heart disease. See Chapter 36 page 485.

Chest pain

Chest pain is not usually caused by heart disease in most developing countries. If pain is from the heart, it is in the centre of the front of the chest but may also be felt in the arms or jaw. It is of a few types. Angina pectoris comes only when the heart is doing more work pumping more blood, e.g. on exertion (see page 381). Myocardial infarction pain is constant (see page 382). Pericarditis pain may be constant but may be worse on breathing or swallowing. Heart pain is usually like a tight band around the chest or a heavy weight on the chest. See Chapter 20 page 381.

Palpitations

Palpitations are present when the patient feels his heart beating faster or harder than normal or irregularly (i.e. out of time). See page 371.

Signs of cardiovascular disease

Pulse rate (PR) and pulse regularity and pulse volume

The normal PR for adults is 60–80/minute. The normal pulse is regular in time.

The normal pulse has a good volume – you can feel it beat strongly. This means that each contraction of the heart pumps the normal amount of blood into the arteries.

In cardiovascular disease the pulse may be

- fast (more than 100/minute), *or*
- slow (less than 60/minute), *or*
- small volume (or 'weak') (this means that each contraction of the heart pumps less blood than normal into the arteries) *or*
- irregular in time.

If the pulse is irregular or has small volume, listen to the heart beat with a stethoscope on the chest to find out the true heart rate. Sometimes the heart beats more quickly than the pulse at the wrist, because you cannot feel some of the small volume beats.

Blood pressure (BP)

The normal BP is

- 100–140 systolic (*but* it can be lower),
- 70–80 diastolic (*but* it can be lower).

Many subsistence farmers and rural people have a BP lower than 100/70. If they feel well, the pulse is not fast, and the systolic BP is over 70 and they are not dizzy on standing and pass urine, there is no problem.

If the patient has a low BP caused by shock, he will also have the other symptoms and signs of shock – pulse fast (over 100) and weak; dizziness and further drop of blood pressure if he sits up; breathlessness; pallor; skin usually cold and moist; etc.

If the BP is higher than 140 systolic or 90 diastolic the patient has high blood pressure or hypertension.

Signs of heart failure (see this page)

1. raised jugular venous pressure (almost always)
2. enlarged liver (almost always)
3. oedema (almost always)
4. fast pulse (usually)
5. cyanosis (often)
6. crackles in the lungs (sometimes)

Signs of shock (see page 371)

1. The patient is dizzy, faint, restless or even unconscious.
2. The pulse is fast (over 100) and small volume (sometimes you cannot feel it at all).
3. The blood pressure is low (less than 100 and often less than 70 systolic) (sometimes you cannot record it at all). If you sit the patient up it will go lower.
4. Shortness of breath (usually deep breaths).
5. Pallor, or paleness.
6. Skin cold and moist (occasionally warm and dry; but only in *some* severe infections).
7. The patient makes little or no urine.

Disorders of cardiovascular function

Heart failure

Definitions and diagnosis

Heart failure is present if the heart cannot pump enough blood around the body quickly enough for the body's need of blood. Heart failure may be acute or chronic, severe or mild.

You can check the amount of blood the heart is pumping round the body by examining these things.

1. *The pulse* – in heart failure it is usually fast (more than 100/minute) and has a small volume (it feels weak). But the pulse could be too slow (less than 40/minute). An irregular pulse can also occur in heart failure.
2. *The blood pressure* – in heart failure it is usually normal or low. But high BP for a long time may cause heart failure and it could therefore still be high.
3. *The colour and temperature of the body tissues, especially the skin* – in heart failure the skin is often cool or even cyanosed (blue).
4. Only a little or no urine made.

Acute severe heart failure can cause shock if the heart can only pump a very little blood round the body (see page 376).

In heart failure blood can return to the right side of the heart from the body more quickly than the right ventricle can pump it out again. This causes the veins behind the heart to become overfilled and they distend (or stretch). Some fluid from the blood leaks (goes out) of the distended veins and causes oedema (swelling) of the organs nearby. You can check for overfilling of the veins by looking for these things:

1. oedema of legs and sacral area (lower part of back),
2. enlargement of the liver (tenderness also if it happened quickly),
3. distension of the veins in the neck (raised jugular venous pressure) (see Figures 27.8 and 27.9).

If the blood returns to the left side of the heart more quickly than the left ventricle can pump it out, then the veins behind the left side of the heart (i.e. the pulmonary veins or the veins in the lungs) are overfilled and distended. Some fluid will leak out causing oedema of the lungs. You can tell if there is oedema in the lungs by listening with the stethoscope for crackles in the lower parts of the lungs.

It is also possible to examine the heart for signs of heart failure. But this is difficult and you should not try to do it unless you have been taught. (Heart murmurs are not signs of heart failure.)

Signs	
• Raised jugular venous pressure • Enlarged liver • Oedema of legs or sacral areas	if right heart failure
• Crackles in the lung bases	if left heart failure
• Pulse often too fast or too slow • Blood pressure often too low or too high • Skin pale and cool or even cyanosed • Decreased or no urine output	decrease in blood pumped out and blood circulation

When you diagnose heart failure, always look for the cause.

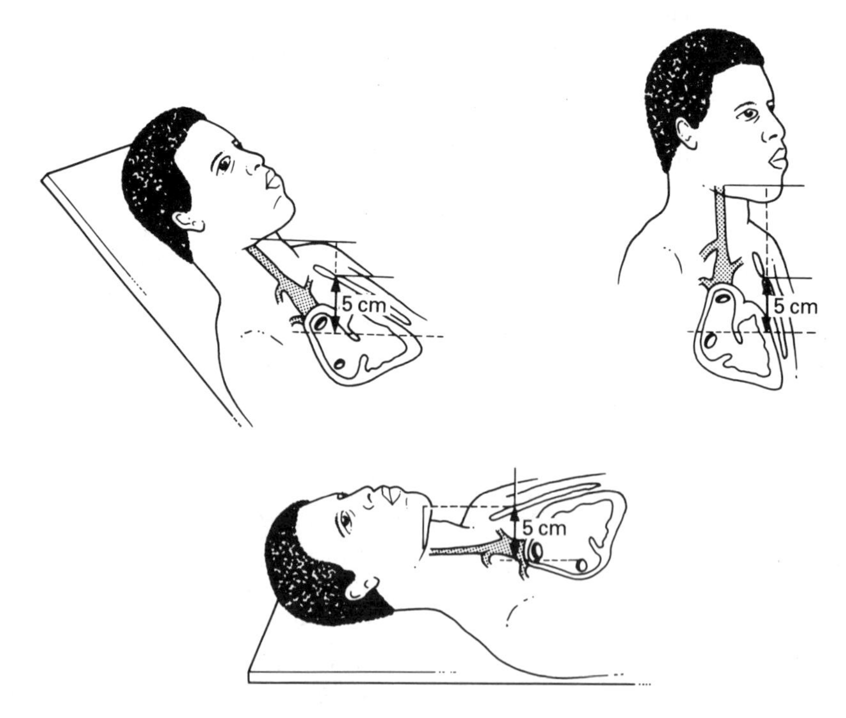

Figure 27.8 Diagrams showing jugular venous pressure. (1) Note that in all positions in all persons (as in this patient), the vertical height of the sternal angle remains 5 cm above the level of the middle of the right atrium. (2) Note that the jugular venous pressure is normally not higher than the level of the sternal angle. (3) Therefore, in a normal person, the jugular veins are full when he is lying flat. You can see the top of the pulsation of the jugular veins of a normal person best when the patient is lying at 45° (i.e. half way up). If he is lying lower the veins are normally full. If he is lying higher the top of the pulsation is behind the clavicle, and too deep in the neck to see. (4) So, as the jugular venous pressure rises, the patient must sit further upright for you to see the *upper level* of the pulsation (otherwise the upper level is in the head). But you can see the venous pulsations of the neck at a higher level that normal (the sternal angle level).

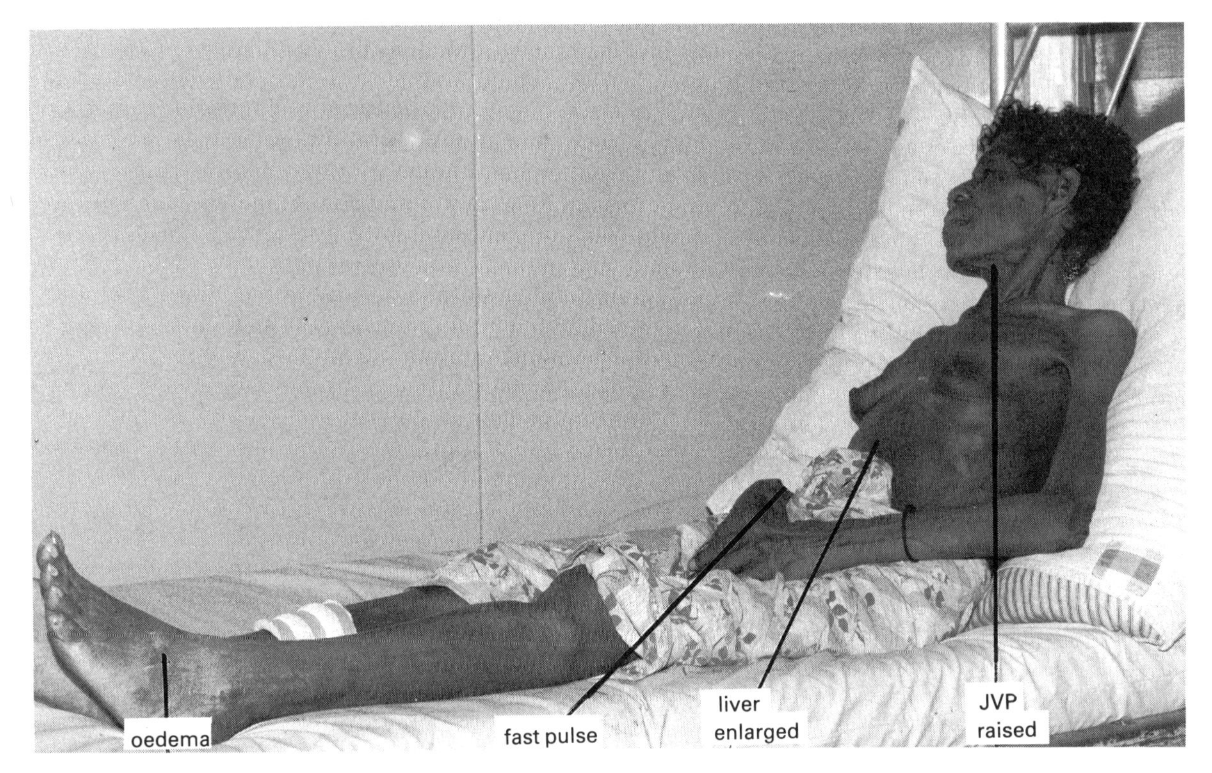

Figure 27.9 A patient with heart failure. Note the usual features of heart failure.

Unfortunately it is not possible to treat many of the causes of heart failure. But you can cure or help some of the causes of heart failure. It is important that you quickly diagnose and treat causes that will result in death unless treated. If you cannot diagnose the cause or if you cannot treat the cause in the health centre, then refer or transfer the patient for the Medical Officer to diagnose and treat. However, if you can diagnose the cause and there is no treatment possible for the cause, then do not transfer the patient.

Common causes of heart failure which you can treat include:

1. *Severe acute pneumonia*. The toxins from the organisms damage the heart muscles. Also the heart does not get enough oxygen from the blood which has gone through the diseased lung. But the heart must pump faster and do more work because of the infection. These things can cause heart failure.
2. *Chronic lung disease* usually caused by chronic obstructive lung disease (COLD) (but in some countries caused by schistosomiasis). Chronic lung disease destroys many blood vessels in the lungs. The remaining blood vessels contract and become narrow. The heart tries to pump the normal amount of blood through these few narrow vessels. The pressure therefore rises and makes the heart work harder. Finally the heart cannot do all this work, and it fails. Little blood then goes through the lungs. Much blood distends the veins behind the heart. This causes congestion (overfilling of the veins) and oedema of the organs behind the heart.

   If acute lung infection (acute bronchitis or pneumonia) then occurs, the toxins damage the heart, less oxygen goes to the heart and the heart failure gets worse. The heart failure may start or get worse during an acute chest infection (acute bronchitis or pneumonia) in a patient with COLD (chronic obstructive lung disease).

> The most common cause of heart failure is an acute chest infection in a person with chronic lung disease.

3. *Other infections* which affect the heart, include:
   - typhus fever,

- trypanosomiasis both acute and chronic (Chagas' disease in South America and East African trypanosomiasis in Africa).
- typhoid fever,
- relapsing fever,
- septicaemia.

4. *Severe anaemia*
   The blood contains a small amount of haemoglobin, so the heart must pump it around the body more quickly to take enough oxygen to the body. But while it does this extra work, the heart gets less oxygen. This can cause heart failure.
5. If you give a *large volume of intravenous fluid* (or a smaller volume too quickly) to someone who already has a condition (such as anaemia) which can cause heart failure, the extra work of pumping this extra fluid can make the heart fail.
6. *Beriberi*. If the diet is poor and there is not enough vitamin B_1 (also called aneurine or thiamine) in it, the heart muscle cannot pump properly. The lack of vitamin B_1 also makes the blood vessels dilate (get bigger) and so the heart must pump more blood to fill the blood vessels. These things cause heart failure. Sometimes the lack of vitamin B_1 also stops the nerves in the legs working properly, and this causes pain and weakness in the legs. Beriberi occurs most often in poor people, in people during a famine or in alcoholics.
7. *Acute rheumatic fever* (see Chapter 29 page 393)
8. *Hypertension* (see page 380)
9. *Coronary heart disease* (see page 381)
10. *Thyrotoxicosis* (see Chapter 30 page 405)
    Often the pulse is fast and irregular; the patient has lost weight despite eating well; the eyes are staring or the patient has exophthalmos; and the skin feels warm.
11. *A patient with heart failure stops his treatment.*
12. '*Epidemic dropsy*'
    If a group of people eat food that contains mustard oil or another poison and then develop heart failure and other symptoms and signs, notify the Medical Officer immediately (and tell the people not to eat mustard oil or that other food until the Medical Officer has it tested for poison).

You can diagnose or treat most of the above conditions at the health centre.

Refer or non-urgently transfer all other cases as there are conditions that the Medical Officer:

1. may be able to diagnose and possibly treat, e.g.
   - thyrotoxic heart disease,
   - hypertension,
   - coronary heart disease,
   - pericarditis,
   - infective endocarditis,
   - syphilitic heart disease,
   - arrhythmias (abnormal heart rate or rhythm);
2. may diagnose, but as expensive surgery or other treatment is needed, may not be able to treat:
   - congenital heart disease,
   - coronary heart disease,
   - hypertension with a treatable cause,
   - valvular heart disease from rheumatic fever and other causes;
3. may diagnose, but there is no specific known treatment at present:
   - endomyocardial fibrosis,
   - cardiomyopathies of various sorts including:
   - 'dilated cardiomyopathy' and
   - 'peri-partum cardiac failure',
   - Chagas' disease.

Differential diagnosis

Check that the patient does not have another cause for the symptoms or signs of heart failure:

- *Oedema* – toxaemia of pregnancy, nephrotic syndrome, chronic liver disease or filariasis, etc. See Chapter 36 page 485.
- *Enlarged tender liver* – especially amoebic abscess. See Chapter 24 page 313.
- *Shortness of breath* – especially pneumonia, acute bronchitis, asthma or tuberculosis. See Chapter 20 page 232.

> If you think the patient could have heart failure always look for raised jugular venous pressure (almost always raised if there is heart failure).

Treatment

1. Treat the heart failure itself.
2. Look for and treat the cause of the heart failure.

Treat the heart failure itself

1. Rest
2. Oxygen if acute and severe
3. Diuretics
4. No salt in food
5. Potassium chloride if necessary
6. Digoxin
7. Aminophylline may sometimes help

1. *Rest*
   Sit the patient up in bed if he is in an acute stage and short of breath. When sleeping or lying tilt the bed 20° (head end up and foot end down). The patient must rest for some weeks if he is in a chronic stage; but do not stop him walking around.
2. *Oxygen if acute and severe*
   Give intranasal oxygen 1–2 litres/minute. Give only in acute heart failure. *Do not* give more than 2 litres/minute if he has COLD. There is not usually enough oxygen available for treatment of chronic heart failure from COLD.
3. *Diuretics*
   Give frusemide 40 mg (4 ml) IVI immediately for acute heart failure. You can repeat this in $\frac{1}{2}$–1 hour if necessary and increase the dose to 60–80 mg (6–8 ml) if necessary.
   Give hydrochlorothiazide 50–100 mg (1–2 tabs) every morning in the acute and chronic stage.
   Give frusemide 40–160 mg (1–4 tabs) also every morning if the hydrochlorothiazide tabs are not effective.

Diuretics are the most effective and important treatment in most cases

However, do not give a diuretic if the patient has shock. If the patient has shock, give digoxin.

4. *No salt in food*
   Tell the patient not to eat salty foods or put any salt in food when it is being cooked or when he is eating it.
5. *Potassium chloride if necessary*
   Give potassium chloride 1200 mg (2 tabs) three times a day if on diuretics *and if*
   (a) the patient is taking frusemide (furosemide) *and* hydrochlorothiazide; or
   (b) he is *not* on a tuber diet (e.g. sweet potato, yam, taro, etc.); *or*
   (c) he *is* taking digoxin.
6. *Digoxin*
   Give digoxin *if*
   (a) there is heart failure in a previously healthy person *or*
   (b) the patient has shock (Do not give diuretics if the patient has shock. Use digoxin instead.) *or*
   (c) all the other treatment for heart failure (above) and treatment of the cause (below) does not control the heart failure.

   Digoxin is not given often in health centres.
   The signs of too much digoxin are:
   (a) loss of appetite or vomiting or
   (b) pulse slow (< 60) or irregular (if the pulse was not slow or irregular before starting digoxin).

   If the signs of too much digoxin develop *then*:
   (a) *stop the digoxin* for 48 hours,
   (b) *after 48 hours* start the digoxin again at *only half of the previous dose.*

   Digoxin dose
   - 0.5 mg ($\frac{1}{2}$ mg) or 500 micrograms (2 ml or 2 tabs) once and repeat one more time only in 6 hours, i.e. 2 doses *for large, young adult* IMI or orally
   - 0.5 mg ($\frac{1}{2}$ mg) or 500 micrograms (2 ml or 2 tabs) once only *for small or old adult* by IMI or orally *then*
   - 0.25 mg ($\frac{1}{4}$ mg) or 250 micrograms (1 tab) daily *for* large young adult orally
   - 0.125 mg ($\frac{1}{8}$ mg) or 125 micrograms ($\frac{1}{2}$ tab) daily *for small or old adult* orally

You must always give potassium chloride (2 tablets three times a day) if you are giving diuretics with the digoxin.

If a patient on digoxin loses his appetite or vomits or his pulse is slow or irregular, **stop the digoxin** for 48 hours and **then** give it at only **half of the previous daily dose**.

7. *Aminophylline or theophylline if* all other treatment fails may sometimes help.
   Give aminophylline by *slow* IVI –

- For a large adult (> 50 kg), give 375 mg (15 ml)
- For a small adult (< 50 kg), give 250 mg (10 ml)
- Give it by *slow* IVI (take 10 minutes by the clock).

Give aminophylline for acute severe heart failure after the frusemide (furosemide) and for acute heart failure that is not responding to all the other treatment.

Also give for chronic heart failure that is not responding to all other treatment.

After this large starting dose, give only a small dose, 100 mg (1 tab) twice daily for a small adult or 100 mg (1 tab) three times a day for a large adult (i.e. about half ($\frac{1}{2}$) of the dose for asthma).

Stop if there is nausea or vomiting not caused by digoxin. Increase the dose every 2–3 days until the heart failure is controlled or nausea or vomiting occurs. Do not give more than 400 mg daily if heart failure.

Look for and treat the underlying cause

1. Chest infections – give antibiotics, etc. See pneumonia (Chapter 20 page 219).

Antibiotics are an essential part of the treatment in most cases of heart failure as chest infection is a common cause.

2. Chronic obstructive lung disease. See Chapter 20 page 226.
3. Other infections and septicaemia. See Chapter 12 page 53.
4. Anaemia. See Chapter 21 page 238.
5. Beriberi – thiamine (aneurine or vitamin B_1) 50 mg (1 tab) immediately and daily for 2 weeks. (If available, 50 mg (1 ml) IMI immediately.)
   Give a good mixed diet.
   Give aneurine to all patients who have no obvious underlying cause for heart failure; especially if the patient is on a poor diet (famine, old, drinks a lot of alcohol or has bad dietary habits), or is anaemic, or has weak or painful legs.
6. IV saline or blood given too fast – stop or slow down the drip.
7. Acute rheumatic fever – start prophylactic treatment with benzathine penicillin and treat any streptococcal infection with benzyl penicillin.
8. Hypertension – start a tablet to lower the blood pressure as well as all the above treatment.
9. Coronary heart disease – start aspirin and start all the lifestyle changes needed.
10. Thyrotoxicosis – transfer for treatment with special drugs
11. A patient on treatment who has stopped his drugs – start treatment again.

Refer or transfer to Medical Officer

1. All cases of heart failure who do **not** have COLD or anaemia or another treatable cause (for diagnosis – because they may have a curable cause) (non-urgent).
2. All cases of heart failure with an irregular pulse (urgent if acute heart failure).

Shock

The medical term shock means collapse because not enough blood is circulating through the body. Shock is always acute and very serious. (Shock, in the medical sense, has nothing to do with the 'shock' people are said to have when they get a big surprise or very bad news and are mentally upset.)

There are two main causes of shock:
(see below for a third cause)

1. There is not enough volume of blood. This can be caused by loss of blood itself through bleeding from broken blood vessels, or loss of just the water and salt from the blood through blood vessel walls (as in dehydration, burns, septicaemia, etc.) or not enough water and salt absorbed into the blood vessels (as in late stages of dehydration especially from gastroenteritis).
2. There is widening of some of the venous and capillary blood vessels. Blood collects in these blood vessels and does not return to the heart. This is often caused by a change in the nervous system control of the blood vessels.

In either case, there is not enough blood for the heart to pump around the body and fill the arteries, and so the blood pressure falls.

The body then tries to keep the blood going to the most important parts of the body (brain, heart and liver) by closing down the blood vessels to the less important parts (skin, muscles, gastrointestinal tract and later kidneys). These parts then become pale and do not work properly. Also the heart pumps all the blood there as fast as it can, i.e. the pulse rate is fast.

If, after this, there is still not enough blood for the heart to pump round to the brain, liver and heart, these organs also do not work properly. If the blood volume is not quickly increased the patient soon dies.

A third cause for shock occurs when the heart itself is weak and cannot pump the blood around the body even when there is enough blood (acute severe heart failure) (see page 371)

Diagnosis

The diagnosis of shock is usually obvious from the symptoms and signs (see Figure 27.10).

1. The patient feels weak, faint and dizzy (especially when he stands up, but often also when sitting). In severe cases, he is restless or unconscious. This is because not enough blood is going to the brain.
2. The pulse is fast (over 100/minute) and has a small volume.
3. The blood pressure is low (less than 100 and usually less than 70 systolic) and lower when sitting.
4. There is shortness of breath (deep breaths).
5. There is pallor or paleness.
6. The skin is cold and moist (sometimes in some infections the skin may be warm and dry).
7. Little or no urine is made.

Cause

The cause of shock is usually obvious. If it is not, find out from the history and examination of the patient (see Chapter 6). *Do this while you are starting treatment* for the shock. The cause is usually one of these things:

1. Loss of blood or fluid from the blood vessels.
   - external bleeding
   - internal bleeding (e.g. from ruptured spleen or ectopic pregnancy)
   - burns
   - gastroenteritis
   - malaria
   - severe infections (peritonitis, septicaemia, typhus fever, relapsing fever, etc.)
   - allergic reactions.

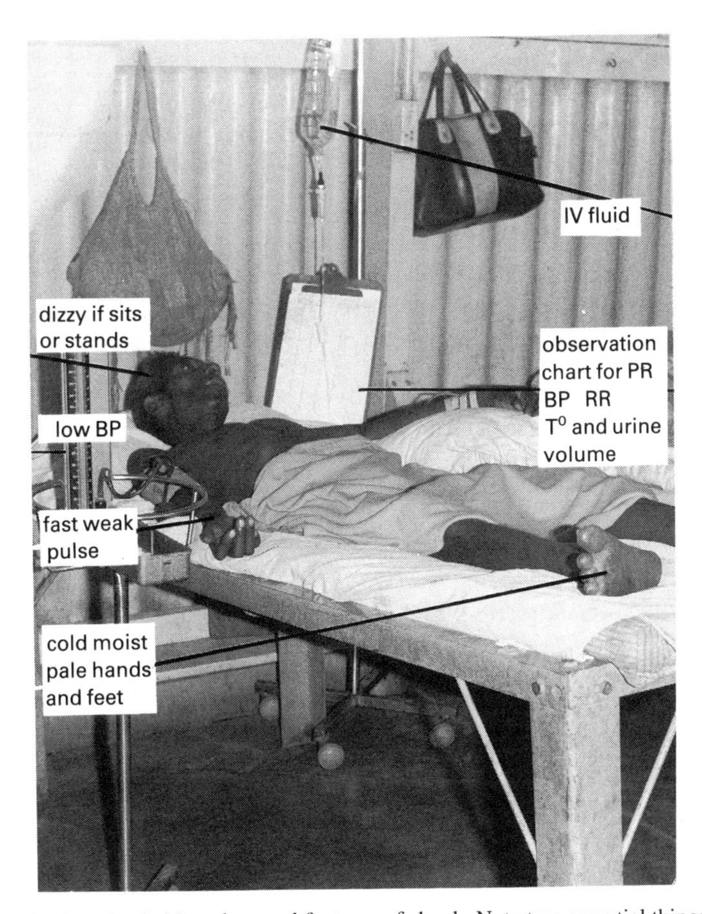

Figure 27.10 A patient who has shock. Note the usual features of shock. Note two essential things in treatment.

2. Dilation of blood vessels.
   - infections
   - allergic reaction
   - severe pain
   - fright or fear
   - standing still for a long time

   } 'fainting' – usually a *slow* pulse
3. The heart not pumping properly.
   - severe infections with toxaemia and low oxygen, e.g. severe pneumonia, malaria, acute trypanosomiasis, typhus fever, relapsing fever
   - chronic trypanosomiasis (Chagas' disease)
   - coronary heart disease with myocardial infarction 'heart attack'

Management of a patient with shock

Immediately put up an intravenous drip of 0.9% sodium chloride (even before you diagnose the cause).

Diagnose the cause. The cause is usually obvious. If it is not, diagnose it from the history and examination of the patient (or from a history given by the patient's relatives or friends). *Do this while you are putting up the drip.*

Shock is usually caused by:

1. loss of fluid
2. loss of blood } (common)
3. septicaemia or infection
4. allergy } (uncommon)
5. heart not pumping properly (very uncommon).

If no cause is obvious, look carefully for internal bleeding (especially ruptured spleen or ectopic pregnancy). If you cannot find the cause, treat for shock from septicaemia.

Management
1. Keep the airway clear. Give artificial ventilation if necessary.
2. Give oxygen.
3. Give analgesics, if severe pain.
4. Keep the patient lying down and warm.
5. Diagnose and treat the cause:
   (a) If loss of fluids – give IV fluids.
   (b) If loss of blood – stop bleeding.
   - give IV fluids and/or plasma volume expander and/or blood.

   (c) If septicaemia – Give IV chloramphenicol, quinine, fluids, digoxin.
   (d) If acute allergic reaction:
   - give IM (or IV) adrenaline,
   - give IV antihistamine,
   - give IV fluids.
6. Look for signs of heart failure. Treat heart failure if it occurs.
7. Transfer patient if necessary.

Treatment depends on the cause (see below). But do the following in all cases,

1. Make sure the *airway* is clear. If the patient is unconscious, give routine care of the airway for an unconscious patient (see Chapter 25 page 332). If he is not breathing enough, give artificial ventilation (see Chapter 37 page 504).
2. Give *intranasal oxygen*, 4 litres/minute.
3. *If there is severe pain give pethidine* (75 mg ($1\frac{1}{2}$ ml) for small adult or 100 mg (2 ml) for large adult *slowly* over 5 minutes by IVI.
4. *Keep the patient lying down flat* with the legs raised. Keep the patient warm but not hot.
5. *Treat the cause* (see below).

(a) When loss of fluid (dehydration) is the cause (usually from gastroenteritis) treat as described below.

- IV 0.9% *sodium chloride* as fast as possible until signs of shock go. Check the patient after each litre. Give up to 4 litres. If the patient is still shocked after 3–4 litres, he needs IV plasma volume expander.
- IV *plasma volume expander* polygeline 3.5% (Haemaccel) or dextran 70, 6% (Macrodex or Gentran 70) or SPPS (stable plasma protein solution) or albumin 4–5%) as fast as possible until the signs of shock disappear. Give 0.5–1.5 litres (1–3 bottles).
- When the signs of shock go, finish that bottle of plasma volume expander, then change back to 0.9% sodium chloride.
- IV 0.9% *sodium chloride* 1 litre every hour until the signs of dehydration go.
- See gastroenteritis (Chapter 23 pagc 285) for details of replacement of continuing fluid losses and maintenance fluids.
- If the 3–4 litres of 0.9% sodium chloride and the 1.5 litres of plasma volume expander do not cure the patient's shock, there is probably also

another cause of the shock, e.g. septicaemia *or* hidden blood loss. See below for treatment.

(b) When loss of blood is the cause (e.g. bleeding peptic ulcer, obstetric bleeding, trauma, etc.) treat as described below.

- Stop the bleeding if possible. If you cannot certainly stop the bleeding arrange an urgent blood transfusion and emergency transfer.
- Give IV 0.9% *sodium chloride* as fast as possible. Give up to 1500 ml. If the signs of shock go, finish off that bag of saline and then change to maintenance fluids (0.18% sodium chloride in 4.3% dextrose, 1 litre every 8 hours – see Chapter 23 page 285).
- If the signs of shock are still present after 1500 ml 0.9% sodium chloride, give: IV *plasma volume expander* (polygeline 3.5% (Haemaccel) or dextran 70, 6% (Macrodex or Gentran 70) or SPPS (stable plasma protein solution) or albumin 4%) as fast as possible. If the signs of shock go, finish that bottle of plasma volume expander and change to maintenance fluids (see above or Chapter 23 page 285).
- If the signs of shock have not gone when you are giving the third bottle of IV plasma volume expander, i.e. 1000–1500 ml, the patient needs *blood.*
- If possible transfer the patient to a Medical Officer before blood is necessary. If you cannot transfer the patient quickly, see a reference book for details of how to crossmatch and give blood.

(c) When septicaemia or other acute severe infection is the cause treat as described below.

Treat for septicaemia if:

- the history, symptoms or signs suggest septicaemia; *or*
- there is no obvious cause for shock.

- Give IV *chloramphenicol* 2 g immediately then 1 g every 6 hours.
- Give 2 g (2 bottles) by IVI immediately. If *immediate* IVI is not possible, give 1 g (1 bottle) by IMI. Then give an IV 1 g dose also as soon as an IVI possible.
- If an IV dose is still not possible 1 hour after the first IM dose, then give another 1 g (1 bottle) by IMI.
- Give 1 g by IVI or by IMI every 6 hours after the first dose.
- Give by IVI if:
  - shock is still present or
  - a drip is necessary.
- For details about antibiotics, see acute severe bacterial infections (Chapter 12 page 53 and Chapter 11 page 46).
- Give IVI *quinine* 10 mg/kg (if unable to weigh patient, 600 mg if large adult and 450 mg if small adult) in 500 ml 0.18% sodium chloride slowly over the first 4 hours in another (a second) drip. Give by IMI if another IV drip is not possible. Complete the treatment course. (See malaria Chapter 13 page 64.)
- Give IV *fluids* as in 'Loss of fluids' (above). But do not give more than the least fluid necessary to correct the shock. Look carefully for heart failure; treat it, if it occurs (stop IV fluids and see page 375).

(d) When acute allergic reaction is the cause (anaphylactic reaction) treat as described below.

- Give IMI *adrenaline* tart. 1:1000 solution 0.5 ml ($\frac{1}{2}$ ml) immediately. (If the patient is about to die, you can give the adrenaline intravenously slowly at 0.1 ml (or $\frac{1}{10}$ ml) every minute, i.e. 0.5 ml (or $\frac{1}{2}$ ml) in 5 minutes). The best way to do this is to mix 0.5 ml ($\frac{1}{2}$ ml) of adrenaline with 4.5 ml of 0.9% saline and give 1 ml each minute).
- Give IVI *promethazine* 50 mg (2 ml) immediately.
- Give IV *fluids* as in 'Loss of fluids' (above).

Watch carefully for heart failure; treat it if it occurs (page 375).

- *Repeat the antihistamine and adrenaline* after 10 minutes if necessary.

6. When you give intravenous fluids, look carefully for signs of heart failure.
   - Signs of heart failure are high jugular venous pressure or shortness of breath and crackles in the lungs that were not present before the IV fluids started. Later the liver enlarges and becomes tender and oedema develops.

- Heart failure is not probable in shock from dehydration or blood loss until the fluid or blood loss is cured.

(a) When mild heart failure occurs:

- Change to 0.18% sodium chloride in 4.3% dextrose and slow the drip to 1 litre every 12 hours.
- Give digoxin 0.5 mg or 500 micrograms (2 ml) IV slowly over 2 minutes immediately *or* 0.5 mg (2 tabs) immediately. See page 375 before you give further doses.

(b) When severe heart failure occurs (patient becomes very breathless or has a lot of crackles in his chest)

- Stop the IV fluids.
- Give frusemide 40 mg (4 ml) IVI immediately once and repeat in $\frac{1}{2}$ to 1 hour if necessary.
- Give aminophylline once. Give 375 mg (15 ml) for a large adult (> 50 kg) or 250 mg (10 ml) for a small adult (< 50 kg) slowly – take 10 minutes by the clock. See Chapter 20 page 226 before you give more doses. See heart failure pages 375–6.
- Give digoxin (see above).

Transfer to Medical Officer care

1. Any case which needs blood transfusion (urgent – emergency).
2. Any case which does not greatly improve with treatment in 3 hour (urgent – emergency).
3. Any case for which you cannot find or treat the underlying cause successfully in a health centre (urgent – emergency).

Prevention

Prevention is by carefully observing and giving proper treatment early to all patients who have a condition that can cause shock.

Systemic vascular hypertension

Hypertension or high blood pressure is said to be present when the blood pressure is 140 systolic or higher and/or 90 diastolic or higher on three separate blood pressure measurements on two separate examinations. However it would not usually be treated in developing countries unless it was 160/95 or higher. Also it is most often discovered when a patient has a stroke or another condition and the blood pressure is taken.

In some parts of Africa up to 20% of adults suffer with hypertension, with blood pressure above 160/95. Causes include kidney disease and abnormalities of many other organs. However, few hospitals are able to do the tests to find these causes and even fewer able to treat any causes found. Even if patients do have lots of tests in hospital, most cases have no cause found and are called 'essential hypertension' (meaning no cause is found). However, we know that there are a number of things which make it more likely for people to get hypertension and for any hypertension they have, to be worse; and these include urbanisation, drinking more alcohol than is healthy (more than two standard drinks for a woman or three standard drinks for a man daily), having much salt in the diet, having body weight above the ideal, smoking and not exercising.

If blood pressure is higher than normal, it can cause damage to the blood vessels (as damage would happen to any hose or tube or pipe which had a pressure in it greater than it was made for). The types of blood vessel damage caused include atheroma (which includes fatty patches in the lining of the artery which partly or completely block the artery), clots in the artery and actual bursting of the artery. These abnormalities in arteries can cause cerebrovascular disease or stroke, damage to the retina of the eye with loss of vision, kidney failure and also coronary heart disease with angina or myocardial infarction (see page 381). As well as this, the heart may not be able to pump all the blood through the narrowed vessels at such a high pressure and blood may collect behind the heart and heart failure develop. Most patients with high blood pressure have no symptoms until one of the above complications occurs.

Treatment

If a patient has high blood pressure you should do the following:

1. Tell him the above risks of hypertension even though he may have no symptoms from the hypertension.
2. Tell him that if he corrects any of the risk factors (above) that he has, over the next 6 months, his blood pressure may fall and the risks from hypertension will be less. He should therefore avoid excess alcohol, not eat salty foods or add salt to cooking or when he is eating food, diet to get his weight to the ideal for his height, stop smoking if he smokes tobacco and start doing regular exercise for at least 20–30 minutes at least four times a week (even walking without stopping is enough).

3. If after 6 months his blood pressure is still high, decide with him if he wants to have drug treatment for high blood pressure.
   First of all find out if there are in fact, drugs available for him for the rest of his life.
   Also, find out if he agrees to take tablets every day for the rest of his life. Send blood tests before starting treatment including for a full blood count, electrolytes, urea and creatinine and also send urine for examination for protein, glucose and microscopy.
   Ask your Medical Officer to review the case before starting treatment to make sure there is no underlying cause easily treated and that he is suitable for treatment.
   Use the lowest dose of the cheapest once daily treatments available. This will be from one of the following groups:
   - Thiazide diuretics, e.g. hydrochlorothiazide 12.5–50 mg daily.
   - Centrally acting alpha agonist, e.g. reserpine 0.1–0.25 mg (no more) or methyldopa (but this needs twice daily treatment and is expensive, 250–750 mg twice daily) These drugs often cause tiredness or depression.
   - Beta-blockers including propranolol 40–160 mg twice daily or atenolol 25–100 mg daily.
   - Alpha-blockers, e.g. prazozin 0.5–5 mg twice daily.
   - Angiotensin converting enzyme (ACE) inhibitors, e.g. captopril 12.5–100 mg daily and trandolapril 0.5–4 mg daily and the newer related angiotensin II receptor antagonists, e.g. losartan and irbesarten.
   - Calcium-channel blockers, including nifedipine 30–60 mg daily and verapamil 120–240 mg daily.
   - Vasodilators although there are unlikely to be any daily ones available.

Black Africans tend not to get the BP lowered by beta-blockers and ACE inhibitors as much as other races.

If drugs are given, the patient needs to be started with a low dose and seen each month and the blood pressure taken and the dose very slowly increased, as long as he does not have any side effects from the drugs. If it is possible, the urea, creatinine and electrolytes should be checked at each visit as sometimes these drugs stop the kidney working properly.

Prevention

The patient should avoid those things which make hypertension more likely, as mentioned above, and good treatment should be given for any conditions which cause kidney disease.

Coronary heart disease or ischaemic heart disease

Coronary heart disease is caused by any condition that narrows the coronary arteries which take blood from the aorta to the heart muscle. The commonest cause of narrowing is atheroma. Atheroma is a condition in which fatty patches form on the inside of arteries. These patches of atheroma can partly block the artery, or if a clot forms on top of one of them, it can completely block the artery suddenly. There are other causes of blocked arteries including syphilis affecting the aorta but this and other causes are uncommon.

Frequency, cause, pathology, symptoms, signs and complications

This condition is uncommon in village people in non-industrialised countries who still live in their traditional ways; but it occurs in middle-aged and elderly town people who have changed to some of the western ways of living, eating, smoking, working and not exercising. It is more common in people with high blood pressure or diabetes, especially if they are not treated properly; and in those who over-eat (especially animal fats), exercise little and are overweight; and in those who smoke. High levels of some fats in the blood (cholesterol and triglycerides) follow the above and seem to be the main cause of the atheroma which causes coronary heart disease. It is common in middle-aged and old people in industrialised countries.

If the coronary arteries are partly blocked, not much blood can get to the heart muscle. When the heart does not have a lot of work to do, such as sitting or sleeping, there is enough blood for the heart muscle. When the heart has a lot of work to do, such as exercising or after a large meal or if the patient becomes cross, then there is not enough blood for the heart muscle. This lack of blood causes pain – like pain in any other part of the body if this part of the body is repeatedly exercised doing something it is not able to keep on doing. This pain is called 'angina pectoris' or just 'angina'. Angina comes on exertion (and after a few other things) and goes once the exertion is stopped within a minute or so, but will come back again when the same amount of exertion is done again. The pain is in the centre of the front of the chest but as well as that can sometimes also be felt in the arms or jaw. It is like a crushing weight or tight band. Sometimes this partly blocked artery can also cause the heart to beat irregularly. Sometimes it can cause heart failure.

If the artery becomes completely blocked, then the part of the heart muscle which it normally supplied will die and eventually be replaced by scar tissue which cannot pump blood. Meanwhile, the patient will have pain like angina, except that it will be there all the time for hours and not go away. The patient is at risk of dying from the pulse being too fast or too slow or heart failure or shock. This is called a 'myocardial infarction' or a 'heart attack'.

Differential diagnosis

Check that there is not another cause of:

- chest pain (see Chapter 20 page 234) or
- heart failure (see page 373) or
- shock (see page 377) or
- irregular heart rate, e.g. thyrotoxicosis.

Treatment

Treatment of all patients

On diagnosis, make sure the patient starts correcting any of those things which caused the condition if they apply to him;

1. reduce body weight to the ideal,
2. do not eat a lot of animal fat but more cereals, vegetables and fruit,
3. treat any diabetes present,
4. treat any hypertension present especially reducing salt in the food,
5. stop any tobacco smoking,
6. exercise regularly at least for 20–30 minutes for at least four times a week (walking, quickly without stopping will do),
7. send blood for serological test for syphilis.

Treat any other condition which may be making the patient worse:

1. Carefully look for and treat any anaemia present.
2. Look for and treat any heart failure present.
3. Look for a fast or irregular pulse and discuss any such patient with your Medical Officer about tests for thyrotoxicosis and other tests and if the patient should have digoxin.
4. Look very carefully for thyrotoxicosis and if possible arrange for tests for this or get your Medical Officer to see the patient.

Treatment of angina pectoris

1. Aspirin 100–150 mg daily (to try to stop blood clots forming in the artery).
2. Glyceryl trinitrate (0.5 or 0.6 mg tabs) dissolved under the tongue slowly if angina or before doing things known to usually cause angina. Side effects include flushing, headaches and dizziness. If the pain stays and side effects do not occur, a second dose can be taken. Isosorbide dinitrate (5 mg or 10 mg tabs) can be used instead.
3. If the patient still continues to have problems refer him to your Medical Officer for consideration for further treatment which could include long-acting nitrates, beta-blocker drugs or calcium-channel blocker drugs.
   Cholesterol lowering drugs and coronary artery dilation, stenting and bypass grafting surgery are not normally available.

Treatment of myocardial infarction

1. Make the patient rest and sit or lie down.
2. Get the patient to swallow 300 mg of aspirin (1 tab) immediately (to help stop more blood clotting).
3. Put glyceryl trinitrate 0.5 or 0.6 mg or isosorbide dinitrate 10 mg under the tongue and let is dissolve slowly. If the pain is still present and the blood pressure over 100 in 15 minutes, give a further dose.
4. If the pain is still present, give morphine 10–15 mg (1–1.5 ml) or pethidine 100–150 mg (2–3 ml) IMI and repeat the dose when necessary.
5. Give metoclopramide 10 mg by IVI or IMI and repeat later if any nausea or vomiting.
6. Treat any heart failure present in the usual way, including oxygen, diuretics and digoxin (see page 375).
7. If the pulse rate and heart rate (listening at the heart apex with the stethoscope) is 40 beats per minute or less, then (a) lift up the legs (feet above hips) and tilt the head end of the bed down and (b) give atropine 0.6 mg (1 ml) IVI then repeat if still needed in 5 minutes and can be repeated in 1 hour and then each few hours to a maximum of 3 mg in

24 hours to try, if possible, to get the heart rate above 60.
8. If the pulse is irregular and fast (over 140) start digoxin (see page 375) and propranolol 40 mg or atenelol 25 mg.

Most deaths occur soon after the myocardial infarction, most in the first hour and most of the rest in the first day. If therefore the patient survives this time, there is a good chance he will slowly get better and you can slowly get him to do more and more activity. However, you should talk to your Medical Officer about what facilities are available at the hospital and what you should do about such cases, and their treatment, transfer, etc.

Prevention

People should not eat too much animal fat or refined carbohydrates (such as white sugar); not get fat; not smoke; exercise regularly; and get proper treatment for hypertension, diabetes mellitus, etc.

28

Disorders of the Bones and Muscles

Anatomy

See Figure 28.1

Osteomyelitis

Osteomyelitis is an infection of the bone.

Acute osteomyelitis is caused by bacteria, usually staphylococci (which may be resistant to penicillin), and, in some parts of the world, salmonellae (which are usually resistant to penicillin).

Chronic osteomyelitis can develop from acute osteomyelitis that is not treated properly. Chronic osteomyelitis can also be a chronic infection from the start and is then often caused by tuberculosis bacteria, usually in the spine. Chronic osteomyelitis in the other bones is usually caused by ordinary bacteria.

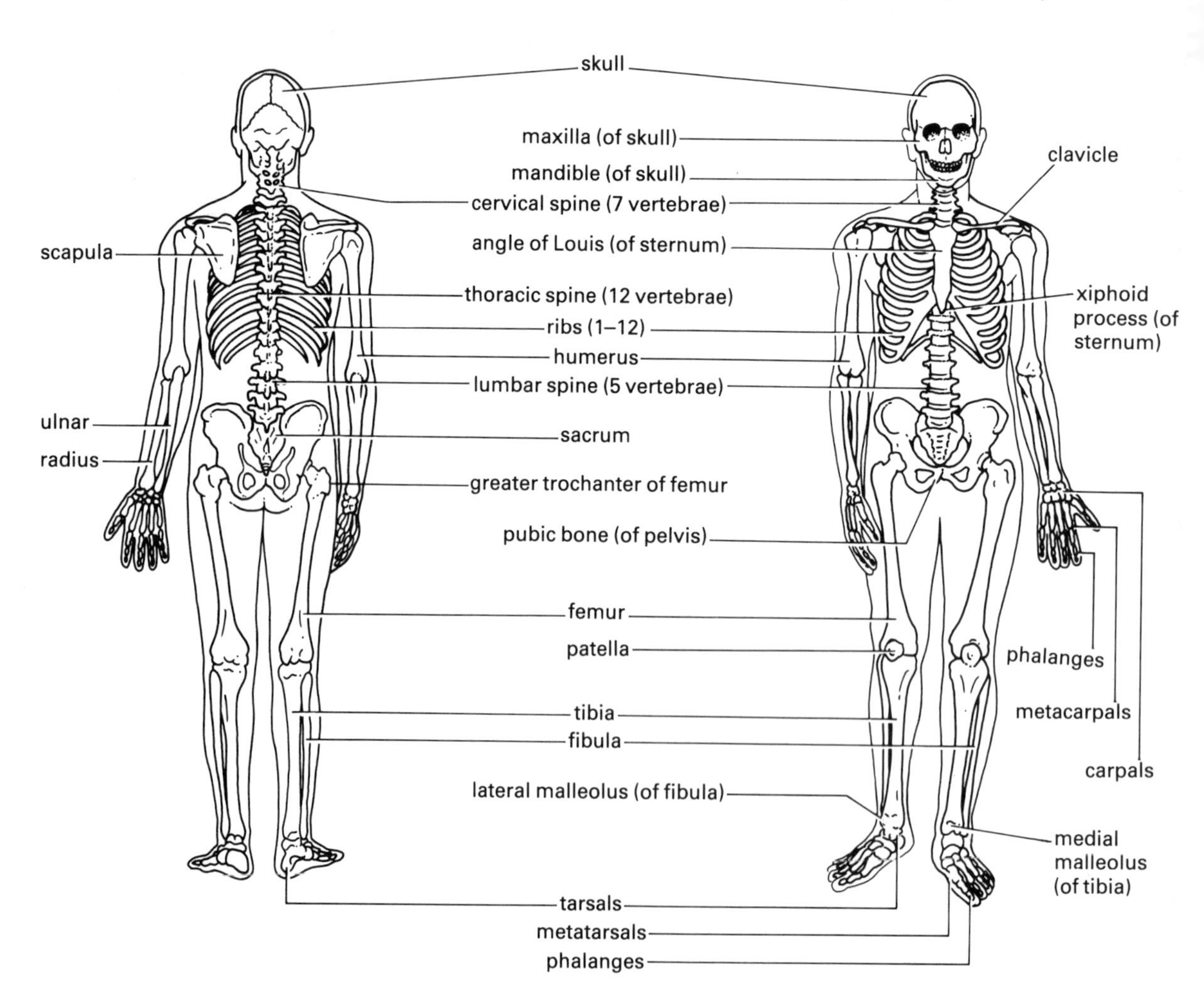

Figure 28.1 Diagram showing the skeleton (or bones of the body).

Acute osteomyelitis

The organism carrying the bone infection usually goes to the bone through the blood.

The *history* from the patient usually includes:

1. A recent skin infection that may be still present (often).
2. A recent injury to the bone (often).
3. The sudden start of symptoms and signs.

Another history suggestive of acute osteomyelitis is

1. A patient with sickle cell disease.
2. The sudden onset of symptoms and signs in a bone (often the fingers or toes, but any bone) which has not improved in 2 days and has settled within 7–9 days after the usual treatment for an infarction crisis (see Chapter 21 page 245).

Symptoms usually include:

1. Sudden start of fever, rigors, etc.
2. Severe pain where the bone infection is, which gets worse quickly.
3. The patient cannot use the affected limb.

On examination you will usually find these signs:

1. Fever, fast pulse, etc.
2. Severe tenderness, swelling, heat and other signs of acute inflammation where the bone infection is.
3. Muscle spasm (the patient cannot use the affected limb).

Complications include:

1. Septicaemia.
2. Acute bacterial arthritis of a nearby joint.
3. Damage to the bone, so that it does not grow properly later.
4. Chronic osteomyelitis, usually with a sinus which discharges pus.

Treatment includes

1. Rest the affected part by splinting it, and putting the patient to bed.
2. Give chloramphenicol or dicloxacillin or flucloxacillin or cloxacillin (see Chapter 11 page 46). You can reduce the dose when the patient appears to be cured; but you must still continue the antibiotic until at least 4 weeks. If you use penicillin and it does not work quickly, change to e.g. dicloxacillin except in sicke cell anaemia, to chloramphenicol.
3. Analgesics (see Chapter 7 page 29).

Transfer the patient for operation if:

1. the affected area is not much improved in 2 days, or
2. it does not appear to be completely cured in 2 weeks.

Chronic osteomyelitis

Symptoms may include continuous or repeated discharge of pus from a sinus over the affected bone.

On examination the bone is usually thickened and there are usually scars or sinuses in the skin over the bone. There is usually chronic tenderness over the affected bone.

Repeated acute attacks of osteomyelitis occur.

Transfer such cases for treatment. Treatment includes antibiotics and rest in the acute stage, but importantly later an operation by a Medical Officer.

Osteomyelitis of the spine

Osteomyelitis of the vertebrae causes a continuous neck or back ache which gets worse slowly and stiffness and tenderness of that part of the spine.

If the condition is acute and the patient also has a fever, the osteomyelitis may be caused by ordinary bacteria. If the condition is chronic, then tuberculosis is a more usual cause (see Chapter 14 page 78).

Transfer all suspected cases of osteomyelitis of the spine to a Medical Officer for diagnosis and treatment. This is very important, as if treatment is not given quickly enough the bone may collapse (squash) and the spinal cord be pressed on and this could cause paralysis.

Other bone and muscle diseases

Neoplasms in bone

Neoplasms in bone may be either primary (benign or malignant) or secondary (malignant).

Symptoms and signs can include:

1. Pain and/or tenderness in a bone which does not improve, and keeps the patient awake at night.
2. A deformity of a bone – most often a lump.
3. A pathological fracture (a fracture after only a small injury or no injury, because the bone was

weak because it had been partly replaced by a cancer).
4. Compression of the spinal cord, if vertebrae affected by the cancer collapse.
5. Anaemia.

Transfer to or consult a Medical Officer in case it is due to an infection which could be treated.

Pyomyositis or tropical myositis

Pyomyositis is an acute bacterial infection of one or more of the large skeletal muscles, usually with *Staphylococcus aureus*. An abscess usually forms in the muscle and general symptoms and signs of infection develop. If you do not give treatment the condition can become chronic.

Pyomyositis is common only in developing and tropical countries.

Symptoms and *signs* include:

1. General symptoms and signs of infection – malaise, fever, fast pulse etc. If a large abscess or septicaemia develop, these become severe.
2. Pain in the affected muscle, which is present at rest and much worse when the patient moves the muscle. The affected muscle is firm and tender and painful if stretched during examination.
3. The general and local symptoms and signs of infection get much worse in the next few days. The muscle may become fluctuant; but only if it is just under the skin.
4. If it is not treated, the affected muscle becomes a bag of pus, and the patient becomes wasted, with anaemia etc. Septicaemia and death can occur.

Differential diagnosis of painful muscles:

1. generalised illness, e.g. malaria, influenza
2. unusual exercise
3. trauma to muscles
4. parasitic diseases of the muscle (e.g. trichinosis)
5. pain in nearby structures
   - joints
   - bones (osteomyelitis or fracture)
   - tendons
6. referred pain
7. others – see a medical reference book.

If the diagnosis is not certain, put a needle into the affected muscle. You can usually aspirate pus if the condition is pyomyositis.

Treatment is simple, if you make the diagnosis.

1. Antibiotics.
   If possible use tetracycline, as it needs no injections and the organisms are usually sensitive to it. Penicillin is often also effective, but needs repeated injections. Chloramphenicol may be needed, though if available one of the anti-staphyloccal penicillins such as dicloxacillin or flucloxacillin or cloxacillin would be best. Do not continue with tetracycline or penicillin if the patient is not quickly getting better. (See Chapter 11 page 46.)
2. Incision and drainage, if pus has formed.
   This is best done under general anaesthetic. Bleeding is sometimes severe and may need packing of the abscess cavity and local pressure to stop it. Incision and drainage is essential once pus has formed, for the patient to get better.

If the abscess is large or the patient very sick or if the patient does not quickly improve, it would be best to *transfer* such cases as soon as possible to your Medical Officer.

29

Disorders of Joints (Arthritis)

Anatomy

There are three types of joints in the body (see Figure 29.1).

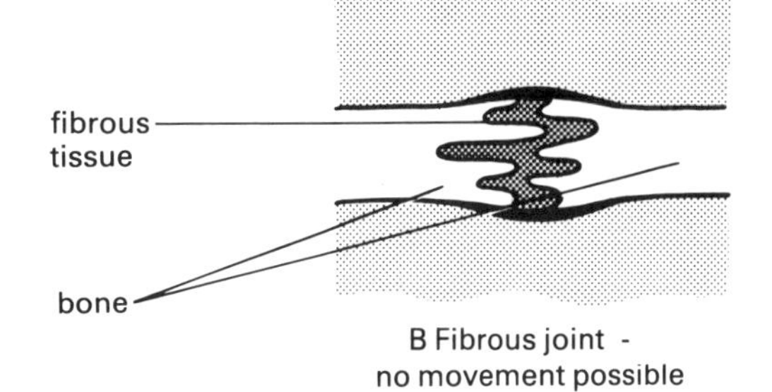

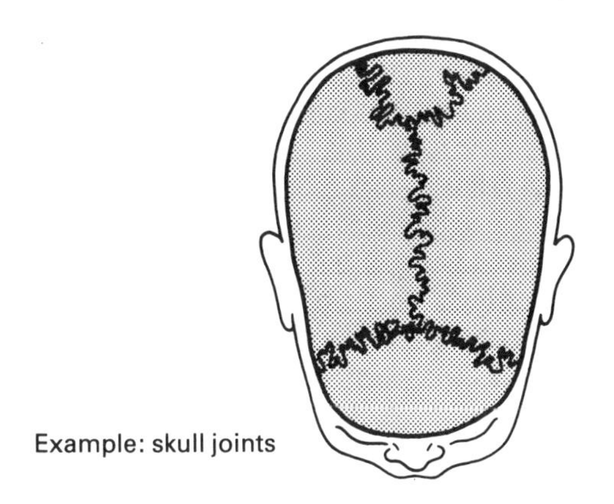

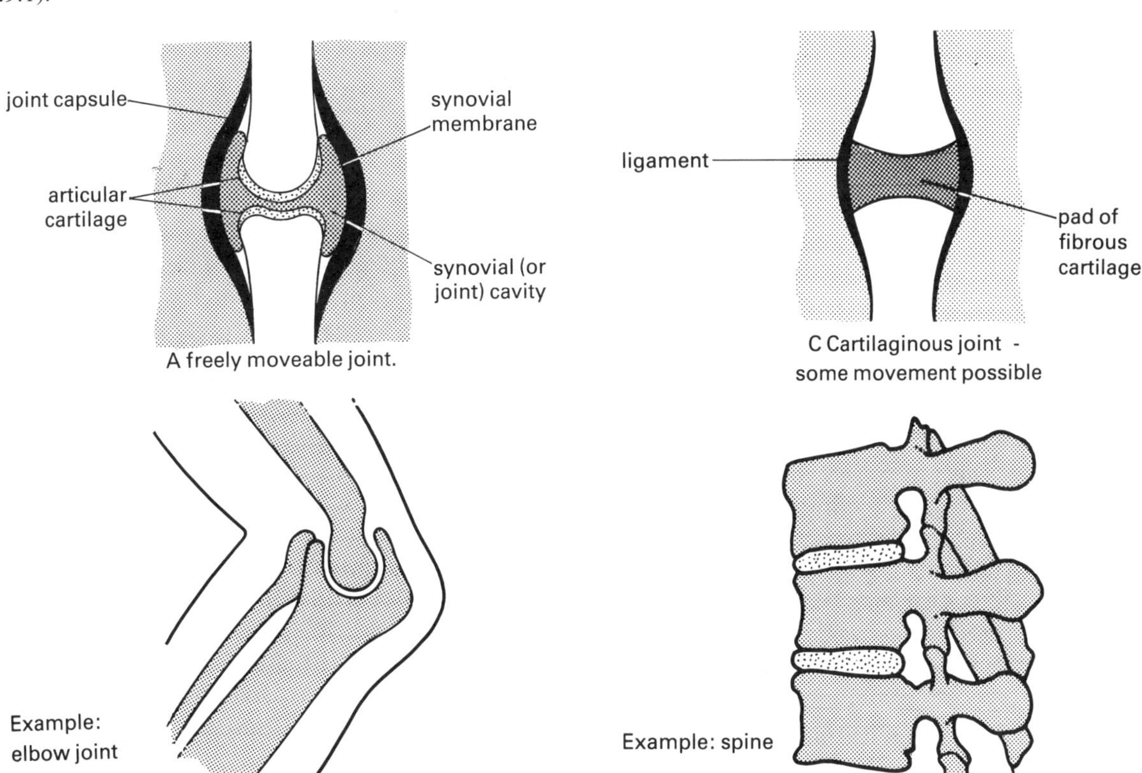

Figure 29.1 Diagram to show three types of joint. Note that in the freely movable type joint the articular cartilage is often not present. (For details of the anatomy of the spine see Chapter 25 page 339.)

Pathology, symptoms and signs

Arthritis is inflammation of a joint. Arthritis may be acute or chronic.

Symptoms and signs in the affected joint itself

The joint can have any of the usual symptoms and signs of inflammation.

1. Pain – acute and chronic cases.
2. Tenderness – acute cases only.
3. Swelling – acute and chronic cases.
4. Heat – acute cases only.
5. Redness and shininess – acute cases only.
6. Loss of function – i.e. not able to move properly (active and passive) and not able to work properly or bear weight – acute and chronic cases.
7. Abnormal fluid in the joint itself (called 'effusion') – acute and chronic cases

The patient complains of:

- pain,
- swelling, and
- loss of function (cannot move or use the joint).

On examination (depending on the type of arthritis);

1. *Inspection*
   - swelling
   - redness
   - deformity
2. *Palpation*
   - swelling
   - fluid
   - bone overgrowth at edges of joint
   - soft tissue swelling
   - tenderness
   - heat
   - movement
   - passive (patient rests and you move the joint), less than normal, painful, sometimes with crepitus (a grating feeling or noise)
   - active (patient moves the joint), less than normal, painful, sometimes with crepitus.
3. *Work or weight bearing*
   - less than normal or not possible

Symptoms and signs in the muscles which move the affected joint

In acute arthritis the muscles go into spasm so that the joint cannot be moved normally (movement causes pain). Later, and in chronic arthritis, the muscles waste and become thin and weak.

Even later, if the patient does not have physiotherapy, the muscles and tendons become shortened and changed into bands of fibrous tissues and cannot be stretched. These hold the joint in abnormal positions. These muscle and tendon changes are called contractures.

General symptoms and signs

These can include fever, fast pulse, malaise, wasting, etc.

1. Some may be the result of the cause of arthritis, e.g. rheumatic fever.
2. Some may be caused by the effect of the arthritis, e.g. toxins from the bacteria causing acute bacterial arthritis.

Disease in other parts of the body may be present and cause symptoms and signs

An example is tuberculosis of the lungs in a patient with tuberculous arthritis.

Note on examination of the spine

Check for:

- deformity (lump or twisting) of the spine,
- tender areas on palpation or percussion of the spine,
- movement of the spine in all directions,
- legs – movement and sensation,
- abdomen – bladder enlargement or incontinence of urine

Tests

The only important test you must do at a health centre is *the aspiration of a joint if the joint may be infected with bacteria (septic arthritis).* (Put a needle into the joint and suck out any fluid with a syringe. If pus is present, you must give antibiotics in high dosage.

Always use careful aseptic procedure when you aspirate a joint. Do not introduce bacteria into the joint and cause acute bacterial (septic) arthritis. Scrub up. Use mask gown and gloves. Prepare the skin carefully with iodine in spirit or another suitable anti septic. Use sterile needles and syringes. Always give a local anaesthetic before putting the large needle into the joint. Suck out all of the fluid that is in the joint. Put a sterile dressing over the needle hole.

Method of aspirating joints

These diagrams show where you can put a needle into the various joints (see Figures 29.2, 29.3, 29.4, 29.5, 29.6 and 29.7). But do *not* try to aspirate a hip joint unless you have had special training. Transfer a patient who needs aspiration of the hip joint to a Medical Officer.

Details of joint conditions

Traumatic arthritis

Traumatic arthritis is an acute arthritis caused by an injury to the joint. There is usually a *history* of an injury.

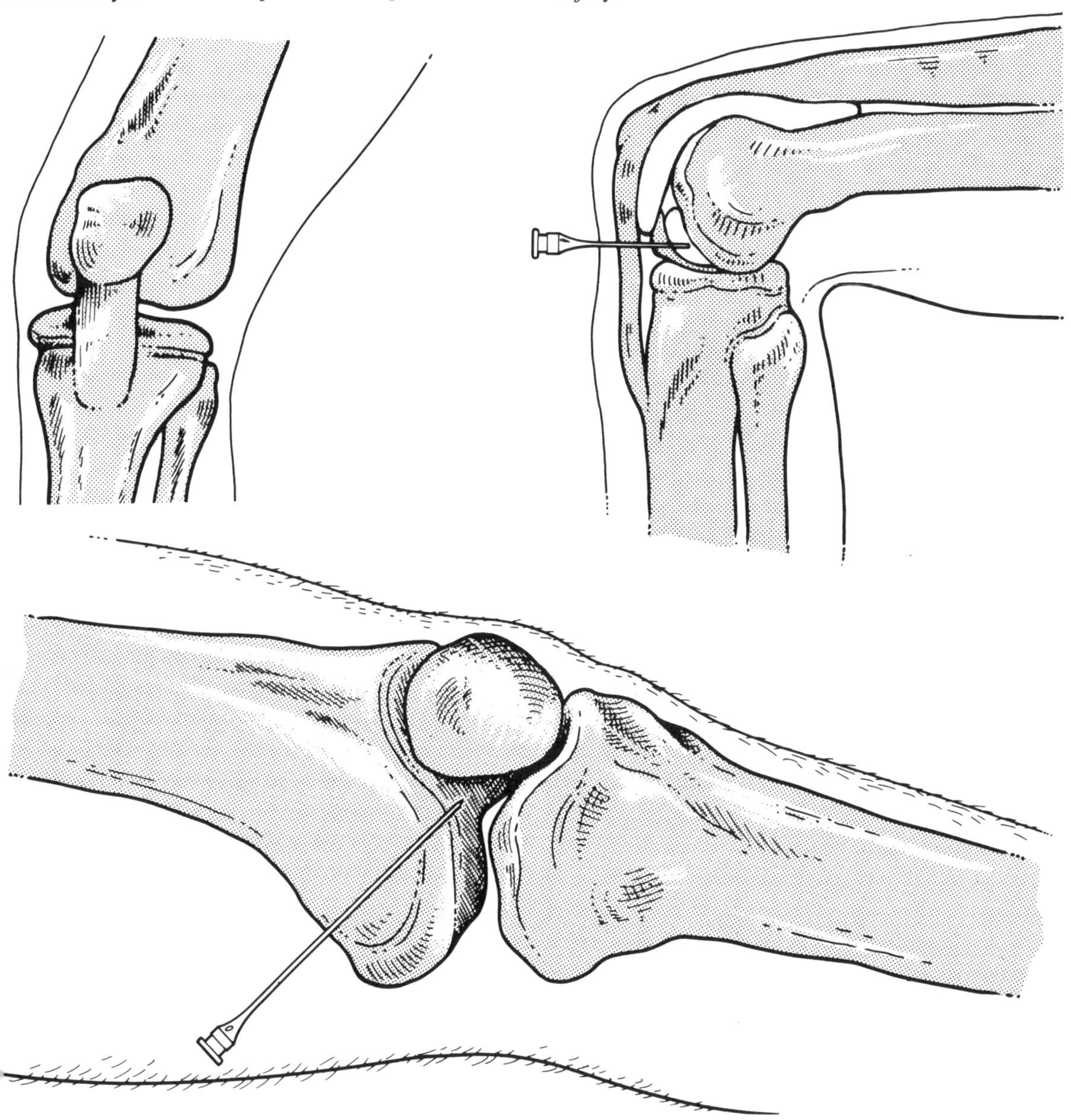

Figure 29.2 Methods of aspirating the knee joint. The top diagrams show an anterior method you can use when the knee is flexed (bent). The lower diagram shows a lateral method you can use when the knee is extended (straight). Usually you will use the lower method as a patient with acute arthritis usually cannot flex (bend) the knee.

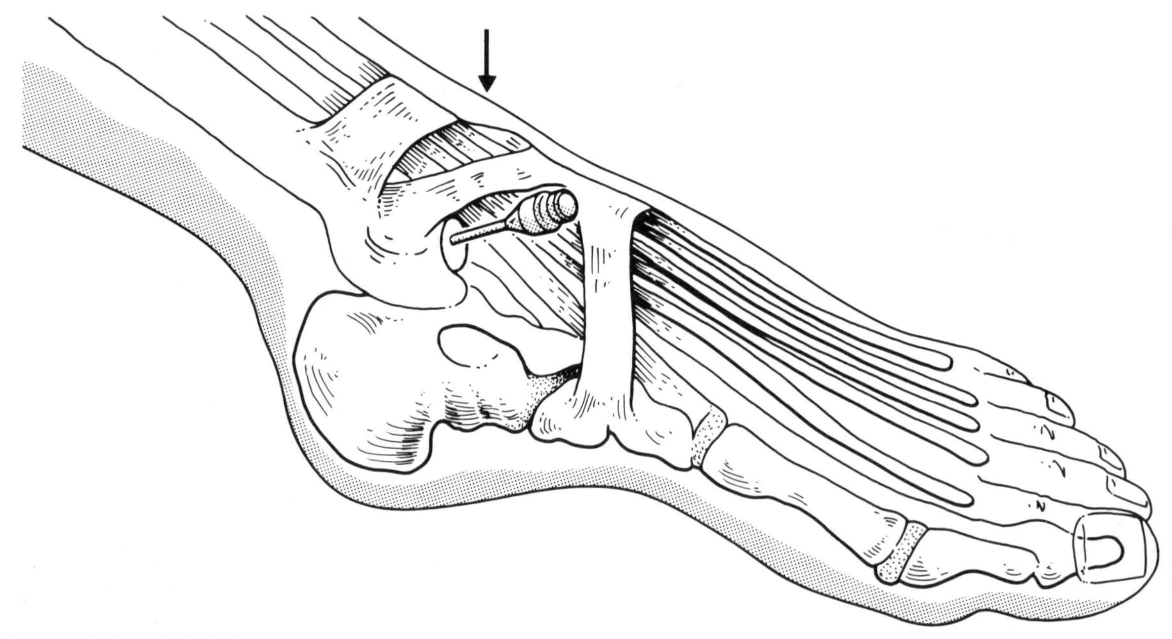

Figure 29.3 Method of aspirating the ankle joint.

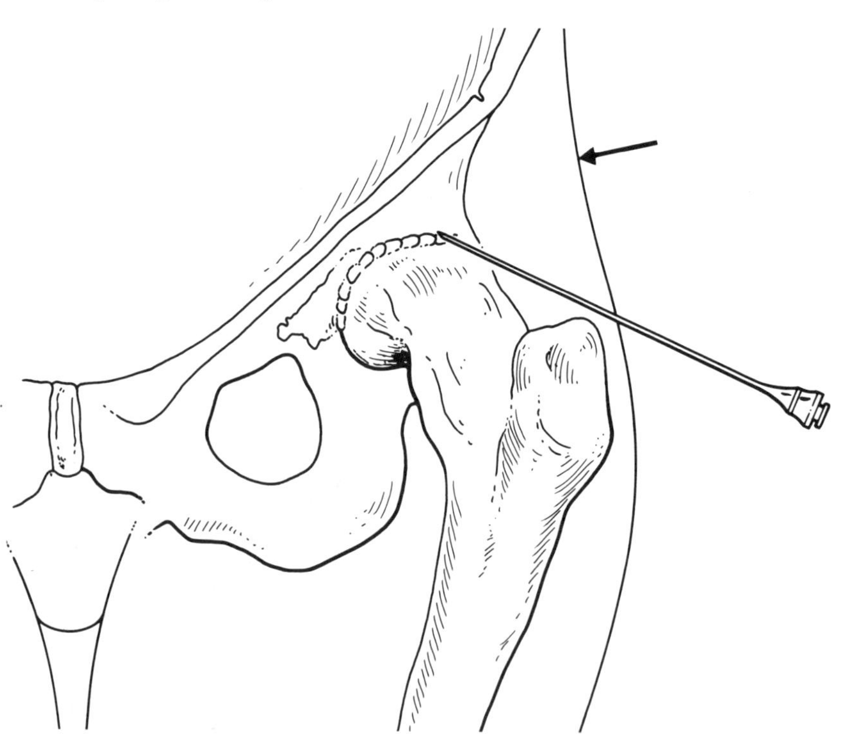

Figure 29.4 Method of aspirating the hip joint. Do not try to aspirate the hip joint unless you have had proper training.

On examination you will find:

1. acute arthritis with tenderness over the damaged area of the joint or of the ligaments around the joint; and usually an effusion;
2. no general symptoms and signs of infection.

Aspiration shows clear yellow fluid or blood.

Treatment includes:

1. aspiration of the joint;
2. splint until the acute stage is finished;
3. exercise muscles in the splint – 10 contractions o the muscles which move the joint in the splint

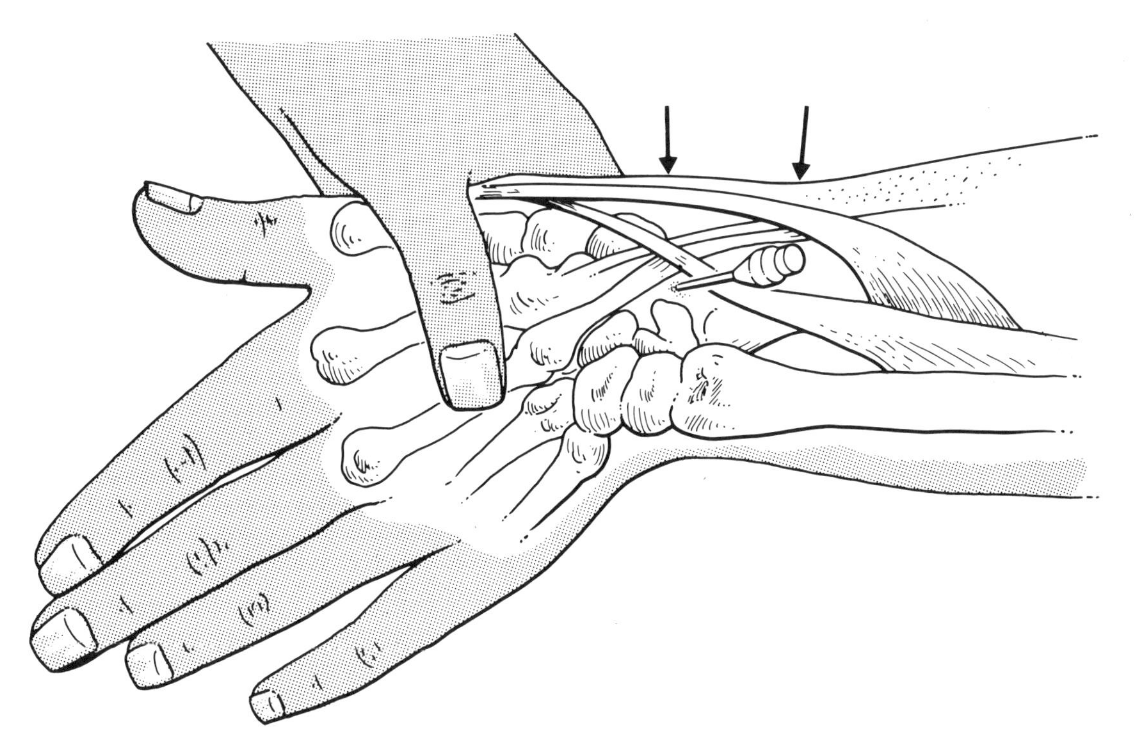

Figure 29.5 Method of aspirating the wrist (radio-carpal) joint.

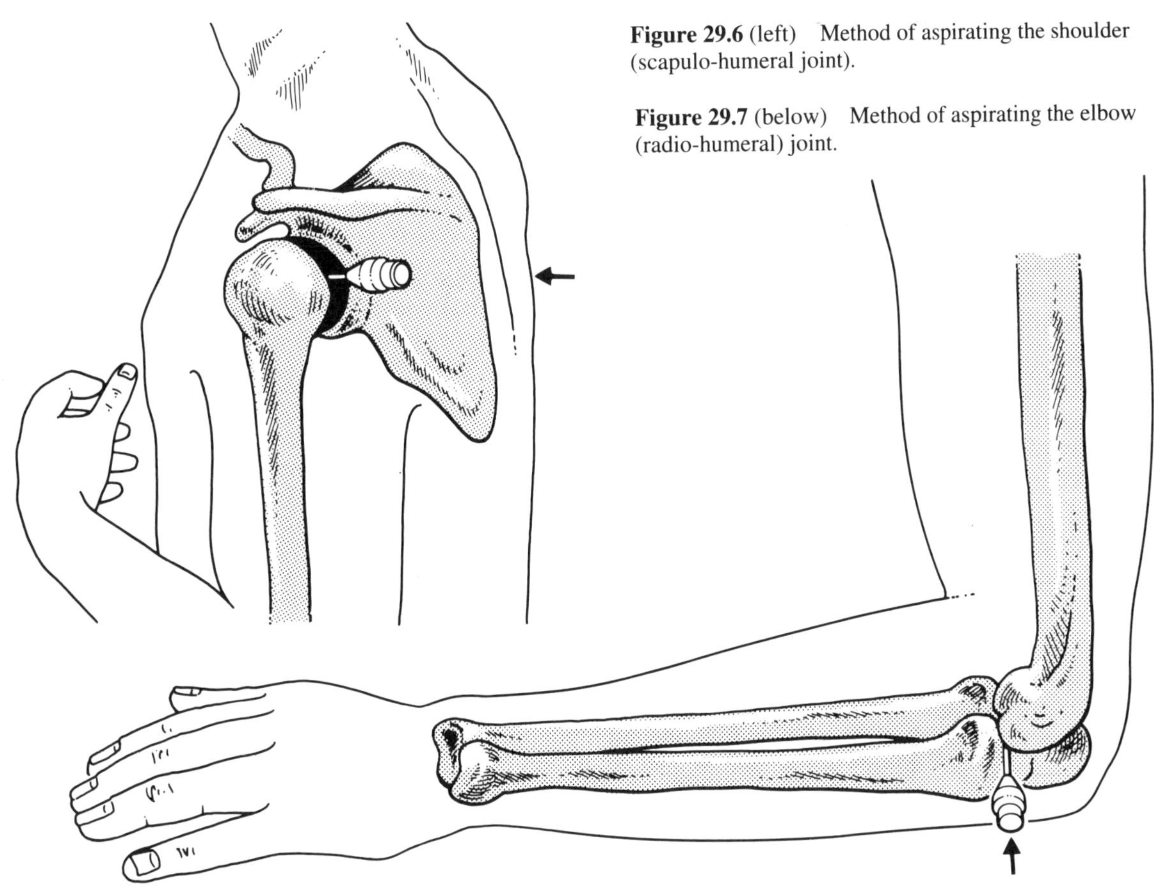

Figure 29.6 (left) Method of aspirating the shoulder (scapulo-humeral joint).

Figure 29.7 (below) Method of aspirating the elbow (radio-humeral) joint.

Table 29.1 The common causes of acute and chronic arthritis

Acute		*Chronic*
1. Traumatic	The most common	1. Oesteo-
2. Acute bacterial (septic)	The most important as (1) treatment cures (2) joint destroyed if not treated	2. Chronic bacterial (septic) 3. Tuberculous
3. Rheumatic fever		
4. Tropical arthritis	Acute, recurrent or chronic	4. Tropical arthritis
5. Rheumatoid	Usually chronic	5. Rheumatoid
6. Others See page 399	Usually acute See page 399 and medical reference book	6. Others See page 399

four times a day (but without letting the joint bend);
4. aspirin if necessary.

Transfer to Medical Officer if:

1. there are signs which may be caused by a fracture; *or*
2. the joint is unstable (ligaments are torn and it bends more than normal in any direction).

Acute bacterial (septic) arthritis

Acute bacterial arthritis is not common; but it is very important. Treatment will cure it. If it is not treated, it will destroy the joint.

Symptoms, signs and tests

Symptoms and signs of infection in another part of the body (especially skin infection but also urethral or lung or other infection, etc.) were often present *before* the arthritis. The infection was carried to the joint by the blood. Sometimes there was a wound that entered the joint. Sometimes there was a soft tissue or bone infection that got bigger and went into the joint. Sometimes there was an aspiration of the joint with an unsterile needle.

Symptoms in the joint are usually extreme pain and swelling of the affected joint, which the patient cannot move.

Signs in the joint (see Figure 29.8) are usually:

- swelling, caused by an 'effusion' made of pus,
- tenderness,
- heat,
- redness or shininess, and
- severe pain on moving the joint with guarding of the muscles which move that joint. This is usually so severe that the patient will not allow any movement of the joint.

General symptoms and signs of infection caused by the toxins from the arthritis are usually severe – fever, rigors, fast pulse etc.

Aspiration of the joint shows pus.

Treatment

1. Aspirate all the pus from the joint. Use strict aseptic precautions. Send pus for Gram stain, culture and sensitivity if possible. Repeat the aspiration when more pus forms (daily or more often if necessary).
2. Give antibiotics as for any acute severe bacterial infection (see Chapter 12). Give chloramphenicol 1 g (4 caps) orally immediately and repeat every 6 hours. Give 1 g (1 bottle) by IMI or IVI if necessary. Continue the antibiotic for at least 2 weeks. Reduce dose when the patient improves.
3. Splint the joint (usually with a well padded plaster-of-Paris (POP) back-slab). Elevate (raise up) the affected limb.
4. Give aspirin 600–1200 mg (2–4 tabs) or codeine compound tablets 2 tabs every 6 hours if needed for pain.

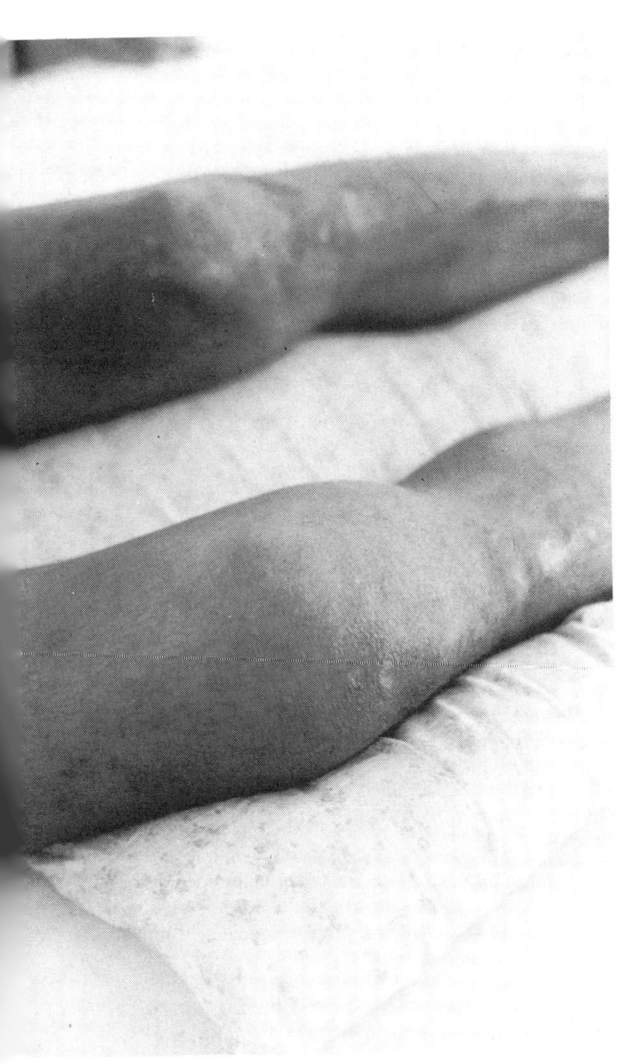

Figure 29.8 Acute bacterial ('septic') arthritis of the right knee. Note the large amount of swelling. Note that because of severe pain the patient is lying with the knee slightly bent over a pillow and would not allow the examiner to bend it during examination. This joint needs *immediate* aspiration. The patient needs *immediate* large doses of antibiotics.

5. Give antimalarial drugs as indicated; usually chloroquine 450–600 mg (3–4 tabs) daily for 3 days, if there is fever.
6. When the acute inflammation starts to improve, begin physiotherapy. Supervise the patient doing active exercises three times a day in the splint (the patient should contract all the muscles which normally move the joint 20–30 times; but without bending the joint). Move the joint through all its movements out of the splint, once daily. Remove the splint and start active exercises of the joint when all the signs of acute inflammation have gone.

Transfer to Medical Officer care:

1. all severe cases (urgent – but not emergency);
2. all cases of acute arthritis of the hip joint (urgent – but not emergency);
3. any case not much improved in 2 days (urgent – but not emergency);
4. any case where you have not aspirated all the pus for 2 days running (urgent – but not emergency); and
5. any case not cured in 2 weeks (non-urgent).

Rheumatic fever

Rheumatic fever is an acute non-infectious inflammatory disease of the joints and heart, and other parts of the body.

It is caused by an abnormal reaction of the immune system of the body to a streptococcal infection (usually a throat infection) the patient had about 2 weeks before.

It usually affects children and young adults.

Symptoms and signs

1. Usually fever is present, with one or more of the other signs and symptoms.
2. Acute arthritis. The arthritis usually:
   - starts quickly,
   - affects a large joint,
   - affects only one or two joints at a time,
   - is a typical acute arthritis,
   - gets completely better in the affected joint after a few days,
   - then affects another joint or joints,
   - lasts for 1–5 weeks moving from joint to joint.
3. Carditis (inflammation of the heart). This causes:
   - fast pulse and at times heart failure (this can get better),
   - damage to the heart valves (this does not cause immediate trouble, but it does not get better, and can slowly get worse and cause heart failure many years later).
4. Chorea or abnormal twisting movements of the body which the patient cannot stop.
5. Skin rash.
6. Nodules under the skin.

Treatment

1. Rest if there is acute arthritis or heart failure.

2. Aspirin in large doses regularly (see Chapter 7 page 30) starting with 600–900 mg 6th hourly.
3. Usual treatment of heart failure if this develops (see Chapter 27 page 375).
4. Procaine benzylpenicillin 1 g or 1,000,000 units IMI for 10 days to kill any of the bacteria left from the infection which caused the abnormal reaction.
5. Routine antimalarial treatment, if in a malarious area.

The arthritis usually gets better very quickly with treatment.

Prevention of further attacks is necessary so that the heart is not damaged again. Give long-acting penicillin injections, e.g. benzathine penicillin, 1.2 million units, every month for 10 years, or until the age of 20–25 years.

If bacteria get into the blood (during operations or dental extractions etc.), they can start to grow on the damaged valves before the body can destroy them. To stop this give all patients with damaged heart valves benzyl (crystalline) penicillin 2,000,000 units (4 ml) and streptomycin 1 g (2 ml) and procaine benzyl penicillin 900,000 units (3 ml) 1 hour before the operation or dental extraction; and after the operation, procaine benzyl penicillin 900,000 units (3 ml) daily for 3 more days.

'Tropical arthritis'

Tropical arthritis is an unusual type of chronic (but sometimes acute) arthritis that occurs in some tropical countries.

The cause is sometimes infection with filaria. Most times the cause is not known.

Clinical features

Young adults are usually affected; but patients can be any age.

It affects one or two (only sometimes more) joints, usually the knees or ankles.

Symptoms include swelling or pain of the joint.

Signs include marked swelling (caused by effusion) and painful movement of the joint (see Figure 29.9). Tenderness and heat may occur in acute cases. Limited movement and deformity may occur in late severe cases. Usually no general signs are present.

Aspiration gives fluid which is green or yellow and clear or cloudy; but the fluid is usually different from pus.

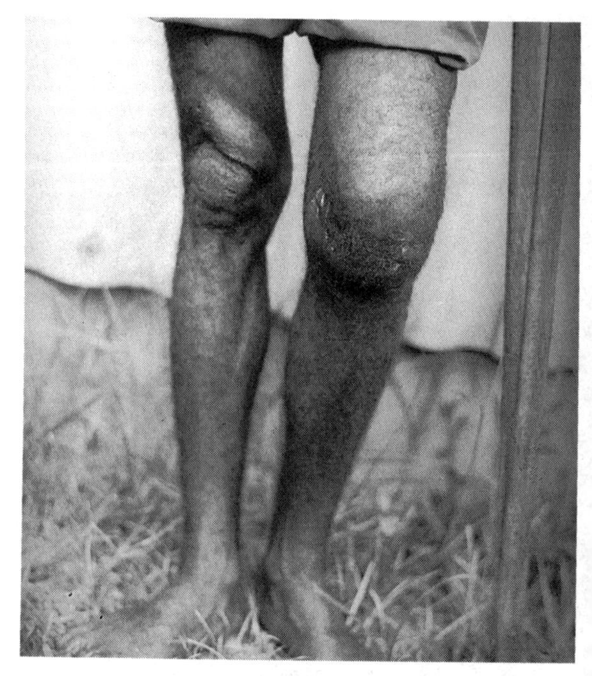

Figure 29.9 Tropical arthritis affecting the left knee. The patient was treated first with chloramphemicol in large doses for 2 weeks (but joint fluid aspirated and examined in the laboratory did not confirm the diagnosis of bacterial infection). He was then treated with diethylcarbamazine for 3 weeks. He had large doses of aspirin during this time, and a splint and physiotherapy. At 6 weeks he still has arthritis with a lot of swelling but not much pain. This is common in 'tropical arthritis'.

Send a serology test for filariasis or *thick smears for microfilaria* (see Chapter 22 page 261) to laboratory for examination for microfilaria.

Sometimes the arthritis goes away without treatment. Sometimes it returns later. Sometimes chronic pain and swelling continue for months or years. In severe or prolonged cases, the joint is destroyed.

Management of a case of tropical arthritis

Always check that it is not:

1. acute infective arthritis, by aspirating the joint;
2. traumatic arthritis and rheumatic fever and rheumatoid arthritis, by history and examination;
3. tuberculous arthritis, if possible, by history and examination (if this is not possible, transfer the patient for investigation).

Admit all suspected cases. Send serology test thick blood smears (taken at midnight on three nights) for examination for microfilaria.

Treatment

1. Aspirate all the fluid from the joint. Use strict aseptic precautions. Send the fluid for Gram stain, culture and sensitivity (if possible). If you think the fluid may be pus, treat as for acute bacterial (septic) arthritis (see page 392).
2. Splint the joint (usually in a well padded POP back-slab) until the acute stage finishes. When you are certain that no further improvement will occur (e.g. after 6 weeks), remove the splint.
3. Physiotherapy.
   Make the patient do active exercises three times a day in the splint. Show the patient how to contract all the muscles which normally move the joint but without moving the joint itself. Tell the patient to do this 20–40 times three times every day.
   Move the joint through all its movements out of the splint once daily; but only after the acute inflammation has started to improve (if it was present).
   Make the patient do active exercises with movement of the joint after all the signs of acute inflammation have gone.
4. Aspirin 900–1200 mg (3–4 tabs) four times a day.
5. Antimalarial drug as indicated usually chloroquine 450–600 mg (3–4 tabs) daily for 3 days, if there is any fever.
6. Diethylcarbamazine 100 mg (2 tabs) three times a day for 3 weeks if the patient is in (or has been in) an area where filariasis occurs. See Chapter 22 page 261 about reactions to diethylcarbamazine and how to start with a low dose and give promethazine.

Transfer to Medical Officer care if:

1. the arthritis may be acute bacterial (septic) arthritis which is not improving with antibiotics (urgent); or
2. the arthritis may be tuberculous arthritis (non-urgent).

Rheumatoid disease

Rheumatoid disease is a chronic disease that affects the whole body but especially the joints. The cause is not known. Often patients are middle-aged adults; but it can affect people of any age.

First, general symptoms and signs of ill health are present for some weeks – malaise, fever, aches and paints, etc. Then there can be anaemia, weight loss, etc.

The arthritis usually:

1. is chronic, but it can start with an acute attack and become acute from time to time;
2. is roughly symmetrical (i.e. same joints on both sides of body);
3. starts in the small joints of hands and feet (especially the first joints of the fingers) see Figure 29.10;

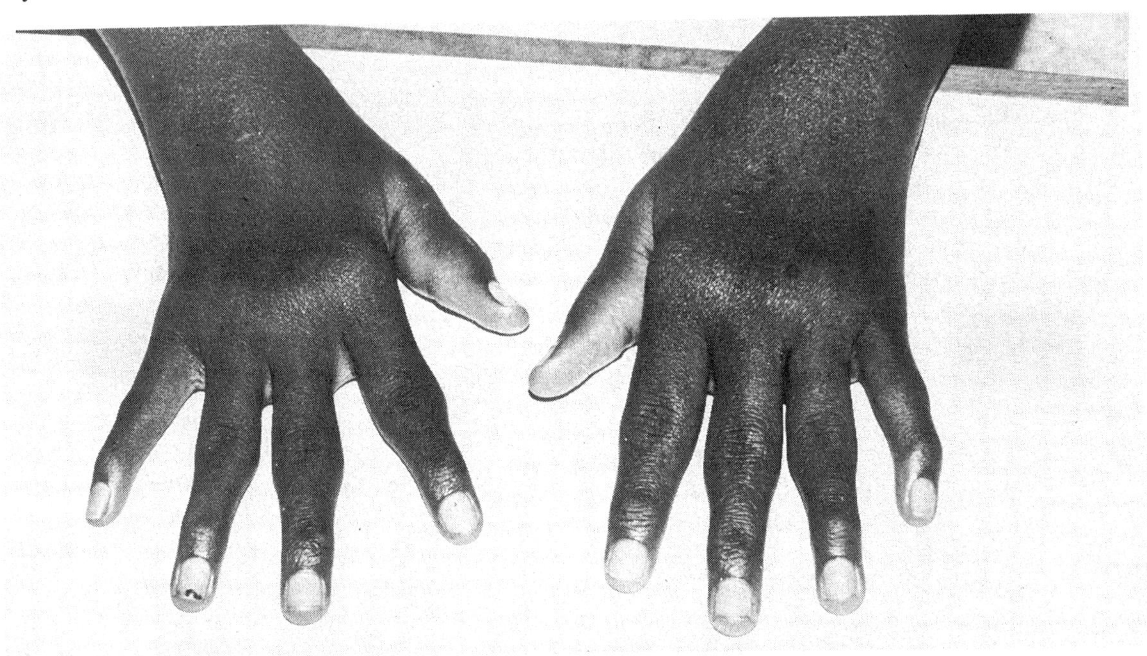

Figure 29.10 Late severe rheumatoid disease affecting hands. Note the swelling of the first joints of the fingers, which suggests rheumatoid disease.

4. then spreads to larger joints (wrists, ankles, knees, etc. and sometimes the spine);
5. has symptoms of pain and stiffness, worse in the morning or after rest and a little improved by use or exercise;
6. has, at first, signs of:
   - swelling of soft tissues around the joint
   - effusion and
   - inflammation;
7. has, later, severe joint destruction with deformity, stiffness and loss of use of the joint, especially if not treated properly.

Aspiration is usually not necessary for diagnosis (as many joints are involved and the arthritis is not very acute); but aspirated fluid is yellow and cloudy if you do this.

Sometimes acute bacterial arthritis can develop in a joint affected by rheumatoid arthritis.

Treatment includes aspirin in large doses, e.g. 900–1200 mg (3–4 tablets) four times a day (maximum 4 g daily) regularly for months or years; the patient should wear splints made to hold the joints in their proper positions at night if deformity is developing and he should also have physiotherapy.

Tuberculous arthritis

Tuberculous arthritis is a chronic inflammatory arthritis caused by infection of the joint with tuberculosis bacteria.

Tuberculous arthritis is not common; but it is important. Treatment will cure it. If it is not treated, it will destroy the joint.

Most often if affects the hip or knee (see Figure 29.11); but it can affect any joint.

Most often the patient is a child or young adult; but it can affect people of any age

Symptoms include pain and stiffness of the joint, or a limp.

Signs include:

1. *Chronic arthritis which slowly gets worse* (swelling, tenderness, warmth, pain on moving joint; limited movement of joint, the patient cannot use joint properly, etc.).
2. *Severe wasting of the muscles* which move the joint.
3. Nearby lymph glands usually enlarged.
4. A sinus discharging pus near the joint late in the disease.

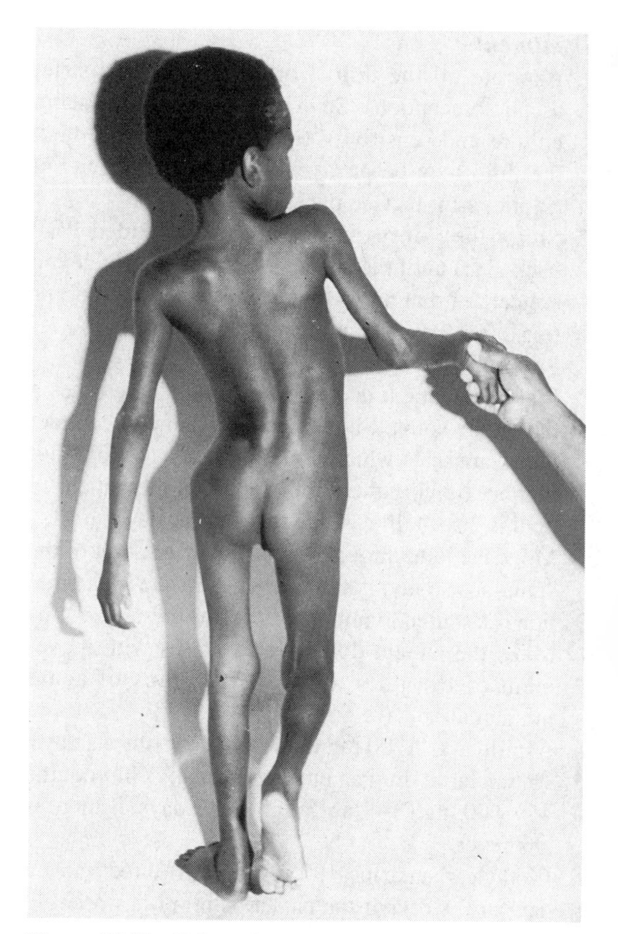

Figure 29.11 Tuberculous arthritis of the left hip. Note that any patient with chronic arthritis of one joint must be transferred for test. Note the typical severe wasting of the muscles of the left thigh.

5. Symptoms and signs of tuberculosis in other parts of the body (e.g. chronic cough or enlarged lymph glands).
6. The tuberculin test is usually positive.

> You should suspect tuberculous arthritis in any chronic arthritis that gets progressively worse over months and refer or transfer the patient for tests. This is especially important if only one joint is affected and if the tuberculin test is positive.

Do not diagnose a case of arthritis as osteoarthrosis if there are signs of *inflammation* which *get slowly worse*. Osteoarthrosis does not usually have inflammation of the joint and it has times when it gets better and times when it gets worse. Think instead of tuberculous arthritis and transfer the patient for tests and treatment.

Vertebral tuberculosis

Vertebral tuberculosis is a special type of tuberculous arthritis. It starts in the joints between the vertebrae and then spreads to the bones of the vertebrae.

Symptoms include:

1. Back pain and stiffness which lasts for weeks or months and does not get better but gets increasingly worse.
2. Later, a lump or deformity in the spine (if some infected bones collapse).
3. Sometimes, weakness or paralysis and loss of sensation in the legs and the patient cannot pass urine properly (if there is spinal cord pressure).

Signs include:

1. Tenderness and stiffness of part of the spine.
2. Later, a lump or deformity of the spine.
3. Sometimes, weakness or paralysis and loss of sensation in the legs and an enlarged bladder or urinary incontinence (if there is spinal cord pressure).
4. There may be symptoms or signs of tuberculosis in other parts of the body, e.g. chronic cough or enlarged lymph glands.
5. The tuberculin test is usually positive.

Transfer the patient for diagnosis by X-ray, if you suspect vertebral tuberculosis. Transfer urgently for treatment, if cord pressure occurs.

Suspect vertebral tuberculosis at the stage of chronic, constant, increasing backache with stiffness and tenderness of the spine, before a lump forms or the spinal cord is damaged. (See Figure 29.12.)

Osteoarthrosis (osteoarthritis)

Osteoarthrosis is a degeneration or 'wearing out' of joints.

It occurs in older adults in the joints they use most – hips, knees, spine, etc. *or* in younger persons in a joint which has previously been seriously injured.

Osteoarthrosis is not an *arthritis*. There is no inflammation of the joint (unless it has been injured

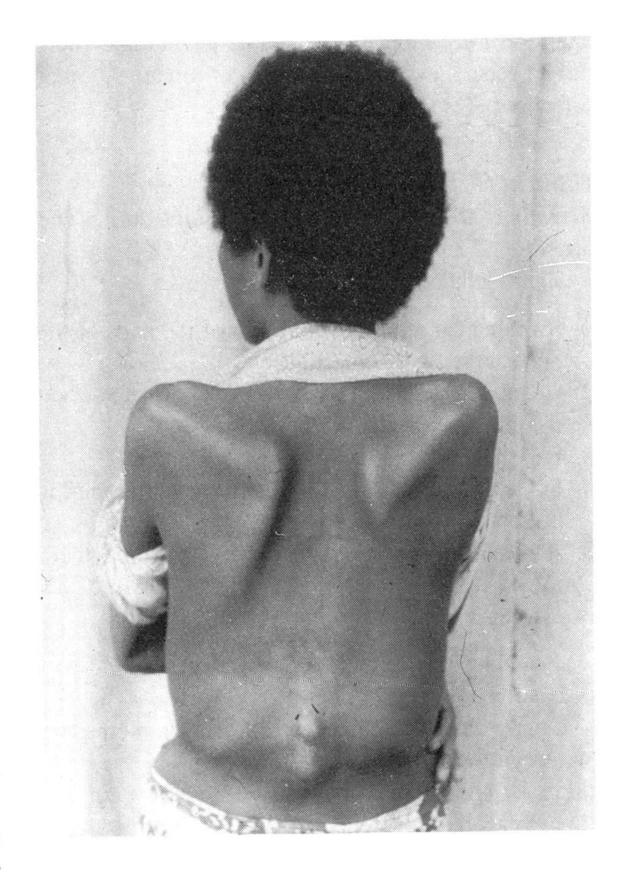

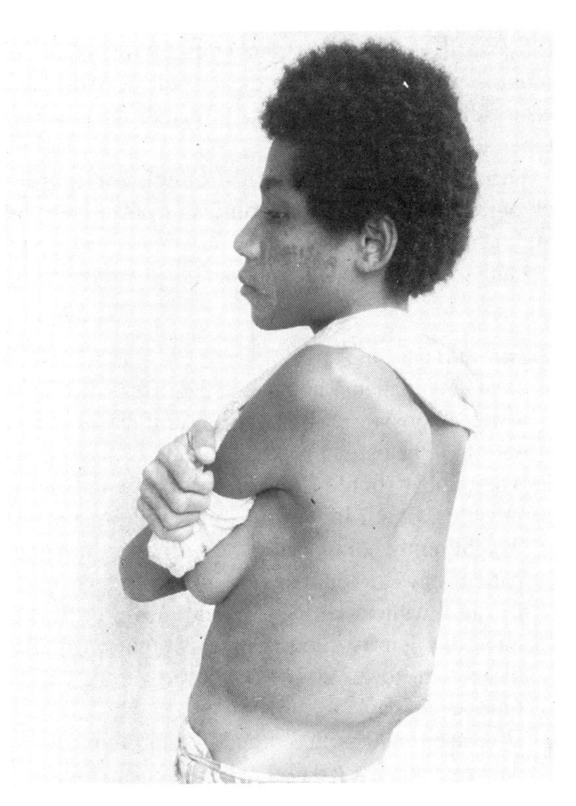

Figure 29.12 Tuberculosis of the spine. Note the deformity of the spine (often called a 'gibbus'). Tuberculosis of the spine is often called Pott's disease. This patient needs urgent transfer before she becomes paraplegic.

again or used a lot, just before examination). There are no general symptoms or signs of inflammation or infection.

Clinical features

Symptoms are usually of pain in a joint during and after use. The pain is improved by rest.

Signs include:

1. Swelling caused by overgrowth of the ends of the bone at the 'worn out' joint.
2. Crepitus (a 'crackling' you can feel or hear) when the joint is moved.
3. Full movement of the joint is not possible.
4. Some wasting of muscles which move the joint is present.
5. *If recent injury or hard work* by the joint, there may be some tenderness and sometimes an effusion.

If you aspirate any effusion present the fluid will be clear yellow. It is not pus.

Usually there is a slow start of the symptoms and signs. Very slowly the condition gets worse. Usually there are times when there is little or no pain and times when the symptoms are much worse.

Always check that the condition is not tuberculous arthritis. If there is inflammation of the joint, and if the arthritis gets worse and worse over weeks or months, and if there is severe muscle wasting, and especially if only one joint is affected, then suspect tuberculous arthritis.

Other diseases you should check for include chronic infective (bacterial) arthritis, 'tropical' arthritis and rheumatoid arthritis.

Outpatient or inpatient treatment is possible.

Treatment

1. Rest. The patient should use the affected joint as little as possible. Tell the patient how to lose weight if the patient is fat.
2. The patient should do exercise to strengthen the muscles which move the joint without putting weight on the joint during the exercises. *Show* the patient how to contract the muscles which move the joint without letting the joint move, or how to move the joint without putting weight on it. *Tell* the patient to do 20–40 of these exercises three times every day.
3. Give aspirin 900–1200 mg (3–4 tabs) four times a day (maximum 4 g daily), when pain is present.

Transfer to Medical Officer care is not necessary unless tuberculous arthritis is a possibility (see page 396).

Osteoarthrosis of spine

Osteoarthrosis of the spine is the same as oeteoarthrosis of other joints, except that it affects the spinal joints. The nerves that go from the spinal cord to the body may *sometimes* be pressed on. This can *sometimes* give pain radiating to the arms, trunk or legs and/or weakness of the muscles of the arms or legs.

Symptoms include:

1. Pain and stiffness in the neck or back, often worse after exercise and improved by rest.
2. Pain radiating to the trunk or the limbs (sometimes).
3. Weakness of some muscles (sometimes).

Signs include:

1. Stiffness of the neck or back (which will not bend properly in all directions); pain on some movements of the spine; and sometimes tenderness on percussion of the spine.
2. Loss of sensation of part of a limb (sometimes).
3. Muscle weakness of part of a limb (sometimes).

The symptoms and signs may be severe, then greatly improve only to return again (i.e. there are good and bad times).

Treatment is as for osteoarthrosis of other joints, and especially 'extension exercises' to strengthen muscles along spine.

Check that the patient has no weakness of the legs, loss of control of the bladder, signs of inflammation of the spine, increasing worsening of the disease, or symptoms and signs of tuberculosis in other parts of the body. If the patient has any of these things, *transfer* the patient for the Medical Officer to check that it is not tuberculosis of the spine.

Deformity of spine

Causes include:

1. fracture,
2. tuberculosis,
3. others – see a specialist reference book.

Acute arthritis of many joints from other causes

The causes of 'tropical arthritis' (see page 394) and rheumatoid disease with arthritis (see page 395) are not known in most cases. But both of these diseases have characteristic clinical features. Even if you are not certain that the patient has one of these when you first see him, the characteristic clinical course usually makes you certain after some weeks.

Sometimes also you will suspect rheumatoid disease or tropical arthritis; but the arthritis gets better quickly or has a course not typical of these diseases.

There are a large number of other conditions which can cause arthritis similar to rheumatoid disease or tropical arthritis; and these are often hard to diagnose in a health centre.

Whenever you see a case of arthritis first *check that it is not acute bacterial arthritis* or *tuberculous arthritis*; although these usually affect only one joint. Other conditions which the patient may have are:

1. *Reiter's syndrome* is a condition which causes arthritis, conjunctivitis, urethritis and other skin and mucous membrane lesions. It often follows a sexually transmitted disease or gastroenteritis. Tetracycline treatment and aspirin sometimes helps.
2. *Virus infections such as hepatitis and rubella* can cause an arthritis that affects several joints. The arthritis is usually not severe. Other signs of the virus infection are present.
3. *Virus infection carried by mosquitoes and other insects* (arbor viruses) can cause both single cases and epidemics of arthritis of several joints. Fever and rashes of various types are often present at first; but the disease gets better after some weeks or months. See Chapter 17 page 129.
4. *Allergic reactions of various types* (see Chapter 10 page 39), especially the 'serum sickness' type and those caused by drugs (including intravenous iron infusions) can cause acute and chronic arthritis of many joints which finally gets better. Reactions in leprosy (Chapter 15 page 103) can also cause arthritis.
5. There are also a large number of *other causes.*

If the patient has arthritis which you cannot diagnose and which continues to get worse, refer or transfer to a Medical Officer for diagnosis.

Diagnosis and management of joint problems

Acute arthritis of one or a few joints

Admit all cases for inpatient treatment.

Find cause by history and examination (see Chapter 6 page 17 and pages 388–92 of this chapter and Table 29.1):

- acute bacterial infection
- trauma
- 'tropical'
- rheumatic fever
- rheumatoid disease (usually chronic and many joints affected)

Do a diagnostic joint aspiration on all cases of acute arthritis unless you are certain that the diagnosis is *not* bacterial infection.

Treatment

1. Aspirate any joint which has fluid in it. Use proper aseptic precautions (see page 389). Aspirate (suck out) any fluid in the joint until no more fluid remains. If you find pus, repeat the aspiration whenever more pus is formed (daily or more often if necessary).
2. If aspiration shows pus, or if aspiration does not get any fluid out, give chloramphenicol 1 g (4 caps) orally immediately and repeat every 6 hours. Continue chloramphenicol for at least 2 weeks. (See Chapter 12 page 53.)
3. Splint the joint (usually with a well padded POP back-slab). Elevate (raise up) the affected limb.
4. Aspirin 900–1200 mg (3–4 tabs) every 6 hours (maximum 4 g daily).
5. Antimalarial drugs as indicated (see Chapter 13 page 61) usually chloroquine 450–600 mg (3–4 tabs) daily for 3 days if there is fever.
6. Give diethylcarbamazine 100 mg (2 tabs) three times a day if the patient is in (or has been in) an area where filarasis occurs and the aspirated fluid is yellow or green but does not look like pus. See Chapter 22 page 261 first.
7. When the acute inflammation improves, start physiotherapy. Make the patient do active exercises three times a day in the splint. Show the patient how to contract all the muscles which normally move the joint without moving the joint itself. Tell the patient to do this 20–40 times three times each day. Move the joint through all its movements out of the splint once daily. Remove

the splint and start active exercises (with the patient moving the joint) when all the signs of acute inflammation have gone.

Transfer to a Medical Officer if:

1. It is a severe case (urgent – but not emergency).
2. The hip joint is affected (urgent – but not emergency).
3. The patient is not greatly improved in 2 days (urgent – but not emergency).
4. Pus is present but you cannot aspirate it for 2 days (urgent – but not emergency).
5. The patient is not cured in 2 weeks (non-urgent).

Chronic arthritis of one or a few joints

Do a history and examination. See Chapter 6 page 17 and pages 388–92 of this chapter to find the cause.

Outpatient or inpatient treatment is possible.

Treatment

1. Rest. (The patient should do things which put weight on the joint, or make it work, as little as possible.) The patient should use the affected joint as little as possible. Tell the patient how to lose weight if he is fat.
2. The patient should do exercises to strengthen the muscles which move the joint without putting weight on the joint. *Show* the patient how to contract the muscles which move the joint without moving the joint, or how to move the joint without putting weight on it. *Tell* the patient to do 20–40 of these exercises three times a day.
3. Aspirin 900–1200 mg (3–4 tabs) four times a day (maximum 4 g daily) when pain is present.

If the joint improves with this treatment and there are no important signs of inflammation of the joint (not warm, red or shiny, tender, etc.), then the condition is probably osteoarthrosis. Repeat the treatment whenever it is necessary.

If:

- there are signs of inflammation of the joint (warm, shiny, tender, etc.) *or*
- there is a sinus near the joint *or*
- the joint does not improve much with treatment, or later the joint gets slowly worse *or*
- muscle wasting becomes severe –

then the arthritis may be caused by tuberculosis or chronic bacterial infection.

Transfer these patients to Medical Officer care.

Arthritis of many joints

Do a history and examination (see Chapter 6 page 17 and pages 388–92 of this chapter) to find the cause:

- rheumatoid disease,
- viral infection,
- serum or drug or allergic reaction,
- rheumatic fever, usually only 1–2 joints,
- leprosy reaction.

Give treatment for any cause

Give aspirin 900–1200 mg (3–4 tabs) four times a day (maximum 4 g daily).

Look carefully for signs and symptoms of acute bacterial arthritis – aspirate any joint which may have bacterial infection (see page 389).

If the patient is not cured in one month transfer to a Medical Officer non-urgently for diagnosis and treatment.

Backache

Look for a disease in the organs listed below.

Do a full history and examination (see Chapter 6 page 17). Test the urine for pus, protein and blood.

> Examine the spine for tenderness and movement. Do a pelvic examination PV if necessary.

1. Spine

   (a) *Direct traumatic injury.*

   (b) *Acute back strain* (muscle or joint damage from lifting something heavy):
   - sudden start during lifting,
   - pain, tenderness and stiffness of part of the spine.

   (c) *Chronic back strain*:
   - the patient is often a student or a clerical worker or a woman,
   - chronic ache,
   - usually lower back or neck,
   - often worse after the back is used,
   - no abnormalities on examination of spine,
   - often improves if patient improves posture and strengthens muscles by 'extension exercises'.

   (d) *Osteoarthrosis of spine* (see page 398):
   - pain, stiffness and tenderness varies from time to time.

(e) *Tuberculosis of spine* (see page 397):

- slow start; but constant and increasing pain and tenderness and stiffness of part of the spine.

2. Kidney

(a) *Ureteric colic* (see Chapter 26 page 360):

- pain from where lowest rib joints spine to genitalia,
- kidney often tender,
- blood in urine often.

(b) *Pyelonephritis* (urinary tract infection) (see Chapter 26 page 353):

- fever,
- urinary pain and frequency,
- kidney tender,
- urine shows pus and protein.

3. Reproductive system

(a) *Pregnancy.*

(b) *Labour or miscarriage.*

(c) *Painful menstrual period (dysmenorrhoea)*:

- on examination, no abnormalities found.

(d) *Pelvic inflammatory disease*:

- pelvic examination PV shows pus in vagina, tenderness on moving cervix and tenderness or masses in pelvis.

4. General diseases

(a) *Malaria* (see Chapter 13).

(b) *Viral diseases, especially influenza.*

Deformity of the spine

See page 398.

30

Disorders of the Endocrine Glands

Anatomy and physiology of the endocrine glands

Glands that make secretions that flow into the blood (and not outside the body or into one of the mucous membrane lined tubes, such as the gastrointestinal tract) are called endocrine glands.

The secretions of the endocrine glands are called 'hormones'. Hormone means messenger.

Endocrine glands find out if something needs changing in the body. They usually do this from finding changes in the blood. The endocrine gland then puts more or less of its hormone into the blood and this hormone goes to other parts of the body with a message for those parts of the body to change their function (and occasionally their structure). See Figure 30.1.

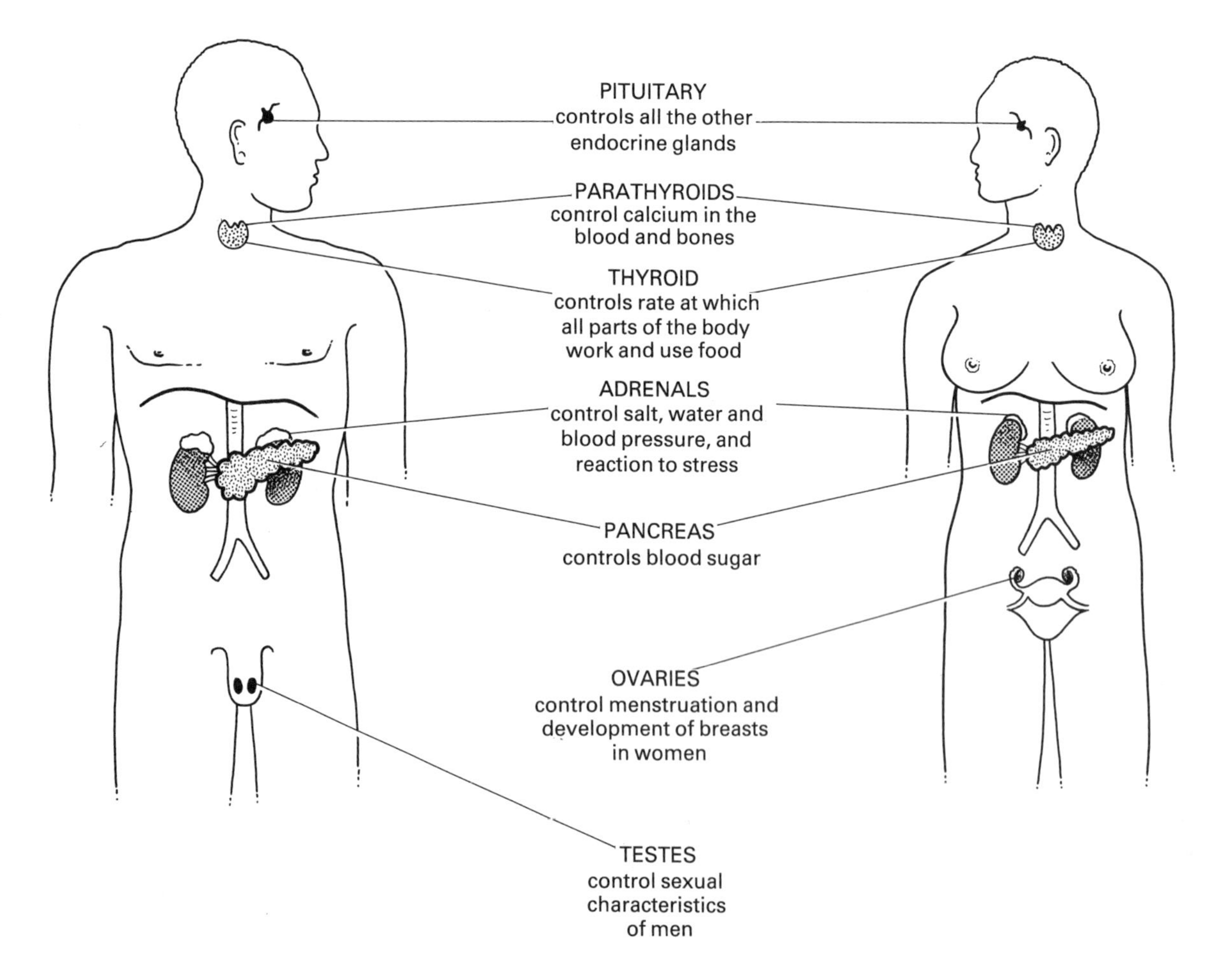

Figure 30.1 Diagram to show the location and function of the endocrine glands.

Pathology of the endocrine glands

Diseases of endocrine glands cause symptoms and signs in three ways.

1. More hormone is secreted than is needed.
2. Less hormone is secreted than is needed.
3. Effects of the disease in the gland – the most common effects are (a) swelling of the gland and (b) spread of any malignant cancer cells from the gland to another part of the body.

Diseases of the thyroid gland

The thyroid gland normally makes the right amount of thyroid hormone to allow all the cells of the body to work normally. (See Figure 30.2.)

Diseases of the thyroid gland which you may see in a health centre include:

1. endemic goitre,
2. endemic cretinism,
3. hypothyroidism or myxoedema, and
4. hyperthyroidism or thyrotoxicosis.

Endemic goitre

A goitre is an enlargement of the thyroid gland from any cause.

There are many causes of goitres including thyrotoxicosis (page 405), cancer of the thyroid, and inflammation or infection of the thyroid. But if there are several people in the community with goitres, the most likely cause is endemic goitre, caused by a shortage of iodine.

Endemic goitre occurs when there is not enough iodine in the food and so there is also not enough iodine in the blood. The thyroid gland grows bigger (i.e. a goitre forms) to try to take more iodine from the blood. This shortage of iodine usually occurs only in mountainous areas.

Usually it affects girls at puberty and women during pregnancy more than others.

Symptoms and *signs* include:

1. swelling in the neck caused by a goitre (see Figure 30.3) – this is usually the only symptom and sign;
2. difficulty in breathing – but not usually;
3. difficulty in swallowing – but not usually.

Many textbooks and many Medical Officers say you should not treat patients with endemic goitre with iodine. But in some parts of the world, iodine makes many endemic goitres get smaller. You must find out the Health Department policy for your area and follow this policy. Do not give iodine if the goitre goes from the neck into the chest or if there is difficulty in breathing. Refer or non-urgently transfer these patients to a Medical Officer.

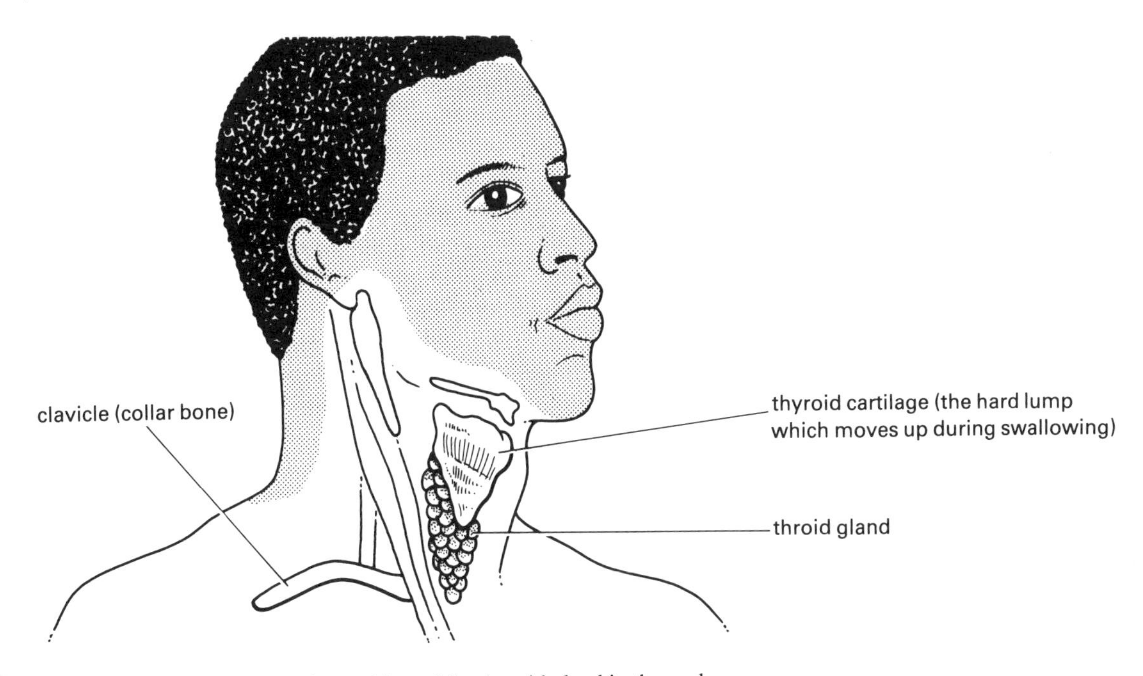

Figure 30.2 Diagram to show the position of the thyroid gland in the neck.

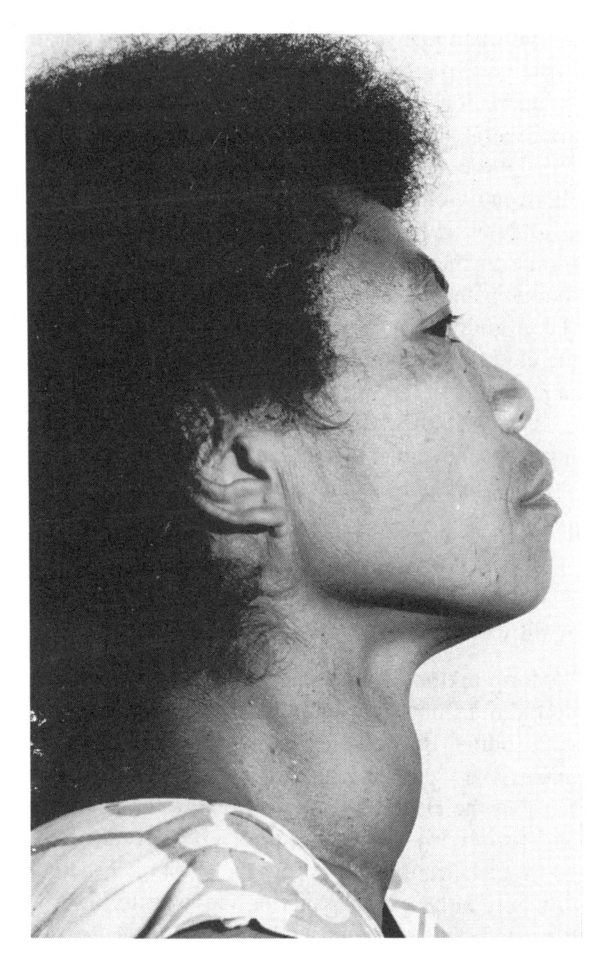

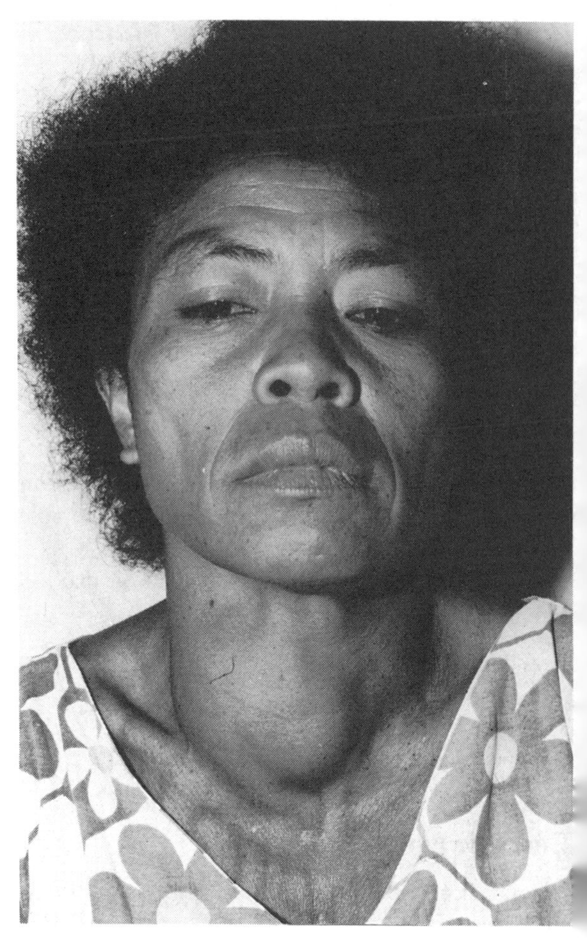

Figure 30.3 An enlarged thyroid gland. This is called a 'goitre'. See Figure 30.2 for normal position and size of the thyroid gland. A normal gland is not usually visible except in some females at puberty and in the child-bearing years; but even then it should not be very large.

Endemic goitre can be prevented by the government passing laws so that all salt sold has iodine in it. If goitres are common in a community, it is possible to treat the whole community (or at least the women and girls) with prophylactic iodised oil fluid injection. The main reason for giving iodine is to stop endemic cretinism occuring in the children of affected women (see below).

If you find a few people with endemic goitre, or if you find only one patient with endemic cretinism (see below) in the community, then notify the Medical Officer so that he can arrange a survey and iodine prophylaxis. Goitres causing difficulty in breathing, swallowing or in general, can be surgically removed.

Endemic cretinism

A patient has endemic cretinism if he has:

1. deafness from birth and cannot speak;
2. spastic legs and was slower than normal children in learning to sit, walk etc.;
3. mental subnormality;
4. squint.

Not all patients with endemic cretinism have all these symptoms and signs – deafness and lack of speech are the most common (see Figure 30.4).

Endemic cretinism is caused by a shortage of iodine in the mother's blood before the child was born. So endemic cretins are born only in areas where adults have goitres.

Notify the Medical Officer if you find any case of endemic cretinism of if you find several adults with a goitre in an area. The Medical Officer will arrange a survey and, if necessary, mass treatment with iodine to prevent more endemic cretinism.

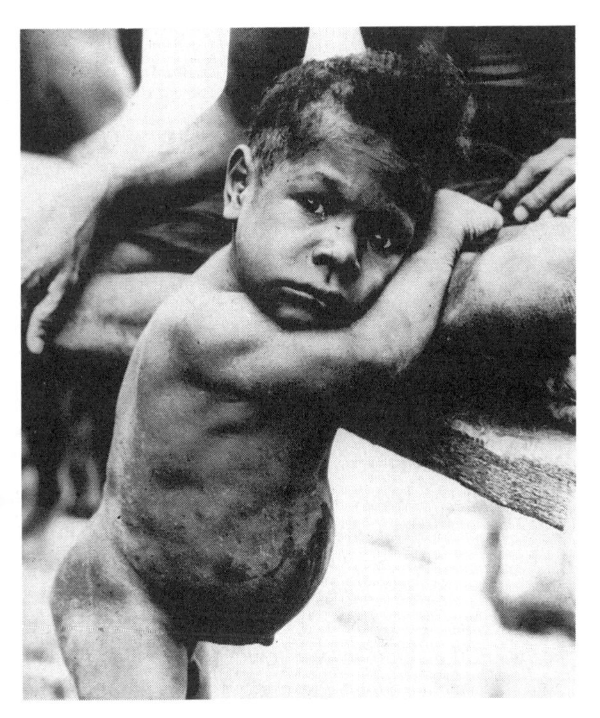

Figure 30.4 Endemic cretinism. Note that the child cannot walk (he has 'spastic' legs). He is deaf, cannot talk and is mentally dull. He has a large abdomen and an umbilical hernia, which are also common in cretinism.

No treatment is possible for cases of cretinism.

Prevention is by everyone eating salt with iodine in it; or, if this is not possible, by giving all girls and women prophylactic iodised oil fluid injections.

Thyrotoxicosis or hyperthyroidism

Thyrotoxicosis or hyperthyroidism is present when too much thyroid hormone is made by the thyroid gland. The most common cause of this is an abnormal reaction of the immune cells of the body which affects the thyroid gland and the eyes and is called 'Graves' disease'.

Thyrotoxicosis is not common, but it is important. It usually affects adults.

Thyrotoxicosis may cause any of these three groups of conditions (all of them need not be present).

1. All parts of the body work faster than normal but not as well as normal. (This is caused by too much thyroid hormone.) Look for:
   - weight loss and weakness of the muscles, although the patient eats well;
   - pulse fast, even while the patient is at rest or asleep, pulse irregular (sometimes with some weak beats so that the heart rate counted with the stethoscope on the chest is more than the pulse rate felt at the wrist);
   - heart failure for no other obvious cause;

   > Always think of thyrotoxicosis in anyone (especially older adults) who have heart failure and you cannot find the cause, especially if pulse irregular.

   - shaking of the hands (look for this when the patient holds his hands out straight ahead of him);
   - nervousness or mental illness;
   - feels hot and sweaty all the time (more than before).
2. The eyes may seem to be staring (i.e. the patient does not blink often; and when he looks up and then down, the whites of the eyes show above the brown). (See Figure 30.5.) The eye or eyes may be pushed out (exophthalmos).
3. A goitre (swelling of the thyroid gland) is present or comes. (But only if there are also some of the other signs.) (See Figure 30.3.)

It is possible to cure thyrotoxicosis. But if it is not treated, it can cause death from heart failure or blindness from exophthalmos.

If you suspect a patient has thyrotoxicosis because of any the above features refer or non-urgently transfer the patient to a Medical Officer for diagnosis and treatment.

Hypothyroidism (myxoedema)

Hypothyroidism is present when not enough thyroid hormone is made by the thyroid gland. Again the most common cause is an abnormal immunological reaction. It can, however, be from iodine deficiency when even the large (goitrous) thyroid cannot get enough iodine from the blood to make thyroid hormone. It can follow hyperthyroidism. There are many other causes. Most of the effects of low thyroid hormone are the opposite to the effects of hyperthyroidism.

1. All parts of the body work slower than normal and not as well as normal:
   - weight gain,

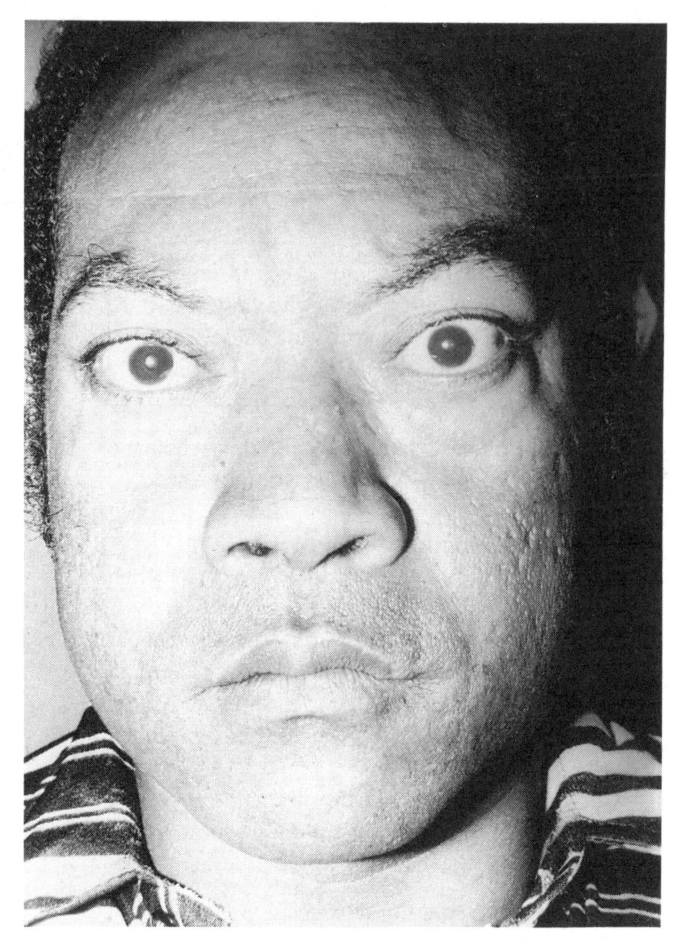

Figure 30.5 The eyes in thyrotoxicosis. Note the whites of the eyes above the corneas. The patient appears to be staring and does not blink often (lid retraction). When you look from the side, you can see that the eyes are pushed out (exophthalmos).

- slow pulse,
- aches and pains and all muscular action slower than normal,
- mentally dull,
- tired all the time,
- depressed and eventually even psychosis,
- feels the cold weather more,
- hoarse voice,
- skin dry and flaky,
- hair dry and can start to fall out,
- the patient can slow down so much that they eventually go into a coma and die.

2. The eyes are not particularly affected but may seem to be puffed up and the tissues around them swollen or oedematous.
3. A goitre may or may not be present.

It is possible to cure hypothyroidism by giving thyroid hormone tablets. If it is not treated it will cause death.

If you suspect the patient has hypothyroidism because of any of the above features refer, or non-urgently transfer, the patient to a Medical Officer for diagnosis and treatment.

Diseases of other endocrine glands

Diabetes mellitus

Diabetes mellitus occurs when there is more glucose (sugar) in the blood than is normal and the blood sugar stays at these abnormally high levels. Rising or high blood glucose would normally make the pancreas make and release insulin into the blood which would cause the body cells to take the glucose out of the blood into themselves, lowering the blood sugar. Diabetes occurs when there is an abnormality of the pancreas so that it cannot make enough insulin. It can also occur if there is an abnormality in the body cells so that they are partially resistant to the action of insulin and need large amounts of insulin in the blood to make them take the sugar out of the blood. If the pancreas has to make these large amounts of insulin for a long time, it can become exhausted and not able to continue to make this amount of insulin.

Lack of insulin affects not only glucose in the body, but also other carbohydrates, fats, protein, water and electrolytes. Sudden changes in these may cause acute disease or death. After some years these changes cause permanent damage in other parts of the body and in particular the arteries, especially the arteries of eyes, kidneys, nervous system and feet. These changes are called the 'complications' of diabetes.

Three types of diabetes are recognised in tropical countries.

1. Type I diabetes, or insulin-dependent diabetes mellitus (IDDM), is not as common as other types and is due to inherited factors, viral infections, immunological abnormalities and other things. As a result of these causes, all the cells of the pancreas that usually make insulin are destroyed, and the body then has no insulin. This type of diabetes occurs in younger people and is not as common as NIDDM because (a) it occurs less often, and (b) the patients often die soon after the disease develops.

2. Type II, or non-insulin-dependent diabetes mellitus (NIDDM), is more common and is again due to inherited factors. It is often associated with obesity, high blood pressure, abnormal fats in the blood, etc. and is due to resistance of the body cells to the effects of insulin. In NIDDM the pancreas still makes some insulin. This type affects 1–4% of the population; but in some areas it is much higher, even up to 50%; although it is relatively rare in Africans. Obesity is the main thing that seems to bring this on.
3. Malnutrition-related diabetes mellitus (MRDM) is more like IDDM, except that a serious complication called 'ketoacidosis', which occurs in IDDM, does not occur in MRDM. It is thought that patients have had a history of malnutrition, which may have damaged cells in the pancreas, or that they have 'chronic fibrocalculus pancreatitis' or 'tropical calcific pancreatitis' where all of the pancreas as well as the insulin producing cells are damaged. They often have attacks of abdominal pain from this.

Diabetes can also occur in a number of other less common situations. Table 30.1 shows the features of the two common types.

If the blood glucose is high, glucose gets through the glomeruli into the urine and holds water with it. This leads to large urine volumes, dehydration and thirst.

When there is no insulin to use glucose, as in IDDM (though not as expected in MRDM and not in NIDDH), large amounts of fat have to be broken down to supply energy. This causes weight loss and excess ketones and acids from the fat in the blood. This 'ketoacidosis' (unless treated with rehydration and insulin) quickly leads to unconsciousness and death.

Some infecting organisms grow better in the body if the glucose is high.

In all types of diabetes complications occur and include the following:

1. Kidney damage with proteinuria or nephrotic syndrome or kidney failure.
2. Damage to the blood vessels in the retina of the eye with progressive loss of vision and blindness.
3. Damage to the nervous system with:
   - peripheral neuritis with permanent loss of sensation in the legs similar to leprosy;
   - sudden loss of function of any nerves which may recover;
   - permanent loss of function of nerves to the internal organs with low blood pressure on standing, abdominal fullness, constipation or diarrhoea, impotence.
4. More infections – some difficult to treat.
5. Damage to blood vessels in the legs, often with death of toes (dry gangrene) when absent pulses may be noted above the affected area.

Think, therefore, of diabetes in any one who:

1. is thirsty, drinking a lot of fluid and passing a lot of urine;
2. has weight loss even though he is eating well; or
3. is obese;
4. has infections:
   - not expected – especially thrush in the mouth or vagina or on the penis or skin, and
   - all cases of tuberculosis.

Table 30.1 Features of the two main types of diabetes mellitus.

Factors	*Insulin-dependent diabetes mellitus (IDDM)*	*Non-insulin-dependent diabetes mellitus (NIDDM)*
Age of onset	Younger	Older
Family history of diabetes mellitus	Not often	Usually
Duration of symptoms	Weeks	Months to years
Body weight	Normal or low	Obese
Ketones in urine	Yes	No
Rapid death without treatment with insulin	Yes	No
Diabetic complications present at diagnosis	No	Sometimes

Also think of diabetes if you see patients with complications that can be caused by diabetes including:

1. Blindness for no obvious reason.
2. Kidney problems including proteinuria, nephrotic syndrome and kidney failure.
3. All sorts of abnormalities of the nervous system.
4. Ulcers on the feet from loss of sensation.
5. Gangrene of the toes or feet with poor circulation and loss of pulses.

In all the cases, test for sugar in the urine (with e.g. Benedict's solution). If the patient is pregnant or breastfeeding a baby, the sugar (lactose) from the breast milk can get into the blood and urine (and give a positive test for sugar with Benedict's solution), even when the patient has no glucose in the urine and does not have diabetes. Test patients who are pregnant or breastfeeding a baby with a stick test, e.g. Clinistix or another test which is positive for glucose only.

If there is glucose in the urine, transfer the patient to Medical Officer care for confirmation of the diagnosis and treatment.

The treatment for diabetes includes:

1. The patient should have a diet containing as little refined sugar and fat as possible. Most traditional village diets, except for sugar cane and sweet fruits, are usually all right. The patient should eat enough food to be at the normal weight for his height and age. Then the patient should eat only enough to remain at this normal weight.
2. The patient should have daily physical exercise.
3. Insulin-dependent diabetes mellitus patients need insulin injections every day. This will be either:
   (a) unmodified or clear or soluble insulin – these injections last for 4 up to 6 hours; *or*
   (b) modified, cloudy or depot insulin – these last for approximately 1 day.
   The Medical Officer will have said what dose to give. Do not stop the insulin if the patient gets sick or has gastroenteritis. If sick or vomiting, continue the insulin and give intravenous 4.3% dextrose in 0.18% sodium chloride.
4. Non-insulin-dependent diabetes mellitus patients may be given tablets such as tolbutamide or glibenclamide, if diet alone does not control their condition.
5. Treat any complications quickly and properly.

If a patient is on treatment for diabetes with insulin or tablets and develops any of these – weakness, sweating, shaking, mental abnormality or unconsciousness – do a blood glucose estimation if possible. If blood glucose low then immediately give two large spoonfuls of sugar in water by mouth or by intragastric tube (or, if available, 50 ml of 25% or 50% dextrose solution for injection by IVI if the patient is unconscious). If blood glucose high, start intravenous 0.9% sodium chloride as for dehydration from gastroenteritis (see Chapter 23 page 285) and give a dose of unmodified or clear or soluble insulin, 10–20 units by IMI. If blood sugar tests are not possible, first of all try the effect of the glucose and if this is not effective, put up the drip but do not give the extra insulin. In all cases then urgently consult a Medical Officer as to what is the next thing to do.

Prevention of diabetes (NIDDM) is by not eating too much (especially refined carbohydrate foods) and not getting fat.

Acute adrenal insufficiency

The adrenal gland of the body normally makes a small amount of cortisone each day and a large amount of cortisone at a time of stress (e.g. acute infection or accident or operation).

Medical Officers give cortisone or cortisone-like drugs called adrenocorticosteroid drugs including hydrocortisone, prednisone, prednisolone and dexamethasone for some conditions.

After some weeks of taking cortisone-like drugs, the adrenal glands of the body stop making cortisone, and cannot make it again even at times of stress. If the patient suddenly stops taking his drug he will have no cortisone in his body and may develop gastrointestinal symptoms, weakness, low blood pressure and then shock and die (acute adrenal failure). Also, if the patient does not take an extra dose of the cortisone-like drug at a time of stress, he may die.

Also the high dose of cortisone makes the patient more likely to get diseases from infections, especially malaria and tuberculosis, amoebae in the bowel and *Strongyloides* may spread out of the bowel into the rest of the body.

If you have a patient who is taking a cortisone-like drug, see a specialist reference book for details. Remember these rules:

1. The patient must take the drug as indicated and not stop it (unless the Medical Officer stops it).
2. If there is a time of stress the patient must take 3–4 times the normal dose of the drug immediately, and then daily. You must consult the Medical Officer urgently.
3. The patient must take prophylactic antimalarials and prophylactic isoniazid, if he is in an area where malaria occurs or if tuberculosis is common.
4. Treat any infection quickly and well with antibiotics and antimalarials.

31

Disorders of the Eye

Anatomy

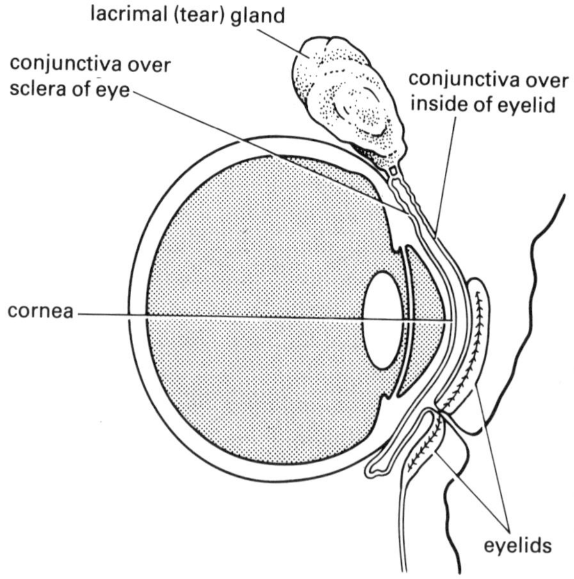

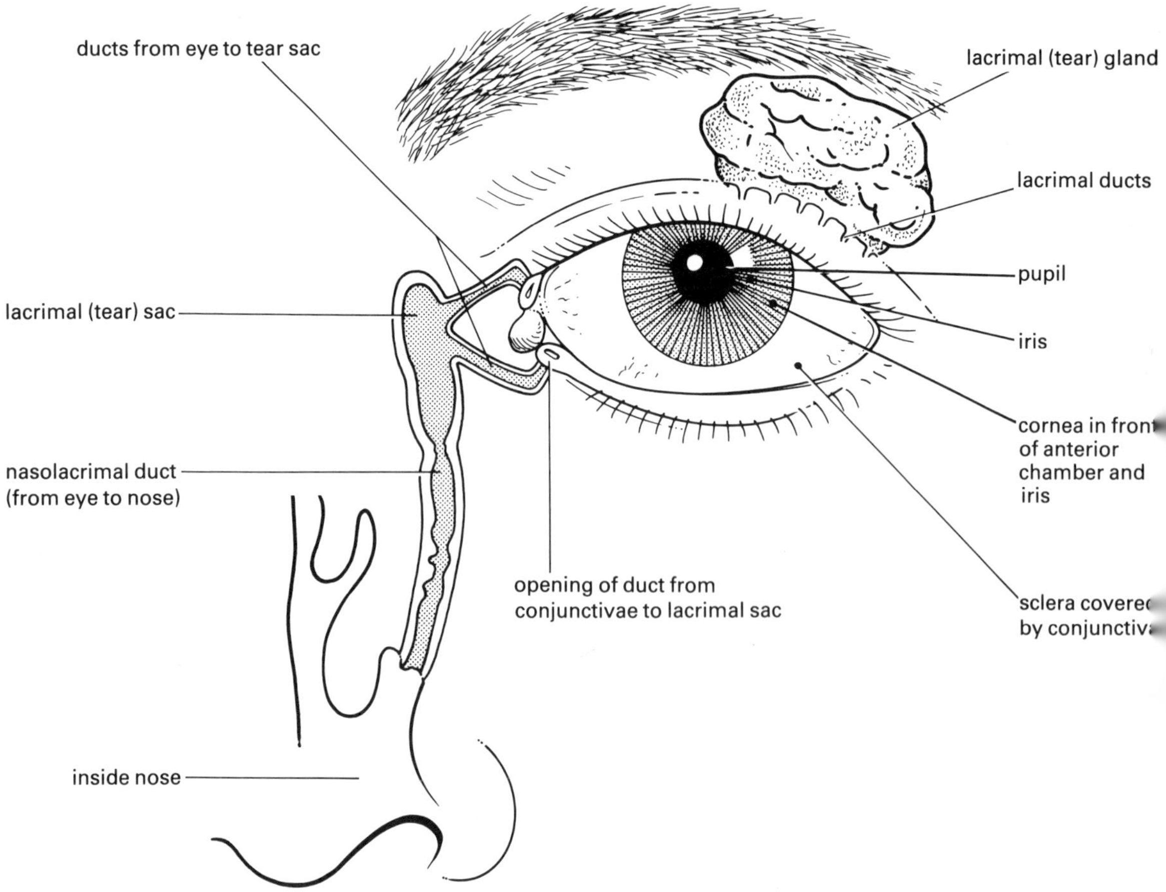

Figure 31.1 Diagrams to show the structure of the eye and the tear gland and ducts.

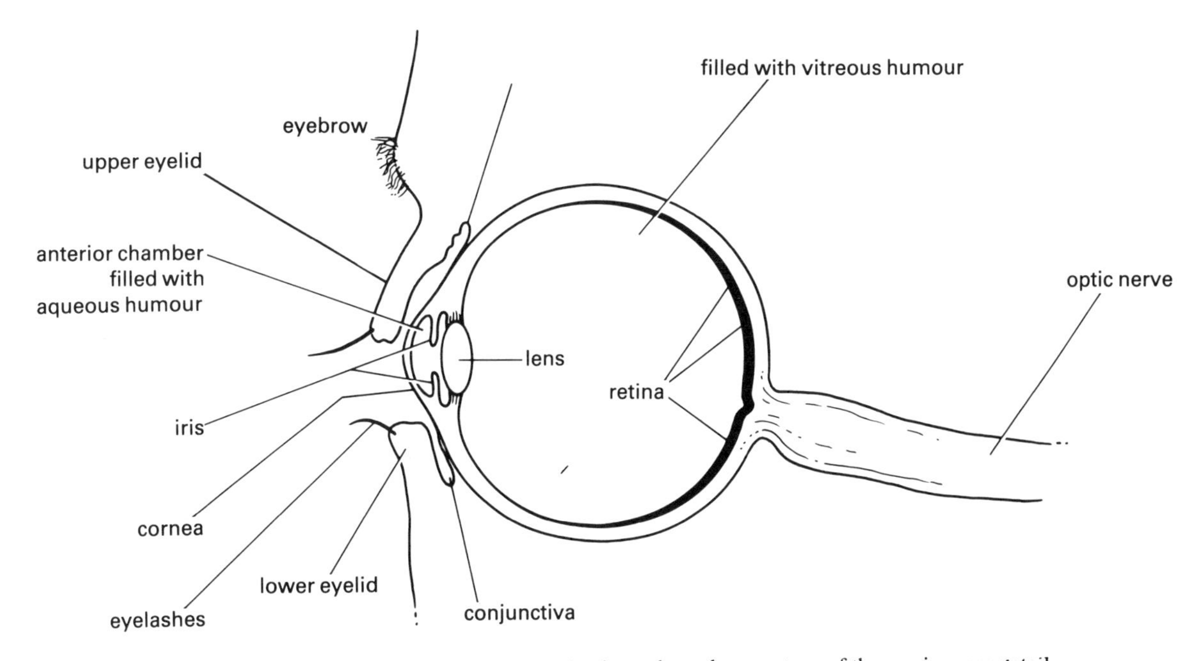

Figure 31.2 Diagram of the eye in section from front to back, to show the structure of the eye in more detail.

History and examination

Symptoms of eye diseases

1. loss of vision
2. pain in the eye
3. eye red; watering; or sticky (from pus)

Signs of eye diseases

Examine structures of the eye from the outside ones to the inside ones to find any signs present.

1. *Look at the site, shape and size etc. of the eyes*
   - exophthalmos?
   - orbital cellulitis?
2. *Look at the eyelids*
   - 'stye'?
   - entropion?
   - infection?
   - oedema?
   - haematoma?

   Ask the patient to open and close his eyes.
   - ptosis?
   - lagophthalmos?
3. *Look at the conjunctiva*

   (a) over the sclera,

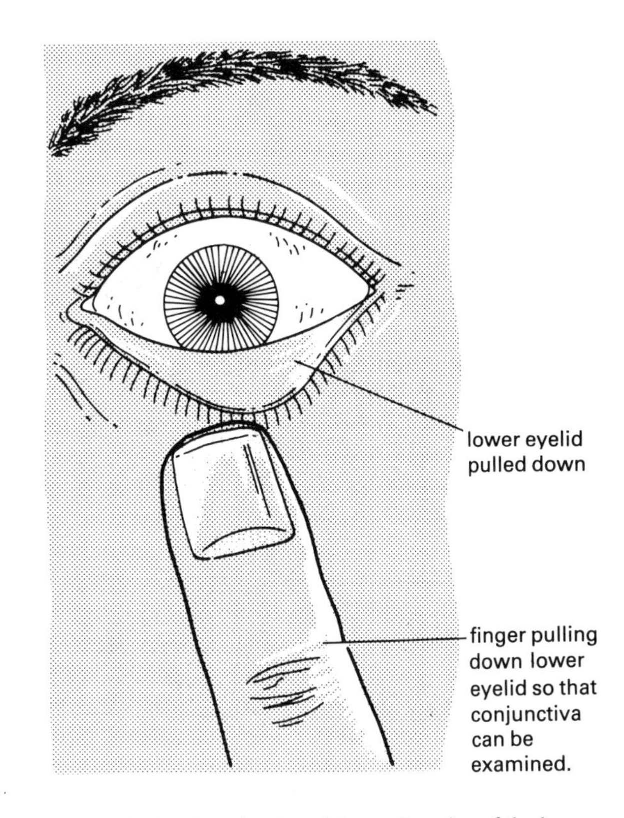

Figure 31.3 Examination of the conjunctiva of the lower lid.

(b) inside the lower lids (see Figure 31.3),
(c) inside upper lids (turn upper lid inside out) (see Figure 31.4).

- foreign body?
- inflammation of all conjunctiva or just around cornea?
- pus?
- nodules?
- pterygium?

4. *Look at the cornea*

(a) Anaesthetise with 2% amethocaine or tetracaine 0.5% sterile eye drops, 2 drops into the outer side of the eye every minute for 2–3 minutes, as necessary (see Figure 31.5) Note that anaesthetic is only needed if the patient has pain.
(b) Stain with fluorescein. Put one drop of sterile solution, or lay the end of a sterile ophthalmic strip on the conjunctiva of the sclera (white part of the eye) on the lateral (outer) side of the eye for a few seconds. Then get the patient to blink. Corneal ulcers will show as green areas.
(c) Shine a light in from side and ask the patient to look up, down, right and left.
(d) Use a torch and a loupe if available. Otherwise use an auriscope without a speculum (see Figure 31.6).

- foreign body?

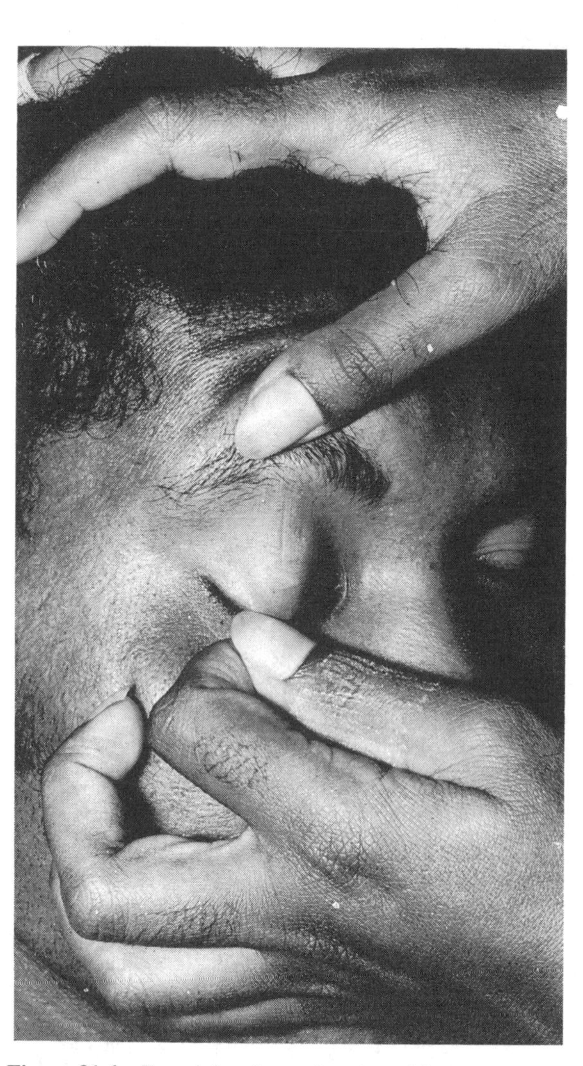

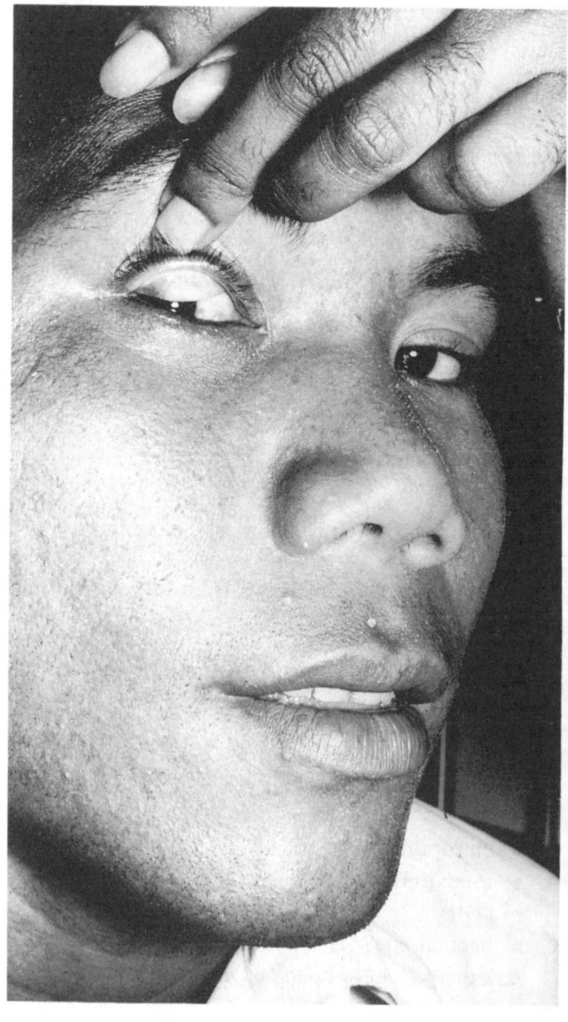

Figure 31.4 Examining the conjunctiva of the upper eye lid. Left photograph, first step. Right photograph, second step. See text for details. The conjunctivae may be red and inflamed all over with or without the formation of pus (conjunctivitis). They may be inflamed just around the cornea (acute iritis). A vascular fleshy growth may be growing across it to the cornea (pterygium). A foreign body may be present.

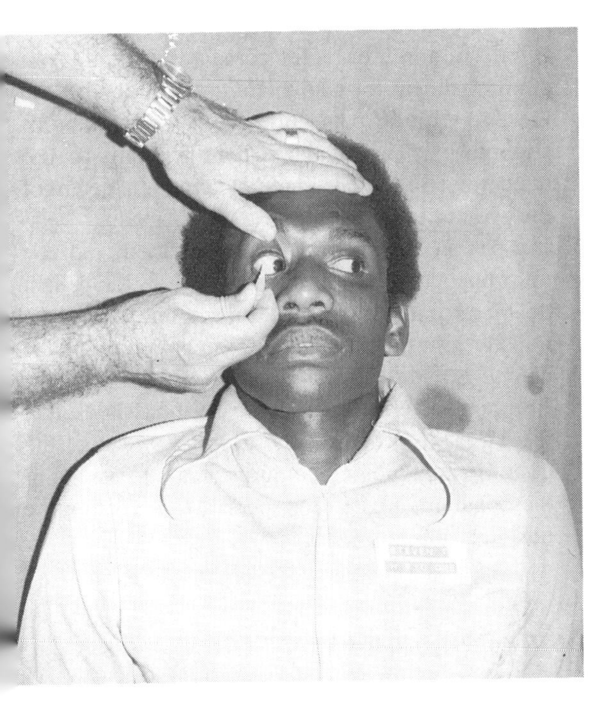

Figure 31.5 Putting local anaesthetic and fluorescein drops into the eye. Local anaesthetic is only necessary if the patient has pain. Fluorescein is necessary in all patients. Note that the drops are put in the outer side of the eye while the patient looks towards the other side.

- ulcer?
- clear or cloudy?
- scar?

5. *Look at the anterior chamber by shining a light into it*
   - clear?
   - cloudy?
   - pus or blood at the lower part?
6. *Look at the iris and the pupil*
   - pupil shape round or irregular?
   - pupil size normal, large or small?

   Shine a light into the pupil
   - pupil constricts (gets smaller) when light goes in and dilates (gets bigger) when light goes away, or not?
7. *Look at the lens*
   - cataract?
8. *Test eye movements*

   Ask the patient to follow with his eyes one of your fingers, which you move up then down then to the right and then to the left
   - double vision?
   - squint?

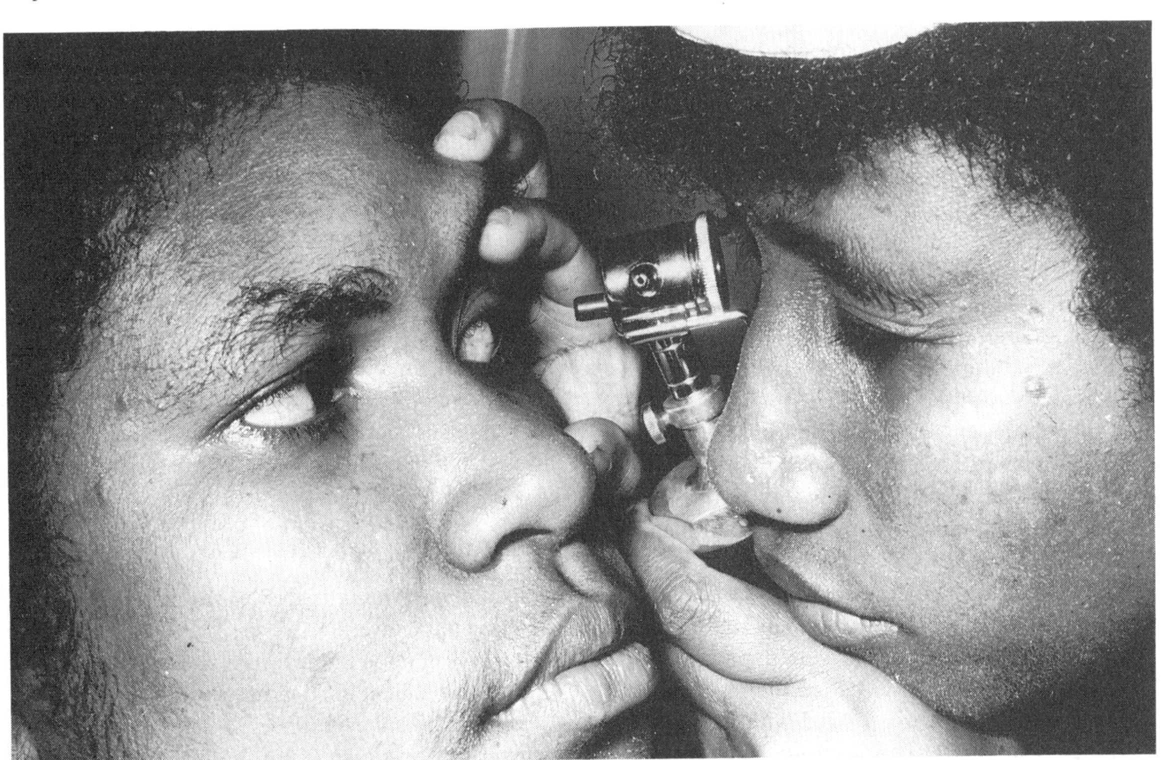

Figure 31.6 If you use an auriscope with a magnifying lens you can examine the eye more closely and accurately.

9. *Visual acuity*
   - check vision with an eye chart at 6 metres (6/6 or less) *or* count fingers *or* see light
   - read small print for close vision

Check for symptoms and signs of disease in the rest of the body, if the eye condition is not just an eye injury.

Using these symptoms and signs, you can easily diagnose the most important eye diseases. See Table 31.1.

Treatment of eye diseases

Most of the important eye diseases are infective or traumatic (and traumatic injuries often get infected), so it is important always to do certain things if a patient has an eye condition.

1. Always look for foreign bodies in the eye. (This is especially important if the eye is red and painful.) Carefully look all over all surfaces of the conjunctiva. Carefully look all over the cornea.
2. Always look for corneal ulcers. Always stain the eye with fluorescein. Then shine a light into the eye from each side, and above and below.
3. If an infection or injury is present, use any antibiotic ointment in the eye. Remember that sulphacetamide is not very strong in killing organisms; but is usually soothing.
4. If an eye infection is serious, chloramphenicol is the most powerful antibiotic usually available. It should be put into the eye at least every 3 hours. If the infection is inside the eye, give chloramphenicol capsules (or injections, if vomiting is present). (Penicillin alone is not very effective for most infections inside the eye.)
5. If there is any injury or infection inside the eye or a severe injury or infection on the cornea, always dilate the pupil with atropine eye ointment or drops. Use atropine 3–4 times daily until the pupil dilates. The pupil will stay dilated for a week, sometimes more. If necessary, continue the atropine once daily. Injuries or infections in the eye may fix the iris, so that the pupil cannot get bigger or smaller. It is better for sight and for other reasons if the iris is fixed with the pupil big rather than small. This is the reason for using atropine.
6. Always put a pad on an eye with a serious injury or infection in it or on the cornea. But a pad is not good treatment for conjunctivitis. Hold the pad on the eye with strip of adhesive cellulose tape or sticking plaster. Put the strips diagonally across the corners of the eye (and not across the centre of the eye).
7. If a patient has only one eye, the patient and you must take great care of this good eye. If the patient develops injury or disease in his one good eye, transfer him quickly, if you are not certain of the diagnosis and treatment.
8. Before transferring any eye case, first check that the Medical Officer at the hospital will take the case. He may prefer a non-urgent case to wait until the ophthalmologist (eye specialist) is visiting the hospital.

Some common eye diseases

The common stye

The common stye is an abscess or pimple in the gland of an eyelash.

Symptoms
Pain and swelling of the eyelid.

Signs
A swollen tender red hot area in the eyelid (see Figure 31.7).

After a few days it points to the edge of the eyelid, then discharges pus, and gets better without treatment.

Treatment
Hot bathing three or four times a day.

Tetracycline 1% or antibiotic compound eye ointment three or four times a day. This does not cure the disease, but often stops the pus starting new styes.

Conjunctival foreign bodies

Conjunctival foreign bodies cause pain, redness and watering of the eye.

Remove foreign bodies from under the lower eyelid with the patient looking up. See Figure 31.3.

Remove them from under the upper lid with the patient looking down. Turn the upper lid inside out over swab stick or a finger. See Figure 31.4.

Table 31.1 Clinical findings of the common eye disorders.

History and examination	*Acute conjunctivitis*	*Foreign body in cornea*	*Corneal ulcer*	*Acute iritis (infection from outside)*	*Acute iritis (from other diseases)*	*Acute glaucoma*	*Cataract*
History of injury	No	Often	At times	Corneal ulcer or penetrating injury	No	No, sometimes yes	Sometimes
Red discharging eye	Yes, pus	Yes, watery	Yes, watery	Yes, varies	Yes, watery	Yes, watery	No
Pain in eye	No	Yes	Yes	Yes	Yes	Yes	No
Loss of vision	No	Often	Often	Yes	Yes	Yes	Yes
Conjunctiva	All inflamed, pus	Inflamed	Inflamed	Inflamed – only around cornea or all	Inflamed only around cornea	Inflamed around cornea only	Normal
Cornea	Normal	Foreign body	Ulcer	Ulcer or injury often	Normal	Cloudy	Normal
Anterior chamber	Normal	Normal	Normal	Cloudy or hypopyon	Cloudy or hypopyon	Not easily seen	Normal
Pupil	Normal	Normal	Normal	Small irregular, will not dilate	Small irregular, will not dilate	Large, oval, will not constrict	Normal
Lens	Normal	Normal	Normal	Normal	Normal	Normal	White
Other disease present	At times	No	No	No	Often yes	No	Not usually

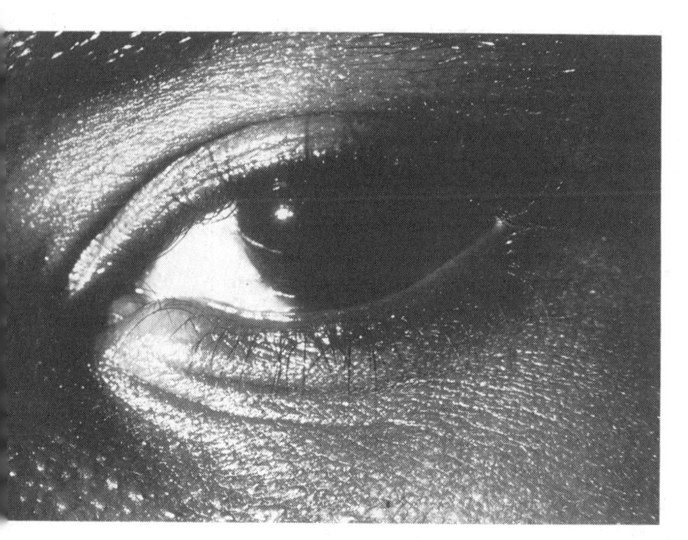

Figure 31.7 A common stye affecting the medial (centre) part of the lower lid.

Chemicals in the eye

Lime is the most common and dangerous chemical that gets into the eye. Chemicals can quickly cause damage to the eye. Give immediate proper first aid.

1. Hold the affected eye open and pour large amounts of water across it for 10–15 minutes, even though this causes pain.
2. Then anaesthetise the eye with a local anaesthetic, see page 412.
3. Stain the cornea with fluorescein, see page 412.
4. Remove any foreign bodies very carefully.
5. Wash the eye with water again if necessary.
6. If the cornea is clear, treat with tetracycline 1% or antibiotic compound eye ointment three or four times a day.
7. If the cornea is not clear, treat as for iritis, (see page 420) but the oral chloramphenicol is not necessary.
8. Transfer the patient to Medical Officer's care if he is not much better in 1–2 days.

Acute conjunctivitis

Conjunctivitis is inflammation of the conjunctiva of the eye with or without the formation of pus.

Causes include:

- gonorrhoea or chlamydia in infants at birth (from the mother's cervix or vagina),
- trachoma, acute stage (see page 417),
- infection with (other kinds of) bacteria,
- viral infections,
- allergic reactions.

Spread of most infectious types of conjunctivtis is by direct contact, or by a vehicle (e.g. towel), or by vectors (especially flies).

Symptoms include:

- red watering eyes,
- eyelids stuck together with pus in the morning, and
- some discomfort (but no pain).

If there is pain, another serious disease is present as well as conjunctivitis

Signs include:

- inflammation of the conjunctivae, over the sclera and under the eyelids of both eyes; and
- discharge, which may be watery, or pus

> You must always stain the cornea with fluorescein and examine it for any corneal foreign body or corneal ulcer. Examine the anterior chamber and pupil for iritis.
> (These things are especially important if the conjunctivitis is only on one side because conjunctivitis almost always spreads to both eyes. If conjunctivitis is only in one eye there is usually a local cause in that eye, such as foreign body, entropion (rolling in of the eyelid) or blocked tear duct, etc.).
> These things are especially important if the inflammation is only around the cornea, because conjunctivitis causes inflammation of all of the conjunctivae. If the inflammation is only around the cornea, then a corneal ulcer or foreign body or iritis or glaucoma is probably present.

A mild chronic conjunctivitis with swelling of the conjunctivae which does not respond to the usual treatment for conjunctivitis can occur from onchocerciasis.

Vitamin A deficiency, especially in children, can cause dry conjunctivae with dry corneas and this can result in painful conjunctivitis. (See page 419.)

Treatment

1. *Show* the patient how to put antibiotic eye ointment under the lower eyelids. *Tell* the patient to do

this four times daily to both eyes. *Give* the patient tetracycline 1% or antibiotic compound eye ointment to take home. Treat for 5 days. Do not pad the eye.
2. If possible, admit the patient for hourly treatment for the first 8–12 hours by member of your staff. This is usually much more effective than the patient giving himself the treatment. The patient can then continue the treatment at home.
3. If infant/newborn. See Chapter 19 page 170.
4. See a specialist reference book for treatment of other acute types of conjunctivitis.

Explain how the infection spreads, and how to stop this spread.

If the patient is not cured, look carefully for foreign bodies, iritis, vitamin A deficiency, onchocerciasis and trachoma and treat urgently.

Trachoma

Trachoma is a chronic inflammation of the conjunctivae and cornea caused by *Chlamydia trachomatis*.

Trachoma is common all over the world. But it is much more common, and causes much more severe disease, in areas that are hot, dry and dusty; where there is rubbish or faeces or cattle which increase fly breeding; and where there is not enough water for people to wash regularly.

Spread of the trachoma bacteria happens when the eye discharge from infected people is passed directly to other people on fingers, towels, clothes or anything used to wipe the face (especially discharging eyes), as well as bedclothes, etc. It is therefore more common in children. Infected people are much more infectious early in the infection. Flies are probably important in spreading the disease. Trachoma can be caused by the STD organism at birth or carried to the eyes on fingers. It is usually children who have active infection. Older children and adults usually have the results of the infection, which is often blindness.

There are four stages in the development of trachoma.

1. *Early trachoma*
   First the eyes are uncomfortable and watery, and the conjunctivae inflamed, like any other conjunctivitis. However the condition is chronic. After about a month, small pink-grey lumps, called 'follicles', develop under the upper eyelid (see Figure 31.8). There is little pus is the eye, unless there is secondary infection by other bacteria.

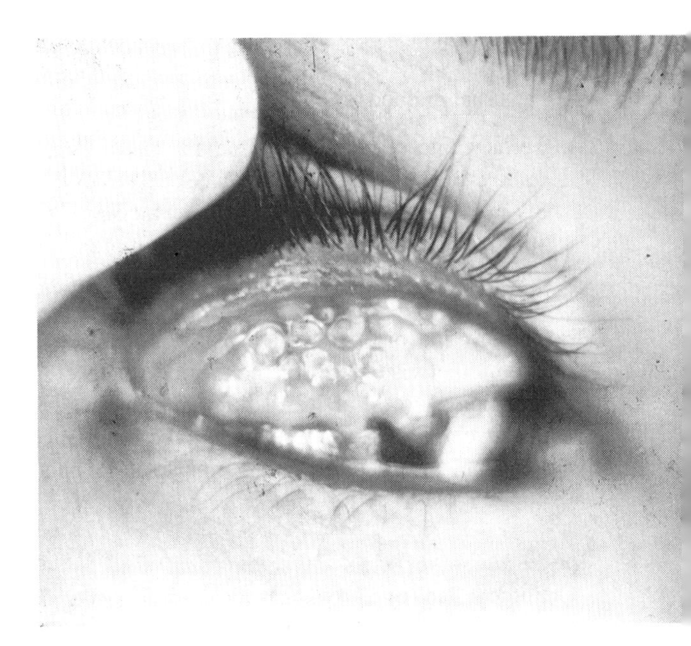

Figure 31.8 Trachoma. Note the follicles on the conjunctiva of the upper eyelid.

2. *Pannus formation*
   Small blood vessels start to grow into the top of the cornea. This is called 'pannus'. Use a loupe or magnifying glass to look for the grey colour of *early* pannus at the top of the cornea.
3. *After some months to years*, especially if there are no repeated re-infections and it is not hot and dusty *the lesions may heal without treatment.*
   The follicles leave white scars on the inside of the upper eyelid. The pannus (which may spread over much of the cornea) leaves a whitish colour and small pits on the cornea (the cornea is normally clear).
4. *Entropion and trichiasis occurs*
   The scarred tissue inside the eyelid, like any scar tissue, becomes smaller over the years. This turns the edge of the eyelid in, and this is called 'entropion'. This makes the eyelashes scrape over the cornea every time the patient blinks. This is called 'trichiasis'. The entropion and trichiasis causes more corneal damage, and finally blindness.

At any stage the patient may get an acute bacterial infection in the eye which can cause a lot more damage to the cornea.

Treatment

In the early stages, before entropion and trichiasis

Treat the patient with tetracycline or sulphonamide or both.

The usual method is:

1. Tetracycline or oxytetracycline 1% eye ointment or oily drops twice daily for 6 weeks. Tetracycline 3% eye ointment (not the usual 1% which does not sting) at least once every day (better if more often) *and* may be more practicable for supervised treatment.
2. Tetracycline or doxycycline if not pregnant or a child, otherwise sulphamethoxazole/trimethoprim (co-trimoxazole) or even sulphadimidine or erythromycin orally for 2 weeks as well as the topical treatment. (For adult doses, see Chapter 11 pages 46–52.)

In the late stages of entropion and trichiasis

1. Remove any eyelashes that are scraping over the cornea. Pull them out with a pair of forceps.
2. Transfer the patient to a Medical Officer for an operation for the entropion, and other operations if necessary.

If there is acute bacterial infection at any stage

Treat quickly, as for corneal ulcer (see this page).

Control and prevention

1. Kill the organism in the reservoir.
   Treat all infected cases early, when they are most infectious. School surveys may be necessary every 6 months, to find cases early. If trachoma is very common, give the teacher enough 3% tetracycline eye ointment to treat all the children once daily for 5 days, every month for 6 months. If more than 20% of the population is affected, it is worth considering treating all of the population.
2. Stop the means of spread.
   It is very important that there is enough water for regular washing of the hands and face. Give education about personal hygiene. Control of flies will help.
3. Immunisation is not yet possible.
4. Prophylactic treatment (see 1 above).

Corneal or scleral foreign bodies

Usually there is a *history* of something going into the eye.

Symptoms include:

1. pain in the eye,
2. the patient cannot open the eye properly, and
3. red, watering eye.

Examination shows:

1. inflammation of the conjunctiva, and
2. foreign body on the cornea if you anaesthetise the cornea and stain it with flourescein and examine with a light and loupe or an auriscope.

Treatment

1. Anaesthetise the eye with amethocaine 2% sterile eye drops (see page 412).
2. Stain the cornea with fluorescein (see page 412).
3. If the foreign body does not penetrate (go right through) the cornea into the eye, remove it. Remove the foreign body with the point of a large hypodermic needle. Hold the needle parallel to the surface of the eye with your hand resting on the patient's face. If the foreign body is iron, also remove any rust stain surrounding it.
4. Then treat as for corneal ulcer (see below).
5. Look for signs of infection inside the eye (pus in the anterior chamber, or the pupil small or irregular). If either of these are present, also treat for acute iritis (see page 420).

Transfer to Medical Officer care

1. If the foreign body penetrates through into the eye. Do not try to remove it (urgent – emergency). Meanwhile treat for acute iritis – see page 420 and give tetanus prophylaxis – see Chapter 25 page 331).
2. If you cannot remove the foreign body (urgent).
3. If you cannot see a foreign body but it may have gone right into the eye and still be there. This is especially important if the foreign body is made of iron.

> Always look for a foreign body in anyone who has a painful or red eye.

Corneal ulcer

A corneal ulcer is present when there is loss of part of the outside surface of the cornea (see Figure 31.9).

Corneal ulcers are caused by foreign bodies, abrasions, drying (when the eyelids will not close, e.g. leprosy), other injuries, bacterial infections, herpes virus infections, onchocerciasis, vitamin A deficiency, chemicals especially lime, etc.

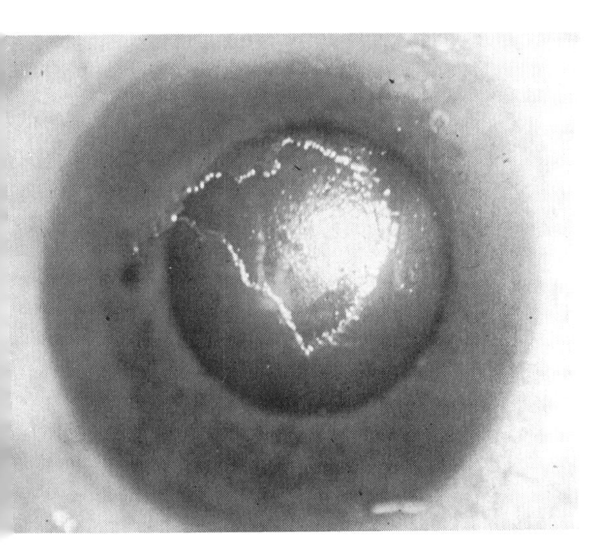

Figure 31.9 Corneal ulcer.

Symptoms include:

1. pain in the eye,
2. red watery eye, and
3. some loss of vision.

Signs:

1. The conjunctiva are inflamed.
2. You can see the ulcer on the cornea but often only if you give a local anaesthetic and stain with fluorescein and use a torch and loupe or an auriscope. In areas where onchocerciasis occurs you may find white areas deep in the cornea (but no surface ulcer); these slowly become bigger.
3. There is some loss of vision, if the ulcer is central.
4. Iritis (small pupil and pus in the anterior chamber) may be present if the ulcer penetrates (goes through) the cornea.
5. Foreign body or trichiasis or other cause sometimes.

Treatment

Admit for inpatient treatment, unless the ulcer is very small.

1. Give tetracycline 1% or antibiotic compound eye ointment four times a day. (Do not use any ointment or drops which contain hydrocortisone or prednisolone or cortisone-like drug.)
2. Keep a firm pad on the eye all the time. But do not pad the eye if there is a discharge from the eye.
3. Examine the eye (after staining with fluorescein) every day.
4. If the ulcer gets worse or iritis develops, treat for iritis – see next page.
5. If there is any possibility of vitamin A deficiency, give vitamin A immediately (see below).

Transfer to Medical Officer care

1. if the ulcer gets worse (urgent);
2. if the ulcer does not improve within 2 days of the start of treatment (urgent);
3. if the ulcer has not almost healed after 5 days of treatment (non-urgent).

Note – There may be a scar for which no treatment is possible. Do not transfer if there is only a scar.

> Always look for a corneal ulcer in anyone with a red painful eye.

Vitamin A deficiency

Vitamin A deficiency, affecting the eyes, is common between the ages of 6 months and 6 years. It is uncommon in adults but can occur in pregnant or breastfeeding women or in both sexes in times of famine or war. Other nutritional deficiencies are often present also and should be looked for and treated.

The earliest symptom or sign (not helpful in young children) is often not being able to see properly at night – night blindness.

Dryness of the conjunctiva and cornea (called 'xerophthalmia') is an important sign. The conjunctiva look dry, roughened and wrinkled. Patches of dry non-wettable conjunctivae can be seen when the child stops crying. Bitot's spots are spots of white material often in groups on the conjunctivae near the cornea. The eyelids can be red and swollen. The eye can become painful and there is pain on looking into the light. The cornea is then not clear and colourless as normal, but looks dry and a little dull and hazy.

In severe disease, a spreading white spot appears on the cornea. A large corneal ulcer may form. The cornea may break open. This can occur suddenly, especially if the patient gets measles.

Prevention is by eating a diet with enough vitamin A, especially fruits and vegetables with orange or dark green colouring including red palm oil and of course if available, liver, meat, fish and eggs. If a good diet is not possible a single oral dose of a capsule of 200,000 IU of vitamin A each 6 months will prevent the condition.

Treatment is by synthetic vitamin A 100,000 IU for those under 1 year old and 200,000 IU for those over 1 year old, immediately and repeated after 1–4 weeks. If vomiting give 55 mg retinol water soluble IMI instead. Pregnant women should be given lower doses, as high doses may cause abnormalities in unborn babies – 5000 IU orally or 1 mg retinol IMI daily. If there is any involvement of the cornea, use antibiotic ointment and after carefully closing the lid, pad the eye. If there is a white area in the cornea or a corneal ulcer, give also oral antibiotic as for corneal ulcer.

Acute iritis

Acute iritis is an acute inflammation of the eye, including the anterior chamber and iris.

Causes include:

1. infection from outside the eye (e.g. after injuries or corneal ulcer);
2. infection which started inside the eye, i.e. taken there by the blood (e.g. leprosy, onchocerciasis);
3. non-infective causes (e.g. rheumatoid disease, leprosy reaction, etc.); and
4. no cause diagnosed (most cases if it is not infection).

Symptoms include:

1. severe pain in the eye, made worse by light, and
2. loss of some vision.

Signs include:

1. inflammation of the conjunctiva around the edge of the cornea only (not under the eyelids);
2. pus in the anterior chamber (cloudy anterior chamber or hypopyon);
3. pupil irregular and small and does not contract and dilate normally;
4. eye tender when touched;
5. loss of some vision;
6. you may find the cause of the iritis (see above).

See Figures 31.10 and 31.11

Treatment

Try to find the cause. Always stain the cornea with fluorescein, and look for foreign body and ulcer – see page 418.

If the cause is obvious, e.g. corneal injury or ulcer, treat as below.

If the cause is not obvious, always look for leprosy, and especially a leprosy reaction, (see Chapter 15 page 103); also look for onchocerciasis (see Chapter 32 page 442).

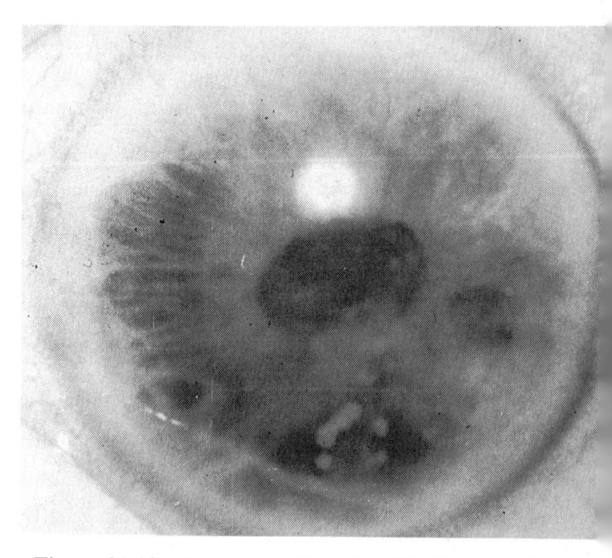

Figure 31.10 Acute iritis. Note that: (1) There are dilated blood vessels in the conjunctiva around the cornea (not present all over the conjunctiva). (2) The anterior chamber is not clear. (3) The pupil is small and irregular – it does not dilate in a dark place.

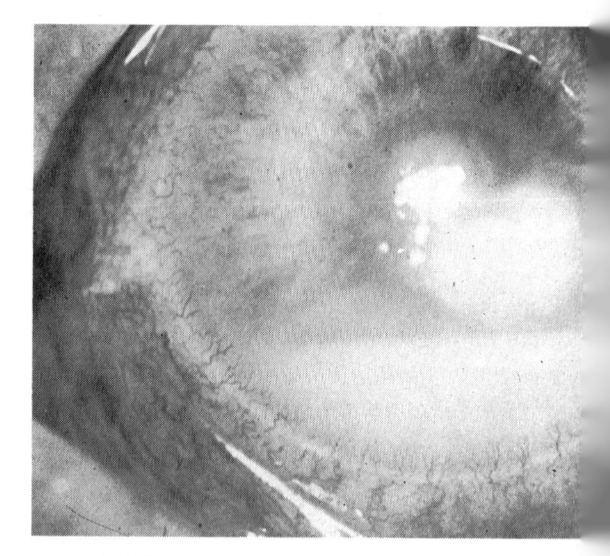

Figure 31.11 Acute iritis with hypopyon. Note that: (1) The circum-corneal conjunctival vessels are enlarged. (2) A corneal ulcer is present (the cause of the iritis). (3) The pus has settled to the bottom of the anterior chamber (called hypopyon). (4) The anterior chamber is all cloudy, so that you cannot see the small irregular pupil clearly.

If the cause is leprosy or you cannot find the cause treat as below, *and* transfer to Medical Officer car (urgent).

1. Antibiotic eye ointment – use chloramphenicol or tetracycline 1% or antibiotic compound ointment, put under the lower lid every 3 hours.
2. Atropine sulphate 1% eye ointment – put under the lower lid four times a day, until the pupil is widely dilated, and then once daily.
3. Keep a firm pad on the eye all the time. But do not pad the eye if it is discharging.
4. Chloramphenicol 1 g (4 caps) every 6 hours – Give by IMI if necessary. Reduce the dose to 750 mg (3 caps) four times a day when the patient improves.
5. Aspirin 600–1200 mg (2–4 tabs) or codeine compound tablets (2 tabs) should be given every 6 hours for pain, if necessary.

Continue the treatment for 10 days, or until all the redness goes and the eye is completely better (up to 3 weeks), whichever is the longer.

Transfer to Medical Officer's care if:

1. It is caused by leprosy (urgent) or onchocerciasis (urgent if acute).
2. You cannot find then cause (urgent).
3. The patient is not improving after 2 days of treatment (urgent).
4. The patient is not completely cured after 2–3 weeks of treatment (non-urgent).

> Always look for acute iritis in anyone with a painful red eye.

Onchocerciasis (river blindness)

See Chapter 32 page 442 for description and treatment.

See also 'Conjunctivitis' (page 416), 'Corneal ulcer' (page 418) and 'Acute iritis' (page 420).

Glaucoma

Glaucoma occurs when the fluid produced in the eye is not absorbed properly and the pressure inside the eye becomes high.

If this happens quickly, as in closed angle glaucoma, the eye becomes inflamed with red conjunctivae around the cornea, cloudiness of the cornea, the anterior chamber difficult to see, the pupil large, oval and dilated, the eye hard and tender to touch and there is great loss of sight.

If this happens slowly as in open angle glaucoma, the patient notices no symptoms until a lot of his sight is lost. There are no other symptoms or signs that you can find without an ophthalmoscope.

Treatment of both is by surgery. In acute closed angle glaucoma, unless the surgery is done quickly, the patient becomes blind. In open angle glaucoma, the surgery is done as the only other treatment is eye drops 2–4 times every day for the rest of the patient's life, which is expensive and not practicable.

Cataract

A cataract has formed if the clear lens of the eye becomes cloudly.

Causes include:

1. rubella infection during pregnancy;
2. a large number of illnesses and drugs including alcohol and tobacco;
3. a large number of eye infections, injuries and conditions;
4. old age;
5. others.

Symptoms: Slow loss of vision which continues to get worse, is usually the only symptom.

Signs include:

1. The pupil seems white not black when you shine a light into it.
2. There is loss of vision which varies from little to total.

Treatment

Transfer the patient to the eye specialist when there are cataracts in *both* eyes and he cannot see enough for normal living. (The eye specialist will operate on the worst eye and, if a lens could not be put back into the eye, give him special glasses.) No other treatment is possible.

Diabetic retinopathy

Diabetic retinopathy is due to changes in the blood vessels in the retina caused by diabetes that has been present for years.

After 20 years almost all IDDM and a half of the NIDDM patients will have diabetic retinopathy. Diabetic retinopathy will be less bad in patients who have good control of their diabetes with blood sugars near to normal.

There may be loss of vision.

It can be diagnosed only with the use of an ophthalmoscope and only after training to be able to recognise it.

It can be treated only with the use of a laser.

If an ophthalmologist (eye doctor) is available or regularly visits and has a laser, then all diabetic patients should be sent to him regularly as he directs, e.g. each year, to see if their diabetic retinopathy has got worse and if it needs treatment to stop blindness developing.

Prevention is by diet and exercise and if needed insulin or oral drugs to keep the blood sugars normal.

Long sight and short sight

The patient slowly loses his vision of things close to the eyes if he has long sight; or of things far away if he has short sight.

Examination shows that the patient cannot see the small part of the eye chart if he has short sight, or small printing if he has long sight. There is no other abnormality. But if you give the patient with short sight a card with a small hole (pin hole) in it to look through, he can see things much better.

If the patient cannot see enough for normal living, refer or transfer him non-urgently to the eye specialist, who will give him glasses to wear.

If this is not possible he could buy glasses to help him see better.

Strabismus (squint)

The two eyes do not look in the same direction at the same time.

Causes include:

1. abnormal development in a child,
2. trauma, and
3. disease of brain or the nerves to the eye.

Treatment

If a child has a squint, refer or non-urgently transfer the patient to the eye specialist. It is essential that this is done before he is 7 years old.

Eye injuries

Bruising of eye lids

No treatment is necessary.

Sub-conjunctival haemorrhage

If you can see all of the edges of the haemorrhage (even if part of the edge goes right up to the cornea or the eyelid edge) then the haemorrhage is probably not serious and probably no treatment is needed.

However if the haemorrhage extends towards the back of the eye and you cannot see where it ends, then the bleeding may be from behind the eye as a result of a skull fracture. This could be serious so the patient should be transferred to a Medical Officer for care.

Corneal abrasions

Treat as for a corneal ulcer.

Hyphaema (blood in the anterior chamber)

Order complete rest in bed and an eye pad until all the blood goes.

Transfer urgently to Medical Officer care if most of the anterior chamber is filled with blood (for urgent surgery).

Iris damage

Treatment does not help. Treat other conditions present.

Cataract after injury

No treatment is possible. If there is severe pain, transfer urgently for surgery.

Wounds of the eyelids

Carefully suture to make the edges of the eyelids level.

All penetrating wounds of cornea and sclera

Urgent transfer to Medical Officer's care is necessary. Meanwhile, treat as acute iritis and give tetanus prophylaxis.

Problems of diagnosis and management

Painful or red eye

Take a history of the present illness and also about the loss of sight, pain, redness and discharge.

Do a full examination of the eye, see pages 411–14.

1. *Find out where the redness is*

If it is all over the conjunctiva (on the undersurface of the eyelids as well as around the cornea) then diagnose:

- conjunctivitis (see page 416) or
- foreign body or chemical in eye (see pages 416, 418).

If it is mainly around the cornea, then diagnose:

- corneal ulcer, or
- corneal foreign body, or
- iritis, or
- acute glaucoma.

(see 2 below)

2. *Put fluorescein into the eye* (see page 412)

If the cornea stains green in some parts, then diagnose:

- corneal ulcer (see page 418) or
- corneal foreign body (see page 418).

If the cornea is normal, then diagnose

- iritis, or
- glaucoma.

(see 3 below)

3. *Find out the size of the pupil*

If the pupil is small, then diagnose iritis. See page 420.

If the pupil is large then diagnose glaucoma. Transfer to Medical Officer (urgent if there is still some sight in the eye).

32

Disorders of the Skin

Anatomy and physiology

The skin has a number of functions:

1. protection of the body from things outside the body – mechanical injury, heat, cold, light, chemicals, organisms etc;
2. keeping salt and water and other things inside the body;
3. keeping the temperature of the body normal, e.g. by sweating when the body is too hot; and
4. taking sensations into the body, e.g. touch, pain, heat, cold etc.

Pathology

There are many different types of lesion of the skin. See Figure 32.2, for illustrations of them.

1. *Macule* (or macular lesion)
   A macule is an area of skin which is different from the surrounding skin. It is not raised above the

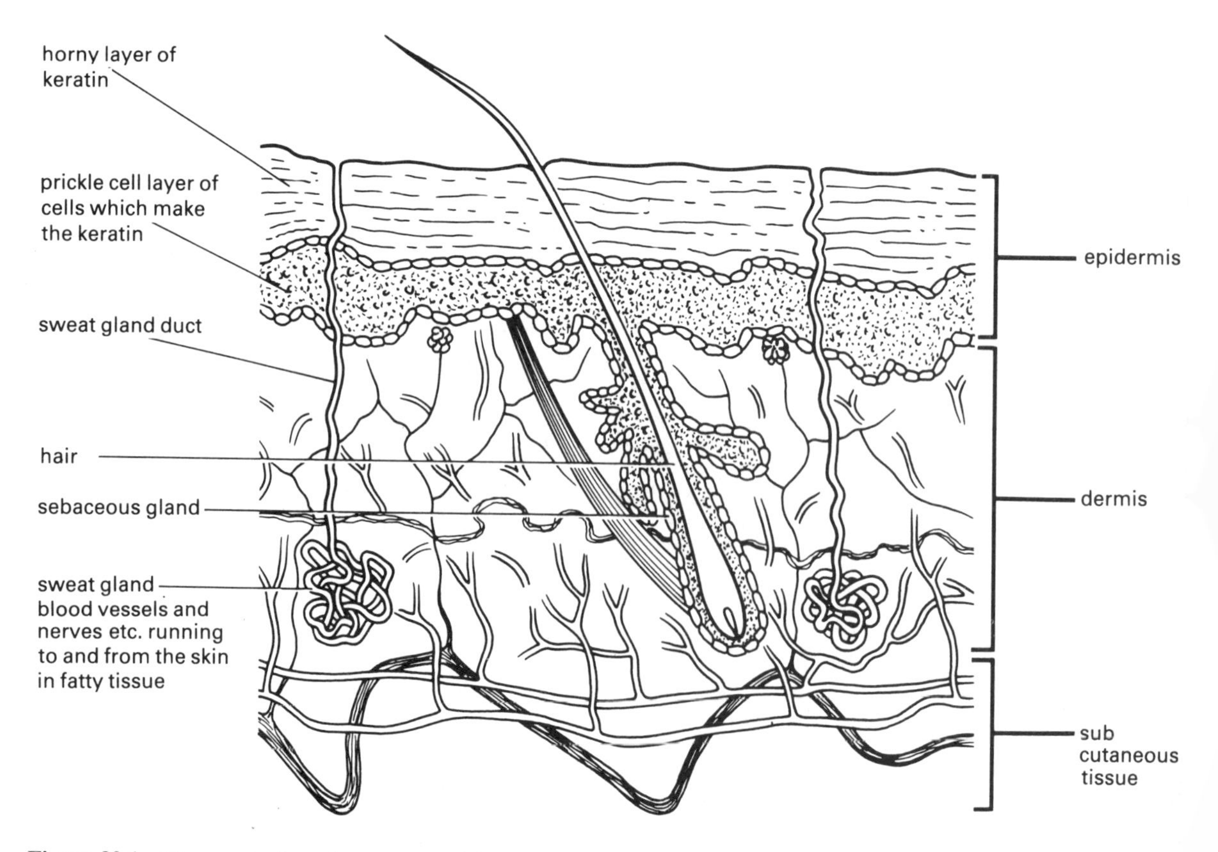

Figure 32.1 Diagram to show the structure of the skin under the microscope. In some parts of the body certain parts of the structure of the skin are more marked than usual (e.g. thick horny layer on the soles of the feet).

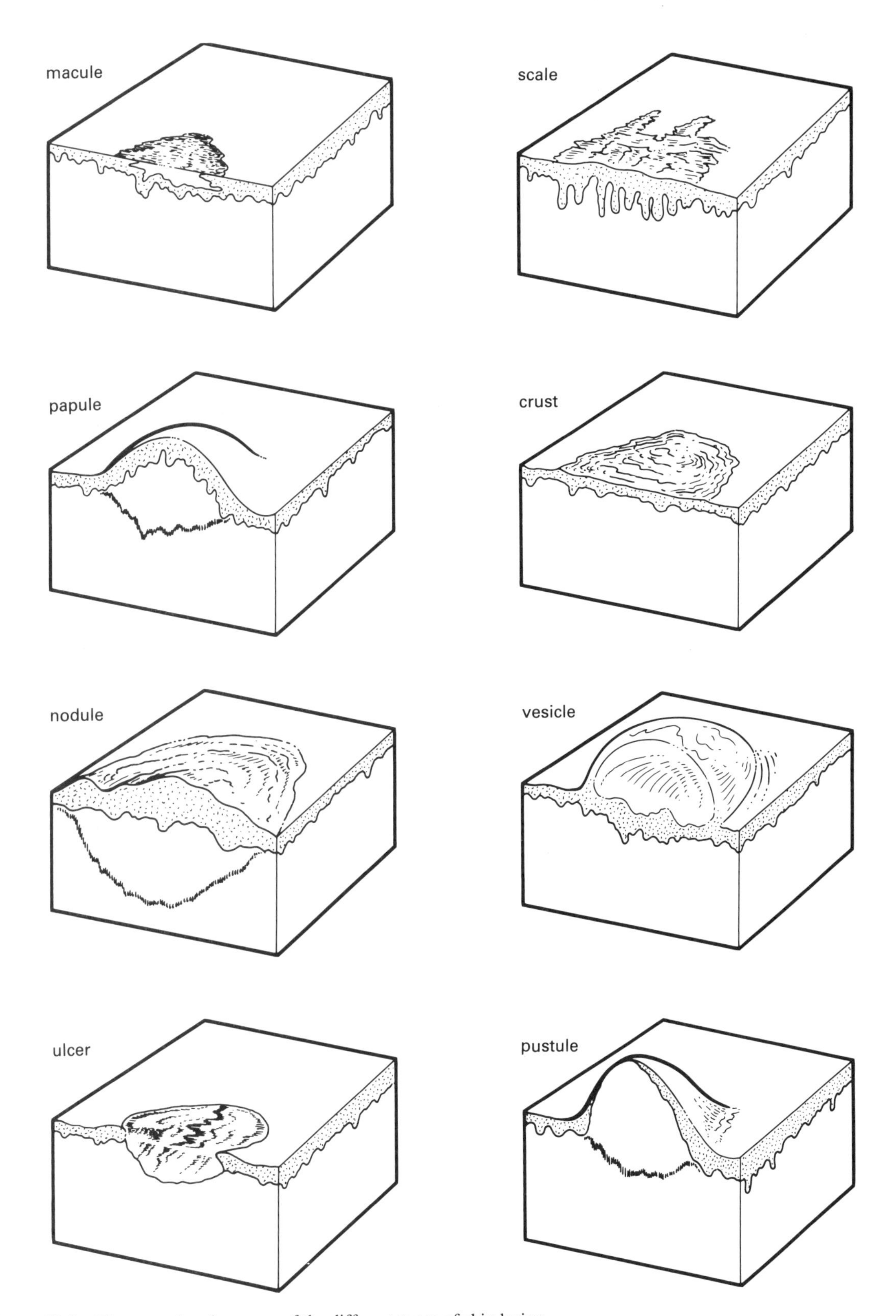

Figure 32.2 Diagrams showing some of the different types of skin lesion.

level of the skin surface. You can see (e.g. different colour) and/or feel it in the skin.

2. *Papule* (or papular lesion)
   A papule is like a macule, but it is raised above the level of the skin surface.
3. *Vesicle* (or vesicular lesion)
   A vesicle is like a papule, but there is clear fluid under the surface of the lesion.
4. *Pustule* (or pustular lesion)
   A pustule is like a vesicle, but the fluid contains pus.
5. *Crust*
   A crust is dried exudate (fluid which comes from the lesion) and may consist of:
   - serum (yellow),
   - blood (red or brown),
   - pus (yellow, grey, green), or
   - mixtures of these.
6. *Scales* are built up surface layers of the skin. They may be:
   - yellow and greasy (e.g. seborrhoeic dermatitis),
   - silvery (e.g. psoriasis), or
   - grey (e.g. eczema)
7. *Ulcers* are areas where the skin has been destroyed.
8. *Dermatitis* is any inflammation of the skin. There are many different types of dermatitis.
9. *Eczema* (or eczematous reaction or eczematous dermatitis)
   Eczema is the most common type of dermatitis (see Figures 32.3 and 32.4). In the acute stage the affected area gets red, shiny and warm because the blood vessels widen. Then small vesicles appear on the surface of the skin. These vesicles soon burst. The exudate dries and forms a crust. Secondary bacterial infection may occur. After some time chronic eczema develops. The affected area may be thick, dry, scaly and the normal lines in the skin become very deep. Cracks can develop deep into the flesh underneath.

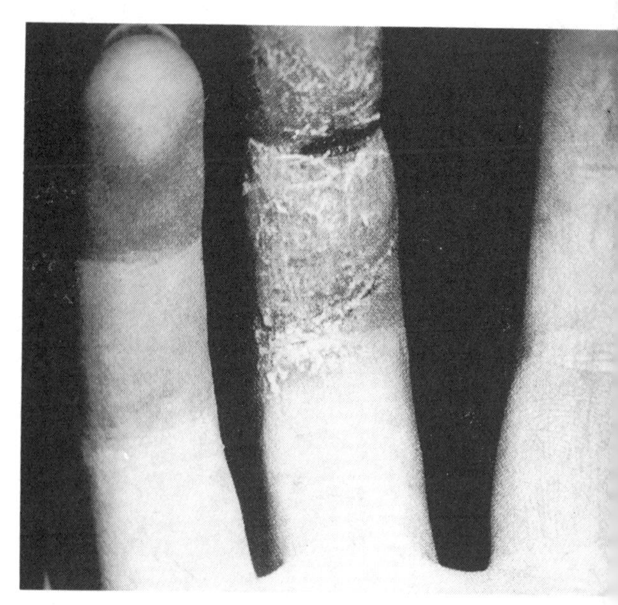

Figure 32.3 Acute eczematous dermatitis.

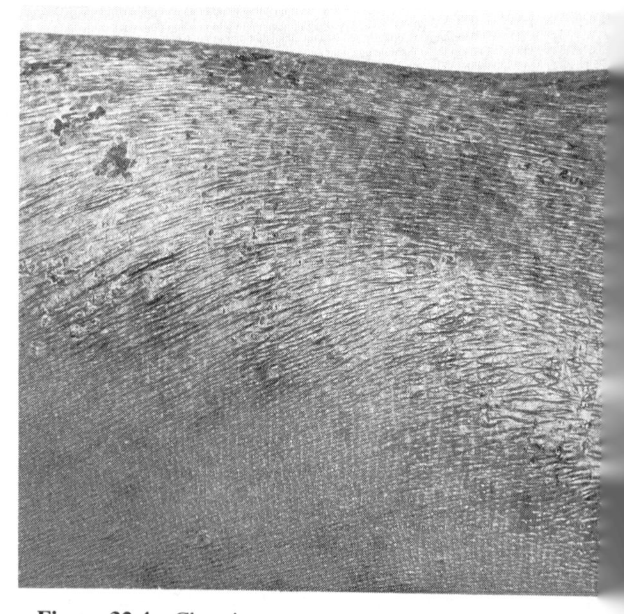

Figure 32.4 Chronic eczematous dermatitis. The area has become 'lichenified' – the skin is thick and dry and the normal creases are deep.

Diagnosis and treatment of skin conditions

Sometimes you can easily recognise the symptoms and signs of a certain disease. If you cannot, then do a full history and examination and test the urine (see Chapter 6). Look at the skin all over the body. Decide which of the two main groups of skin conditions your patient is in:

1. *Generalised illness with a skin condition*, e.g. chickenpox, measles, syphilis, yaws, leprosy or other infections; malnutrition; allergic reaction to a drug; etc.

2. *Localised skin conditions*, i.e. conditions affecting only the skin.
   Important causes include:
   (a) external parasites, e.g. scabies, lice;
   (b) fungal infections, e.g. tinea;
   (c) bacterial infections, e.g. impetigo;
   (d) eczematous dermatitis which has many causes;
   (e) itching which causes scratching which causes damage to the skin (i.e. dermatitis) which causes more itching …

Localised skin conditions are very common and important, and so you should know about:

1. the preparations that are available to treat localised skin conditions; and
2. how to use these skin preparations.

Preparations often available for treatment of skin conditions

You do not need all of these preparations.

1. *Antibacterial preparations*
   - Eusol[1] solution
     – use for dressings if there is much pus or dead tissue
     – stop when the lesion is clean
   - Antiseptics
     – hexachlorophene 3% emulsion (e.g. Phisohex) – use with water to clean the skin or a lesion
     – chlorhexidine compound solution (e.g. Savlon) in either water or spirit (alcoholic) solution – use to clean the skin or a lesion
   - Antibiotics
     – antibiotic compound ointment (e.g. neomycin and bacitracin ointment)
     – antibiotic compound powder
     – powder from inside a tetracycline capsule (use no other antibiotics like this)
     – silver sulphasalazine 1% or silver sulphadiazine 1% (usually with chlorhexidine) cream (often kept just for patients with burns)
   - Methylrosanilinium chloride usually called crystal violet or gentian violet 0.5% in either water ('aqueous') or alcohol (spirit or 'tincture') solution. Use only the water solution and never the alcohol solution on mucous membranes
   - Iodine 2.5% solution in spirit (alcohol) – use to clean a lesion of the skin
   - Acriflavine emulsion (use only with strong 3% saline[1] dressing); stop when infection goes or it will stop healing
   - Potassium permanganate (Condy's crystals) 1:10,000 solution[1] in water

   Give also an oral or injected antibiotic (see Chapter 11 page 46) if there is a severe infection.
2. *Antifungal preparations*
   - Benzoic acid compound ointment (Whitfield's ointment) or benzoic acid 6% and salicylic acid 3% cream or ointment.
   - Salicylic acid 10% paint
   - Gentian violet 0.5% solution (methylrosanilinium chloride) in water or spirit (alcohol), but is useful for only *Candida* ('thrush')
   - Potassium permanganate (Condy's crystals) 1:10,000 solution[1] in water
   - Iodine 2.5% solution in spirit (alcohol)
   - Sodium thiosulphate 15% solution (for tinea versicolor only)
3. *Anti-inflammatory preparations*
   These are used for eczema and other dermatitis and to help healing.
   - Potassium permanganate (Condy's crystals) 1:10,000 solution[1] in water
   - Aluminium diacetate 10% solution (Burow's solution) in water – dilute before using
   - Weak 1% saline[1] solution
   - Calamine lotion
   - Zinc cream
   - Glycerine and ichthammol
   - Cod liver oil ointment
   - Wool fat anhydrous (lanoline)
   - Ammoniated mercury ointment 2.5% (Ung. HAD)
4. *Anti-itch preparations*
   - Weak 1% saline[1] solution
   - Potassium permanganate (Condy's crystals) 1:10,000 solution[1] in water
   - Calamine lotion
   - Give also an antihistamine orally or by injection if required
5. *Anti-external parasite preparations*
   - Benzyl benzoate 25% solution
   - Iodine solution 2.5% *Dilute immediately before use* with an equal volume of water
   - Carbaryl 0.5% or 1% lotion and 1% shampoo
   - Malathion 0.5% lotion and 1% shampoo
   - Permethrin 5% (50 mg/g) cream

1 For details of how to make this, see page 428.

- Permethrin 1% (10 mg/g) lotion
- Gamma benzene hexachloride (lindane 1% solution) no longer recommended
- DDT 2% emulsion – not recommended and usually not available.
- DDT 10% powder – not recommended and usually not available.

A number of preparations have more than one function and can be very useful if the diagnosis is not certain, or if two or more conditions are present e.g.:

- Potassium permanganate solution
  - anti-inflammatory
  - anti-itch
  - antifungal
  - antibacterial
- Crystal violet (methylrosanilinium chloride)
  - antibacterial
  - antifungal (for *Candida* ('thrush') only)
- Iodine solution
  - antibacterial
  - antifungal
  - antiscabies
  - (but this can itself cause a rash)

How to make simple useful skin preparations

Eusol solution

Mix chlorinated lime 12.5 g (20 ml) with enough water to make a paste. Add a little more water and shake. Add boric acid 12.5 g (20 ml) and shake. Add enough water to make 1 litre. Shake well. Leave overnight. Filter. Store in a dark coloured bottle. Note that Eusol is a clear solution with the smell of chlorine. It does not store well and you should use it within a week. If the solution is more than a week old, or does not smell of chlorine, throw it away.

Potassium permanganate 1:10,000 solution

Dissolve $1\frac{1}{4}$ ml or $\frac{1}{4}$ of a teaspoonful (not heaped) of potassium permanganate (Condy's crystals) in 10 litres ($\frac{1}{2}$ bucketful) of clean water. It is a dark pink colour.

Strong (3%) saline

Dissolve $7\frac{1}{2}$ ml ($1\frac{1}{2}$ teaspoonful, not heaped) of salt in 200 ml (1 cup) of clean water.

Weak (1%) saline

Dissolve $2\frac{1}{2}$ ml ($\frac{1}{2}$ teaspoonful, not heaped) of salt in 200 ml (1 cup) of clean water.

Dressings

Use a *wet gauze bandage* for all painful conditions on legs, arms, feet, hands, and head, especially if you think it will heal slowly.

Use *adhesive plaster* for all small painless conditions on rounded parts of the body, joints, etc.

Use *crepe bandages* for all painful conditions on joints and thighs, and for large deep ulcers, wounds, etc. anywhere.

Use *elastic plaster bandage* on soles, palms and early boils.

Use dry *gauze bandages* only for tinea of the feet. (See Table 32.1)

Table 32.1 Dressings for skin conditions.

		Cost	*Pain relief?*	*Helps healing?*	*Stays on?*	*Pain when removed?*
Gauze bandage (WOW)	Wet	Cheap	Good	Good	Good	No pain
	Dry	Cheap	Some	Some	Poor	No pain
Adhesive plaster		Very cheap	None	None	Good in dry weather	A little painful
Elastic plaster bandage		Expensive	Some	Some	Good	Very painful
Crepe bandage		Expensive	Very good	Very good	Good	No pain

Note these things about treatment

1. Do not make a dermatitis worse by treatment which irritates the already damaged skin. (For example, do not immediately use Whitfield's ointment on an acutely inflamed fungal infection. It is better to use potassium permanganate solution wet dressings to start with until the condition is not acute. Then you can use the Whitfield's ointment (see Figure 32.7).)
2. You must treat any bacterial infection.
3. Always look for signs of scabies and lice if there is (a) an itch or (b) if there is skin infection, especially if more than one area is affected and especially if it returns after treatment.
4. Always treat an itch which causes scratching. If you do not treat the itch, the scratching causes dermatitis and the dermatitis causes more itch and more scratching …
5. Always think of the possibility that drugs or skin treatment have caused the skin problem. Treatment for a condition, which has gone, may have caused a new skin condition.

The common skin conditions

Tinea

Tinea is an infection of the skin with one of many fungal organisms.

Complaints include itching and worry about the appearance of the skin.

Examination usually shows affected areas that are roughly circular. The edges are often a little raised and a little inflamed. Sometimes there are small papules, vesicles or pustules at the edge. The skin in the rest of the lesion is often peeling. The centre of the lesion may appear to be healing.

There are many other types of tinea – see Figures 32.5, 32.6, 32.7 and 32.8.

Make sure the lesion is not caused by leprosy. Do tests for loss of sensation, etc. If you have real doubts, do a biopsy (but not on face). Scrapings of skin and cut off pieces of nail can be sent to the laboratory with a request for examination for tinea or fungal organisms.

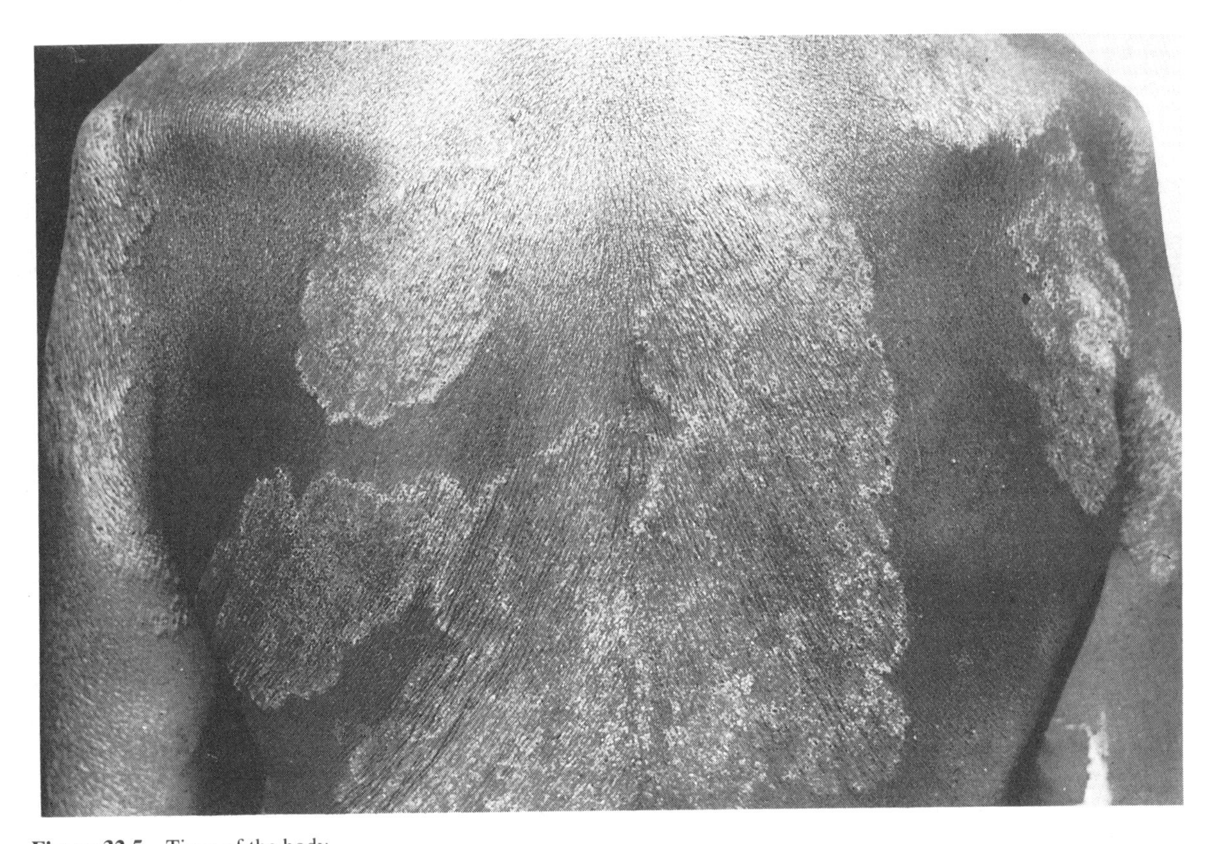

Figure 32.5 Tinea of the body.

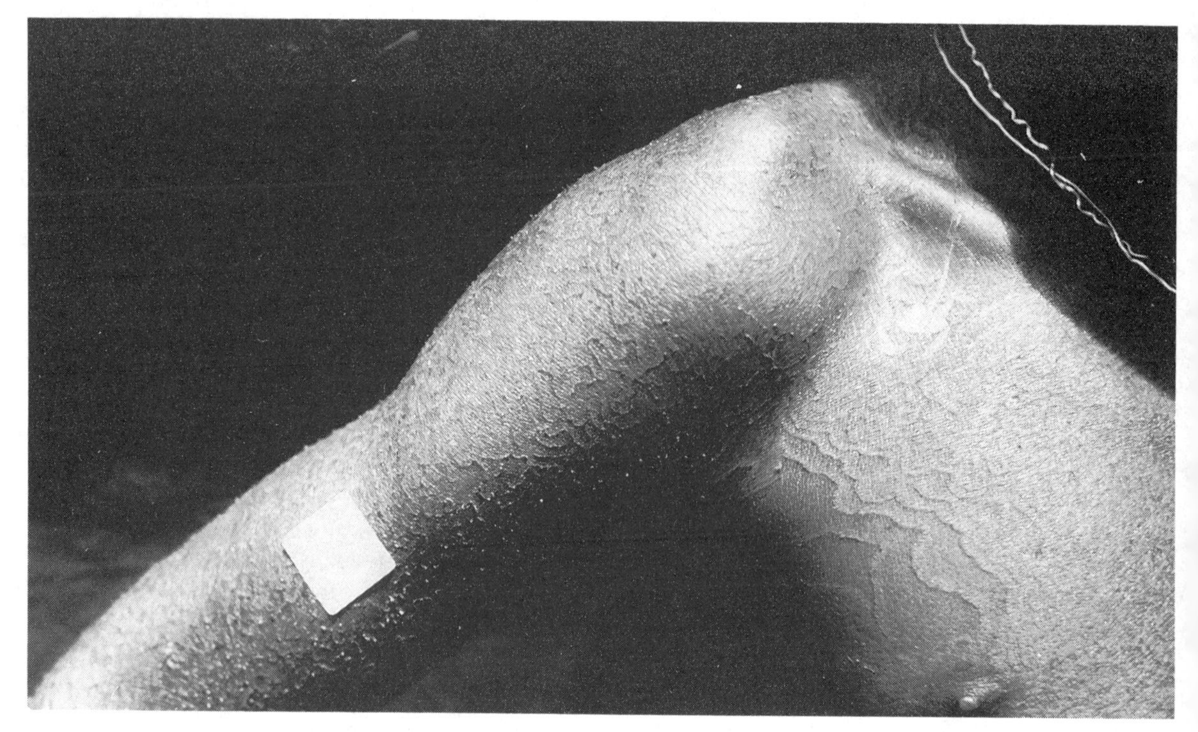

Figure 32.6 Tinea imbricata. There is an abnormality in the immunity of many of these patients. This is probably inherited, because the disease is common in certain families. The disease usually returns, even after successful treatment.

Routine treatment (but *not* for an acutely inflamed area)
Treat as an outpatient.

1. Remove any hair from the affected area.
2. Wash the affected area with soap and water every day. Rub off any scales. Dry the skin well after washing. Keep the skin as dry as possible.
3. Put either salicylic acid paint *or* benzoic acid compound ointment (Whitfield's ointment) (or other benzoic acid and salicylic acid paint, cream or ointment) on the affected area twice daily. Also put it on the normal skin for 2 cm round the edge of the affected area. Do not cover more than one-quarter of the body every day.
4. Change and wash the clothes every day.
5. Continue the treatment every day until all the tinea goes and then for 2–4 weeks after this.

Treatment of an acutely inflamed area of tinea

1. Do not treat with Whitfield's ointment or salicylic acid paint at first.
2. Bathe the area with potassium permanganate 1:10,000 solution and then put on a *little* acriflavine emulsion on a dressing soaked in strong 3% saline.
3. Also give sulphamethoxazole 800 mg/trimethoprim 160 mg (co-trimoxazole) orally twice daily or tetracycline 250 mg (1 cap) four times a day or doxycycline 100 mg (1 tab) daily for at least 5 days for infection if necessary.
4. Give routine treatment (as above) only when the acute inflammation improves.

The above treatment by itself will not cure:
- tinea of the nails,
- most cases of tinea of the scalp or
- many cases of tinea of the skin.

Talk to your Medical Officer about further treatment.

There are now many new more effective, but much more expensive, antifungal skin drugs including miconazole, tolnaftate, ketoconazole, clotrimazole, econazole and others. If the above treatment is not effective, the patient may decide to purchase one of these; but make sure the diagnosis of fungus infection is correct before he spends the money and make sure the patient does not have HIV infection.

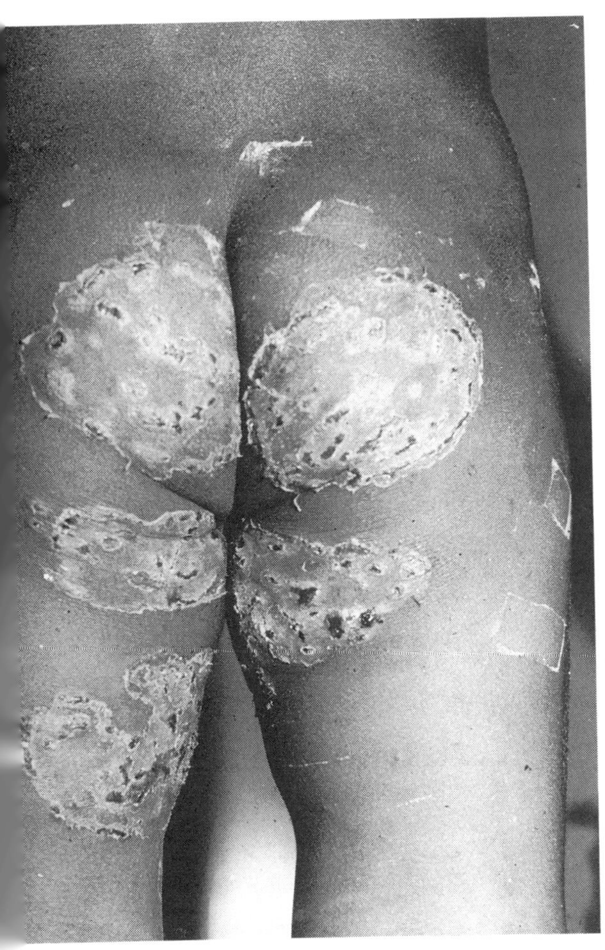

Figure 32.7 Tinea of the body, with secondary bacterial infection. You must treat the bacterial infection and the skin inflammation before you treat the tinea infection.

None of the above will cure tinea of the nail. However, ciclopirox olamine and amorolfine nail laquer applied for 6 months for fingernails and 12 months for toenails may well cure this condition.

Cases of tinea of the nails and even some cases of tinea of the scalp and beard and body are not cured by even the above new drugs and systemic oral treatment is needed. Terbinafine 250 mg daily is effective but very expensive and would have to be used for 6–12 months for tinea of the nail, although only for a couple of weeks for other skin fungus infections.

Griseofulvin (only the ultra microsize preparation 330–375 mg once daily, or, if unavailable, the less effective microsize griseofulvin 500 mg) once daily with the main meal of the day can be tried. Again, make sure the diagnosis of fungal infection is correct by laboratory examination and consultation with your Medical Officer and that the patient does not have HIV infection, before these very expensive drugs are purchased.

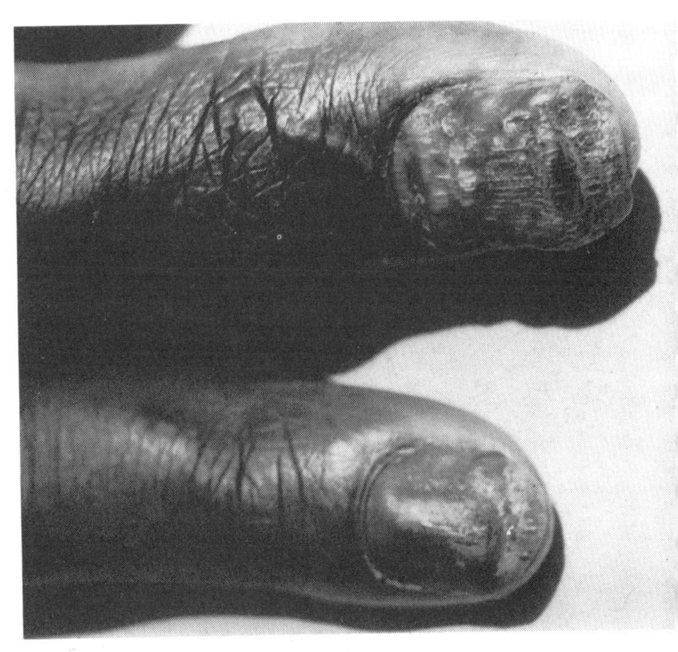

Figure 32.8 Tinea of the nails.

Tinea versicolor (white spot)

Tinea versicolor is a different fungus infection which causes many small lesions which are pale and covered with powdery skin (see Figure 32.9). The patient may complain of the appearance or of the itch.

Treat with 10–20% sodium thiosulphate solution ('hypo' or X-ray fixer) on the whole body daily for 3 weeks or Whitfield's ointment (benzoic acid and salicylic acid) daily on the affected areas (but not more than $\frac{1}{4}$ of the body daily).

If this is not successful, the patient may be willing to buy selenium sulphide 2.5% solution as a shampoo and use it as a skin preparation, putting it on at night and not washing it off until the next morning, but being careful, as it is a poison.

Griseofulvin tablets do not help at all. However ketoconazole tablets may cure the tinea versicolor but have occasional side effects including hepatitis.

Mycetoma ('madura foot')

Mycetoma is a fungus infection which spreads to deep structures (such as the bones). It is common in dry areas of Africa, the Middle East and parts of

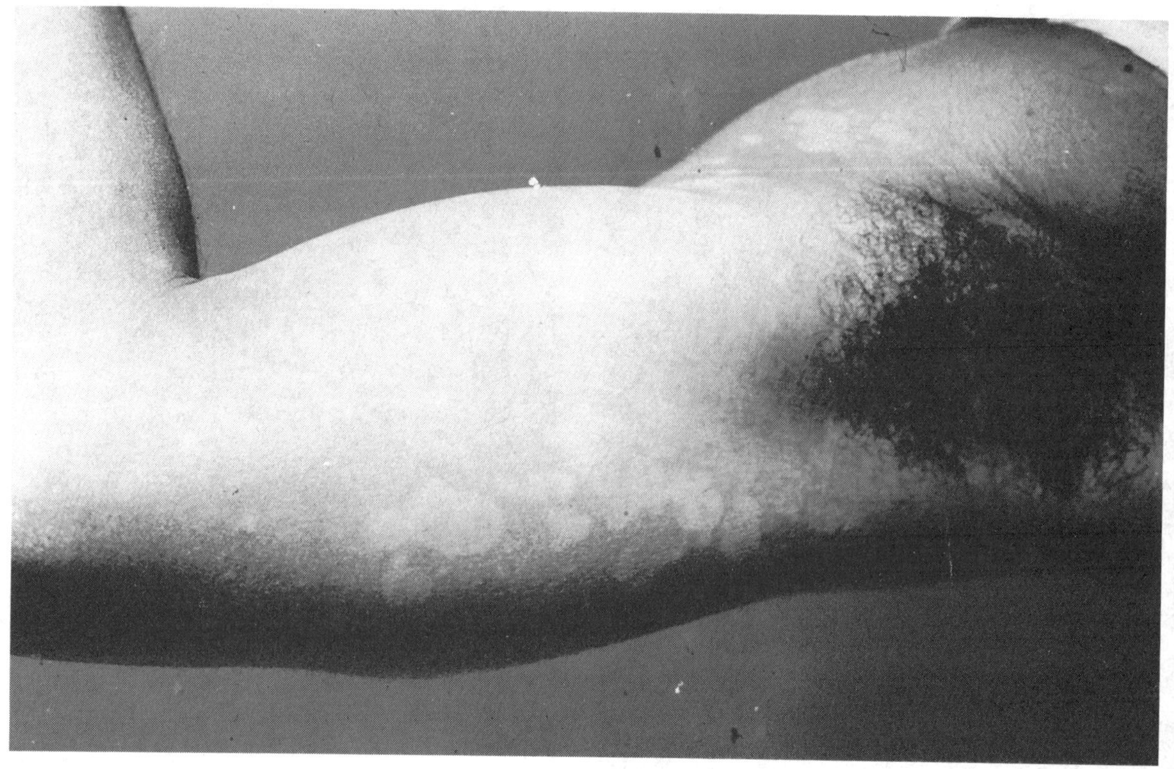

Figure 32.9 Tinea versicolor.

Asia. It is common in people who do not wear shoes, especially farmers. Most often it affects the patient's foot but can affect scalp or back, etc.

First there is a painless swelling of the area. The area affected slowly becomes larger. Lumps may appear on the swollen area. The lumps may burst and sinuses may form. Pus, with little lumps of coloured material (e.g. black, red, yellow), comes out of the sinuses. There is still no pain or fever, and the patient can still use the affected area. But over months or years the affected area becomes larger. The infection does not often spread to the lymph glands or to other parts of the body.

After many years the infected area (usually the foot) is so badly affected that the patient cannot use it. (See Figure 32.10.)

Treatment of some of these infections with drugs is possible. However surgery is usually necessary. Refer or non-urgently transfer affected patients to a Medical Officer.

Prevention may be possible if you can get people in the areas where the disease is common to wear shoes.

Impetigo

Impetigo is a bacterial infection of the skin, usually caused by staphylococci or streptococci. It is very infectious and spreads to others by direct contact or by vehicles, such as towels.

First a blister forms. This bursts and leaves a red wet surface. A thick yellow crust forms. Then new blisters form. There are other types of impetigo. (See Figure 32.11.)

Management

1. Gently rub off the scabs and crusts with antiseptic solution (see 2 below.).
2. Wash the whole area with antiseptic solution twice a day, and then daily, when it improves. Suitable antiseptics include chlorhexidine comp. antiseptic in water (e.g. Savlon) or hexachlorophene emulsion (e.g. Phisohex).
3. Put a dressing over the affected area especially if it is large or has pus coming from it.
4. Put antibiotic compound ointment *or* a *little* acriflavine emulsion on a dressing wet with strong

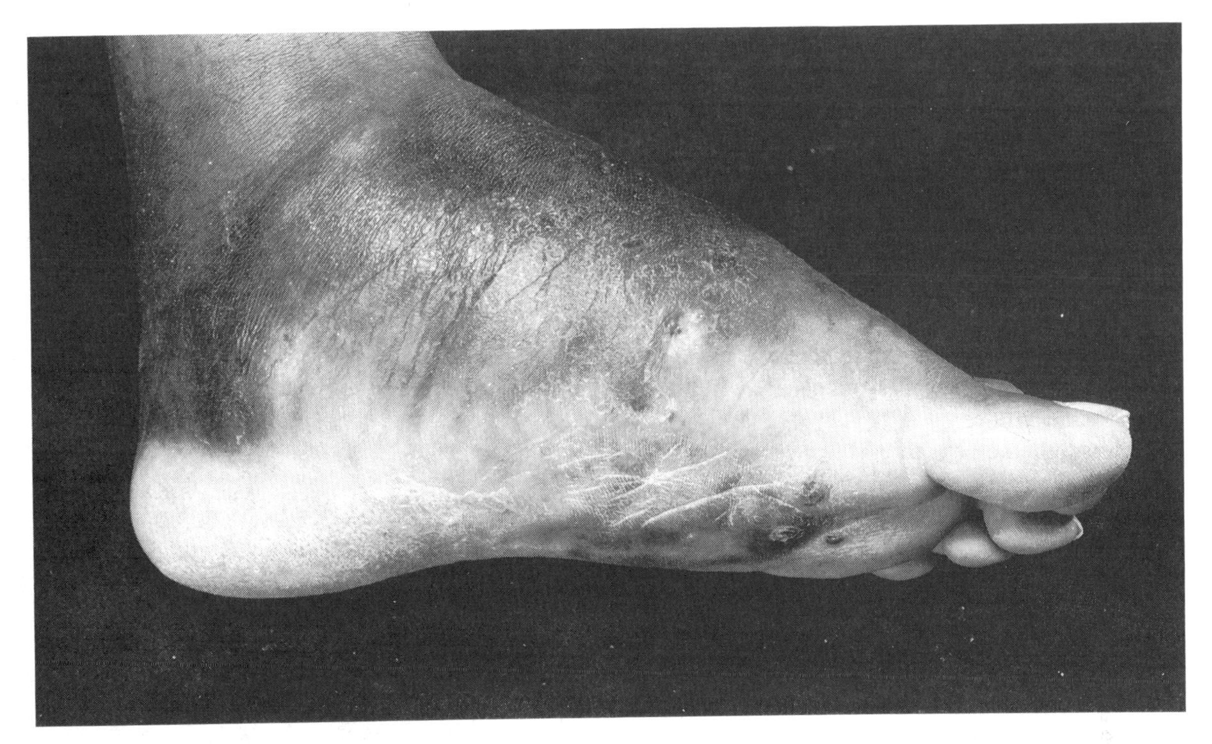

Figure 32.10 Foot affected by mycetoma.

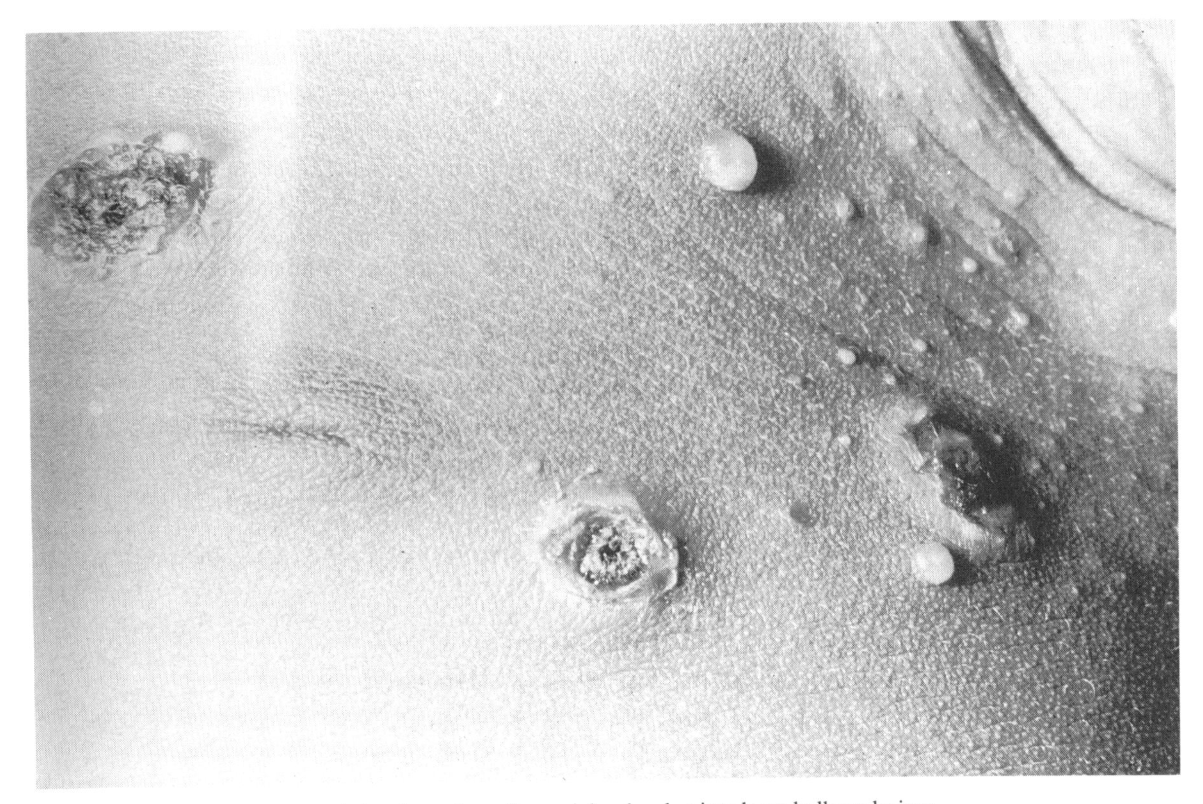

Figure 32.11 Impetigo with vesicles. Sometimes the vesicles develop into large bulbous lesions.

3% saline on to the affected area. Do this three times a day at first; and then daily, when it improves.
5. Change and wash the clothes daily.
6. Give antibiotics for 5–10 days *if*
   - the patient develops general symptoms and signs of infection *or*
   - the skin lesions are very large or inflamed *or*
   - the condition does not respond to the above treatment *or*
   - the condition continually returns *or*
   - you are not certain that the patient will do the treatment properly.

   Give sulphamethoxazole 800 mg/trimethoprim 160 mg (co-trimoxazole) twice daily or tetracycline 250 mg (1 cap) four times a day or doxycycline 100 mg (1 tablet) daily but not if pregnant, when you give erythromycin 500 mg three to four times a day or if not available, penicillin.
7. Look very carefully for scabies and lice, especially if there is an itch. (The lesions of scabies and lice are not always typical.) Treat if present (see pages 440–1).
8. If the condition appears in new areas, or returns after it was cured and treatment was stopped, then wash the *whole body* (including the perineum and inside the nose) with the antiseptic solution daily. Then give all the above treatment, especially 6 and 7.
9. Tell the patient that the infection spreads by pus from the infected areas taking germs to new areas. He should not touch the infected areas. He should wash his hands often. He should not allow others to touch his towel and clothes until he is cured.

Furuncle or boil

A boil is an infection (usually caused by staphylococci or streptococci) of the skin in the place where a hair grows. A boil starts as a small tender lump in the skin. It becomes bigger over some days, and has all the signs of acute inflammation. It then 'points' – softens in the centre as pus forms. The skin bursts and the pus comes out. A day or two later the 'core' comes out – the dead part of the skin which made the hair. (See Figure 32.12.)

In an area where myiasis occurs, check that any slowly developing 'boil' is not caused by the myiasis (see page 442)

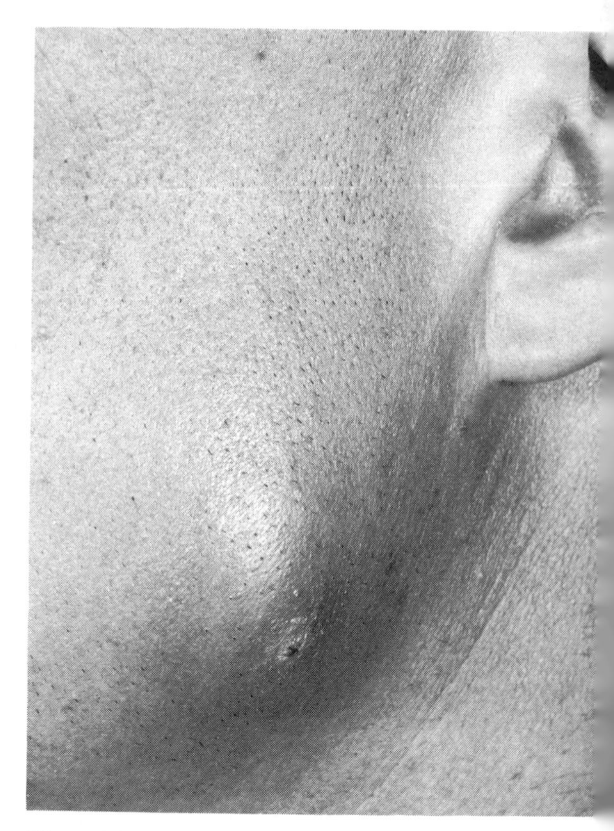

Figure 32.12 Furuncle or boil.

Treatment

At early stage (only inflamed swelling)
1. Paint the lesion (and several cm all round it) with iodine solution 2.5%.
2. Cover the area with a large square of elastic plaster bandage (e.g. Elastoplast). Stretch the elastic plaster as you stick it on to the skin. (This will 'splint' the area.)
3. Give aspirin 300–900 mg (1–3 tabs) four times a day for pain, if necessary.
4. Test the lesion under the elastic plaster for fluctuation every day.
5. If the lesion goes, remove the plaster; but only when it has *completely* gone.
6. If *definite* fluctuation develops, remove the elastic plaster with one quick pull. This will probably also pull off the thin skin over the surface of the boil and allow it to drain – incision will then not be necessary.

At other stages
See Chapter 11 about antibiotics and a surgery book about incision (cutting open) to drain the pus.

Antibiotics will not cure the condition once pus has formed. The lesion needs incision to let the pus drain out.

If repeated boils
Treat as for repeated impetigo (see page 432).

Tropical ulcer

Tropical ulcer is a skin infection with special types of bacteria, (*Bacillus fusiformis* and spirochaetes), which cause an acute severe infective ulcer, which may become a chronic ulcer.

The special bacteria that cause tropical ulcer may be spread by direct contact and by flies or other insects.

A tropical ulcer usually comes on exposed areas, usually below the knee. First a painful vesicle (blister) forms. This bursts and leaves an ulcerating, dirty surface. The ulcer spreads very quickly. It is painful and itchy. The edge is slightly raised but not undermined. The surface is covered with a smelly grey-green or bloody membrane. (See Figure 32.13.)

The patient has no general symptoms and signs of infection. After about a month, the ulcer stops spreading. It may heal. If it does not heal, the base slowly becomes scarred and skin cannot then grow over the surface as there are no blood vessels from underneath to keep it alive. The ulcer may then be present for life. If at any time it does heal it has a very thin skin over it which is often broken by minor injury and forms an ulcer again.

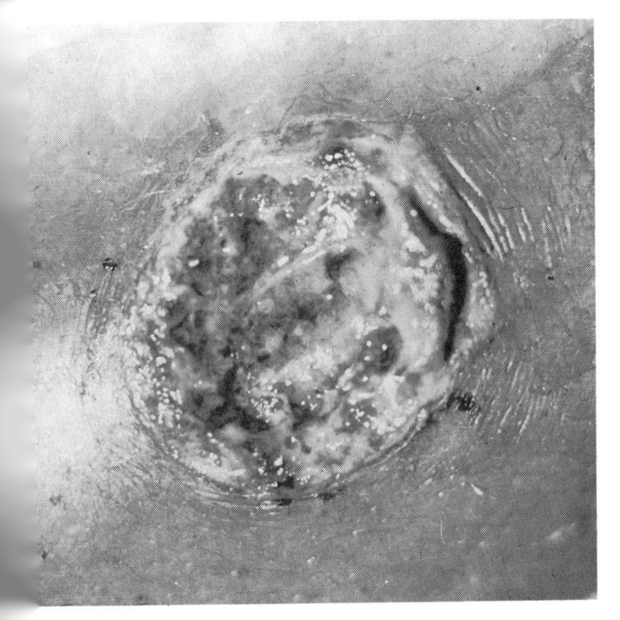

'igure 32.13 Tropical ulcer. You can diagnose the ulcer y its very quick growth, its typical appearance (raised dge, a grey bloody membrane on the surface). There are ery few general symptoms and signs.

Treatment

If the ulcer is severe or large, or has been present for more than 2 months admit for inpatient treatment. If it is small, treat as an outpatient.

1. Give procaine benzylpenicillin 1 g or 1,000,000 units IMI daily until the ulcer is healing well or at least 7 days (this is very important if it is a true tropical ulcer).
2. Give tetanus toxoid if needed.
3. If possible, rest the affected area. Keep the leg with the ulcer on it higher than the rest of the body. If this is not possible, firmly bandage a cotton wool pad over the dressing (see 3 and 4), using a crepe bandage if possible.
4. Dress the ulcer twice daily (or more often if necessary) with Eusol, or strong (3%) saline solution, until the ulcer is clean. The dressing should stay wet. Cover it with a sheet of plastic if needed.
5. When the ulcer is clean, dress with any non-irritating non-sticky dressing, e.g. cod liver oil ointment or antibiotic compound ointment or vaseline or even something such as coconut oil on gauze, as long as it will come off without sticking to the underlying healing ulcer. Change the dressing only when it is really necessary. You must not make the ulcer bleed when you take the dressing off. Keep the ulcer covered until it is completely healed.
6. Skin graft the ulcer if it is larger than 3 cm in diameter, and does not heal with treatment.
7. The resultant scar may always need protection from injury with a dry dressing.

Transfer to Medical Officer's care non-urgently if:

1. The ulcer has not healed with treatment in 6 weeks.
2. You cannot do a skin graft, if needed.
3. The ulcer is very large, or there is bone at the base (bottom) of the ulcer.

Yaws

Yaws is a bacterial (a spirochaete, *Treponema pertenue*) infection spread by direct contact or by flies.

It affects children much more often than adults. The first (or primary) lesion is a sore, on an exposed area, often on the leg (see Figure 32.14). It begins as a macule and becomes a papule. It is not painful but it is itchy and usually becomes an ulcer 1–5 cm wide and is raised at the edge. It has an irregular white-yellow crust and if you remove the crust, it leaves a bleeding surface with yellow spots. After some months it heals. The nearby lymph nodes are enlarged but not tender.

Secondary skin lesions are similar to the primary lesions (see Figure 32.15). There may be many of them all over the body and they appear when the primary lesion is getting better or has gone. If a lesion appears on the sole of the foot, it is painful and the patient limps. Lesions in moist areas of the body may look like condylomata lata. Skin on the hands and feet may become thick and crack. Bones and joints may become painful, tender and thickened at this stage. The forearm and lower legs and especially the fingers, may become swollen and tender. After some weeks or months, all these things may go; but

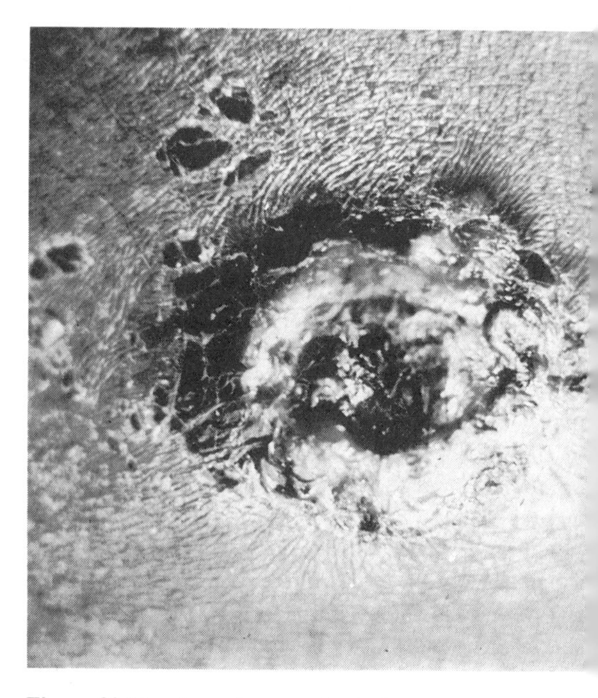

Figure 32.14 An early yaws skin lesion.

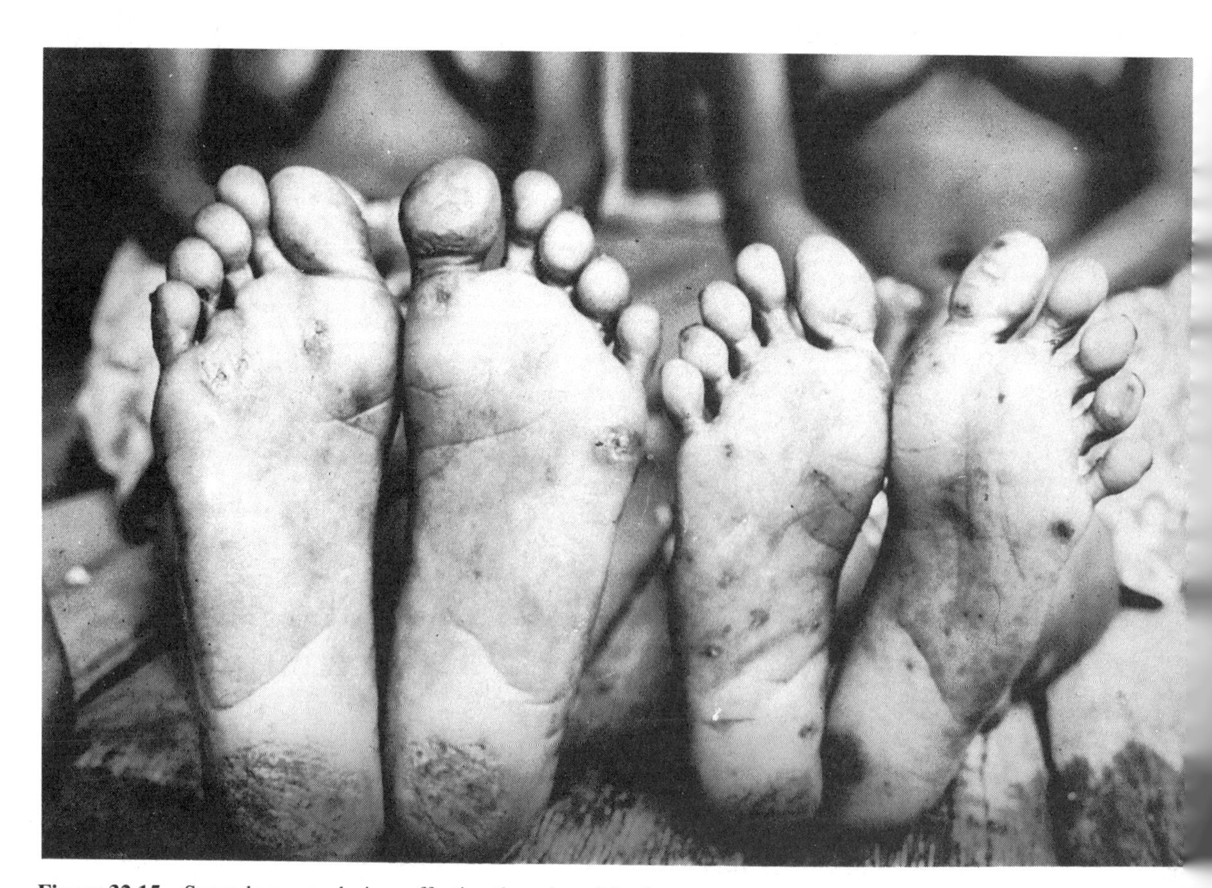

Figure 32.15 Secondary yaws lesions affecting the soles of the feet.

they may often return again and again for some years.

Late yaws develops in some patients. This can cause deep large skin ulcers (gumma); thickening and cracking of the skin of the feet; curving of the long bones; and destruction of the bones of the nose and face (see Figures 32.16 and 32.17).

Syphilis serology becomes positive in yaws. Penicillin cures yaws. But if you find a case, arrange for a survey to find out if control measures are necessary. If a survey shows only a low frequency (less than 5% of the population) you only need to treat the family and obvious contacts of a case. If there is medium frequency (5–9%) treat all children in the community. If there is high frequency (more than 10%), treat everyone in the community. For prophylactic treatment one dose of procaine penicillin of 1,200,000 units for adults and 600,000 units for children is very effective (especially procaine penicillin with aluminium monostearate (PAM)).

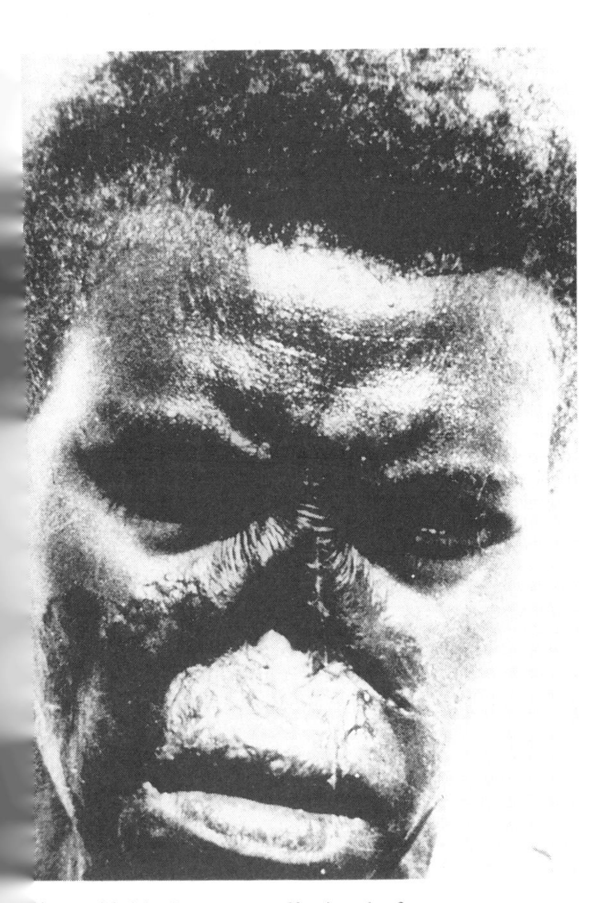

'igure 32.16 Late yaws affecting the face.

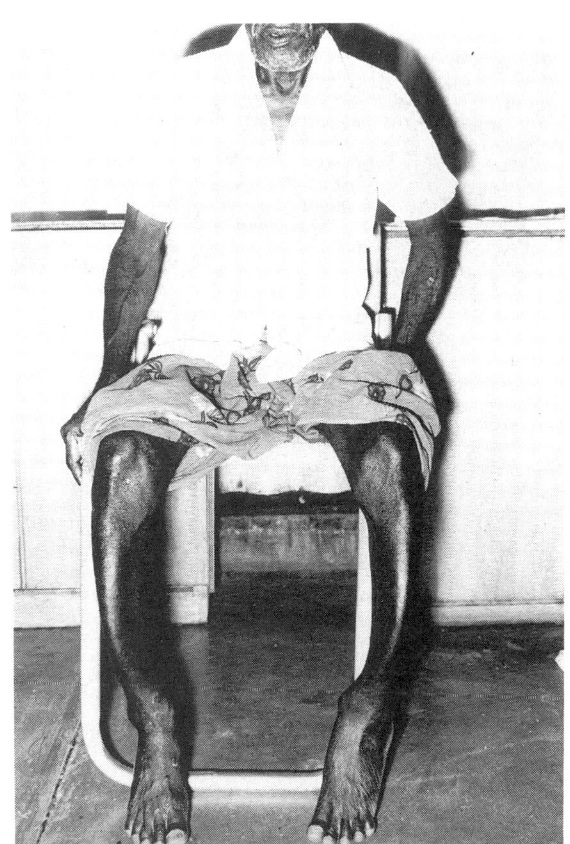

Figure 32.17 Late yaws affecting the bones.

Bejel (endemic syphilis) and pinta

Endemic syphilis (called bejel or other local names) occurs in the Middle East and Africa and is caused by non-sexually transmitted syphilis in childhood. Spread is by close personal contact, and by cups etc. Children can develop all the lesions of secondary syphilis (see Chapter 19 page 171) and sometimes skin lesions, which are the same as yaws (see above). After some years these conditions go; but after some more years, severe destruction of the skin and the bones of the face can occur as in late yaws. Late lesions as in syphilis do not occur. The serological test for syphilis is positive. (See Figure 32.18.)

Treatment is with penicillin, as for syphilis (see Chapter 19 pages 172–3).

Pinta (which has other local names) occurs in Central and South America and perhaps the Middle East. It is caused by an organism related to the syphilis and yaws bacteria. Spread is by non-sexual transmission, like yaws. First there is an itchy scaly

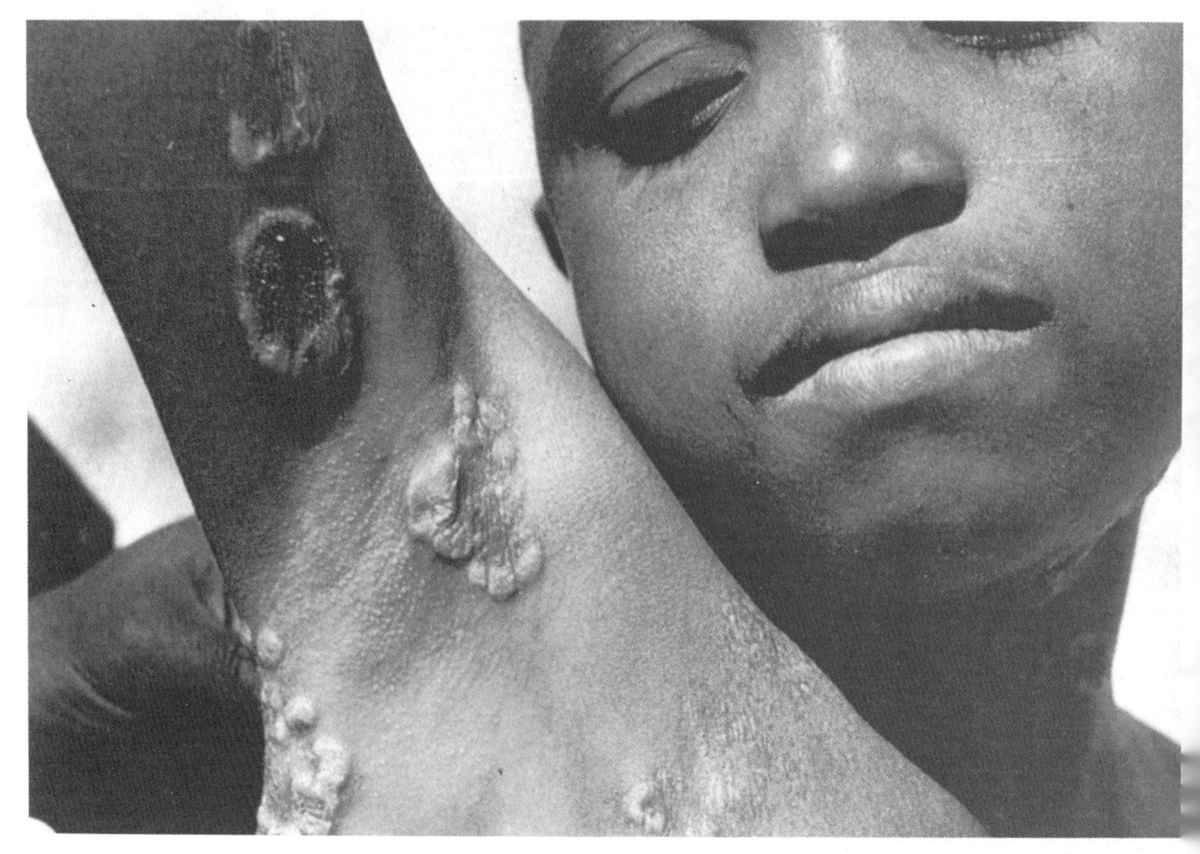

Figure 32.18 Secondary rash caused by bejel (endemic syphilis).
(Source: W. Peters and H.M. Gilles. *A Colour Atlas of Tropical Medicine and Parasitology*. London, Wolfe Medical Publications, 1981) (Dr A. Buck)

papule. This slowly enlarges and joins with new papules which continue to appear around its edge. The papule becomes up to 10 cm in diameter. Nearby lymph nodes are enlarged. This lesion often remains, but later many other lesions appear on the exposed parts of the skin. These lesions are most often dark. After many years, the lesions on the limbs become symmetrical (i.e. the same on both sides) depigmented (pale) and thin. The serological test for syphilis is positive. (See Figure 32.19.)

Treatment is with penicillin, as for syphilis (see Chapter 19 pages 172–3).

Anthrax

Anthrax is normally a bacterial infection of cattle and sheep etc. It can infect people on exposed parts of their skin, most often on the face. A papule forms quickly. This soon becomes a vesicle filled with blood-stained fluid. Small vesicles appear around the original vesicle. The area around the lesion becomes very swollen, and looks inflamed; but it does not pit on pressure, and it is not very tender. After some days the vesicle dries, becomes black, and starts to heal.

Usually there is some enlargement of the nearby lymph glands, but few general symptoms and signs of infection. But the infection can spread and cause septicaemia and death. Other more severe forms of the disease can occur.

If you suspect a patient has anthrax, immediately start treatment with penicillin, and check with your Medical Officer for methods of control and prevention.

Mycobacterium ulcerans ulcer

Mycobacterium ulcerans is a bacterium which can cause a chronic skin ulcer. The reservoir and means of spread is not certain.

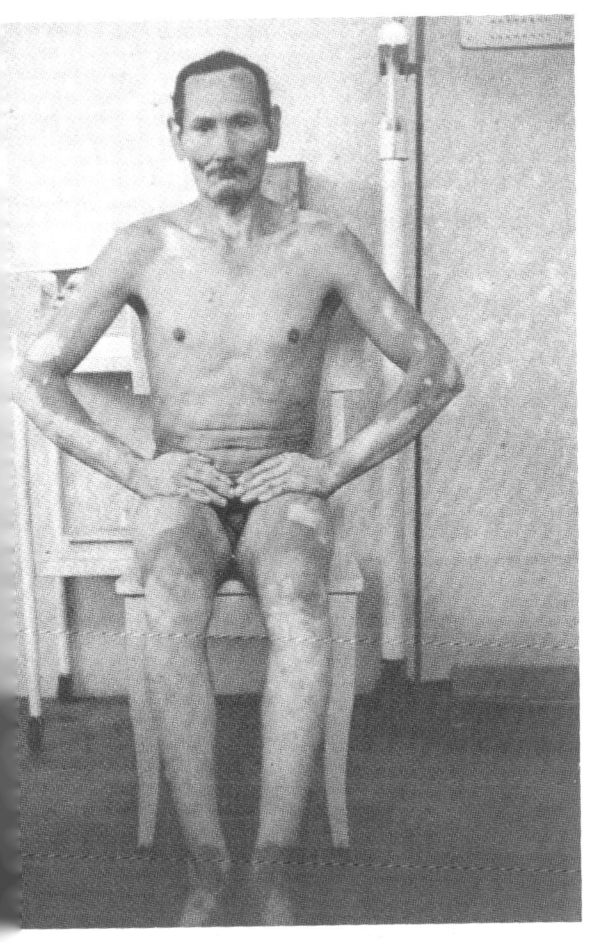

Figure 32.19 Depigmented lesions caused by pinta. (Source: W. Peters and H.M. Gilles, *A Colour Atlas of Tropical Medicine and Parasitology*, London, Wolfe Medical Publications, 1981)

The lesion usually starts as a firm painful nodule which may be itchy. As it grows it bursts to form an ulcer. The ulcer grows slowly over weeks or months. It goes down to the muscle, and sideways underneath the skin. This causes a very typical appearance, where the skin overhangs the edge of the ulcer, sometimes by several centimetres (see Figure 32.20.) Surrounding ulcers may start and soon be joined under the skin. It remains painless. It eventually stops but by then may have caused severe scarring or even loss of all the skin of an arm or leg.

Diagnosis is by the typical appearance of the ulcer/s and AFBs seen on a smear or by a biopsy sent for examination in the laboratory.

If you diagnose this condition, non-urgently *transfer* the patient for surgery to make flaps out of remaining skin, clean under these flaps and in the

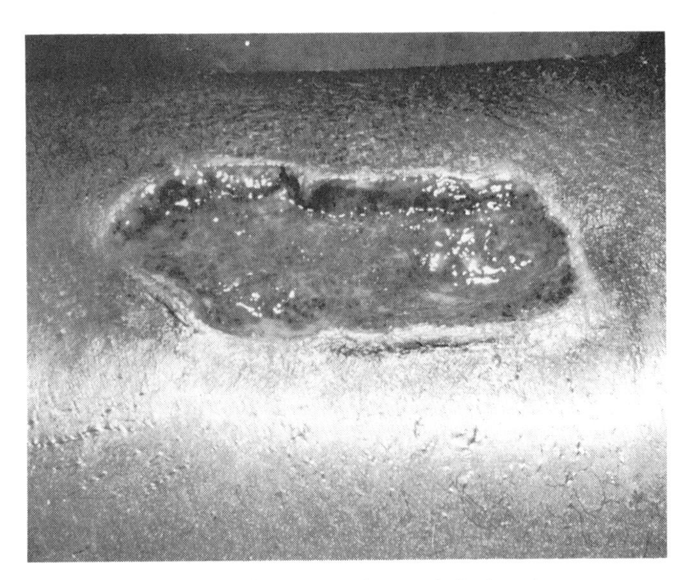

Figure 32.20 A *Mycobacterium ulcerans* infection. A probe can go several centimetres under the apparently normal skin at the edge of the ulcer.

base of the ulcer with antiseptic such as silver nitrate 0.5%, do skin grafts if needed and consider special drugs. Clofazimine and rifampicin may sometimes help; but only if the above surgery is also done.

Cellulitis

Cellulitis is an inflammation of the cellular and other tissues underneath the skin. These tissues normally join the structures under the skin. The inflammation in cellulitis usually spreads along the divisions between the organs under the skin. If cellulitis is not cured quickly, pus can form. Abscesses can then form and even gangrene of the skin can occur.

There is usually pain in the area, but not at one definite place. There is swelling, redness and tenderness of the affected part of the body, but again it is not usually in one particular place. Blisters can form on the skin. There is usually malaise, fever, fast pulse, etc.

Treatment is by rest and antibiotics. Benzyl (crystaline) penicillin, 1,000,000 units by IMI every 6 hours until the condition improves and then procaine benzyl penicillin 900,000 units daily by IMI is usually enough. If the condition gets worse, the antibiotic should be changed to chloramphenicol 1 g (4 caps) orally every 6 hours and if pus has collected in any area, and it can be drained easily without risk of damaging any important structure, incision should be made over the area. Should pus be deep, however, or should the inflammation be in an area where there are many important structures, such as the neck or hand, *transfer* the patient urgently to a Medical Officer.

Cutaneous leishmaniasis ('oriental sore' and 'espundia')

See Chapter 18 page 139.

Scabies

Scabies is an infestation of the surface layer of the skin by an insect, the scabies mite. The scabies mite spreads from one person to another during close personal contact. It usually infests all people who live in the same house as a person with scabies.

The patient usually complains of an itch in part of the body or of repeated sores in part of the body.

The usual lesion of scabies is a dark papule, several mm in diameter (Figure 32.21). You can sometimes see the path the mite made through the skin. The patient scratches the lesions and often causes an eczematous reaction or a bacterial infection (such as impetigo) in the area.

Most often it affects the areas between the fingers, the front of the wrists, the elbows, the breast, the penis, the pubic region and, in babies, the sides of the feet (Figure 32.22).

Treat as an outpatient.

1. Apply permethrin 5% (50 mg/g), *or* benzyl benzoate 25% *or* tetmosol 5% *or* malathion 0.5% (*or* if none of the other treatments is available, gamma benzene hexachloride 1% emulsion, but *not* for babies) lotion or cream like this:
   (a) Wash all the body with soap, using a cloth. Rinse and dry the skin.
   (b) Shake the bottle very well, and put the lotion on all the body except the face especially in the folds of the skin. Scabies does not often affect the skin of the face. The medicine must remain on the skin for 24 hours.
   (c) After 24 hours, wash the lotion off and put on clean clothes.
   (d) Four days later, repeat the treatment as in (a), (b) and (c).

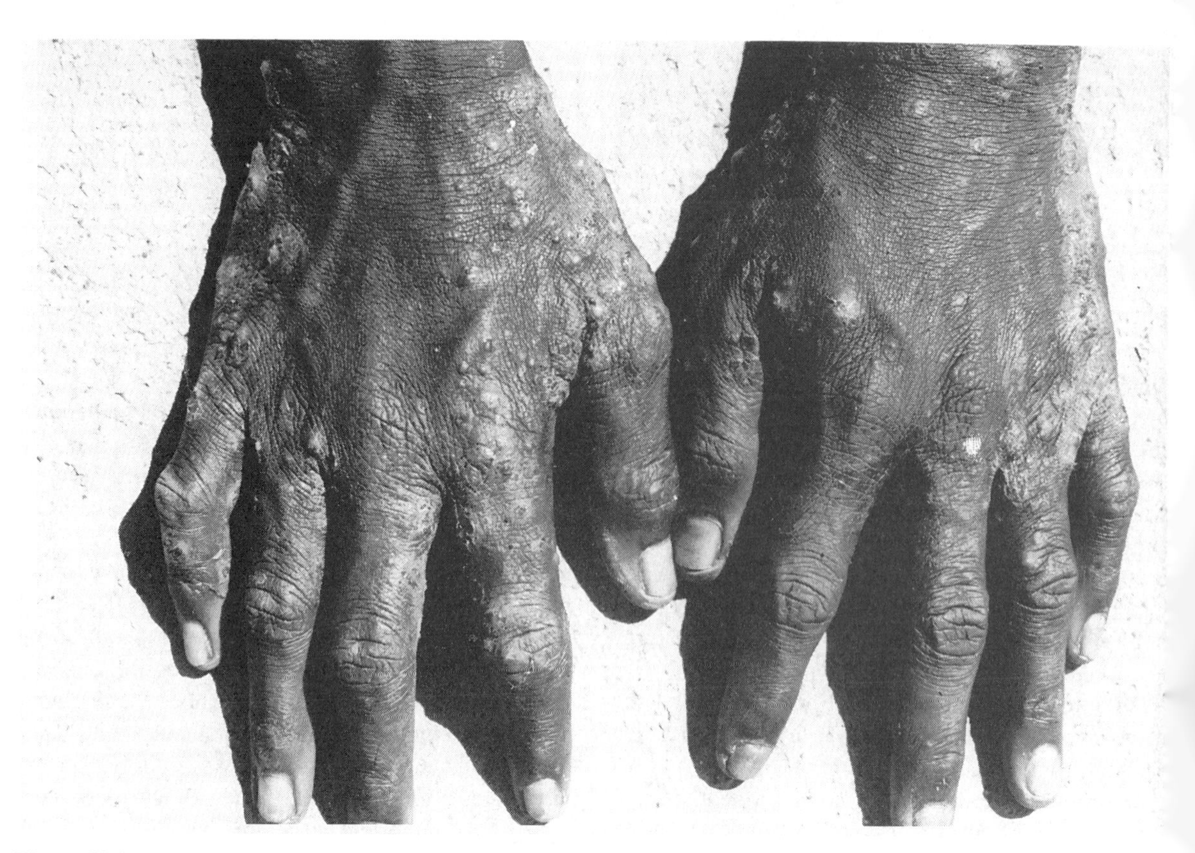

Figure 32.21 Scabies

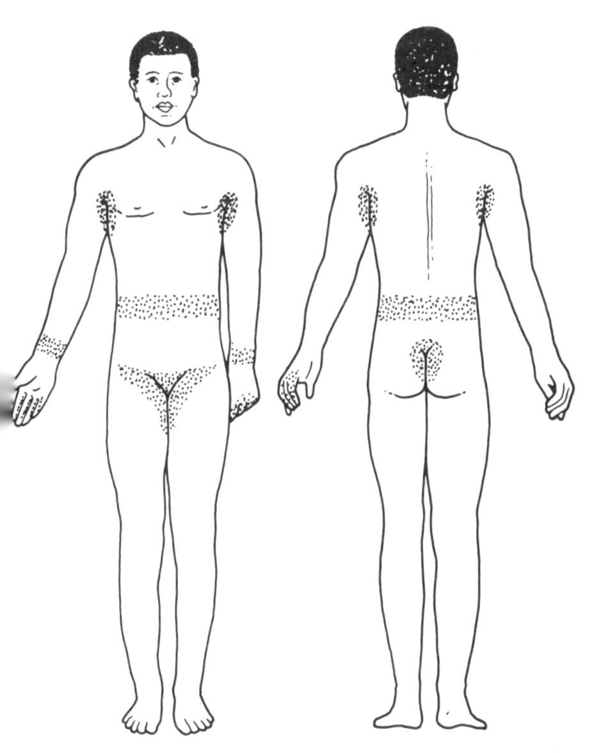

Figure 32.22 Diagram to show the usual distribution of scabies lesions.

> Give the patient a private room where he can completely undress. The patient can wash himself. **But a health worker must apply the lotion** to all the skin of the patient (except the face). The patient cannot do it well enough.

If the patient is a mother, wash the breasts before breastfeeding. After breastfeeding, put the application on again.

2. If the lesions are infected, give procaine benzylpenicillin 1 g or 1,000,000 units IMI or if not pregnant, sulphamethoxazole 800 mg/trimethoprim 160 mg (co-trimoxazole) or tetracycline 250 mg (1 cap) four times a day or doxycycline 100 mg (1 cap) daily starting on the day of the first permethrin or other lotion treatment until the infection goes. If impetigo is present, treat this first (see page 432) before giving the insecticide treatment.
3. Treat (or show the patient how to treat) all members of the patient's family, and anyone else who lives with him. Other people with early infection may not know they have it as the itch may take one month or so to start.
4. Change and wash the clothes and bedclothes, and put them in the sun, at the end of every 24 hour treatment.
5. Educate the patient about the cause and prevention of the disease. Encourage the patient and his family to wash regularly with soap. Encourage the patient to keep clean and regularly wash his clothes, bedclothes, and house.

   Tell the patient to come for treatment when any new lesions appear (before they are bad or there are many).

In resistant cases talk to your Medical Officer about possible other treatment including ivermectin.

Lice (pediculosis)

Lice are insects that can infect people. They can carry dangerous disease (e.g. typhus). But usually they only cause itching and skin rash. There are three types of lice.

Head lice live on the scalp and put their eggs on the hair ('nits'). Lice cause severe itching of the scalp. Scratching often causes eczema or results in bacterial infection of the scalp. The glands in the neck are often enlarged. You can diagnose lice by finding them or their eggs on the scalp or hair.

Body lice cause itching, scratching and eczema or bacterial infections of the body; especially around the waist. You will find the lice and eggs in the clothes (especially under the edges).

Pubic lice affect the pubic area, and also the eyelashes.

Treatment is with permethrin 1% (10 mg/g) or benzyl benzoate 25% or gamma benzene hexachloride 1% cream, lotion or emulsion.

Put one of these insecticides on the hair and scalp. Cover the hair with a cloth for some hours. The next day wash and carefully comb the hair to remove all the eggs. Repeat the treatment a week later.

For body lice, boil or iron the clothes and bedclothes during each treatment. Treat the patient and his clothes with insecticide. See Chapter 17 page 128 for methods of mass treatment in epidemics.

For pubic lice, it may be necessary to shave off the pubic hair. But do *not* shave or cut the eyelashes.

Control and prevention is by treatment of cases, good personal hygiene, and using repellents in epidemics of typhus.

In resistant cases talk to your Medical Officer about treatment with temephos or ivermectin. In some countries some (not all) ordinary shampoos and hair conditioners seem to suffocate and kill head lice.

Tungiasis

Tungiasis occurs mostly in South America and Africa. It is an infestation with the chigoe or jigger flea, which affects man and pigs.

Most often it affects the feet. The flea goes into the skin, and grows to the size of a small pea. It then pushes eggs out through the skin lesion. First there is itching. Later there can be secondary bacterial infection. Tetanus can occur.

In treatment you must remove the whole flea in one piece with a sterile needle and prevent and treat secondary bacterial infection and give tetanus prevention. If there are very many lesions, soak the affected area in a 5% solution of benzene hexachloride.

Myiasis

Myiasis is an infestation with the larvae (maggots) of flies. The larvae can go into the skin and make a lesion like a furuncle or boil. In areas where myiasis occurs, always think of this condition when a patient has an inflamed swelling of the skin.

In treatment put oil (such as liquid paraffin) on the lesion so that the larvae cannot breathe and start to come out of the skin to get air. If you put more oil on and press the sides of the lesion this will usually remove the larvae. Sometimes surgery is necessary. Treat any secondary infection with antibiotics.

Onchocerciasis ('river blindness')

Onchocerciasis is a chronic disease of the skin and eye. It is caused by an infestation with a filarial worm. The adult worm causes nodules in the skin. The larvae (microfilaria) cause dermatitis and blindness.

Onchocerciasis is common only in parts of Africa, the Middle East and in Central and South America. (See Figure 32.23.)

The bite of an infected *Simulium* (a small black fly) injects infective larvae of the worm. These flies breed only in fast flowing rivers; but some types can fly many kilometres from the rivers.

The larvae develop into adult worms in the skin of the infected person. The adults cause painless nodules under the skin. These may become large lumps and are most common where bones are just under the skin (e.g. around joints, hips, ribs, back of head). The adults make many larvae (called microfilaria) which travel around the body in the tissues of the skin and eye (but not in the blood).

At first the microfilaria cause a very severe itch although the skin can look quite normal. Later, they cause dermatitis with severe itching and form macules and papules. The skin loses its elasticity and looks like an old person's skin. The skin can become lichenified (or thickened) and wrinkled. This is sometimes called 'lizard' or 'elephant' skin. After some years of severe itching and scratching, the skin can become thin and loose (called 'tissue paper' skin) and patches of the skin become pale (called 'leopard' skin). Folds of skin can form in the groin ('hanging' groin). (See Figures 32.24, 32.25 and 32.26.)

The microfilaria can cause many sorts of damage to the eyes, which can lead to blindness ('river blindness'). They can causes conjunctivitis or a chronic oedema of the conjunctivae and eyelids. They can also cause whitish spots on the cornea and later a thickening and loss of clearness of the cornea, often with blood vessels growing in the affected area. This change starts at the bottom of the cornea and grows up over the cornea so that the patient cannot see through it. Microfilaria can also cause iritis and later glaucoma and cataract. The retina of the eye may be damaged. From any one or more of these things the patient often becomes blind.

You can *diagnose* onchocerciasis like this:

1. remove a nodule, cut it across and see an adult worm in it; *or*
2. take a 'skin snip', put it into saline for $\frac{1}{2}$–24 hours then look at the saline under the microscope to see microfilaria.

Treatment is with a new drug called ivermectin (Mectizan) given each year. Ivermectin kills all the microfilaria and makes the adult worm not able to produce more microfilaria for 6–12 months. It does not kill the adult worms so treatment may need to be continued until they die (5–20 years). The dose is 150–200 micrograms (0.15–2 mg)/kg body weight which usually means two of the 6 mg tablets for an adult. The drug manufacturers Merck Sharp and Dohme supply this drug free to any government who uses it in an onchocerciasis control programme. It has been found that distribution by properly organised community programmes is the best way of getting it

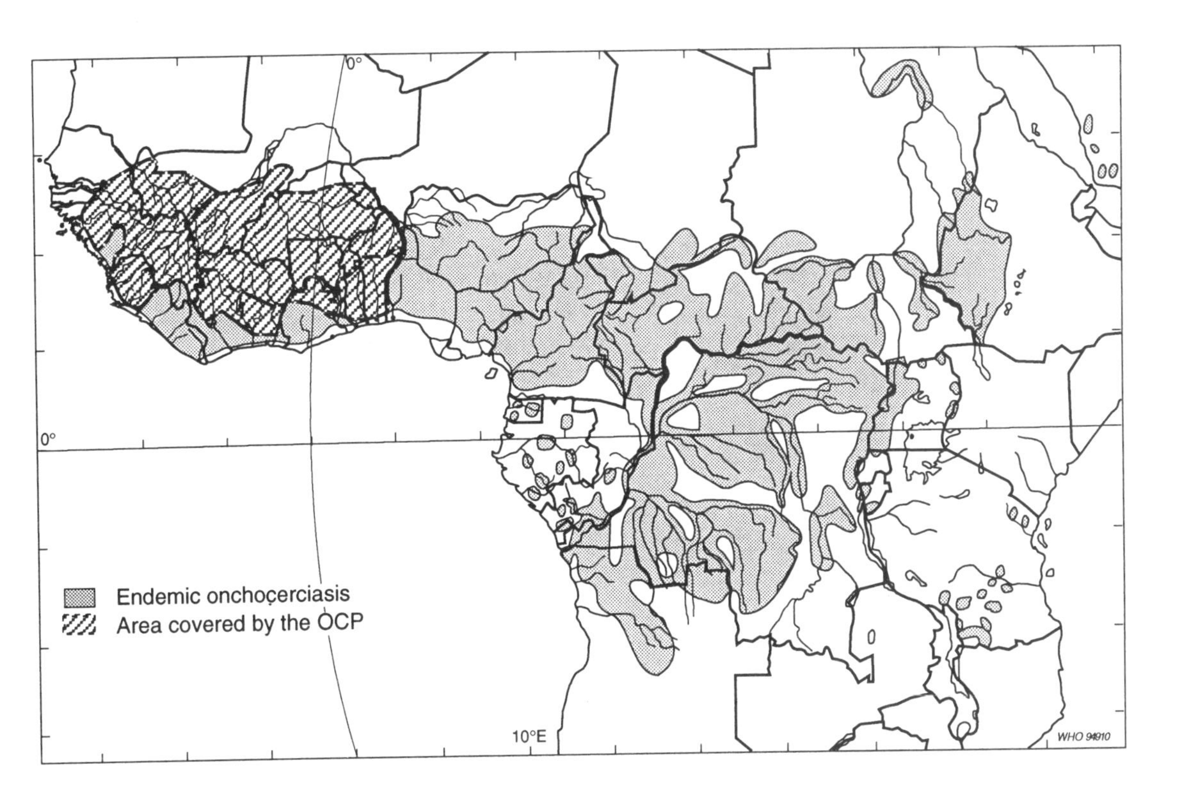

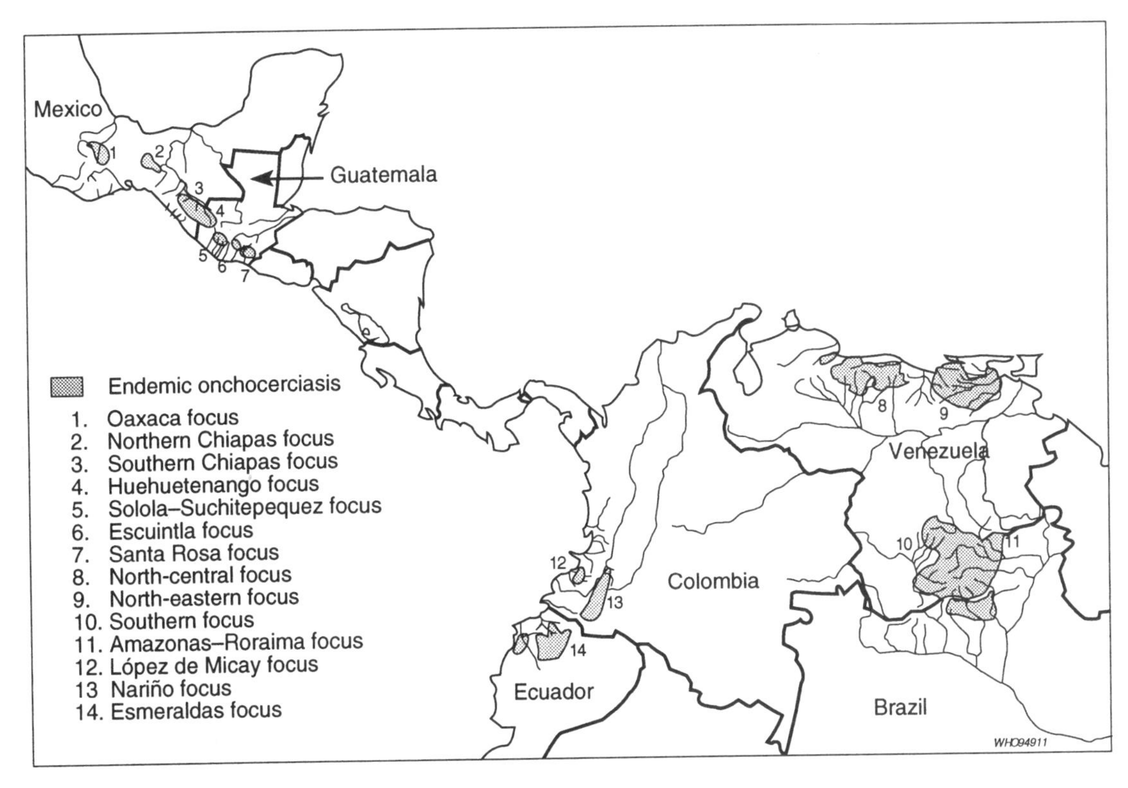

Figure 32.23 The distribution of onchocerciasis. (Source: WHO Technical Report Series No. 852, 1995 (Report of a WHO Expert Committee on Onchocerciasis Control))

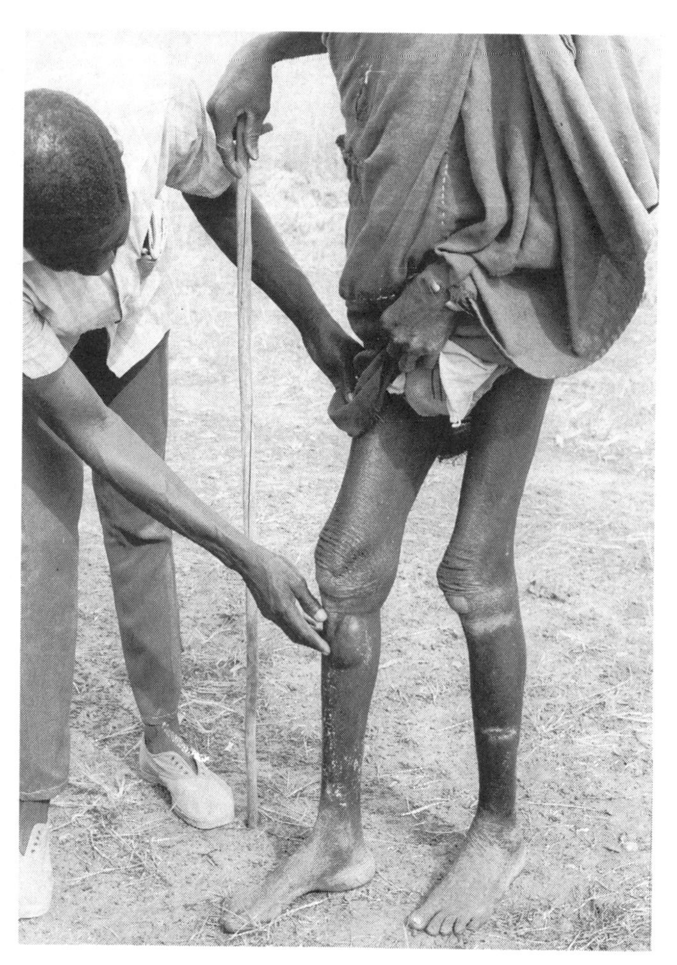

Figure 32.24 Nodules of onchocerciasis. If you remove and cut a nodule you can see the adult worms lying inside.

to all of the population. It is not given during pregnancy.

Otherwise, treatment is not necessary in patients who do not have symptoms or signs other than lumps.

Treat if there are eye lesions, or severe dermatitis, or many nodules.

Treatment, which may at times be done by a Medical Officer, may include:

1. surgical removal of the nodules which contain adult worms especially those that are on the head near the eyes and whose microfilaria may damage the eyes;

   or
2. treatment with diethylcarbamazine and an antihistamine but with careful small doses of diethylcarbamazine first.

The only present treatment which will kill the adult worm is suramin. However, it is an extremely toxic drug but is not given now that ivermectin is available.

If there are eye lesions, see the appropriate parts in Chapter 31.

Control and *prevention* is by the following:

1. Kill the microfilaria in the bodies of all the people in affected areas with ivermectin so that they cannot infect *Simulium* flies (now the major method of control).
2. Stop the means of transmission by stopping the breeding of flies (previously the major method of control). Flies can be stopped from breeding by spraying things into the river systems to kill their larvae. This often has to be done from aeroplanes. Previously insecticides such as temephos, carbamates and pyrethroids were used; but now a specific microbial larvacide *Bacillus thuringiensis* H14 has been found to be the cheapest and most effective. Protective clothing and repellents can be used to stop the flies biting people.
3. Raising the resistance of potential new hosts by immunisation is not at this time possible.
4. Prophylactic treatment of the whole population is being done with ivermectin, although the real reason it is being given is to kill the microfilaria so that the flies cannot be infected.

Loiasis

Loiasis is an infestation of the subcutaneous tissue with a filarial worm *Loa loa*. It occurs in Africa.

The adult worms are up to 7 cm long. They can cause areas of oedema, and often pain, in the skin ('Calabar swellings'). The swellings are often many centimetres in diameter and may last for a number of days. Sometimes the adult worms are seen wriggling under the skin or crossing the conjunctiva of the eye.

The adult produces microfilaria which circulate in the blood. These infect *Chrysops* ('mango' or 'softly-softly' flies) which then give the infection back to man.

Treat people who have repeated swellings as for onchocerciasis (see above).

Prevention, by fly control and stopping the *Chrysops* fly biting people, is difficult. Mass treatment of the population with diethylcarbamazine is usually not warranted especially as the patient may also have onchocerciasis and may develop side effects to large doses of diethylcarbarnazine.

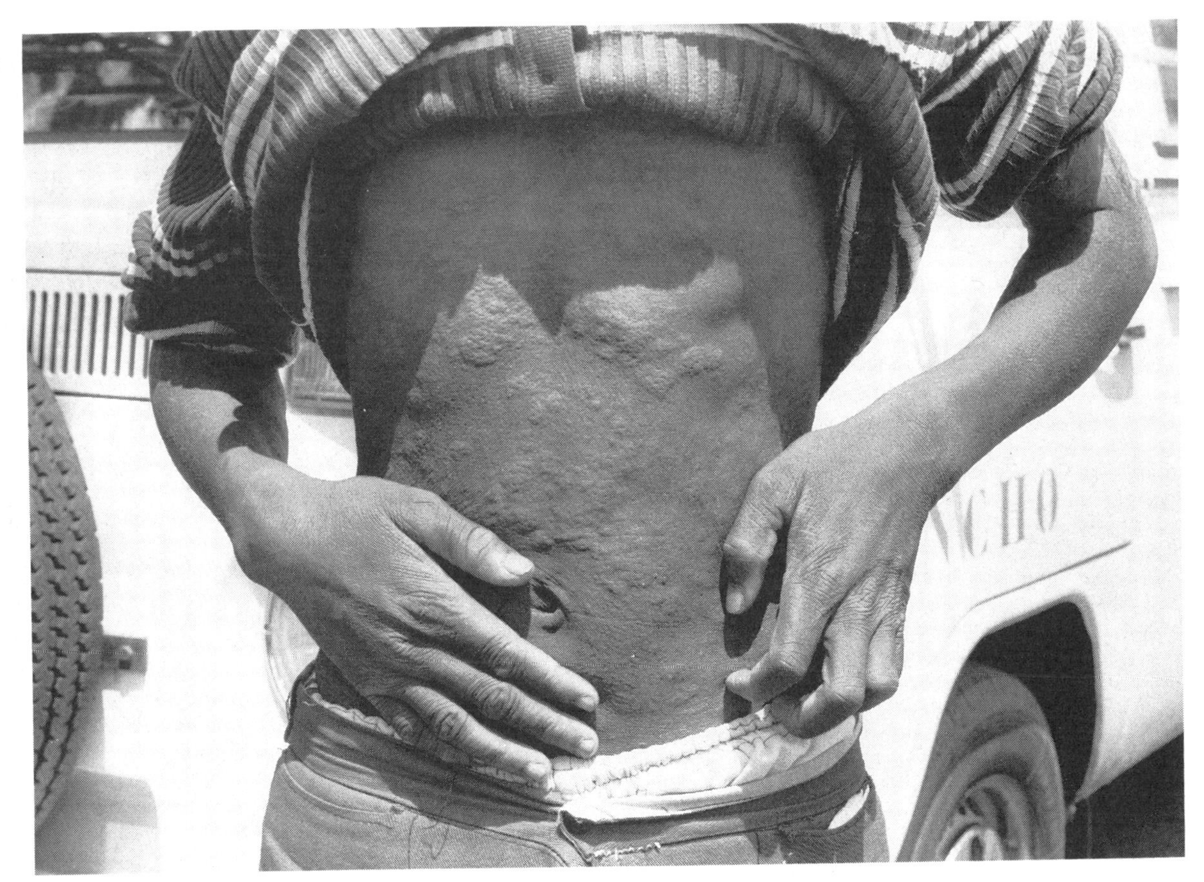

Figure 32.25 Skin changes and itching caused by onchocerciasis.

Guinea worm

Guinea worm infestation occurs in parts of Africa, the Middle East, India and South America.

The Guinea worm is a long (e.g. 1 metre) worm which lives under the skin of people and dogs and cats. Adult worms cause irritation of the skin in one area, usually a leg. A painful blister forms. The blister bursts and a very itchy ulcer forms, see Figure 32.27. The itch is helped by putting the leg in water. When the patient puts the leg in water, the end of the worm comes out through the ulcer and passes its larvae into the water. The worm larvae go into water fleas, and develop into larvae which are then infective for people. If people drink water with these infective larvae in it, the larvae develop into new worms under their skin; and the cycle starts again.

Symptoms and *signs* include:

1. There are allergic reactions, fever or vomiting as the worm starts to go through the skin.
2. A painful blister forms where the worm goes through the skin. This is usually on the foot or leg or part of the body that is cool and often wet. The blister bursts and an itchy ulcer forms. You can see the end of the worm passing white larvae when the ulcer is in water.
3. After 3–4 weeks the worm dies or leaves the body.
4. If the worm goes into another part of the body, or if it dies, or if other infections go into the ulcer, the patient may develop
   (a) abscess,
   (b) arthritis, or
   (c) tetanus.

Treatment includes:

1. Treat any bacterial infection with antibiotics (see Chapter 11 pages 46–52).
2. Give metronidazole 400 mg three times a day. This helps symptoms but does not kill the worm or stop it producing larvae. However metronidazole

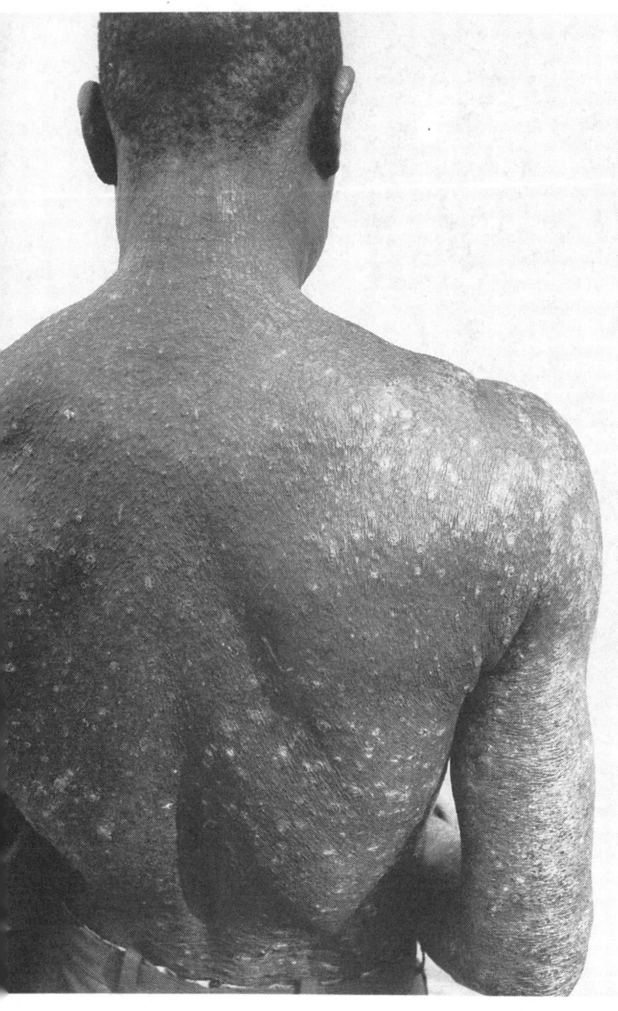

Figure 32.26 Characteristic pale patches on the skin caused by scratching. Early in the disease the itchy skin may look normal.

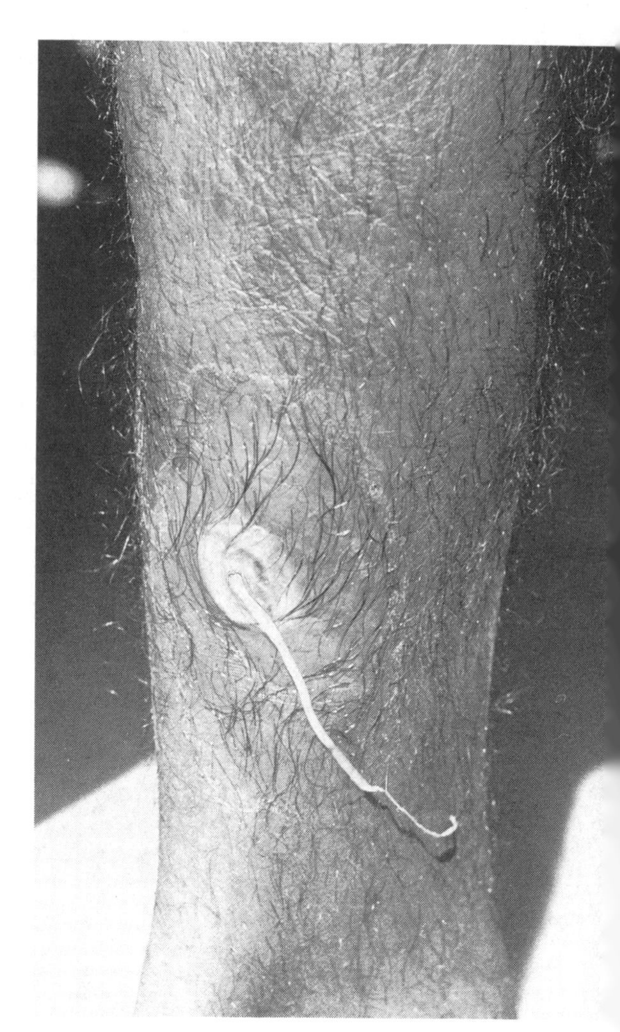

Figure 32.27 A Guinea worm emerging from an ulcer in the patient's leg.

weakens the worm's attachment to the patient's tissues so that it is easier to pull out. Mebendazole can also be used.

3. Prevent tetanus (see Chapter 25 page 330).
4. Put the affected part into cold clean water for half an hour daily for a few days, so that the worm will pass all its larvae. Then tie the end of the worm to a sterile stick with sterile cotton. Slowly wind the worm out of the ulcer round the stick until it becomes tight. Do only a little each day, and take care not to break the worm. Cover with antiseptic and a sterile dressing.
5. Check to see if tests have shown if albendazole or ivermectin would help in your area or not.

Control and *prevention* is by supplying safe drinking water; or if this is not possible, by boiling drinking water; or if this not possible, filtering all drinking water through two layers of fine clothing material (such as is used for making shirts), to remove the infected water fleas.

Skin rashes due to worms – including cutaneous larva migrans

Human hookworm and other worms can cause a mild itch or rash when they enter through the skin; but are then carried from the skin to other parts of the body where they complete their life cycle and the skin symptoms stop.

Hookworm of other animals, e.g. the dog hookworm (*Ancylostoma braziliense*) after entering the skin of a person cannot get carried away to complete its life cycle. The worm (larva) then travels (migrates) through the skin (cuta), leaving a slow moving inflamed irritated path or line across the skin of the legs or buttocks (where it entered). It can be killed by freezing it by spraying the head of the track with ethyl chloride for a few seconds; or by giving thiabendazole 40 mg daily for 2 days, though albendazole may be better.

Warts (verrucae)

Warts are caused by a virus infection of the skin.

The virus makes the cells which make the surface layer of the skin grow too much. They make too much skin in that place and cause a lump. The surface is often rough, or even like cauliflower (see Figure 32.28). If warts develop under the feet, they are pressed flat and make a hole in other tissues of the foot. This can be painful. In other areas they do not usually cause symptoms.

Most warts eventually go away without treatment. If you cover warts with sticking plaster they often go away more quickly. If you decide that the warts need treatment, apply salicylic acid (e.g. 12% in collodion) to the wart once a day until the wart falls off. It is important that you do not put this treatment on nearby normal skin because it will cause severe damage.

Molluscum contagiosum

Molluscum contagiosum is an infectious disease caused by a virus (Figure 32.29).

It is passed from a patient to another person by close contact or sexual intercourse. It is common in children. It is now common in patients with HIV infection.

The lesions may occur anywhere on the body. There are almost always many of them. They may vary in size from 2 mm up to 2 cm although large ones are uncommon. They are small white tumours of the skin tissue, but the centre is sunk in and is darker. If you press the larger lesions, a white discharge comes out of the centre.

Treatment is not usually necessary as the lesions go away in time. If the lesions are covered with sticking plaster and this is left on and not taken off for a couple of weeks, the lesions are often gone when the

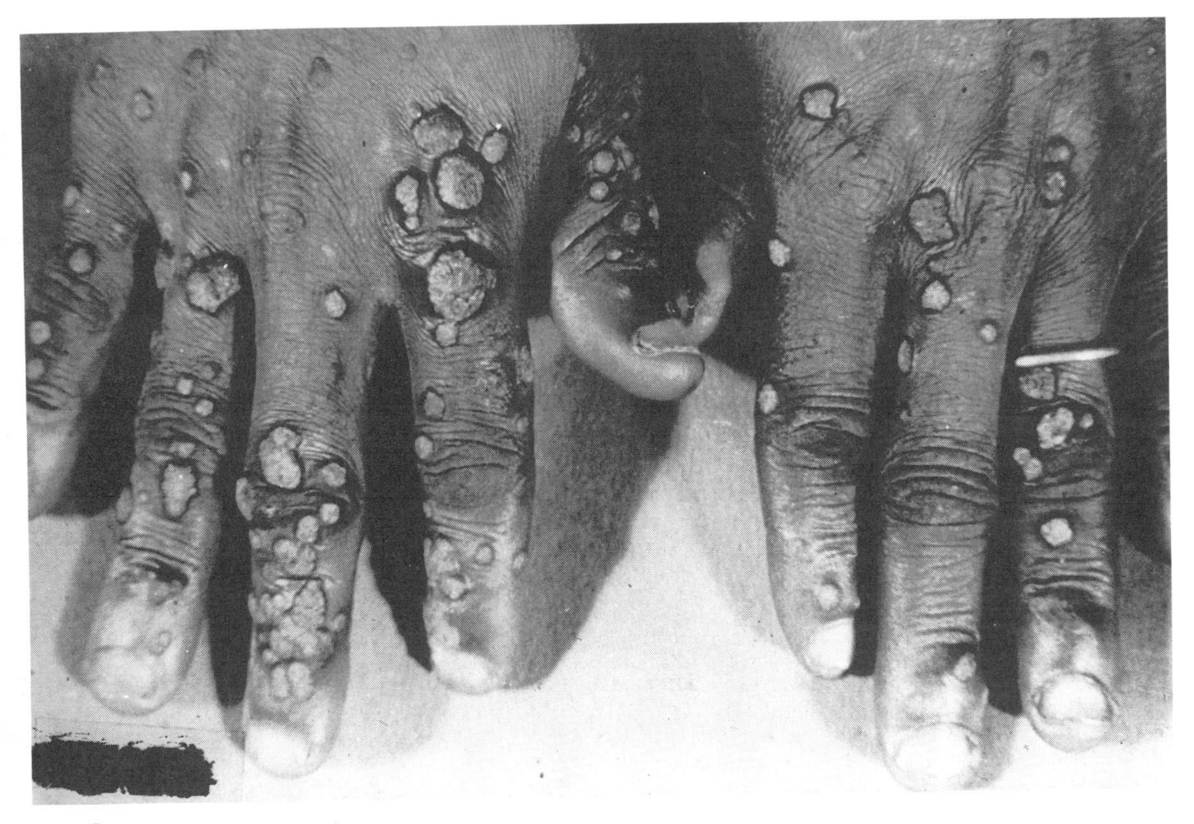

Figure 32.28 Warts on the hand.

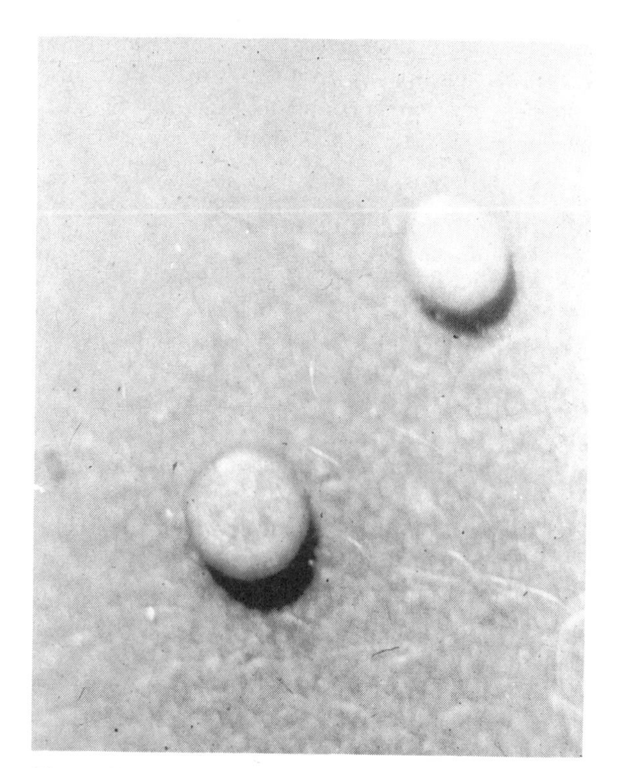

Figure 32.29 Molluscum contagiosum. (The dark centre is often more obvious than in the photograph.)

plaster is taken off. If treatment is necessary make a small incision in the centre of the nodule. Then squeeze out the white contents. Then put on tincture of iodine 2.5% solution. Use gloves and mask and goggles if the patient may have HIV infection.

Prevention is by avoiding contact with infected persons.

Pellagra

Pellagra is a condition caused if there is not enough group B vitamin in the food. It is only common in places where maize (corn) is the main food, and little else is eaten (e.g. some parts of Africa) or in times of famine or war.

Pellagra causes three conditions:

1. dermatitis – the most common condition;
2. diarrhoea – often with a sore tongue and other gastrointestinal symptoms; and
3. dementia – more often only anxiety and depression; though dementia and even coma can occur.

The dermatitis of pellagra occurs in areas exposed to sunlight – usually the face and arms. At first there is redness, swelling and discomfort (like sunburn). In acute cases the skin cracks, crusts and ulcerates, and may become infected. In chronic cases the skin becomes dark, thick, dry, rough and scaling. By this stage dermatitis of the vulva, perineum and perianal area is usually also present. (See Figure 32.30.)

In *treatment*, give vitamin B compound tablets (containing nicotinamide) three or four times a day until the patient improves; but more importantly, improve the diet by including as many animal products and legumes (peas etc.) as the patient can afford.

Eczema or eczematous dermatitis

The patient usually complains of an itch or rash. Examination shows an acute or chronic eczematous reaction (see page 426).

You must then find the *cause* of the eczematous reaction. *Always* think of these four things:

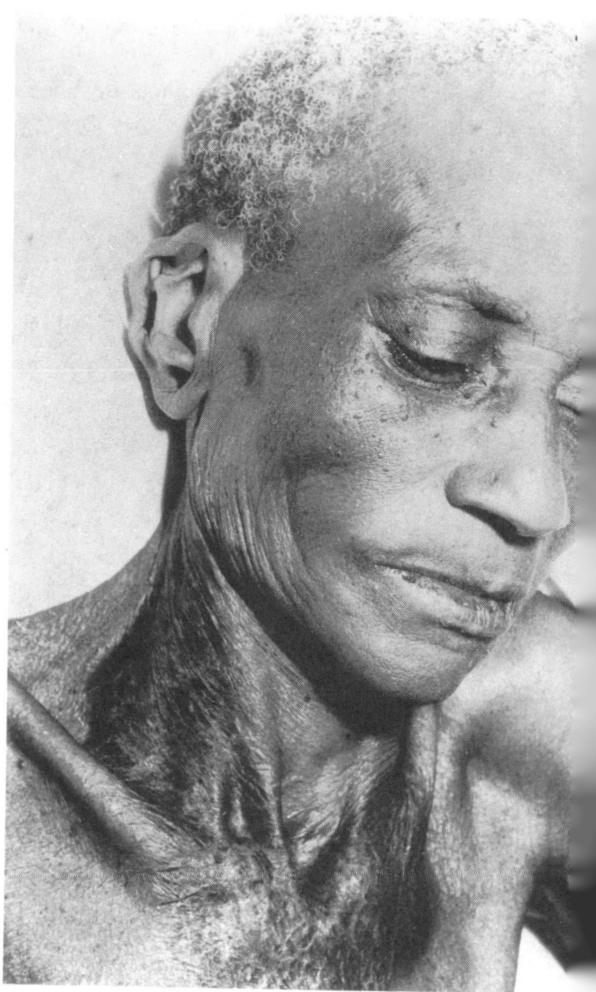

Figure 32.30 A severe case of acute pellagra.

1. contact, especially with chemicals, drugs, cosmetics, metal of jewellery and clothing,
2. infections or infestations, specially with scabies and lice,
3. drugs, and
4. scratching.

There are also two special types of dermatitis for which the cause is not known:

1. *Atopic dermatitis* occurs in allergic patients. Usually it affects areas behind the knees and in front of the elbows but in adults can be on the face and trunk (like infants).
2. *Seborrhoeic dermatitis* affects the scalp, eyebrows and eyelids, the sides of the nose and the front of the chest. There are usually thick greasy scales on the affected area.
   Note that seborrhoeic dermatitis can get worse with HIV infection.

Treatment – see pages 426–9 and find and stop or treat the cause above. If this is not successful, and hydrocortisone 1% cream is available, this could be added to the treatment. If this is not available or successful, *refer* the patient to your Medical Officer non-urgently.

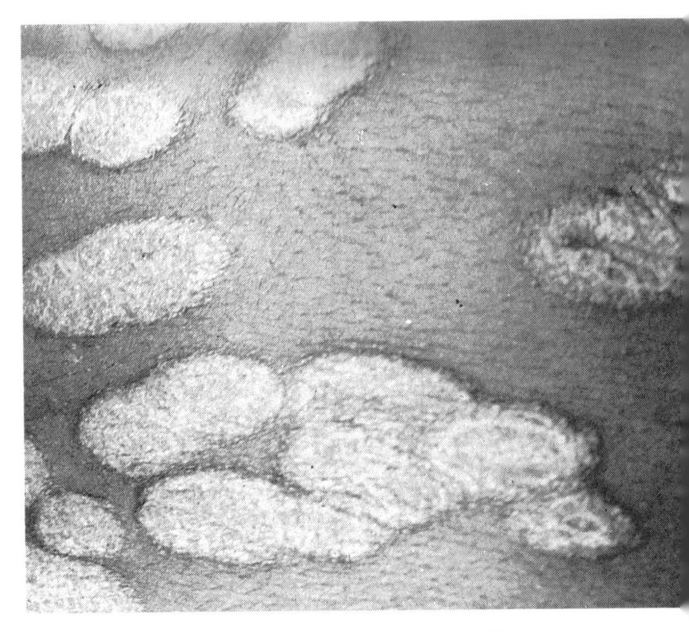

Figure 32.31 Typical skin lesions of psoriasis. Note the definite edge. These patches are covered by scales.

Psoriasis

In psoriasis, patches of redness and inflammation of the skin covered by silvery scales appears. The lesions do not itch or cause pain. The edges of the patches, where they join the normal skin, are very definite (see Figure 32.31). The finger nails are often pitted.

Treatment – try 10% strong coal tar solution or 4% coal tar paste, preferably with 1–2% salicylic acid to be put on to the lesions themselves once or twice daily. If this is not effective, *refer* to your Medical Officer.

Acne vulgaris

In acne, blackheads and pimples form in the skin. Some may become infected and cause boils. Scars and keloids may occur. (See Figures 32.32 and 32.33.)

Treatment includes regular washing with soap and water and, if not pregnant, oral doxycycline 100 mg daily or tetracycline 250 mg 4 times a day for several months. Special treatment, which is expensive and the patient may buy, is with lotions of benzyl peroxide and retinic acid. There is a very special very expensive (and dangerous if pregnant) oral drug,

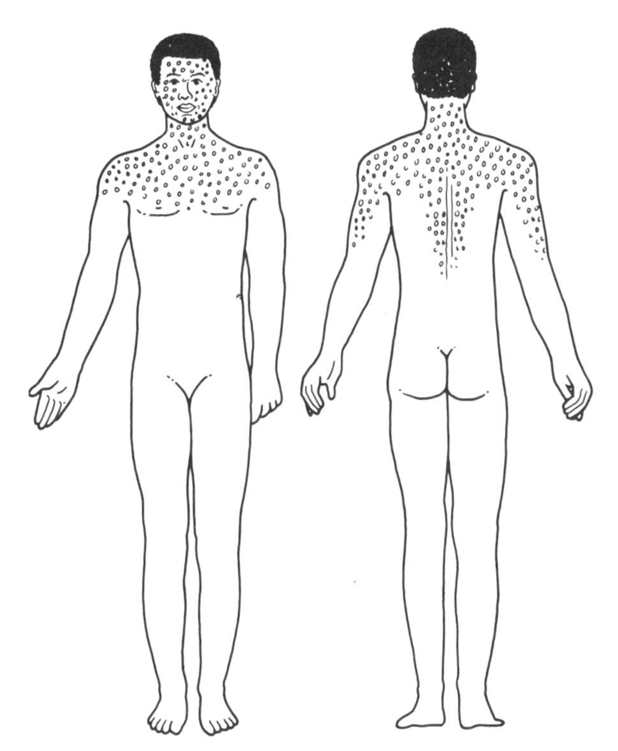

Figure 32.32 Diagram to show the parts of the body where lesions of acne vulgaris most commonly occur.

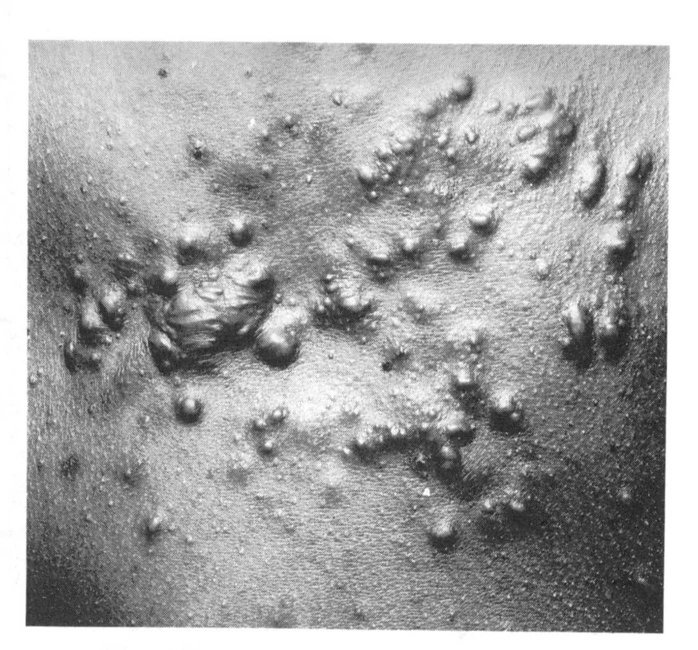

Figure 32.33 Photograph showing a close up view of skin affected by acne. You can usually see 'blackheads' on the patient more easily than in this photograph.

isotretinoin, which could be ordered by the Medical Officer if the patient were willing to buy it, if the above were not effective.

Vitiligo or leucoderma

In vitiligo patches of normal skin lose their pigment and become white (see Figure 32.34). The skin is otherwise perfectly normal. There is no loss of sensation over the patches.

Do not mistake leprosy, late yaws, late onchocerciasis, etc. for vitiligo.

No treatment for vitiligo is necessary or possible at the health centre, except to protect the skin from sunburn. Vitiligo is not dangerous and is not infectious.

At the time of writing even the latest treatment, which is very expensive, helps (and does not cure) at the most only 20% of patients. It is important to encourage patients to accept the problem and not waste a lot of money on treatment that is of little use.

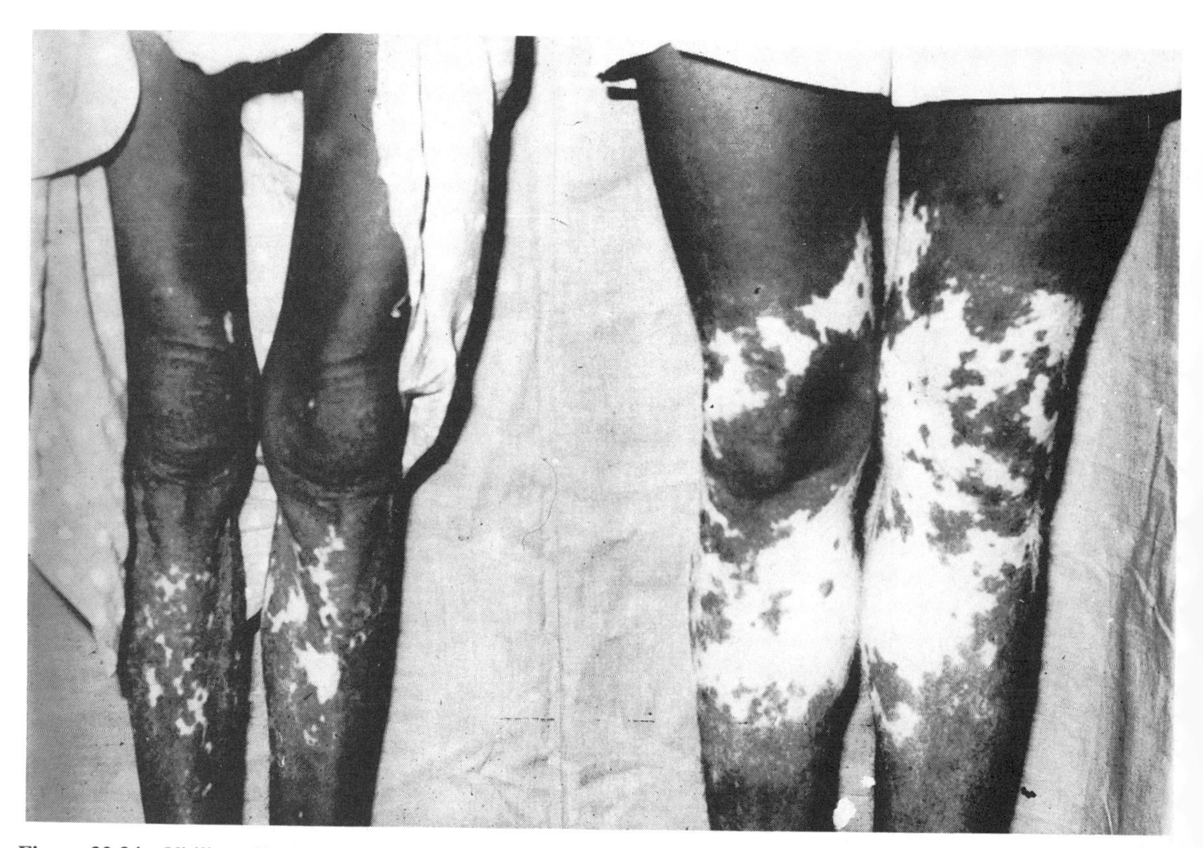

Figure 32.34 Vitiligo affecting the skin of the legs. The skin is normal except that it is milky white.

Albinism

Albinism is a hereditary condition in which there is not enough pigment formation in the body (Figure 32.35).

The irises of the eyes are pink or red, and the hair and the skin are white. The skin does not become darker in the sun.

The main complication is skin cancer caused by the sun continually burning the skin, which is not protected by pigment.

This is no cure for this condition.

Treatment includes wearing clothes to keep the sun off the skin – hat, long sleeved shirt and long trousers or dress, etc. all the time during the day. The person should keep away from the sun as much as possible. He should put a sunscreen on (e.g. 5% para aminobenzoic acid in ethanol or 'UV Cream') twice daily or more often, before going in the sun.

If the patient develops any sores that do not heal, *refer* or *transfer* him non-urgently for biopsy and probable excision of lesion, in case it is a skin cancer.

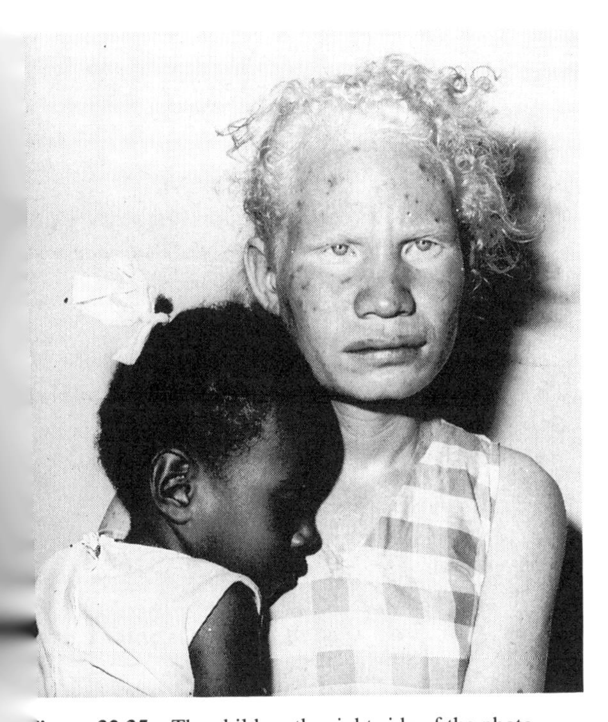

Figure 32.35 The child on the right side of the photograph is an albino. Note the sun-damaged white skin. She looks older than her age because the sun damage to her skin is the same as for a much older person with normal skin.

Common skin symptoms and signs

Itch (with or without rash)

Do a full history and examination (see Chapter 6 page 17)

Test the urine for protein, sugar and bile.

Note especially:

1. where the itch is, and
2. the details of any skin lesions (rash) present. *Diagnosis* depends on where the itch and rash is. *Treat* as in this book (see Index) or see a specialist medical reference book.

Rash between fingers or on wrists or on elbows or on genitalia; but not on face, then

- scabies – see page 440.

Rash in hair or around waist or in eyelashes or in pubic area, then

- lice – see page 441.

Rash only on uncovered areas (arms, legs, face), then

- insect bites, or
- contact with irritants (contact dermatitis), or
- sunshine and a drug taken or put on skin (e.g. tetracycline) (photosensitive dermatitis).
- HIV infection – itch usually in other places also and small lumps usually develop which become dark.

Itch around anus, then

- tinea – see page 429, or
- enterobius (threadworm) – see Chapter 23 page 279, or *Strongyloides* – see page 280, or
- haemorrhoids or anal fissure, or
- diabetes mellitus (glucose in urine) – see Chapter 30 page 406.

Itch of vulva, then

- all conditions as for anus, or
- *Candida* (thrush) or *Trichomonas* infection, or
- after menopause – needing hormone treatment.

Itch all over, then

- onchocerciasis if there are skin nodules over bony areas and especially if there is trouble with the eyes – see page 442, or
- HIV infection – see Chapter 19 page 186, or
- drugs and other causes of allergy – see Chapter 10 page 39, or
- jaundice – see Chapter 24 page 313, or
- chronic kidney failure – see Chapter 26 page 359.

Itch where there is a rash of round patches which are worse at the edges, anywhere on the body, then

- tinea – see page 429.

Itch where there is a rash on face or behind knees and in front of elbows and is either

1. *lesions which are thick and very dry or*
2. *small blisters which burst leaving moist red areas*, then
   - eczematous dermatitis – see page 448.

Rash (for rash and itch – see also itch)

Do a full history and examination (see Chapter 6 page 17).

Note:

1. where the lesions are, and
2. the type of the lesions they are.

Test the urine for protein, bile and sugar. *Diagnosis* depends on the features below. *Treat* as in this book (see Index) or see a specialist reference book.

Acute start; fever; general rash (face, trunk and limbs) then

- chickenpox – see Chapter 16 page 117, or
- measles – see Chapter 16 page 116, or
- other viral diseases – see Chapter 16 page 118

Vesicules, pustules, yellow crusts, then

- impetigo – see page 432.

Dry skin patches:

1. *no loss of sensation; itching, healing in centre*, then
   - tinea – see page 429.
2. loss of sensation and thick nerves, then
3. • leprosy – see Chapter 15 page 95–103.

Nodules

1. *severe itchy dermatitis and eye trouble*, then
   - onchocerciasis – see page 442.
2. *other signs of leprosy*, then
   - leprosy – see Chapter 15 page 95–103.
3. drugs given recently or other causes of allergy, then
   - allergic reaction – see Chapter 10 page 39.
4. other signs of leprosy and patient is sick or has tender nerves or iritis, then
5. • leprosy reaction – see Chapter 15 page 103

Eczematous reaction (small blisters which burst leaving moist red areas with itch or thick dry areas). Then

- eczematous dermatitis – see page 448.

Skin ulcer

Do a full history and examination (see Chapter 6 page 19).

Test the urine for protein, sugar and bile.

Note especially where the ulcer is – there are three common places:

1. genitalia,
2. breast, and
3. leg.

But ulcers can occur anywhere.

Diagnosis depends on the features of the ulcer (see below).

Ulcer on genitalia

Then most likely syphilis or other STD – see Chapter 19 pages 156 and 165.

Ulcer on breast

Acute start in young woman, then

- most likely breast abscess see Chapter 36 pages 488–9 and a surgery book. Transfer if needed.

Chronic start in old woman, then

- most likely cancer. See a surgery or gynaecology book. Refer to Medical Officer.

Ulcer on leg or foot but also anywhere

Ulcer started acutely and spread very quickly and was itchy and painful and smelly. Ulcer becomes chronic, if untreated, then

- tropical ulcer – see page 435.

Ulcer started after injury or infection.
Ulcer is like an ulcer anywhere but is slow to heal then

- bacterial infection (treat as for tropical ulcer).

Ulcer started as nodule which ulcerated.
Ulcer has undermined edges.
Ulcer spread quickly and surrounding ulcers may have developed.
AFB in smear from edge of ulcer or positive biopsy then

- *Mycobacterium ulcerans* ulcer – see Chapter 3 page 438.

Painful ulcer or ulcers on feet.
Papillomas or ulcers in other areas also.
In area where yaws occurs.

Serological tests for syphilis positive.

- yaws – see Chapter 32 page 435.

Ulcer started as a vesicle which ruptured and quickly became 2–3 cm across.
Edges are inverted and slightly undermined.
The ulcer is deep and covered with gray exudate or a dark crust. Surrounding skin is erythematous or blue.
May be paralysis of limb or food swallowed comes back through nose, then

- diphtheritic ulcer (see also Chapter 20 page 216).

Treat with penicillin and dressings as for tropical ulcer (see Chapter 32 page 435).

If paralysis transfer urgently for anti-toxin.

Ulcer started as a blister with general allergic reaction, fever and often vomiting. Blister burst and itchy ulcer developed, relieved by cold water.

Outline of worm under skin or end of worm seen in ulcer, then

- guinea worm – page 445.

Ulcer after chronic anaemia, often jaundice, no bile in urine, infarction crises and especially attacks of bone pain, then

- sickle-cell anaemia ulcer (Treat as for tropical ulcer; but eusol and antibiotics are not necessary if there is no infection.)

Ulcer most often under foot.
Loss of sensation under foot.
Enlarged nerves or patches with loss of sensation, then

- leprosy – see Chapter 15 pages 111–13.

Ulcer most often under foot.
Loss of sensation under foot.
No enlarged nerves or patches with loss of sensation.
Sugar in urine, then

- diabetes mellitus – Chapter 30 page 406.

Ulcer under foot.
Loss of sensation under foot.
Painless.
Not due to leprosy or diabetes.
Serological test for syphilis positive.

- syphilis (see Chapter 19 page 171).

Ulcer anywhere (see leg or foot also)
Ulcer anywhere and keeps on getting larger despite treatment

- possibly cancer – biopsy or transfer to Medical Officer.

Punched out looking ulcer
No pain
No inflammation
Not healed despite treatment
Serological test for syphilis positive

- gumma (from syphilis or yaws) (see Chapter 19 page 171 and page 435).

Ulcer anywhere

Ulcer anywhere, you can see pus and bone, then

- chronic osteomyelitis – see Chapter 28 page 385.

Ulcer anywhere, in an area where dermal leishmaniasis occurs, then

- dermal leishmaniasis (oriental sore) – see Chapter 18 page 139.

33

Bites and Stings

Snakebite

When a snake bites a person, in only about half of the cases does the snake inject enough venom (its poison) to cause any significant harm. However, sometimes enough venom is injected to cause death, even when the place where the snake bit cannot be seen. If a patient claims to have been bitten by a snake, always believe him and give proper first aid. Admit him to the health centre for 24 hours for observation to see if symptoms and signs of injection of the venom develop and if he needs treatment or not.

If a snake injects its venom when it bites the effects of the injected venom may include any or all of the following three groups of conditions.

1. Poisoning of certain body cells.
   - Pain where the bite occurred may appear almost immediately and not long after in nearby lymph glands and later in the abdomen also.
   - Allergic type reactions with swelling of parts of the body, shock, asthma, etc. may occur within minutes or an hour or two and occasionally can keep on coming back.
   - Inflammation where the bite occurred. Swelling may start in 2–3 hours and become very large by about 2–3 days and may eventually involve half or more of a limb; blisters may come on the surface, cellulitis may develop and eventually there may be large ulcers.
   - Shock or heart failure from fluid leaking out of damaged blood vessels or from the heart not pumping well because of damage to its muscle, may occur.
   - Haemolysis (breaking open of red blood cells) in the blood vessels with dark urine from haemoglobinuria and kidney damage may occur.
   - Damage to muscle cells, with aching, stiffness and weakness of the muscles occurs. Also muscle cells die and the myoglobin from inside the muscle cells makes the urine dark and can damage the kidneys.
   - Unconsciousness from damage to the nervous system may occur.
   - Acute inflammation of the conjunctivae and cornea may occur if the snake spat the venom into the eye.
2. Paralysis of the motor part of the nervous system so that muscles become weak or paralysed.
   - If the throat muscles become paralysed, the patient's airway may become blocked. The patient cannot breathe and dies.
   - If the swallowing muscles become paralysed, the patient aspirates (breathes in) saliva into his lungs and gets severe pneumonia or even 'drowns in his own saliva'.
   - If the breathing muscles become paralysed, the patient cannot breathe and suffocates.
3. The blood will not clot.
   - The patient can bleed to death.

If early signs of any of these conditions develop (called 'envenomation') then *give antivenom*. Antivenom is made from the blood of a large animal, e.g. horse or sheep. The animal is at first injected with very small and safe doses of venom, to which it will make antibodies. Then increasing and eventually very large doses of venom, from which it is protected by the previous antibodies, are given. These large doses make the animal produce even more and more antibodies. Blood is then taken from the animal and antibodies taken out of the blood and this is what we call 'antivenom'. Some antivenoms can now be made in the laboratory. Antivenom, then, contains antibodies which, if given to a patient with envenomation from a snake, will destroy the venom in the patient and stop more symptoms and signs of envenomation and death occurring.

If signs of envenomation do not occur, *do not give antivenom*. Often when snakes bite people, they do not inject enough venom to cause envenomation, and the patient does not need antivenom.

The type of antivenom you give depends on which type of snake bit the patient.

You must find out for your area:

1. What types of snake are present.
2. What the effects of their bites are.
3. What antivenoms are available.
4. When you should give these antivenoms.
5. What doses of these antivenoms you should give.

In Papua New Guinea, for instance, on the Papua side of the country, all of the venomous snakes that occur in PNG are found. Usually therefore, in Papua, CSL polyvalent antivenom is given. On the New Guinea side however, almost all serious bites are due to the death adder. Occasionally a significant bite may be from a small-eyed snake. In New Guinea therefore CSL death adder antivenom is used. If this antivenom is not effective, or if it is known that the snake was a large one (death adders do not grow to more than one metre), CSL polyvalent antivenom is given.

If kits are available to determine what kind of venom is on/in the patients then use these kits to tell you what kind of antivenom to use.

First aid

1. Stop any panic. Make sure no further bites occur.
2. Comfort the patient. The patient should not move. Tell the patient to lie down, keep still and rest. The patient must not walk. Take transport to the patient, or carry the patient to transport or the health centre.
3. Wash the wound; but only if there is water available immediately. Gently wipe away venom on the skin. If the venom was spat into the eye, wash out the eye with a lot of water.
4. Do not cut the wound or treat the wound in any other way.
5. If the patient comes to you with something tied round the limb just above the bite, do not remove it, as long as you can feel a pulse below it – but remove it if the pulse cannot be felt.
6. Bandage and splint the limb. Remove any other thing tied around the limb. Bandage from the end of the limb across the bite area and then, as far up the whole limb as possible (tightly as for a sprained ankle). Use a bandage or torn up clothing. Then put all the limb in a splint. If the limb cannot be bandaged, put it in a sling or splint. If you are in an area where snake bites cause swelling of the bite area, check the colour and temperature and pulse of the limb, below the bandage, every half hour. If the limb becomes cold or white or blue, or if the pulse becomes weak or is not present, or if there is a lot of swelling of the bitten area, and the bandages become too tight, then remove the bandages. Bandaging the limb stops the venom being absorbed until antivenom is available.

> The patient must not move the bitten limb or walk. Bandage the bite area and then all the limb firmly. Then put all the limb in a splint.

7. Do not give anything to eat or drink.
8. If there is any problem with unconsciousness, paralysis, difficulty in breathing, or vomiting, lay the patient on his side and give routine care for an unconscious patient, and if needed, artificial ventilation (see Chapters 28 page 333, and 37 page 504).

Management

> Management includes:
>
> Admit all patients who say they have been bitten.
>
> 1. Comfort the patient.
> 2. Make the patient rest.
> 3. Set up an IV drip.
> 4. Take blood. Test it for the time it takes to clot.
> 5. Examine to see if there are signs of envenomation. Repeat the examination every hour. Look for:
>   - paralysis,
>   - abnormal bleeding, and
>   - poisoning of other body cells.
> 6. Give antimalarial drug if you are in a malarious area.
> 7. Give antivenom carefully, but ONLY if signs of envenomation are present or develop. Look carefully for reactions. Treat any reactions quickly.
> 8. Treat any complications in the usual way.
> 9. Do not give aspirin, morphine or pethidine.
> 10. Give tetanus prophylaxis.
>
> Transfer to Medical Officer, if envenomation is probable or present and if there is no antivenom available; or you cannot give antivenom because a reaction occurred; or if another complication occurs.

Admit all patients who say they have been bitten by a snake (for observation and treatment if treatment becomes necessary).

You cannot always tell if envenomation is probable by looking at the bite area.

1. Comfort the patient. Tell him that you can save him.
2. Make the patient rest in bed.
3. Set up an intravenous drip of 0.9% sodium chloride (1 litre every 12 hours).
4. Put 5 ml of venous blood in a clean glass test tube or bottle and let it stand still. Note the time. Tilt the tube after 20 minutes to see if the blood has clotted or not (it should have). If the blood has not clotted, check it again in 4–6 hours.
5. Examine for any clinical signs of envenomation (see below). Repeat and write down these observations:
   - hourly for 12 hours if suspected snakebite,
   - hourly for 24 hours if a definite snakebite,
   - $\frac{1}{4}$-hourly if signs of envenomation are present or develop.

Write the headings on the observation chart so that your staff know what observations to take.

Observations include:

(a) Symptoms and signs of *paralysis*, which are:
- ptosis (drooping of eyelids),
- double vision or paralysis of movements of the eyes,
- speech 'thick', or like a drunken man,
- jaw hanging open, by more than one inch,
- cannot swallow properly, or saliva collects in the throat, and
- cannot take a deep breath and cough.

(b) Symptoms and signs of *abnormal bleeding*, which are:
- venous blood put in a test tube does not clot in 20 minutes (do this once only on admission; but repeat it later if you suspect abnormal bleeding),
- bleeding from the place of the snakebite,
- blood in the sputum, vomit, urine, stool, nose, etc., and
- bleeding into the skin.

(c) Symptoms and signs of *poisoning* of other body cells, which are:
- pulse fast or irregular,
- BP low,
- shock or heart failure,
- respiratory rate fast,
- level of consciousness below normal,
- swelling and tenderness of lymph glands,
- abdominal pain and vomiting,
- swelling and blisters at the place of the bite, and up to the knee or elbow (if the bite was on the foot or hand), or swelling of more than half of the limb, and
- urine is pink or brown or black from haemolysis or muscle damage (examine urine every time it is passed).

6. Give an antimalarial drug as indicated (usually chloroquine) if you are in a malarious area (see Chapter 13 page 61). If a rigor occurs later, then it will probably not be caused by malaria.
7. Give antivenom only if needed.
   Once a drip is running and antivenom is available, take the bandages off the limb.
   Give antivenom only if:
   (a) any signs of envenomation are already present when you first see the patient – give 2 full dose ampoules of the type indicated;
   (b) signs of envenomation develop while you are observing – give 1 full dose ampoule of the type indicated;
   (c) signs of envenomation are the same (including the blood taken on admission still not clotted) or are getting worse 4 hours after you gave antivenom – give 2 full dose ampoules of polyvalent antivenom.
   You must find out the *type of antivenom* indicated for your area.

Dose of antivenom

You must find this out for your area. The dose of antivenom in one CSL ampoule neutralises the amount of venom injected by one usual snakebite. The size of the dose in ampoules in your area may be different.

(a) One usual bite – give one full dose ampoule.
(b) If more than the usual amount of venom was injected and there was more than one bite – give more than one full dose ampoule (usually two; but more than two may be necessary).
(c) Children – dose as for adults.

How to give antivenom

(a) Make sure the antivenom is clear. If it is cloudy it is probably not active, and may be dangerous.

(b) Give antivenom by IV drip.
(c) Put the antivenom into a side drip in a drip that is running.
(d) First inject promethazine 25 mg (1 ml) IV. Keep the syringe at the bedside with another ampoule of promethazine.
(e) Then inject adrenaline tart. 1:1000 solution one half ($\frac{1}{2}$) of the usual dose given for asthma (i.e. 0.25 ml ($\frac{1}{4}$ ml) for an adult) subcutaneously. Draw up into the syringe 0.5 ml ($\frac{1}{2}$ ml) of adrenaline tart. 1:1000 solution and keep this syringe at the bedside with another ampoule of adrenaline.
(f) Draw up the antivenom, and inject it into another 500 ml bag of IV fluid, (e.g. normal saline or 5% dextrose) and run this, as a side drip, into the original IV drip and commence at 1 ml/minute for 5 minutes.
(g) Wait 5 minutes. Take PR and BP, look for skin rash or itch, look for swelling of the face or neck and listen for cough and rhonchi.
(h) If there is no reaction after 5 minutes, inject the rest of the antivenom, slowly over 30 minutes (never in less than 10 minutes).
(i) Observe as in (g) every 15 minutes for 1 hour.
(j) Remove the bandage and splint from the bite area when you have given the antivenom.

If a reaction to the antivenom occurs:
(a) stop giving the antivenom,
(b) give the adrenaline tart. 1:1000 solution 0.5 ml ($\frac{1}{2}$ ml) IMI immediately, and
(c) give the promethazine 25 mg (1 ml) IVI and 25 mg (1 ml) IMI immediately.

If a severe reaction to the antivenom occurs and if the patient looks as if he may die:
(a) give adrenaline tart. 1:1000 solution 0.5 ml ($\frac{1}{2}$ ml) diluted to 5 ml IV slowly over 5 minutes, i.e. 1 ml/minute immediately,
(b) give promethazine 50 mg (2 ml) IV with another syringe immediately,
(c) give hydrocortisone 100–300 mg intravenously if it is available, and
(d) repeat the adrenaline after 5 minutes if necessary.
(e) See the instruction paper with the antivenom and a specialist reference book for further management.

8. Treat any complications in the usual way.
   If paralysis occurs after you have given a repeat double dose of antivenom, or if you cannot give antivenom because of a reaction,
   (a) nurse the patient on his side (head down if necessary),
   (b) suck out the airway every hour (or more often if necessary – noisy breathing or snoring means a blocked airway), and
   (c) give artificial ventilation if necessary.
   If bleeding occurs, give fresh, whole blood; *but first give* a repeat double dose of polyvalent antivenom. Arrange urgent (emergency) transfer to hospital while you do all this.
   If shock occurs, if it is soon after the bite, give an antihistamine and adrenaline as for anaphylactic shock, although if it is when the bitten area is very swollen, give fluids as for dehydration. If in any doubt, treat both ways. (See Chapter 27 pages 378–9.)
   If a lot of swelling or inflammation of the bitten area occurs, treat it as you would treat a burned area and give antibiotics.
   If vomiting occurs repeatedly, give chlorpromazine 25 mg IMI.
   If the eye shows corneal ulcers or iritis, treat in the usual way. (See Chapter 31 pages 418 and 420.)
9. Do not give aspirin (which may make bleeding worse) or morphine or pethidine (which could reduce breathing). If the patient is frightened, restless or in pain, give explanation and comfort and intranasal oxygen. If a drug is really necessary, give paraldehyde and/or paracetamol. If there is no paralysis after 24 hours and pain is severe, morphine or pethidine could then be used.
10. Give tetanus toxoid 0.5 ml ($\frac{1}{2}$ ml) SCI, and finish the course later if the patient is not immunised. If someone has cut the wound, and it may be infected (and the patient is not immunised), then give also tetanus immunoglobulin 250 units (1 ml) IMI.

Transfer to Medical Officer care

Urgently (emergency) if:

- there is a definite bite of a known poisonous snake; or
- there are symptoms or signs of envenomation (weakness or bleeding etc.);

and if also

- there is no antivenom available; *or*
- you cannot give antivenom because the patient is allergic to antivenom (more than just an itchy swelling of the skin which you can treat with adrenaline and promethazine); *or*

- the patient is not cured by a repeat dose of 2 ampoules of polyvalent antivenom.

Non-urgent transfer is necessary if other complications which you cannot manage at the health centre occur.

Prevention

Teach people to be careful in areas where snakes are common. Children must not collect or play with *any* snakes. Discourage young men from climbing trees after snakes. Encourage people to wear shoes and tap the ground when walking at night.

Seasnake bite

The effects of a bite by a seasnake are as for landsnakes; but cell poisoning of muscle is more common. Pain and stiffness of the muscles; then severe pain if the muscles are moved; and then paralysis can occur. The urine becomes red or brown or black from myoglobin (like haemoglobin but from inside a damaged muscle).

If there are real signs of envenomation (especially if there is red or brown or black urine or paralysis), give seasnake antivenom. If there is no seasnake antivenom available, give polyvalent antivenom and other treatment, as for landsnakes, (see page 454), and transfer to a Medical Officer urgently.

Stonefish and other fish stings

Stonefish sting causes:

1. Severe cell poisoning in the stung limb, with very severe pain; oedema; weakness; sometimes necrosis; and later, abscesses.
2. Sometimes, paralysis of all the muscles, including those used for breathing, can occur.

Treatment includes:

1. Put the affected limb into very hot water (45–50°C). The heat destroys the venom. This is very effective treatment.
2. If hot water is not available apply a firm bandage and splint (see page 455) immediately.
3. Infiltrate the sting area with lignocaine (lidocaine) 1% or 2% solution, 5–10 ml. This is also very important.
4. Put up an intravenous drip.
5. Give stonefish antivenom (with precautions as for snake antivenom – see page 456) if there is still severe pain or if general signs are present *after* the above treatment.
6. Treat any other complications in the usual way.
7. Remove any remaining barb or foreign body from the wound.
8. Give tetanus prophylaxis (see Chapter 25 page 331).
9. Treat any secondary bacterial infection with antibiotics.

Stings from jellyfish (and similar sea stings)

Box jellyfish cause the most severe types of stings:

1. very severe pain,
2. severe skin inflammation, like third degree burns,
3. sometimes paralysis of breathing, shock and stopping of the heart.

Other jellyfish and other stingers, e.g. 'blue bottles', cause less severe similar conditions or instead severe body pains after some minutes and sometimes high blood pressure, fast and irregular pulse, rapid breathing, severe anxiety and later sometimes heart failure.

Treatment includes:

1. Immediately get the patient out of the water.
   The rescuer must take care not to be stung (as the tentacles may trail 3 metres behind the jellyfish).
2. If the patient's breathing is not enough, or if it stops, give artificial ventilation (see Chapter 37 page 504).
   If shock develops, treat as for shock caused by acute allergic reaction (see Chapter 27 page 379).
   If the heart stops, give external cardiac massage (see Chapter 37 page 506).
3. Immediately 'disarm' the tentacles on the patient (i.e. stop them injecting more venom).
   Pour 2–10% acetic acid in water, e.g. household vinegar (any brand) over the affected parts and the tentacles. Pour more on as it runs off. Leave the area covered with vinegar for at least 30 seconds.
   In parts of the Atlantic a mixture of sodium bicarbonate (baking soda) and water in equal amounts is said to be effective.
   If no vinegar (i.e. 3–10% acetic acid) is available dry the tentacles by throwing dirt, etc. on them before removing them.

Do not put spirit or alcohol (of any sort) on to the affected area (as used to be recommended). *Do not put any water on to the affected area for 2 hours.*

4. Pull the tentacles off the affected area. This can be done safely with the fingers even if the tentacles have not been disarmed by acetic or by drying with dirt. Do this as soon and as quickly as possible. Do not rub the stung area.
5. Apply a compression dressing as for snakebite (see page 455) as quickly as possible once the tentacles have been either disarmed by vinegar or pulled off.
6. Give analgesics. Try lignocaine (lidocaine) or other local anaesthetic jelly or cream and cold packs. Usually repeated small doses of IV pethidine (10–20 mg) or morphine are also necessary, because of the severe pain. If a nitrous oxide–oxygen mixture (e.g. 'Entonox') (often used at childbirth) is available, give the patient this to breathe. A general anaesthetic with ketamine may be better for the pain than large doses of morphine (which may stop breathing).
7. Give antivenom, if available, if there are problems with breathing, shock or cardiac arrest or if there are still significant symptoms and signs after the above (see page 456).
8. Treat the skin as for burns.

Octopus stings

Stings can cause complete paralysis and stop breathing, but usually they cause no pain. Treat with artificial ventilation (see Chapter 37 page 504) until the patient starts to breathe again.

Coneshell stings

Coneshell stings can cause:

1. pain,
2. strange sensations in the body, and
3. paralysis which can stop breathing.

Treatment:

1. Wash the wound and put on a firm bandage and splint (see page 455).
2. Infiltrate the sting area with 1–2% lignocaine (lidocaine) to relieve the pain.
3. Give artificial ventilation (see Chapter 37 page 504), if the patient stops breathing, until he starts to breathe again.

Scorpion stings and centipede stings

The effects of scorpion stings can be different from place to place. The effects are usually much more severe in children than in adults.

1. Most stings cause severe pain, often with swelling, and sometimes bleeding, at the place of the sting.
2. Some stings cause many types of severe unusual symptoms and signs due to stimulation of the parasympathetic and then sympathetic nervous systems. There may be increased temperature, sweating, increased production of saliva, diarrhoea, vomiting, incontinence, penile erection and abnormalities of blood glucose and slow pulse, high blood pressure, heart failure, etc.
3. Some stings cause unusual signs in the nervous system – fitting, paralysis and death by stopping breathing.
4. Some stings cause heart failure and shock.

Treatment will depend on what type of scorpion is present in your area. For pain, local anaesthetic injections are often very helpful. Pethidine or morphine, however, may be needed. In shock, besides giving the usual treatment, if the pulse is slow, give atropine 0.6 mg repeated as necessary until the pulse is over 60 and if peripheral blood vessels are contracted and the skin is cold, try the effect of sublingual glyceryl trinitrate 0.6 mg repeated if necessary but not if the blood pressure is less than 100. If the patient fits, give paraldehyde or diazepam. If the patient stops breathing, give artificial ventilation.

If antivenom is available, then give this as soon as possible if there are serious signs of envenomation, as well as the above. See page 456 for method and precautions.

Spider bites

Only a few spiders cause severe or fatal bites. *Effects* may include:

1. There may be severe pain at the place of the bite with swelling and redness developing quickly. Later on an ulcer may form.
2. The pain may soon spread all over the body and cause muscle spasm (muscles contract and are then tight all the time) and pain. Shaking and fits can occur.
3. Many different types of general symptoms and signs can occur.
4. Shock may occur.

Treatment includes:

1. Wash or clean the bite.
2. Bandage and splint as for snake bite (see page 455).
3. Give analgesics as necessary for the pain (see Chapter 7 page 29).
4. Give diazepam for severe muscles pain and spasm or for fitting (see Chapter 25 page 336). Calcium gluconate 10 ml of a 10% solution given slowly over 10 minutes intravenously is said to be helpful for muscle spasm.
5. Give atropine 0.6 mg (1 ml) if the pulse is very slow.
6. Treat shock if it occurs (see Chapter 27 page 378).
7. Give spider antivenom if indicated and if available (see page 456).

Insect stings

Insect stings can cause

1. Severe pain at the bite area.
2. General symptoms and signs of cell poisoning but usually only if there are many stings.
3. Allergic reactions, which are usually much more common and dangerous than either of the above two. These reactions may cause death from swelling of the bitten area especially if it is the face, tongue or neck which could block the airway; asthma; shock; etc.

Treatment includes:

1. Give analgesics.
2. Comfort the patient.
3. Remove sting with the point of a needle, if it is from a bee, and take care not to squeeze the sting sac as this will force more venom into the tissues.
4. Wash the affected area.
5. If there is an allergic reaction, give antihistamine orally or IM or IV if necessary, and adrenaline SC or IM if necessary (see Chapter 10 page 39).

Tick paralysis

The bites of some ticks can cause paralysis, if the tick stays in the body for a few days.

Remove the tick. Give artificial ventilation (see Chapter 37 page 504) if necessary. Transfer the patient urgently to a hospital if artificial ventilation is necessary.

The patient will get better if you give artificial ventilation until the paralysis goes.

34

Poisoning

Acute poisoning is almost always caused by a poison that a person swallows and absorbs through the gastrointestinal tract. Sometimes acute poisoning is caused by a poison that a person breathes in and absorbs through the lungs; or caused by a poison that a person gets on the skin and absorbs through the skin; or caused by a poison that a person has injected.

The commonest chemicals that cause poisoning are drugs, petroleum products such as kerosene, weed killers and insecticides.

The poisoned person often takes the poison accidentally, e.g. children find and eat coloured tablets or a person drinks kerosene or weedkiller from a bottle which normally has a drink in it.

The poisoned person sometimes takes the poison to commit suicide (kill himself). People often take poisons not to really commit suicide, but to influence another person (to make him feel sorry or guilty, or to make him behave in a different way). This is called 'self-poisoning', (and *not* 'attempted suicide') and is a form of neurotic mental abnormality or acting out (see Chapter 35 page 475).

When a person says they have been poisoned you *must always* admit and treat the patient, even if you do not know it is true; or even if you think it is not true.

The treatment of poisoning is an emergency. *Treat the patient immediately.* If he has to wait for treatment to start, the patient is more likely to die.

You cannot treat acute poisoning by giving an antidote, because there are no antidotes for most poisons. (An antidote is a chemical that will work against a poison and stop the effects of the poison.)

But you can treat most patients who have been poisoned. You must always do two things when a patient is poisoned. If you do these two things quickly, most poisoned patients get better.

1. Stop the patient absorbing any more poison into his body.
   If the patient swallowed the poison, empty the patient's gastrointestinal tract by making him vomit and giving him diarrhoea (see exceptions later). If available, activated charcoal given after vomiting or gastric lavage has finished, may join or bind with poisons still in the gastrointestinal tract and stop any more of the poison being absorbed.
   If the patient absorbed the poison through his skin, remove all his clothes and wash him all over with soap and water. Wear gloves.
   If the patient breathed in the poison, immediately take the patient into fresh air; and give artificial ventilation and oxygen if necessary. Do not breathe in the poison yourself.
   If the poison was injected, put a firm bandage and a splint on the limb that was injected. The patient must not move the injected limb or walk around (see Chapter 33 page 455).
2. Keep the patient alive by treating any symptoms and signs that develop, until his body removes the poison already absorbed.
   If the patient stops breathing, give artificial ventilation.
   If the patient develops shock, treat shock, etc. *See page 378* for more details.
   You may need to transfer the patient to Medical Officer care for the treatment of some symptoms and signs.

If you do these two things:
1. stop the patient absorbing any more poison, and
2. keep the patient alive, by treating any symptoms and signs which develop,

then you can cure most poisoned patients.

There are two other things which you must do:

1. Give antidotes if there are any.
   The only antidote you probably have in a health centre is naloxone or nalorphine, which you give

for an overdose of morphine, pethidine or codeine. The Medical Officer has only a few other antidotes.

2. Stop the poisoning occurring again.
   If the patient poisoned himself then you must give social or psychiatric help.
   If the patient was poisoned accidentally, then you must give health education about the storage of drugs and poisons. The most common kind of poisoning is a patient who has swallowed a poison.

Poisons (and drug overdoses) swallowed

Admit for inpatient treatment all cases of suspected poisoning. Find out:

1. what the patient has swallowed, (tell a relative to bring a sample and the original container);
2. how much he swallowed; and
3. when he swallowed it.

Treatment of swallowed poisons

For *petroleum products* (e.g. kerosene) see page 463.
For *strong acids or alkalis* see page 464.
If the patient is unconscious see page 464.
For other cases treat as follows:

1. Immediately make the patient vomit (to remove the poison from the stomach), *but not if he is unconscious or has swallowed a petroleum product (e.g. kerosene) or a strong acid.* (Rub the back of the tongue and pharynx with several wooden tongue depressors held together.)
2. Make the patient drink 200 ml (1–2 cups) of milk or water, *but not if unconscious.*
   Then make the patient vomit again. *But not if the patient has swallowed a petroleum product (e.g. kerosene) or a strong acid.*
   Do this many times until he vomits only water or milk and no food or poison. (The milk or water also dilutes the poison and slows its absorption.)

> For chloroquine or quinine poisoning, the most important part of the treatment is to make the patient vomit ***immediately*** and then again many times (or wash the stomach out – see 3 below).

3. Wash out the stomach if patient will not vomit. Lay the patient on his side with his head lower than the rest of his body. Put a large diameter (1.5 cm or $\frac{3}{4}$ inch) tube into the stomach. Then siphon out (by putting the end of the tube lower than the end of the tube in the patient's stomach) or aspirate (suck out with a large syringe on the end of the tube), the stomach contents. Then wash out the stomach, by putting 200 ml (1 cup) of milk or water down the tube and then aspirating it again. Do this at least 20 times, until the aspirated fluid is clear and contains no food or drugs. (It may need over 100 times.)
4. Give activated charcoal (if available) 50 g immediately and then 25 g four hourly. Make the patient drink this after vomiting is finished, or put it down the tube if the stomach is washed out.
5. Give a laxative e.g. magnesium sulphate (Epsom salts) 30 g (30 ml of crystals in a measuring glass or 1 tablespoonful) in two cups of water. Make the patient drink this when the vomiting is finished, or put it down the tube after the stomach is washed out. (This causes diarrhoea and removes the poison from the intestines.) Repeat the dose in $\frac{1}{2}$ hour if there is no diarrhoea.
6. Give an antidote, if there is one (usually there is not).
7. Observe the patient every hour for level of consciousness, RR and depth of respiration, PR, BP, and any other complications which the poison may cause. Note any complications that are developing before they become severe (especially loss of consciousness, not breathing properly and shock).
8. Treat any complication in the usual way, e.g.
   - fitting – anticonvulsants (see Chapter 25 page 335)
   - unconsciousness – routine care of unconscious patient (see Chapter 25 page 335)
   - cyanosis – intranasal oxygen 2–4 litres/minute
   - not breathing – artificial ventilation after clearing the airway (see Chapter 37 page 504)
   - shock – elevate the legs and give IV plasma volume expander (see Chapter 27 page 378)
   - pain – use *small* doses of pethidine or morphine if there is a risk of depression of respiration (usually only give for swallowed acid)
9. Transfer the patient to Medical Officer care if complications which you cannot treat at the health centre may occur (see page 463).
10. Use any case of poisoning to give health education on the proper storage and use of drugs and poisons (see page 463).

11. Check the patient's mental state. Treat any psychiatric condition. Help to solve any problem (see Chapter 35 page 470).

Transfer

Transfer a patient who has swallowed poison or drug overdose (but only after previous treatment) if:

1. You think dose of the poison he has swallowed is more than:
   - aspirin – 300 mg/kg, (50 tablets in adult),
   - chloroquine, amodiaquine (Camoquin) and quinine – twice the normal treatment dose (*but* contact Medical Officer first) (see below),
   - corrosive acid (e.g. battery acid) – anything more than a little,
   - ferrous sulphate (iron) – 100 tablets (but small doses, e.g. 10 tablets are very poisonous to children),
   - methanol (methyl alcohol) – 10 ml, or methylated spirits – 200 ml,
   - paracetamol – 150 mg/kg (or 15 or more tablets in an adult), or
   - phenobarbitone – 20 mg/kg.
2. If poisoned with
   - phenolic weed killers (e.g. dinitro-ortho-cresol (DNOC), dinitrophenol (dinoseb)), after give chlorpromazine 100 mg IMI and cool the patient,
   - paraquat weed killer (e.g. Gramoxone, Gramixel, Priglone, Weedol),
   - arsenical poisons,
   - organophosphorous insect killers (e.g. parathion, TEPP, malathion), after give oxygen and atropine 2 mg IMI.
3. The patient has a dangerous level of consciousness, or respiration, or pulse or BP.
4. The patient's level of consciousness, respiration *or* BP gets worse every hour for 4 hours. Transfer the patient then before the levels of consciousness, respiration and BP etc. become dangerous.
5. Complications occur that you cannot treat properly in the health centre (especially unconsciousness that continues for more than 24 hours).
6. If you think the patient may try to commit suicide again and that you cannot stop him in the health centre.

> Always check the patient's mental state if he tried to commit suicide

Treat with chlorpromazine and transfer the patient if he has severe psychotic depression, or you have another good reason to think that he may try to commit suicide again.

If not, try to solve the patient's problems and treat in the usual way. Do *not* supply phenobarbitone as the patient may take it as another overdose.

Prevention of poisoning

Use any case of poisoning to teach people:

1. Always store all poisons and drugs away from children.
2. Never put poisons, especially kerosene, in drink bottles (soft drink or beer or wine bottles, etc.).
3. Always put a label on all bottles that contain drugs and poisons.
4. Always throw away (into the toilet) any old medicines, tablets or the contents of any bottle that has no label.

Chloroquine, amodiaquine (Camoquin) and quinine overdose

More than the proper treatment dose is dangerous. More than twice the proper treatment dose will probably cause death.

These drugs are absorbed very quickly and cause death usually within 1–6 hours.

The most important part of the treatment is to empty the stomach and intestines *as quickly as possible. Immediately* make the patient vomit many times or wash out the stomach. For other treatment see page 462.

If the dangerous dose of these drugs has already been absorbed, there is not much the Medical Officer can do, unless he has special equipment and drugs. Urgently contact the Medical Officer and ask if you should transfer the patient urgently (emergency).

Treatment if the patient has swallowed a petroleum product (e.g. kerosene)

1. Do *not* make the patient vomit.
2. Give 1–2 cups of milk or water to drink.
3. Do *not* wash out the stomach.
4. Give 30–60 g (30–60 ml) magnesium sulphate crystals (Epsom salts) in water or milk.
5. There is no antidote.
6. Make routine observations (see page 462).
7. Treat pneumonia when it occurs. Give oxygen if it is severe.

8. Transfer if severe pneumonia develops, especially if you do not have oxygen.
9. Use the case to give health education that kerosene should never be stored in drink bottles and should always be stored away from children.
10. Treat any mental disturbance in the usual way.

Treatment if the patient has swallowed strong acids or strong alkalis

1. Do *not* make the patient vomit.
2. Give 1–2 cups of milk or water to drink.
3. Do *not* wash the stomach out.
4. Do *not* give a laxative.
5. Do *not* try to give an antidote (e.g. alkali if acid swallowed).
6. Make routine observations (see page 462).
7. Treat any complication in the usual way.
8. Transfer all patients who have swallowed any strong acid or alkali to Medical Officer care (urgent). Meanwhile, the patient must not eat at all or drink large volumes of fluid.
9. Use the case to give health education that no poison should be stored in a drink bottle, and that all poison should be stored away from children.
10. Treat any mental disturbance in the usual way.

Treatment if the patient is unconscious

1. Do *not* make the patient vomit.
2. Do *not* give fluids to drink.
3. Do *not* wash out the stomach.
4. Do *not* give laxatives.
5. Give naloxone 0.5–1 mg or nalorphine 5–10 mg for pethidine, morphine or codeine overdose. Do not give other antidotes or stimulants.
6. Make routine observations (level of consciousness, size of pupils, RR and depth of respiration, PR, BP).
7. Treat complications in the usual way.

   (a) Give special nursing care for an unconscious patient (see Chapter 25 page 333).

   (b) Check that there is a good urine output (125 ml/hour). Give IV fluids if necessary.

   (c) Treat shock if it occurs (raise legs, give plasma volume expanders and see 'Shock', Chapter 27 page 378).

   (d) Give artificial ventilation and arrange urgent (emergency) transfer if the patient is not breathing enough, or stops breathing (see Chapter 37 page 504).
8. Transfer any patient whose level of consciousness or whose respiration or BP becomes dangerous. Also transfer any patient who is getting continually worse, before the levels become dangerous.
9. Use the case to give health education that no drugs and poisons should be stored in drink bottles and that all drugs and poisons should be stored away from children.
10. Treat any mental disturbance in the usual way.

Poisoning from seafoods

Fish or shellfish can cause poisoning, even though the food looks good and tastes normal. Symptoms and signs include:

1. gastroenteritis,
2. strange sensations in the body,
3. weakness which can develop into complete paralysis and death from paralysis of breathing, and
4. other symptoms and signs.

Treatment is as in the 10 principles for other types of poisoning above.

If weakness of the respiratory muscles develops, treat with artificial ventilation (Chapter 37 page 504) and *transfer* urgently to Medical Officer care.

35

Psychiatric Conditions

Mental disorders and mental diseases

A person in good mental health can think, feel and act in a way his own community expects and understands. He accepts himself, is comfortable with other people and is satisfied carrying out the normal duties of life.

> A mental disorder or disease is present when a person cannot think, feel and act in the way his own society expects or understands.

Remember that:

1. What may be abnormal in one society may be normal in another society.
2. A criminal can behave in a way society expects; but he chooses not to.

There are two groups of psychiatric conditions:

1. conditions with an organic cause, i.e. an alteration in the structure or function of part of the body which causes the psychiatric condition (see page 466); and
2. conditions without an organic cause, i.e. there is no diagnosable alteration in the structure or function of any part of the body (which has so far been found) that causes the psychiatric condition (see page 467).

There is also an important difference between:

1. psychotic conditions or diseases (psychoses) (see page 468); and
2. non-psychotic conditions or disorders (see page 469).

The above two classifications of mental disorder and disease were the basis of a previously fairly simple classification of all mental conditions, which is still used by many (see Table 35.1).

The new ICD-10 (International Classification of Diseases 10th edition) classifies these, however, as shown in Table 35.2 (greatly simplified). We do not have to learn this classification or know all the conditions in it but it will help us in understanding mental diseases and disorders.

Table 35.1 A simple classification of mental conditions

1. Organic	All psychotic (organic psychoses)	Acute Chronic
2. Non-organic	Psychotic (psychogenic psychoses)	Schizophrenia and delusion states (but also drug abuse in some individuals) Manic depressive psychoses (including postpartum depression)
	Non-pyschotic (neuroses)	Anxiety states Reactive depression Hysteria etc.
	Personality disorders	

Table 35.2 Classification of mental disorders according to the 10th edition of the *International Classification of Diseases* (ICD-10)

F0	**Organic**
	Acute, e.g. delirium
	Chronic, e.g. dementia
F1	**Substance misuse**
F2	**Schizophrenia and delusional disorders**
F3	**Mood (affective) disorders**
	Depression
	Mania
	Recurrent affective disorders
F4	**Neurotic, stress-related and somatoform disorders**
	Anxiety disorders:
	Generalised anxiety
	Phobic anxiety
	Panic disorder
	Obsessive compulsive disorder
	Reaction to severe stress:
	Acute stress disorder
	Post-traumatic stress disorder
	Adjustment disorder
	Dissociative (conversion) disorder
	Somatoform disorder
	Neurasthenia
F5	**Behavioural syndromes associated with physiological disturbance**
	Eating disorders
	Sleep disorders
	Sexual dysfunction
	Puerperal mental disorders
F6	**Personality disorders**
F7	**Mental retardation**
	and others

Adapted from: World Health Organization *ICD-10. International Classification of Diseases,* 10th edn. Geneva, WHO.

Mental disorders and diseases are very common. Up to 2% of the population may have psychotic disorders, up to 15% have less severe mental disorders and up to 25% of patients in outpatient clinics may be there because of mental problems. Increasing use of alcohol and drugs by the population increases these numbers.

Causes of psychiatric conditions

Organic causes of psychotic diseases[1]

1. *Any disease of the brain especially*
   - head injury
   - meningitis (all types)
   - cerebral malaria
   - HIV infection
   - viral encephalitis of other types
   - African trypanosomiasis
   - syphilis
   - encephalitis of other types
   - cerebral tumour of any type
   - cerebrovascular disease/stroke
   - malnutrition and in particular:
     - vitamin B_1 or thiamine deficiency (Wernicke's encephalopathy)
     - niacin deficiency (pellagra)
     - vitamin B_{12} and/or folic acid deficiency
   - epilepsy and the postepileptic state
   - damage to the brain at birth (mental subnormality)
   - wearing out of the brain in old age (senile dementia)
   - Alzheimer's disease
   - and others (see a specialist reference book)
2. *Abnormalities in the blood going to the brain*
   - alcohol, drugs and poisons – both intoxication with or withdrawal from
   - low oxygen from any cause, e.g. shock, heart failure, severe anaemia, etc.
   - dehydration from any cause
   - toxins from severe infections in the body especially malaria, septicaemia, pneumonia and typhoid, etc.
   - toxins from the body when organ failure – liver failure, kidney failure
   - blood glucose too high (diabetic ketoacidosis) or too low (diabetic hypoglycaemia from some illnesses or from insulin)

Organic psychoses caused by a disease of the brain or an abnormality of the blood going to the brain can be of two types:

---

1 *Note* that these two lists of causes of organic psychoses are almost the same as the two lists of causes of unconsciousness or of convulsions etc. (see Chapter 25 page 332). An organic psychosis is only another way the brain does not work properly when there is a disease of the brain or abnormality of the blood going to the brain.

1. an acute organic psychosis, or
2. a chronic organic psychosis.

1. *An acute organic psychosis*

   (a) Has started recently – hours or days and not over a month ago.

   (b) Patient on examination:
   - not fully conscious;
   - memory poor for recent events;
   - not orientated in time and place;
   - intelligence usually cannot be tested, i.e. confused or delirious.

   Has a lot of other abnormalities too, including features of a psychosis but the above four features are diagnostic of his illness being 'organic'.

   (c) Usually this type of psychosis can be treated successfully if cause found and correct treatment for cause given.

   (d) Often patient will die if cause not found and correct treatment for cause not given.
2. *A chronic organic psychosis*

   (a) Has been present for a long time (at least one month).

   (b) Patient on examination:
   - may or may not be fully conscious;
   - memory poor for recent events;
   - not fully orientated in time or place;
   - intelligence not as it should be for the person's education and previous position in society, i.e. demented (loss of previous intelligence when fully conscious) and confused.

   Has a lot of other abnormalities too including features of psychosis but the above four are diagnostic of it being 'organic'

   (c) Often this type of psychosis does not have a cause that can be easily found and successfully treated even if found.

   (d) Patient not likely to die quickly so urgent diagnosis and treatment not essential.

Always:

1. Take a full history from the patient and his family or friends.
2. Do a full physical examination.
3. Take a malaria smear and give antimalarial drugs.
4. Do a lumbar puncture and treat for meningitis if present.
5. Look carefully for evidence of any infection. Treat if infection possible with antibiotics or other drugs.
6. Do blood sugar. Give glucose intravenously or orally if blood sugar low or cannot be done.
7. Look carefully for head injury. Transfer urgently to Medical Officer if possible.
8. Smell the breath. Ask if there is any possibility of alcohol or drug overdose or withdrawal or the taking of poisons. Treat if needed.
9. Look for evidence of malnutrition. Give thiamine 50 mg IVI and multivitamin B tablets or injection if malnutrition possible.
10. Test the urine.
11. Send blood for serological test for syphilis and if needed for HIV infection and any other special tests needed.

Always think of an *organic* cause first in every patient who has *any* mental disturbance.
Especially always think of an acute *organic* cause first in any patient with an *acute* mental disturbance who was not mentally abnormal before.
Always consider first that the *cause is organic if*:
1. level of consciousness decreased
2. recent memory poor
3. not orientated in time and place
4. intelligence not normal or not able to be tested

Non-organic causes of psychiatric conditions

Non-organic causes include the experiences the patient has had. Most important are the relationships he has had with his family (especially as a child), friends, girlfriends, wife, etc. Also important are events at home, school, work, etc.

These *relationships and events can cause stress.* Two things especially cause stress. (1) Separation from people important to him. (2) A decision which the person cannot or does not make.

Stress causes anxiety. In anxiety, the brain stimulates certain nerves and the adrenaline producing gland. This causes dry mouth; sinking feeling in the abdomen; nausea and diarrhoea; palpitations; sighing or deep breathing; urinary frequency; sweating, cold hands and feet; a feeling of weakness; tightening of muscle groups (tension which can cause headache or backache if it remains for some time), etc. Anxiety is unpleasant but normal. The best way to remove the anxiety is to solve the problem causing the stress; or if this is not possible, to cope with it in a healthy mature way. If anxiety continues for a long time or if the anxiety is very great, then the stress and anxiety can cause mental disorders and diseases.

Stress and anxiety can cause non-organic non-psychotic conditions. These are called *'Neurotic stress-related' and Body-related disorders* (or by many people just 'Neurotic disorders').

Specific neurotic disorders are:

1. Anxiety disorders
   - Generalised anxiety
   - Phobic anxiety
   - Panic disorder
2. Obsessive compulsive disorder
3. Reaction to severe stress
   - Acute stress disorder
   - Post-traumatic stress disorder
   - Adjustment disorder
4. Dissociative or conversion disorder of 'acting out'
5. Somatoform disorder
6. Neurasthaenia or chronic fatigue syndrome

Stress and anxiety can also start some other, very serious psychotic diseases.

1. An *acute psychotic reaction* occurs when a person's anxiety and fearful thoughts completely take over his normal thoughts.
2. *Schizophrenia and manic depressive psychoses* may occur in people who have an inherited likelihood to get them. But they may not develop the disorder until they reach a stressful time in their lives, e.g. schizophrenia starting at a time of great stress – young person going to school or getting married etc.

Experiences help to form a person's personality. The personality is the characteristic or normal way in which a person thinks, feels, acts. Personality depends on what the person has inherited from his parents; anything that has happened to his brain; and the experiences that he has had, especially as a child. Some people have *abnormal personalities*, such as antisocial personalities, sexual deviations, and alcoholism or drug abuse. The experiences a person has are non-organic causes of the psychiatric condition of abnormal personality. A person's life experiences are the cause of the following disorders.

1. Behavioural syndromes associated with physiological disturbance
   - Eating disorder
   - Sleep disorders
   - Sexual function disorders
   - Puerperal mental disorders
2. Personality disorders

Psychotic or non-psychotic disorder?

Psychotic diseases (or psychoses)

Psychoses have some important typical features. In a psychosis there is a *severe disturbance of the patient's personality.*

The patient's *personality* is the way he thinks, feels and acts. (His acts include his appearance, his behaviour and his speech or talk.) A normal person feels and acts in a way that other people expect him to and that they understand. In a normal person, thinking, feeling and acting are all co-ordinated.

In a psychosis, there is a change in the way the patient thinks, feels and acts. The person is now different. He does not think and feel and act as normal. Also thinking, feeling and acting may not be co-ordinated, e.g. a person may act in a happy way but feel sad.

1. Most commonly there is a *disorder of thought*. The patient *cannot organise his thoughts* or get them 'straight'. His thoughts may suddenly stop or jump from one thing to another. He may have *hallucinations* (see, hear, feel, smell and taste things which are not there). He may have *delusions* (false beliefs which cannot be corrected by logical argument). These delusions are often that a person or something is trying to hurt or kill him. This delusion of persecution is called a 'paranoid delusion'. In organic psychoses (when the patient may not be fully conscious and cannot completely understand or remember what is happening) he may have *illusions* (wrongly understand and interpret real events and physical sensations) and may become *confused* and *delirious.*
2. There may be a *disorder of mood* (the usual 'feelings' of the person).
   He may be *manic* (too happy) or *depressed* (too sad) or seem to have *no feelings*, or the *mood may not be the usual one for the circumstances* (e.g. happy when very bad things are happening).
3. Because of the disturbance of thought and mood the *actions* (appearance, behaviour and speech) may be very *abnormal.*

4. Because of one or more of these things, the patient *loses contact with reality* (does not live in the real world; but lives in his own private world of unreal and strange thoughts and feelings).
5. The patient loses *insight* (to a small or large degree), i.e. he does not know what is really happening. The patient may not know he is sick. You may not be able to convince him he is sick. The patient may think he is normal and everyone else is abnormal. However there is not always loss of insight (or at least this complete loss of insight) in psychotic illnesses.

Non-psychotic disorders

Non-psychotic disorders are different from psychoses. There is *no change in the patient's personality* (or the way he thinks, feels and acts). The person's anxiety causes feelings that are stronger or continue longer than in a mentally healthy person. This results in an exaggeration or lengthening of thoughts and actions. This can also occur in mentally healthy people but they can control it.

1. The patient does not have a thought disorder. He does not have *hallucinations* or *delusions*. He is not confused. His thoughts are often not normal; but you can understand them and they 'make sense' if you know about the stresses and anxiety.
2. The patient's *mood* is appropriate to his thoughts and circumstances. The mood is often not normal; but you can understand it, and it 'makes sense' if you know about the stresses and anxiety and thoughts.
3. The patient's *actions* may not be normal and they may be very disturbed; but you can understand them and they 'make sense' if you know about his stresses and anxiety and his mood and thoughts.
4. The patient *does not lose contact with the real world.*
5. The patient does not lose *insight* and he knows that he is sick. However, he may deny this; but you can usually eventually convince him by logical explanation.
   In some non-psychotic patients, however, there is some or at least temporary loss of insight.

> When you see a patient with a psychiatric disorder, you must find out
> 1. Is there an organic cause or not? page 466–7.
> 2. Is this a psychosis or not? page 468–9.
> 3. Is there a cause for stress and anxiety? page 467–8.

You must do a routine history and examination of *both* physical *and* mental states to find the answers to the three questions:

1. Is there an organic cause or not?
2. Is this a psychosis or not?
3. Is there a cause for stress and anxiety or not?

Psychiatric history and examination

Psychiatric history

When you take a normal history, also take this special psychiatric history *from the patient and other witnesses.*

1. *Admission note*
   (a) Reason for admission. (If the police bring the patient, they must give a signed statement saying why they brought the patient.)
   (b) Names and addresses of those who referred the patient.
   (c) Names and addresses of patient's relatives *and* the people who were with the patient when the illness started.
2. *Complaints and duration*
3. *History of present illness*
   (a) What does the patient say has happened? What does the patient say is the cause?
   (b) What do other people say has happened? What do other people say is the cause?
   (c) What do *you* think really happened? What do *you* think the cause really is?
4. *Specific interrogation*
   Usual questions (see Chapter 6.)
5. *Past history*
   Any previous psychiatric disorder?
   - When did it occur?
   - How long did it continue?
   - What form did it take?
   - Did the patient get completely better?
   - Has the patient been taking any treatment?

   Note especially head injury, drugs, alcohol and the usual questions (see Chapter 6).
6. *Family and contact history*
   Any mental illness and the usual questions (see Chapter 6).

Psychiatric examination

When you do a normal examination of the patient, make these eight observations instead of just the level of consciousness.

1. Check if the patient can *communicate* physically (find out if he can hear, see, talk, move, etc.).
2. Check the *level of consciousness*.
3. *Memory*
   (a) recent events – e.g. What did you eat today?
   (b) long past events – e.g. Ask a fact of local importance,
4. *Orientation*
   (a) person – e.g. Who are you? What are you?
   (b) time – e.g. Is it morning or afternoon? What day is it?
   (c) place – e.g. What is this building? Where is the toilet?
5. *Intelligence* – Ask a problem suitable to the patient's education.
6. *Thoughts* by
   (a) speech
   (b) appearance and
   (c) behaviour
   Especially
   (a) clear logical thinking or muddled up thinking?
   (b) delusions, e.g. Do people treat you normally or in some special way?
   (c) hallucinations, e.g.
   - Are any strange things happening?
   - Do you hear voices when you can see no one there?
   - Do you see people when no one else can?

   (d) any special thing the patient thinks about all the time.
7. *Mood* by
   (a) speech
   (b) appearance
   (c) behaviour
   Especially
   (a) manic (too happy) } e.g. How do you feel in
   (b) depressed (too sad) } yourself?
   (c) co-ordinated with the patient's thoughts and actions or not?
8. *Insight*
   (a) does he think he is sick?
   (b) does he know the *real* cause of the illness?

In examination of the appearance, behaviour and speech note the points listed below.

1. *Appearance*
   - facial expression – happy, sad, or worried
   - posture
   - clothing
   - hygiene
   - anything odd or unusual
2. *Behaviour*
   - overactivity
   - underactivity
   - aggression
   - odd or unusual
   - sensible under the circumstances
   - care of bodily needs – does he eat and drink? does he rest and sleep?
3. *Speech*
   - fast
   - slow
   - none

   (shows what thoughts are and what stream of thoughts is like)

Important psychiatric conditions

Acute organic psychoses

In an acute organic psychosis the brain does not work properly as there is an *acute* (i.e. started recently) *underlying disease of the brain or abnormality of the blood coming to the brain* (see page 466).

This causes a disturbance in level of consciousness.

The typical features of an organic psychosis are therefore:

1. Disturbance of level of consciousness, which causes:
2. Poor memory (especially for recent events), and } These are called 'Confusion'.
3. Loss of orientation, and }
4. Loss of normal level of intelligence, also
5. The patient cannot understand things that are happening and has illusions and hallucinations. } This may be called 'Delirium'.

> A patient who has recently become confused or who is delirious has an acute organic psychosis.

Disturbance of the level of consciousness can be from just a little less alert than normal to drowsy to coma. This means the patient cannot pay the usual attention to what is happening. He therefore cannot remember what has happened, how he came to be where he is, or what time it is.

Also, as the brain does not work properly, he sees things but thinks they are different things from what they really are, e.g. illusions, where a shadow on a wall may be thought to be a rat or spider. He also has delusions where he may see or hear things that do not exist. His thoughts by then are all mixed up and he has difficulty in thinking. He is usually quiet. If he is frightened, however, from delusions or hallucinations, he may become violent. (Visual hallucinations are common during drug intoxication or withdrawal).

The mood is usually in keeping with what he is thinking. His appearance will get worse as he does not remember to take care of his bodily needs.

Typical features of an acute organic psychosis are therefore:

- Level of consciousness decreased
- Memory poor
- Orientation in time and place decreased

} 'Organic'

- Thinking mixed up
  - illusions
  - hallucinations
  - delusions
- Mood variable
- Speech rambling
- Appearance not cared for
- Behaviour quiet, but can be aggressive

} 'Psychotic'

You can treat most causes of acute organic psychosis, and often you can cure them. But, if you do not give proper treatment quickly, then these conditions either cause death or permanent damage to the brain. A good example is acute bacterial meningitis causing acute organic psychosis. See pages 466–7, for the list of the common causes of acute organic psychoses, and of the diagnostic procedures you must do on all patients with acute organic psychosis.

If a patient has an acute organic psychosis you must quickly find the cause and give effective treatment.

Chronic organic psychoses

In chronic organic psychosis there is a *chronic* (i.e. did not start recently) underlying *disease of the brain*. So the brain does not work properly.

This causes the typical features of chronic organic psychosis:

1. Level of consciousness in psychoses that develop after acute attacks may be abnormal. However in those that develop very slowly and are usually called 'dementia', the level of consciousness is at first normal.
2. Poor memory, especially for recent events, is the earliest and most typical feature. Recent things are not remembered but far past things are. Family members may notice these things first. The patient forgets where he puts things and what he is doing or talking about.
3. Some loss of orientation follows as the patient does not remember what has brought him to the present time and place.
4. Loss of previously good intelligence and not being able to learn new things are typical. The patient is no longer be able to do what he previously was able to do or to hold his previous position in society or the family.
5. Thinking gets less and less and the patient does not seem to think of the results of his actions. He may be rude when previously he was polite. He may steal things. He may use bad language. He may be incontinent without being worried about this. He does not think about new things. He does not take interest in what is going on.
6. Mood changes are common. Often the patient is irritable but may suddenly change from one mood to another. Eventually he does not seem to be affected by anything that goes on.
7. Insight is to a smaller or greater extent lost so that the patient does not really understand what is happening.

The patient has 'dementia'. There is a long history of the condition. Most of the causes cannot be treated or cured. See pages 466–7 for a list of the causes of chronic (and acute) organic psychoses and the diagnosic procedures you must do.

Patients with organic causes for their mental disorder do have disorders of thought and mood and insight and therefore have a psychosis, either acute or chronic organic psychosis.

In every case of a mental disorder always first look for an organic cause (disease in brain or abnormality in blood going to the brain). This is especially important if

1. The level of consciousness is not normal. 2. Orientation is not normal. 3. Memory for recent event is not normal. 4. Intelligence is not normal. 5. There are sudden changes in mood.	i.e.	Delirium or Confusion or Dementia

These signs do not occur in non-organic mental disease.

If these signs occur the patient has an organic psychosis.

You must find and treat the cause of the organic psychosis if possible. If the condition started recently urgent diagnosis and treatment are essential.

If the patient does *not have*:

- decreased level of consciousness, and
- recent memory loss, and
- loss of orientation in time and place, and
- abnormality of intelligence;

but *does have*:

- disorder of thought,
- disorder of feeling or mood,
- loss of insight,

then that patient has a so-called non-organic psychosis of which there are only two important groups:

1. Schizophrenia – a disorder of thinking
2. Manic depressive psychosis – a disorder of feeling or mood.

It is important to remember:

1. A schizophrenic-like state can be brought about by the misuse of certain drugs or substances (see p. 473).
2. A depressive state (also others) can be brought on by childbirth and the few months after it.

There is some evidence now that patients with the so-called non-organic psychoses may in fact have very specific or particular types of organic change in parts of their brain which do not affect the whole of their brain (as the conditions which cause organic psychosis do). Although these cannot be found by normal tests now, some abnormalities in the brain chemistry, which in fact have been shown to be present, may be the cause. The fact that schizophrenic-like states can be temporarily caused by misuse of drugs and other substances, would fit with this idea too. However, we do have to wait to find out if these non-organic psychotic patients do have a particular localised or specific type of organic lesion or not.

A patient with:

- level of consciousness decreased,
- memory for recent things decreased,
- orientation and time and place decreased,
- intelligence decreased,

must be assumed to have an organic condition and will be psychotic.

A person who has:

- level of consciousness normal,
- memory normal,
- orientation normal,
- intelligence normal,
- thought disorder or
- mood disorder, and possibly
- loss of contact with reality, and possibly
- loss of insight,

has a psychosis which is not organic and is probably either:

- schizophrenia – a disorder of thinking, or
- substance or drug misuse, or
- manic depressive psychosis – a disorder of mood.

Schizophrenia

Schizophrenia is a non-organic psychosis. You will not find an underlying disease of the brain or abnormality of the blood going to the brain.

There are *abnormal thoughts often with delusions and hallucinations* even though *the patient is fully conscious and orientated.* Mood is also often disturbed and feelings may not be co-ordinated with thoughts and actions, or the patient may appear to have no feelings. So appearance, behaviour and speech etc. may be very abnormal. The patient may have little or no insight and often says he is not sick at all.

In the acute stage the thought disorders may be very severe with strange hallucinations and delusions. Especially important are paranoid delusions (thoughts that someone is trying to hurt the patient when this is not true).

The main problem seems to be that the patient cannot tell the difference between experiences coming from the world outside him and those coming from inside his body and his mind.

The following disorders of thought are common in people with schizophrenia all over the world. There are changes in mood which may follow. The patient may tell you, or you will find out on questioning, that he has some of the following:

1. His thoughts have been put into his mind by another person; or he is thinking someone else's thoughts (thought insertion).
2. His own thoughts are just suddenly taken away from him (thought withdrawal).
3. His thoughts are known to other people – he may be broadcasting them like a radio transmitter or sending them some other way (thought broadcasting).
4. His body movements and feelings are being controlled by another person or thing, not himself (passivity feelings).
5. He can hear voices talking about him, sometimes just saying all he is doing but at other times making critical remarks about him. The voices may also be talking all of his thoughts out loud (auditory hallucinations).
6. He can tell the significance of certain actions although others do not agree on what they mean, e.g. he saw a child with a dog and this meant that the world would come to an end today.

Other less common disorders of thought include:

1. Thoughts become mixed up and one thought does not follow on from the previous one.
2. Newly made up words are used.
3. Delusions become marked and of special kinds, e.g. paranoid (someone or something is trying to kill him (and the patient may attack that person to protect himself)), grandiose (that he is an important person), sexual (that he is capable of extraordinary sexual feats), religious (that he is a religious person or god).
4. Hallucinations of tasting, smelling, feeling, touching things that are not there.

The patient may also have:

- mood changes where he appears not to understand what is happening to him, or
- mood changes which are inappropriate to his thoughts, e.g. laughing at terrible things.

Some patients adopt very strange positions or postures and remain in these for hours or longer. Others at times become aggressive and wild.

Eventually, if the disease proceeds, the patients seem to have:

- few thoughts and just tend to sit there,
- do not seem to have any feelings,
- scarcely speak.

Proper treatment helps especially in acute cases. It seems about 20% of patients make a full recovery and never have any more attacks. About 35% recover completely, but they do have further attacks with full recovery between attacks. About 35% have repeated attacks but after each attack are not quite as well as before that attack and therefore gradually get worse. About 10% quickly get worse without getting better at any time.

In *acute schizophrenia*, the patient is fully conscious, fully orientated, but has abnormal thoughts (especially delusions and hallucinations) and possibly abnormal feelings.

In *chronic schizophrenia* (after many years) the patient may appear to have few thoughts, very little feeling about anything, and may behave like a child.

If a patient:

1. is fully conscious and orientated with a good memory and reasonable intelligence, but
2. has abnormal thoughts especially hallucinations or delusions, and
3. possibly has inappropriate or no feelings

then the patient probably has schizophrenia or a drug or substance misuse.
Check, however, that the patient does not have an acute organic psychosis.

Drug and other substance misuse including withdrawal (including alcohol)

The most commonly abused drug is alcohol. Any more than three standard drinks for a male and two for a female in 24 hours, or 21 for a male and 14 for a female in a week, can have significant effects of health. (A standard drink contains 9–10 g alcohol and is contained in 1 glass (425 ml) of beer or 1 wine glass of wine or 30 ml of spirits.)

Other sedative drugs (besides alcohol) are benzodiazepines such as temazepam and diazepam; barbiturates; opiates including morphine, codeine and heroin; and organic solvents such as found in glues.

If the above sedative drugs are taken regularly, they not only have a bad effect on a person's health and behaviour but the nervous system gets used to being depressed by them and has to, as it were, be more stimulated to keep the person going. If these drugs are suddenly stopped, this excess stimulation, which is no longer needed, can cause a psychotic state ('withdrawal symptoms') something like schizophrenia but usually with frightening visual hallucinations and also shaking and shivering and sometimes even fitting.

There are other drugs which are not sedatives but stimulants. These include cannabis (marijuana or hashish), amphetamines such as dexamphetamine and a drug made from it called Ecstasy; cocaine and another drug made from it called Crack; and hallucinogenic drugs such as lysergic acid diethylamide (LSD) and psilocybin ('magic mushroom') which themselves stimulate the nervous system and can produce psychotic states like schizophrenia.

Manic depressive psychosis

Manic depressive psychosis is a non-organic psychosis. You will not find an underlying disease of the brain or abnormality of the blood going to the brain. However a specific chemical or other abnormality of part of the brain controlling only mood may yet be found.

There is a *disturbance of the mood*. The patient has a definite feeling which he thinks will not stop. It may be of great happiness (mania). It may be of great unhappiness (depression). There is no real cause for this feeling in what is happening to the patient. The patient appears fully conscious and orientated with a normal memory, but he thinks and acts in co-ordination with the feelings he has; so there may be some delusions usually of being a very important person or god, in mania, or of being a very bad person or of having a terrible disease, in depression. Sometimes there are vague hallucinations. So appearance, behaviour and speech may be very abnormal. The patient has little insight and often says he is not mentally abnormal.

The abnormal mood of the patient often goes after some weeks. Sometimes the patient can change from one mood to the other, i.e. from being too happy for no reason to being too sad for no reason. (This change does not happen quickly.)

Depression is more common than mania and often occurs by itself. Mania tends to occur in younger people and become less common as they get older.

The characteristic features of depression are:

- Depressed mood most of the day,
- Not interested in the events of normal living.
- Weight loss (as not eating). Occasionally weight gain.
- Cannot sleep properly especially waking in the early hours of the morning and not being able to go back to sleep.
- Feeling worst in the morning and a little better as the day goes on.
- Tired and no energy all the time and does little.
- Feels unworthy and guilty.
- Can't concentrate or decide on things.
- Thinks of death and often of suicide.

Sometimes patients who feel very depressed try to commit suicide (and sometimes also try to kill their families as they feel they also would be better off dead).

People who are manic often make quick and bad decisions as they feel and think everything will be all right. They may lose their money or their lives because of these decisions.

If a patient:
1. is fully conscious and orientated with a good memory and reasonable intelligence
2. has abnormal feelings (he is too happy or too sad) for which there is no real cause
3. possibly has abnormal thoughts co-ordinated with the abnormal feelings

then the patient probably has manic depressive psychosis.
Check that the patient does not have acute organic psychosis.

In the non-organic psychoses there is a disturbance in thoughts or mood. The patient *does not have*;

1. disturbance in level of consciousness,
2. disturbance of recent memory,
3. disturbance of orientation,
4. disturbance of intelligence, or
5. sudden swings in mood.

} i.e. Delirium or Confusion or Dementia

It the patient has any of these things, look for a disease of the brain or an abnormality of the blood going to the brain.

Neurotic, stress-related and somatoform disorders

All neurotic stress-related disorders

If a patient diagnosed with a neurotic stress-related disorder:

- is not fully conscious,
- has poor memory for recent events,
- is not fully orientated,
- does not have normal intelligence for him,
- has disorder of thought especially
  - abnormal thoughts,
  - hallucinations,
  - delusions,
- has disturbance of mood not in keeping with his circumstances,
- has lost contact with reality,
- has no insight into what is going on;

then

- the diagnosis is incorrect and the patient does not have a neurotic stress related disorder;
- look for organic causes if not fully conscious or not fully orientated or poor memory or intelligence not normal (especially if confused or delirious or demented);
- look for disorders of thought or mood or substance misuse if none of the features of organic disease present.

Anxiety disorders

Generalised anxiety

The cause of anxiety is stress (see page 467). The symptoms of anxiety are the physiological results of stimulation of parts of the patient's body by the nervous system and adrenaline (epinephrine) which are normal for everyone at the time of stress. They include both physical and mental effects.

The effects of generalised anxiety are:

1. Physical:
   - shaking
   - sweating
   - heart beating fast
   - chest pain
   - shortness of breath
   - headache
   - dizziness
   - diarrhoea
   - urinary frequency
   - not able to go to sleep when go to bed
   - not able to concentrate
2. Mental:
   - feeling that something terrible is about to happen
   - worry about everything
   - irritable
   - feeling as if not in their own body

If the patient has excessive or continuing stress, then some or all of these symptoms will continue. Sometimes only one symptom will continue when the others are no longer noticed by the patient. The patient may then be particularly aware of this symptom and not remember how it started and then he will start to worry that he has a disease problem, i.e. there is another cause of stress and anxiety. The anxiety can then keep itself going. Of course if the patient does not solve the cause of the original anxiety, this can also keep the anxiety state going.

Phobic anxiety

When anxiety occurs only in certain situations, it is called a phobia. Agoraphobia occurs when there are anxiety symptoms which come on only when people go out into open spaces and see people. A social phobia occurs when people have to meet other people. Animal phobias are when a patient has a particular fear of a particular animal such as a spider. Other specific phobias include fears of flying, heights, etc.

Panic disorder
When all of the anxiety symptoms happen suddenly in a certain situation, the patient is said to have a panic attack.

Obsessive compulsive disorder
This is said to exist when a special thought or impulse to do something repeatedly pushes itself into the patient's mind despite their trying to stop it. For instance, a patient may know that they have washed their hands and that they are clean, but they have to get up and wash their hands again and then the tap in case their hands got dirty from the tap when they turned it off, and then the door handle in case their hands got dirty from this, etc. Eventually they may have to spend hours washing their hands, taps, handles, etc. Other such rituals can also develop.

Reaction to severe stress
1. *Acute stress disorder* at the time of an event, can cause confusion, anxiety, anger, depression and extreme over-activity or extreme withdrawal.
2. *Post-traumatic stress disorder* occurs weeks or months after a severe stress such as occurs in wars, murders, torture, etc. The patient may suddenly get memories they do not want of the event (flashbacks), not be able to sleep, get episodes of acute anxiety, have nightmares, avoid any situation which reminds them of the traumatic event, tend to use alcohol, drugs, etc.
3. *Adjustment disorders* occur as a reaction to a normal stressful life event and are the processes whereby people get over death by grief reactions, etc.

Dissociative or conversion disorder (hysteria)
It is thought that if a patient has stress and anxiety that they cannot solve, they may unconsciously (without realising it) develop symptoms in their body which mean that their cause of stress and anxiety is solved. However there is nothing really wrong with the part of their body that has the symptoms. For instance, a student who has not studied enough to pass an examination, may develop paralysis of his writing hand and thus solve the problem of possibly failing an exam. Patients may appear to develop disturbance of walking, loss of function of a limb, loss of voice, epilepsy, loss of sensation, blindness and even loss of memory. For the diagnosis to be made, there must be a symptom that usually does not fit with anatomical or physiological organic disease but rather with non-medical ideas of function and disease; there must be no evidence of organic disease; and there must be a cause for the stress and anxiety which development of this problem solves.

One problem about this diagnosis is that it can be incorrectly made and the patient then go on to develop severe disability or death because they have had the mistaken diagnosis of 'hysteria' made when in fact they have an organic disease. Always be very unwilling to make this diagnosis until the patient is cured.

Somatoform disorders
Patients are said to have these disorders when they come for repeated consultations for physical symptoms for which no cause can be found. In many cases history will show that there has been a close relationship with some stressful life event in the past or the start of a continuing conflict when these physical symptoms started. They include pains, nausea, vomiting, diarrhoea, headache, dizziness, urinary symptoms, sexual difficulties, etc. At times there may be a collection of symptoms; at other times it may relate just to one thing (such as heart beating faster than usual, having to take deep breaths or having diarrhoea). The characteristic thing about these patients is that they remain well for years despite having serious symptoms and that tests never show any significant change. However, the symptoms are characteristic if care is taken to find out about them.

Chronic fatigue syndrome or neurasthenia
Numerous causes for this condition probably exist. Some may follow viral infections. Some may be a form of mild depression. Some, however, may be due to anxiety from stress.

Acute psychotic reaction (with no organic cause)

This is any type of severe mental disturbance when these things occur:

1. The patient (who is usually young) has a problem which he cannot solve and which causes great anxiety.
2. Fear replaces clear thinking and controls the thoughts, feelings and actions of the patient. Any type of psychotic (or non-psychotic) behaviour may result. The patient may appear to have schizophrenia or mania (i.e. a non-organic psychosis). Singing, shouting and other disturbing behaviour are common. Irritable answers to all questions are

common. But hallucinations and delusions are not common.
3. Once the problem is found and solved the patient becomes normal again within days or weeks.
4. There may be repeated attacks with repeated problems; but after each attack the patient gets completely better. But the patient may never cope well with problems.
5. The behaviour may be, in that particular society, a socially acceptable and understood way of behaving if a person is under excessive stress.

An acute psychotic reaction is different from a non-organic psychosis (schizophrenia or manic depressive psychoses). In most cases of non-organic psychoses:

1. the patient does not become completely normal even when his problems are found and solved, and/or
2. if the patient had a previous attack he was not completely normal before this attack.

This acute psychotic reaction is presumably a form of the neurotic stress related disorders 'Acute stress disorder' or 'Dissociative or Conversion or Hysterical Reaction'.

> In every patient who has very disturbed behaviour, you must try to find out if the patient has a big problem. If he does, you should try to solve it. Until you do this, you cannot know if the patient's mental disorder is caused by an acute reaction to anxiety or caused by a non-organic psychosis.

You cannot make a diagnosis of acute reaction when you first see the patient. You can only make it when the patient gets better. If the patient does not get completely better, he must have schizophrenia or another condition.

Management of patients with psychiatric conditions

Principles of management of patients with psychiatric conditions

1. Treat symptoms and signs (i.e. give symptomatic treatment).
   Control the patient, if necessary (see page 478).
   Look after the patient's bodily needs.
2. Change the patient himself by
   (a) treatment of any organic cause,
   (b) 'counselling' (talking to the patient),
   - first try to find out any cause of stress and anxiety,
   - then try to solve this cause of stress and anxiety,
   - teach the patient to talk to others about his needs and worries,

   (c) drugs, especially chlorpromazine, and
   (d) electroconvulsive therapy.
3. Change the patient's environment by:
   (a) 'counselling' (talking to the patient's family, friends and the people he lives and works with),
   - first try to find out any cause of stress and anxiety,
   - then try to solve this cause of stress and anxiety,
   - show the people how they can help the patient,

   (b) sometimes change the patient's school, work, etc.,
   (c) sometimes send the patient back to his home area, if he is away from it,
   (d) sometimes send the patient to a rehabilitation village if a suitable one is available.
4. Follow up the patient to see if he needs further treatment or help.

Management of a psychotic patient

This includes patients with schizophrenia, schizophrenic state due to drug or substance misuse, mania, depression, acute reaction, organic psychosis.

> Management includes four things
> 1. *Treat the cause*
>   (a) Treat any organic cause in the usual way.
>   (b) Try to solve any cause of stress and anxiety.
>   (c) Give chlorpromazine for thought, mood and behaviour disorders, diazepam for drug withdrawal psychosis and amitriptyline for depressive psychosis.
> 2. *Treat the psychotic behaviour*
>   (a) Admit with a helpful friend or relative. Educate the friend (see below).

(b) Check that the patient cannot hurt himself or others (see below).
(c) Give chlorpromazine or amitriptyline or diazepam (see below).
Reduce the dose of chlorpromazine when the patient improves. But, if it is a non-organic psychosis continue a maintenance dose (see below).
(d) Give benzatrophine or promethazine or diazepam if muscle side effects of chlorpromazine develop (see below).

3. *Transfer some patients*
   Most patients are best treated in the health centre.
   A few patients need transfer (see below).
   Before transfer, make special arrangements (see below), and give special treatment (see below).
4. *Change the patient's environment if necessary*
   See 'Principles' No. 3 page 477
   Follow up the patient regularly to check that he takes any chlorpromazine necessary, and to find out if he needs more treatment before the condition becomes severe again.

Treat the cause

1. *If organic psychosis* – treat the underlying disease affecting the brain, or the condition affecting the blood going to the brain.
2. *If acute reaction* (to stress and anxiety) – try to solve the problem causing stress and anxiety.
3. *If non-organic psychosis* – treat with
   - chlorpromazine for schizophrenia and manic depressive psychosis, especially manic phase and substance misuse,
   - diazepam for drug withdrawal psychoses,
   - amitriptyline for depressive psychoses.

Treat the psychotic behaviour (the main treatment of non-organic psychoses too)

1. *Always admit the patient with a responsible friend or relative.*
   Tell the friend how to care for and comfort the patient. Check that the staff and other patients do not tease the patient.
2. *Check that the patient cannot hurt himself or anyone else.*
   - Nurse the patient on the floor if he is throwing himself around.
   - Do not leave articles which the patient could use as a weapon, (e.g. knife, piece of wood, etc.).
   - If necessary, get four men to put the patient into a chair. Two strong men can then hold him until the drugs make the patient quiet or he goes to sleep.
3. *Give chlorpromazine* (25 mg *or* 100 mg tablets) and solution for injection 25 mg/ml (50 mg in 2 ml amps) *to produce the neuroleptisation syndrome.*

Choose a suitable oral dose (see below)
- Give this dose regularly 6-hourly and hourly if necessary.
- Give twice this dose immediately and last dose at night.

Choose a suitable IM dose if the patient refuses to take any of these oral doses. (Give the oral dose too when the IM dose settles the patient, see below.)
Increase the dose if necessary (see below).

(a) *Give chlorpromazine tablets regularly every 6 hours.*
- Choose the dose that will probably be necessary (from 50 mg to 200 mg).
- Try 50 mg for a small, old or sick patient, and for a patient who is quiet and is not very disturbed by hallucinations or delusions.
- Try 200 mg for a large or young patient, and for a patient who is violent or very active, and for a patient who is very disturbed by frightening hallucinations or delusions.
- Most patients need between 50 and 200 mg.

(b) *Give an extra dose of chlorpromazine tablets (use the same dose as above)*:
- when you first see the patient,
- with the last regular dose at night,
- every hour *if necessary* for violent behaviour or very disturbed speech and thoughts that are not controlled by the regular doses.

(c) *Give chlorpromazine by injection every time the patient refuses to swallow ANY ONE of the regular 6-hourly or the 'if necessary' doses*
- Choose the dose that will probably be effective (50–100 mg (2–4 ml)).
- Give the oral dose that was refused *also*, when the patient starts to settle after the IM dose.

(d) *Every day, note the total amount of oral and IM chlorpromazine* given the day before, and divide this by 4 (and add to the previous 6-hourly dose to give the new 6-hourly regular dose (which is also the 'as necessary' and night dose).

(e) *If the patient has schizophrenia or manic depressive psychosis*

- Leave him on the dose which settled him for 1 week (after he has settled well).
- Then slowly reduce the dose by 100–200 mg every week to 100–200 mg every night.
- Discharge the patient on 100–200 mg each night.
- It may be possible to stop the chlorpromazine after 3 months but usually it is given for 1 year.
- Follow up the patient every month.
- If the disease comes back soon or often after the treatment stops, then continue the treatment all the time.
- Follow up the patient and give him a supply of chlorpromazine every month, (or at the least each 3 months).

(f) *You can stop chlorpromazine quickly if*:

- the psychosis is a reaction to a problem that has been solved, or
- the psychosis is caused by an organic disease that has been cured.
- the psychosis was due to substance misuse that has stopped.

(g) *If the patient is not reliable in taking chlorpromazine himself*, chlorpromazine-like drugs are now available in long-acting injections, e.g. fluphenazine decanoate 25 mg/ml, the dose being 12.5–25 mg each 5–14 days depending on effect and side effects. This is very useful if the patient has stopped chlorpromazine himself and had a relapse.

4. *Treat any side effects of chlorpromazine*
   If the patient has shaking, muscle spasms, tongue or face spasms, eyes turned up, head bent back, limbs held in unusual positions, etc.
   then biperiden (Akineton) 5 mg or benzatrophine 0.5 mg or benzhexol (or if these are not available, promethazine 25 mg) IMI or IVI; then biperiden 2–4 mg (1–2 tablets) 2–4 times daily or if not available promethazine 25 mg twice daily. If none of the above is available, try diazepam 5 mg IVI slowly over 5 minutes then 5 mg orally twice daily *and* continue the chlorpromazine.
   Other side effects include low blood pressure, especially if chlorpromazine is given by injection. (Do not give larger first doses than recommended and do not give by IMI if blood pressure already low for other reasons.) Excessive sedation with increased appetite and weight gain can occur. Encourage friends and relatives to make the patient physically active. Some problems with dry mouth, blurred vision, constipation, urinary difficulty and impotence can occur but usually can be accepted until the dose is decreased. Some allergic type reactions with hepatitis or skin rash occasionally occur. Stop chlorpromazine if allergic reactions occur.
5. *If the patient is psychotic because of the effect of alcohol or drugs being stopped*, the most helpful other treatment would be diazepam 5–20 mg orally regularly, this dose being slowly reduced every day to zero by 5–7 days. Much less chlorpromazine would then be needed.
6. *If the patient has depression*, amitriptyline or other antidepressant drug would be better than chlorpromazine. Chlorpromazine might be needed as well for other symptoms. Amitriptyline would be given, 25–50 mg three times a day when started, but at home the whole dose of 150 mg would be taken at night. It may take up to 3 weeks to improve the depression and the drug should be continued for several months before being stopped. If the patient is not very depressed and is started on treatment as an outpatient with amitriptyline, start with 25 mg at night and slowly increase the dose each 3–4 days. If the patient is an inpatient, warn about side effects and start 25 mg three times a day and increase to 50 mg three times a day in a couple of days. Side effects include dry mouth, dizziness, difficulty passing urine (in an old man with the urethra partly blocked by the prostate or stricture). Do not use amitriptyline if the patient has glaucoma.

If the patient has repeated attacks of depression, the usual drug used, lithium, cannot be used for treatment at a health centre because blood levels cannot be measured. Ask your Medical Officer if a trial of carbamazepine taken all the time would be worth while.

Transfer

Transfer only these patients to Medical Officer care:

1. an organic psychosis; but you cannot find or treat the cause (urgent);
2. a patient who is not better after 200–800 mg chlorpromazine every day for 3 weeks (non-urgent);
3. a patient who is very depressed and wants to kill himself and does not quickly improve (urgent);

4. side effects of chlorpromazine are not controlled by drugs as on page 478;
5. a patient who has committed a serious crime (the police are responsible for transfer);
6. a patient with schizophrenia, who has not settled back into normal life even with treatment, can be accepted into a special psychiatric rehabilitation village (which is often very successful in improving people enough to get them home again).

Make the following special arrangements when transferring a psychiatric patient:

1. Always send a letter to the Medical Officer with details about the patient and the reasons for his transfer.
2. Always send a reliable friend or relative who can speak the patient's language and whom the patient trusts.
3. For medico-legal reasons, send a letter from the patient's nearest relative requesting the patient's transfer, admission and treatment.
4. Control the patient's behaviour with drugs before transfer (see page 478 and below).
5. Send also a health worker, who can physically manage and treat the patient.

Before transferring a psychiatric patient by air:

1. Make sure the patient's behaviour has been controlled by chlorpromazine.
   - Give another *extra* dose of chlorpromazine 150 mg orally $1\frac{1}{2}$ hours before departure.
   - Fifteen minutes before departure, check the patient again.
   - If the patient is not *very* quiet, give chlorpromazine 50 mg (2 ml) IMI.
2. If you are worried the patient may still not be controlled, also give paraldehyde 0.2 ml/kg (usually 10 ml) IMI or diazepam 5 mg IMI.
3. *Never* transfer the patient alone. There must be a health worker (and, if necessary, another person) with the patient, who can physically control the patient, if he behaves abnormally, and who has chlorpromazine and paraldehyde injections and can give them.
4. Always explain all the details to the pilot.

Management of a non-organic non-psychotic disturbance

This includes patients with anxiety state, acting out, reactive depression, etc.

1. Do a full history and examination (see Chapter 6) and any tests necessary. Check that you look for all the causes of the patient's symptoms. If you find no cause for the patient's symptoms, think of a mental disorder and do these things;
2. Find out if the patient has a cause for stress and anxiety. See the patient often to find out. Also see relations, friends, etc. You can only diagnose mental disorder as the cause of the patient's symptoms, if you find a cause for stress and anxiety (as well as no organic cause).
3. Try to *solve the cause of the stress and anxiety*. This is the most important part of the treatment. You may need the help of a social worker, police, pastor, employer, teacher, family, etc. to do this.
4. Then explain to the patient how the stress and anxiety can cause the symptoms he has. (e.g. If a headache, explain how the tightening of the forehead and neck muscles for a long time causes pain in the head, just as exercising the arm or leg muscles for a long time causes pain in them.)
5. If necessary, give drugs to help reduce the anxiety. Use diazepam 5 mg (1 tab), or if not available phenobaritone 30–60 mg (1–2 30 mg tabs) three times a day for 1–2 weeks. If diazepam is not successful, try chlorpromazine 25–50 mg (1–2 × 25 mg tabs) three times a day for 1–2 weeks.
   Do not keep the patient on drugs. Only give the drugs for a few weeks and then stop. The patient must solve his problem to stop the anxiety. The patient must not depend on drugs (or alcohol) to control the symptoms of his anxiety.
6. Show the patient how to relax and encourage him to do this.
   Tell the patient how exercises and sports will help. Encourage him to do these.
7. If the problems cannot be solved, the patient may improve just by talking to you about how he is.
8. Refer or non-urgently transfer a patient to a Medical Officer when all this does not help the patient, or you cannot be certain that there is no organic cause for the symptoms. There are special psychiatric types of treatment which may be very helpful and which the Medical Officer can organise.

Prevention of psychiatric conditions

1. You can:
   - help to improve family life in the community;
   - help to educate parents and community leaders in good ways of bringing up children;

- help to improve the environment in which the families live; and
- help to meet the other real needs of families.

These things will help children to grow up with normal ways of thinking, feeling and acting and to reduce the possibility of developing psychiatric conditions.

You can co-operate with others in doing things to improve family life.

2. Give help to people at times of stress and anxiety.

   Important times of stress and anxiety include:
   - leaving home – going to school,
   - getting a job,
   - tertiary education,
   - getting married,
   - having children, and
   - sickness or death in the family.

   If a person's problems can be solved or helped at such times, then the mental disease which may be caused by these will not develop.

   You can co-operate with others in giving this help.
3. Early diagnosis and early effective treatment of psychiatric conditions will stop mild cases from becoming severe cases.
4. Effective rehabilitation of patients into the family and the community after treatment will reduce the effect of the condition on the patients, the families and the whole community.

36

Some Common Symptoms and Signs

Pyrexia of unknown origin (PUO)

(fever of unknown cause)

There are many causes of a fever. But there are usually other symptoms or signs, or positive results of tests, in the patient with the fever. These other things usually show you the diagnosis for the patient. You (and the patient) then accept the fever as part of the disease and do not worry about the fever. You treat the cause of the disease and the fever goes away with the rest of the illness.

Sometimes when you first see a patient with a fever you can find no other symptoms and signs or abnormal tests to show you the diagnosis. If you ask the patient every day about his symptoms, and if you carefully examine the patient every day, you can usually find the cause of the fever and make a diagnosis when new symptoms or signs or tests come.

Sometimes you can only find the cause of a fever after all these things:

- history repeated many times,
- examination repeated many times,
- blood tests at a hospital,
- urine tests at a hospital,
- biopsies at a hospital,
- laparotomy at a hospital,
- therapeutic trials of drugs, etc. at a hospital but this is *very* unusual.

Causes of fever include:

1. infections of all types in all organs – these are the most common and important causes of a fever;
2. non-infective inflammatory diseases including:
   - rheumatoid disease and other similar diseases,
   - trauma, and
   - allergic reactions of certain types;
3. neoplasm;
4. drugs and chemicals;
5. inherited diseases; and
6. many other causes.

Infections that cause fever

There are three groups of infections that cause fever:

1. Infection of *a particular part of the body which is caused by one of many different organisms*. The disease is often named after the part of the body infected (e.g. pneumonia when the lung is infected; hepatitis when the liver (hepar) is infected: enteritis when the intestine is infected). There is no one specific organism that infects these places. The organisms may be viruses or bacteria or worms etc. *These infections occur in all parts of the world*. See Chapters 19–32, and septicaemia in Chapter 12.
2. *A specific organism that causes a specific disease which often affects more than one part of the body*. The disease is often named after the specific organism (e.g. measles, chickenpox). No other organism causes the same disease as this specific organism does. *These types of disease occur all over the world*. See specific viral diseases in Chapter 16, malaria in Chapter 13, tuberculosis in Chapter 14, leprosy in Chapter 15, HIV and some of the diseases in Chapter 19.
3. Another group of diseases is similar to group 2. *One particular organism causes disease*, which may affect *more than one part of the body*. But *these diseases occur only in certain parts of the world*. Diseases in this group which cause a short fever (a fever present for a week or less, although it may return) are in Chapter 17. Diseases in this group that cause longer fevers are in Chapter 18. If some of the diseases in Chapter 17 and Chapter 18 do not occur in your country, or where the patient has travelled, do not think of them. Think only of the diseases that the patient can possibly have.

Always include these infections in the differential diagnosis of a patient with a fever

1. A non-specific infection of a part of the body which can occur anywhere in the world
   - meningitis
   - septicaemia
   - upper respiratory tract infection, especially otitis media and sinusitis
   - influenza
   - pneumonia (especially in an upper lobe, where it is more difficult to find on examination)
   - gastroenteritis (see the many possible causes)
   - intra-abdominal abscess, especially pelvic inflammatory diseases, appendix abscess, and liver abscess
   - urinary tract infection
   - osteomyelitis
   - acute bacterial ('septic') arthritis
   - abscess in another place, especially pyomyositis and injection abscess
2. A specific infection which can occur anywhere in the world
   - malaria
   - tuberculosis
   - leprosy with reaction
   - measles
   - mumps
   - chickenpox
   - HIV infection
   - glandular fever
   - typhoid fever
   - brucellosis
3. A specific infection which occurs in your area. If any of these occur in your area, they are likely to be the cause of your patient's fever
   - relapsing fever
   - typhus fever
   - plague
   - bartonellosis
   - dengue and other arbor virus fevers
   - yellow fever, and other arbor virus infections which cause haemorrhagic fevers
   - haemorrhagic fevers caused by other virus infections which are spread man-to-man or rat-to-man or monkey-to-man
   - leishmaniasis
   - trypanosomiasis
   - allergic reactions to schistosomes and other worms or parasites in the body

The management of a patient with a fever of unknown cause

1. Do a full medical history
2. Do a full clinical examination
3. Do routine tests
   - haemoglobin estimation,
   - urine test in *all* cases for protein, pus and bile,
   - others as indicated.

   Take tests to send to the laboratory, depending on which diseases occur in your area:
   - blood slide, for malaria and relapsing fever in all cases,
   - blood or lymph gland or other aspirate for leishmania and trypanosomes if these occur in your area,
   - others as indicated.
4. Write down a differential diagnosis of all possible causes. See list on this page for common infectious diseases.
5. Look for symptoms and signs to check for these diseases in 4.
6. Do tests to check for these diseases in 4, e.g.
   - tuberculin test (but positive test does not mean the patient has fever due to tuberculosis),
   - lumbar puncture (if any signs of meningitis).

   Take tests to send to the laboratory to check for these diseases in 4, e.g.
   - sputum for AFB,
   - blood for HIV,
   - others as indicated.
7. Treat any cause you find *and/or* give *all* patients antimalarial drugs as indicated (see Chapter 13) if the patient is in or from an area where malaria occurs.
8. See the patient daily.
   - Ask for new symptoms daily until the patient is cured. Examine for new signs daily until he is cured. Remember to examine the ears and do a pelvic examination at least once more.
   - Test the urine again.
   - If not cured in 2 days, treat as in 9 or 10.
9. *If you find no other abnormalities and the patient looks 'sick' and does not improve after 2 days (antimalarials for 2 days)*
   - Transfer to Medical Officer care.

   If transfer is not possible, and the patient gets worse:
   - Give IV (slow drip) or IMI quinine then pyrimethamine with sulfadoxine (Fansidar) or

alternative drug if the patient is from or in an area where malaria occurs (see Chapter 13).
- Give IVI fluids.
- Give IVI antibiotics as for septicaemia (see Chapter 12).
- If patient is not greatly improved in 2 days, transfer.
- If transfer is still not possible, and patient may die before transfer is possible, start antituberculosis treatment (see Chapter 14). (Transfer is essential later, even if the patient improves, unless positive sputum proves the diagnosis of tuberculosis.) If treatment for tuberculosis is started, the patient must complete the full course.

10. *If you find no other abnormalities, and the patient does not look 'sick' but does not improve after 3 days (antimalarials for 3 days).*
    - Repeat the course of antimalarials. Observe carefully to check that the drug is swallowed and absorbed (no vomiting or diarrhoea).
    - If the patient still has fever at the end of 1 week, take another malaria smear and send it to the laboratory to find out if the patient has drug resistant malaria.
    - Then treat the patient for chloroquine resistant malaria, and observe the result.
    - If the patient still has fever after a treatment course for chloroquine resistant malaria, transfer is essential.
11. If the fever goes after a 3-day course of chloroquine, but returns within the next 2 weeks:
    - Take a blood smear and send it to the laboratory to find out if the patient has chloroquine resistant malaria or relapsing fever.
    - Treat for chloroquine resistant malaria and observe while waiting for the result.

Malaise (Patient feels unwell)

1. Do a full medical history.
2. Do a full clinical examination
3. Do routine tests: (a) Hb if pale, (b) urine test in *all* cases.
   Take tests to send to the laboratory for the common infectious diseases in your area (see page 483).
4. Write down a differential diagnosis of all the possible causes.
5. Look for symptoms and signs to check for these diseases in 4.
6. Do or send tests to check for these diseases in 4. Especially remember
   - tuberculin test,
   - sputum for AFB,
   - lumbar puncture,
   - blood slide for malaria and relapsing fever,
   - blood or lymph gland or other aspirated material for examination for leishmaniasis or trypansomiasis,
   - blood test for HIV infection.
7. Treat any cause you find *and/or* give *all* patients antimalarial drugs as indicated, if the patient is in or from an area where malaria occurs.
8. See the patient daily.
   - Ask about new symptoms daily until he is cured. Examine for new signs daily until he is cured. Remember to examine the ears and do a pelvic examination at least once.
   - Test the urine again.
   - Manage as in 9, 10 or 11.
9. *If it is an acute illness and you find no abnormalities and the patient looks 'sick',*
   - If it is an acute illness and does not improve after 2 days (and antimalarials for 2 days), transfer the patient.
   - If transfer is not possible and the patient gets worse, treat as for pyrexia of unknown cause. 9. See page 483.
10. *If it is a chronic illness and you find no abnormalities and the patient does not improve after 2 weeks.*
    - Transfer the patient.
    - If transfer is not possible, send blood for Hb white cell count (total and differential), liver function tests, urea and serology tests for HIV infection. Send sputum for AFB. Send urine for full examination. Do a tuberculin test Send the appropriate tests for any other diseases common in your area.
    - Ask for a Medical Officer to send you a *report on what the tests mean.*
11. *If you find no abnormalities and the patient does not look 'sick'.*
    Think of a mental disturbance. Find out if the patient has a problem or a cause for stress and anxiety. But diagnose a psychiatric cause only if:
    - you find *no* organic cause and the patient does not look 'sick' *and*

- a *real* cause for stress and anxiety *is* present, *or*
- positive signs of a non-organic psychosis (see Chapter 35 pages 476–7) are present.

Generalised oedema (swelling of the whole body)

Do a full history and examination (see Chapter 6). Test the urine for protein, sugar, blood and pus.

1. Check that the *whole* body (legs *and* back and sometimes face) has oedema.
   Lymphoedema or elephantiasis usually affect only the limbs (usually legs) and the lymph glands are usually enlarged.
   If localised oedema, see page 486.
2. If the urine contains protein, look for:
   (a) nephrotic syndrome (*much protein* (> $\frac{1}{8}$ or +) *and much oedema*),
   (b) pre-eclamptic toxaemia (*female, pregnant, BP higher than 120/80, protein in urine*),
   (c) chronic kidney failure (*nausea, wasted, anaemic, BP high*),
   (d) acute nephritic syndrome or acute glomerulonephritis (*blood in the urine, BP high, fever*),
   (e) heart failure (*see below*).
3. Look for heart failure
   (a) The signs of heart failure are:
   - *raised jugular venous pressure* } almost
   - *enlarged liver* } always
   - *oedema*
   - *fast pulse* – usually
   - *cyanosis* – often
   - *crepitations* – sometimes

   (b) You can usually find the cause of the heart failure, e.g.
   - *chronic obstructive lung disease*
   - *pneumonia*
   - *severe anaemia*
   - *IV fluids given too quickly*
   - *other* see Chapter 27 pages 373–4
4. Look for severe anaemia.
5. Look for malnutrition (unusual in an adult) or chronic disease of the gastrointestinal tract (especially chronic vomiting or chronic diarrhoea or dysentery).
6. Look for cirrhosis (chronic liver disease)
   (a) *you can find no other cause and*
   (b) *ascites that is worse than the oedema*
   (c) *very thin arms and shoulders, very swollen abdomen, moderately swollen legs* } the typical appearance of cirrhosis see Figure 24.5

Management

Give diuretics

Do not give diuretics if it is toxaemia of pregnancy or malnutrition.

Give hydrochlorothiazide 25–50 mg daily. Increase the dose to 100 mg daily if necessary.

Also give frusemide 40 mg (1 tab) daily if necessary. Increase the dose slowly to 160 mg (4 tabs) daily if necessary.

Give potassium if necessary

1. If the patient is not eating a tuber diet (i.e. sweet potatoes, etc.), *or*
2. he is taking digoxin and diuretics, *or*
3. he is taking frusemide and hydrochlorothiazide,

then give potassium chloride slow release tablets 1200 mg (2 tabs) three times a day.

Treat the cause if possible and transfer to Medical Officer care if necessary

Nephrotic syndrome

- Give prophylactic antimalarials (see Chapter 26 page 358).
- Give treatment for intestinal worms (see Chapter 23 pages 277–82).
- Refer to Medical Officer if the patient is not cured in 6 weeks (as some cases can be cured by other drugs).

Pre-eclamptic toxaemia

The patient must rest in bed.

If the patient not cured in 2 days or if she gets worse at any time or if she has fitting, treat (see an obstetrics book) and transfer urgently.

If she is cured, keep her in the health centre on observation or tell her to return every week for examination, until delivery.

Chronic kidney failure

The patient must drink 3 litres of fluid daily. Give chlorpromazine 25 mg every 6 hours if necessary IMI (1 ml) if there is vomiting or orally (1 tab) if there is nausea.

The patient must take as much salt as possible without causing oedema or heart failure – if these develop, reduce salt until these go.

No high protein foods.

See Chapter 26 page 359.

Other kidney conditions
See a medical reference book.

Heart failure
Diuretics are the most important treatment in most cases (see Chapter 27 page 375). If there is acute, severe heart failure give frusemide 40 mg (4 ml) IV.

Give oxygen if there is acute shortness of breath or cyanosis.

If there is chronic obstructive lung disease, see Chapter 20 pages 227–8.

If there is pneumonia, see Chapter 20 pages 220–1 and give digoxin (see Chapter 27 page 375)

If there is anaemia, see Chapter 21 pages 240–2 and transfer for blood transfusion.

If IV fluids were given too quickly, stop or slow the drip.

If there is no cause obvious, give thiamine 50 mg immediately and daily for 2 weeks (the first dose IMI if available).

If other treatment is necessary (e.g. aminophylline, digoxin) see Chapter 27 pages 371–5.

Transfer to Medical Officer care *if*

1. you have not diagnosed a cause which cannot be treated, especially if the pulse is irregular, *or*
2. you have diagnosed a cause that you can treat but proper treatment does not cure it.

Severe anaemia
See Chapter 21 pages 240–2 and transfer for blood transfusion.

Malnutrition or chronic gastrointestinal disease
Check that the patient has a good mixed diet of enough food, at least three times a days.

Give drugs for intestinal worms (see Chapter 23 pages 277–82).

Treat any cause of vomiting or diarrhoea (see Chapter 23 pages 282–3, 297 and 299).

Diuretics are not necessary.

Transfer the patient if he does not improve.

Cirrhosis
Check the patient has a good mixed diet with high protein but no salt (tinned meat and fish have too much salt).

Give treatment for intestinal worms.

Diuretics are often necessary for the rest of the patient's life (usually a smaller dose after the ascites goes). See Chapter 24 page 310.

Transfer if the diagnosis is not certain, especially if there are masses or tenderness in the abdomen.

Localised oedema (Swelling of one part of the body)

1. *Check for swelling of the rest of the body.* If generalised oedema, see page 485.
2. *Check that the swelling is oedema* and not a lump from another cause.

Types of lump include

(a) Congenital (the patient was born with it)
(b) Traumatic (caused by injury)
(c) Inflammatory
- infection
- trauma
- allergy
- bites, stings, toxins

(d) Neoplastic (cancer)
(e) Degenerative. Remember especially:
- hernia
- prolapse
- thrombosis (clotting) in a blood vessel
- calcification
- swelling caused by a blocked duct

3. *Look for causes of localised oedema* especially:

(a) Injury. *History. Type of lesion. Haematoma often present (bruise).*
(b) Infection. *If acute* – red or shiny; swollen; tender; hot; the part cannot work properly.
(c) Lymph vessel and lymph gland disease (see Chapter 22 pages 257–65) especially:
- acute bacterial infection
- acute filarial inflammation
- chronic bacterial infection
- chronic filarial inflammation
- tuberculosis
- cancer

(d) Snakebite. *History.*
(e) Allergic reaction. *Swelling and often redness and itch but little tenderness.*
(f) Varicose veins
(g) Clots in main deep veins. *History of little recent leg movement (e.g. operation, illness, lon*

trip) or of injury to limb or of IV injection or of infection; you can find no other cause.

4. *Treat any cause you find.*
   (a) Injury. See a surgery book.
   (b) Infection. See Chapter 11 page 44.
   (c) Lymphatic disease. See Chapter 22 page 254.
   (d) Snakebite. See Chapter 33 page 454.
   (e) Allergic reaction. Give promethazine 25 mg (1 tab) 1–3 times daily and, if necessary, adrenaline tart. 1:1000 0.5 or $\frac{1}{2}$ ml each 6 hours.
   (f) Clots in the main deep veins. If it is in the leg, transfer urgently to Medical Officer care. In other cases treat with sling, aspirin, heat and antibiotics.
5. *Treat the affected part.*
   (a) Keep it higher than the rest of the body if possible, e.g. blocks under the foot of bed; arm in sling.
   (b) protect from further injury, especially if chronic, e.g. wear shoes if the leg or the foot is affected.

Generalised wasting

Do a full history and examination (see Chapter 6). Test the urine for protein and sugar.

Send sputum for AFB if there is a cough. Look for signs of these conditions:

1. Malnutrition (history of eating – what? and how often?).
2. Chronic disease of the gastrointestinal tract, especially if there is chronic vomiting (usually transfer) or chronic diarrhoea (possibly treat with pyrantel and metronidazole and tetracycline (Chapter 23) and transfer if this does not cure it).
3. Chronic infections, especially
   (a) tuberculosis (*chronic cough or enlarged lymph glands*),
   (b) HIV infection usually with diarrhoea,
   (c) malaria (*attacks of fever, anaemia, large spleen*),
   (d) hyperreactive malarious splenomegaly or tropical splenomegaly syndrome (*anaemia, very large spleen*),
   (e) visceral leishmaniasis (*fever, very enlarged spleen, enlarged lymph nodes, anaemia, diarrhoea, skin infiltrations sometimes*),
   (f) trypanosomiasis (*history of skin lesions at first, fever, enlarged lymph glands, enlarged spleen, enlarged liver, anaemia, fast pulse, nervous system disease*).
4. Repeated attacks of ordinary infections.
5. Chronic, non-infectious diseases, especially:
   (a) chronic obstructive lung disease (*chronic cough, sputum AFB negative*),
   (b) chronic kidney failure (*protein in urine, anaemia, nausea, BP high*),
   (c) cirrhosis (*thin shoulders, some swelling of legs and back, severe swelling of abdomen, no protein in urine*),
   (d) thyrotoxicosis (*eating much, staring eyes, shaking hands, fast pulse*),
   (e) diabetes (*eating and drinking much, passing much urine, sugar in urine*).
6. Cancer of any organ (*often lumps or bleeding*).
7. Others (see a specialist medical reference book).

Dehydration

Dehydration is present when there is not enough salt and/or water in the body.

The body normally contains 60% water.

If 0–5% of the body weight is lost (3 kg in 60 kg person, i.e. 3 litres) there is mild dehydration.

If 5–10% of the body weight is lost (6 kg in 60 kg person, i.e. 6 litres) there is moderate dehydration.

If 10–15% of the body weight is lost (9 kg in 60 kg person, i.e. 9 litres) there is severe dehydration which will probably soon cause shock and death.

Causes include:

1. Too much fluid lost from
   - intestines (vomiting, diarrhoea)
   - skin (sweating)
   - urine (diabetes, chronic kidney diseases)
   - lungs (fast breathing in high fever)
2. Not enough fluid taken in
   - too sick to drink
   - unconsciousness
   - woman in labour
   - no water to drink

The most important *signs* in adults are:

- fast pulse,
- low BP,
- inelastic skin,
- little urine passed and urine dark colour,
- sunken eyes, and
- dry mouth.

Do not mistake inelastic skin from weight loss (wasting) or old age, for the inelastic skin of dehydration.

For *management* of patient with dehydration, see Chapter 23 page 285.

Loss of weight

Find out *how long* the condition has taken to develop.

1. In a few hours
   - loss of fluid (dehydration), from any cause (see Chapter 23 page 285).
2. In a few days
   - loss of fluid (dehydration), from any cause (see Chapter 23 page 285).
   - not taking in fluid (dehydration), from any cause (see Chapter 23 page 285).
   - not eating
3. In a few weeks or months
   - wasting condition, from any cause (see page 487).
   - malnutrition

Note only loss of fluid can cause rapid (in a few hours or days) loss of weight.

Lumps (masses)

Examination of lump

Note especially:

- Site
  - in that tissue or organ?
  - where in that tissue or organ?
- Size
- Shape
- Surface
- Consistency
- Fluctuancy
- Tenderness and other signs of inflammation
- Fixed to surrounding tissue or not
- Function of the affected tissue or organ
- Regional (or nearby) lymph nodes

Types of lump

1. Congenital
2. Traumatic
3. Inflammatory
   - infection
   - trauma
   - allergy
   - bites, stings, toxins
4. Neoplastic
5. Degenerative – remember
   - hernia
   - prolapse
   - thrombosis (clotting) in a blood vessel
   - calcification
   - swelling caused by a blocked duct

If a lump is neoplastic, these signs will usually help you to find out what type of neoplasm it is:

If it is a simple or benign lump it –	If it is a malignant lump, it –
has clear regular edges	has irregular edges
is not hard	is hard
can be moved	is fixed to other tissues
grows slowly (years)	grows fast (weeks or months)
does not grow into surrounding tissues	grows into surrounding tissues
does not spread to lymph nodes	spreads to lymph nodes
does not spread to other organs	spreads to other organs
does not form ulcers	often forms ulcers

Abscess

An abscess is a collection of pus in one part of the body.

Diagnosis of an abscess

1. There are general symptoms and signs of infection.
2. There are local symptoms and signs of inflammation.
3. There are signs of fluctuation in *two directions* at right angles; but only if the abscess is near the surface of the body. Place the index and middle fingers of one hand on the swelling. Then press down quickly between the two fingers with a finger of the other hand. If fluctuation is present, you will feel the 2 fingers being lifted. Then put the 2 fingers at right angles (or 90°) to the first position and do the test again. If fluctuation is *again* present, then there is fluid (e.g. pus) under

the 2 fingers. Note that fluctuation in one direction only does *not* mean there is fluid under the fingers (normally muscle 'fluctuates' in one direction).

Treatment of an abscess

1. Give *antibiotics* only if:
   (a) There are severe general symptoms and signs of infection (fever, fast pulse, etc.).
   (b) The infection is spreading into the surrounding tissue (cellulitis) or lymph vessels or lymph glands.
   (c) The bone may be infected (osteomyelitis) (continue for at least 4 weeks).
   (d) It is a breast abscess.
   (e) It is a hand or finger abscess.
   (f) It is a pyomyositis.
   See Chapter 11 pages 46–52 for choice of antibiotic.
2. *Incise and drain* the abscess if:
   (a) Pus is definitely present (i.e. if fluctuant in two directions at right angles; or soft).
   (b) A breast abscess has not improved after 2 days of antibiotics or has already been present for 4 days when you first see it.
   (c) It is a hand abscess and patient cannot sleep for 1 night after you start antibiotics (transfer to Medical Officer is usually necessary).
   d) It is pyomyositis or osteomyelitis. Incise immediately if it is very swollen; or after 2 days if it is not almost cured by antibiotics.
   - Use anaesthetic topical spray if it is a small superficial abscess (except hand).
   - Use general anaesthetic (ketamine) or lytic cocktail or regional block if it is a large or deep abscess or in the hand.

> Use these anaesthetics only if you have had special training and have all the necessary resuscitation equipment available.

   - Do not cut or damage other structures.
   - Cut the skin and subcutaneous tissues with a scalpel.
   - Push a closed pair of artery forceps into the abscess, and then open the forceps.
   - Make a hole big enough to insert your finger (except hand abscess).
   - Destroy all walls inside the abscess with your finger (inside a sterile glove). Feel if the bone is affected.
   - Leave a rubber drain in the abscess, that comes out through the skin.
   - Pack the wound with gauze soaked in Eusol or strong 3% saline if it bleeds much.
   - Apply a Eusol dressing.
3. Give *drugs for pain* if necessary See Chapter 7 page 29.
4. *Dress after incision*
   Dress when necessary (at least daily, but more often if necessary).
   - Use either a little acriflavine emulsion smeared on an absorbant pad soaked in strong (3%) saline or an absorbant pad soaked in Eusol.
   - Remove any pack in 1 day.
   - Remove the drain when there is only a little discharge (2–3 days).
   - When the sore is clean and there is no more pus and slough, dress with a weak (1%) saline dressing or a vaseline gauze dressing.

   Transfer to Medical Officer any case where the abscess is deep, or near important structures in the neck, chest, abdomen, or in the hand (usually).

Abdominal pain

1. *Take a full history* (see Chapter 6). Ask about the pain, especially
   - is it a colic? (if colic, see below and page 490)

   or
   - is it a constant pain? (if constant pain, see below and page 490)
   - where exactly is the pain?

   Remember to ask about
   - recent trauma to abdomen,
   - the date of last normal period.
2. *Do a full examination* (see Chapter 6). Remember to check carefully for:
   (a) temperature (? infection)
   (b) PR; BP; skin elasticity; hands and feet warm or cold; (? dehydration, ? shock)
   (c) colour (? anaemia, ? bleeding)
   (d) abdominal
   - distension
   - movement on respiration
   - hernia and scars
   - tenderness – guarding – rigidity
   - masses
   - enlargement of organs
   - intestinal bowel sounds

- pelvic examination 'PR' or 'PV' for tenderness, masses or enlarged organs

(e) chest disease (pain referred to abdomen)

(f) spinal disease (pain referred to abdomen)

3. *Test urine for protein, pus, bile, sugar.*

> Look at any vomit or abnormal stools or vaginal discharge to see what it contains.

The pain is a colic (If pain is constant, see below)

Colic is caused by obstruction or inflammation of:

- the GI tract (stomach or small intestine or large intestine), *or*
- the female reproductive tract (tubes or uterus), *or*
- urinary tract (ureters) (often more a constant pain with times when it is worse), *or*
- biliary tract (bile ducts) (unusual).

See Figure 36.1.

Causes of colic in these organs include:

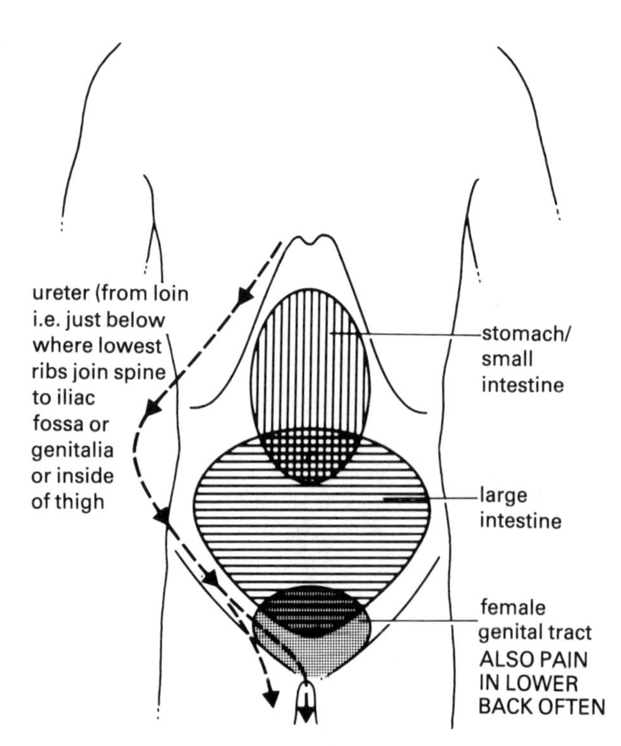

Figure 36.1 Diagram to show the place in the abdomen where the patient feels colic from the various organs that can cause colic.

1. GI tract

   (a) Gastroenteritis (*diarrhoea, central abdominal colic, sometimes vomiting; no definite abdominal tenderness; often dehydration and fever*).

   (b) Intestinal obstruction (*constipation; central abdominal colic; vomiting; no abdominal tenderness; no fever*).

   (c) Enteritis necroticans ('pigbel') (*signs of obstruction and peritonitis* (see Chapter 23 page 292).

   (d) Others

2. Genital

   (a) Labour (*large, non-tender uterus; no fever or shock*).

   (b) Antepartum 'accidental' haemorrhage (*large, tender uterus; often anaemia and shock*).

   (c) Miscarriage (*PV bleeding; uterus enlarged; no abdominal or pelvic masses or tenderness*).

   (d) Ectopic pregnancy (*1–2 periods late or missed; some dark red PV bleeding; usually also constant lower abdominal or general abdominal pain and tenderness; often fainting;* often pale or shocked (see an obstetrics book).

   (e) period pains (dysmenorrhoea) (*history of similar pain with periods; on examination NAD*).

3. Ureters

   Stones (*pain in typical place* (see Figure 36.1); *kidney sometimes tender; often blood in the urine*).

> If the pain is a colic
> 1. Where is the pain? What organ is probably causing it? (see Figure 36.1)
> 2. What condition is probably affecting this organ? (see Figure 36.3)

The pain is constant

(If the pain is a colic, see above.)

Constant pain is caused by:

- inflammation or swelling or stretching,
- of the organ or of the peritoneum,
- at the place of the pain (see Figure 36.2 for position of organs; the peritoneum is around the whole abdomen).

Tenderness in one area means:

- inflammation or swelling or stretching,
- of the organ or the peritoneum,

- under the place of the tenderness (see Figure 36.2 for position of organs; the peritoneum is around the whole abdomen).

Tenderness all over the abdomen (generalised), often with guarding and rigidity means:

- inflammation or irritation of the whole peritoneum by,
- pus (peritonitis), or
- blood from trauma or ectopic pregnancy.

Note. Tenderness over an area is more accurate than pain over that area for diagnosing inflammation or swelling or stretching of the organ or peritoneum under that area.

Note *also* these four causes of constant abdominal pain.

1. All over
   - pus in peritoneum (peritonitis)
   - blood in peritoneum (trauma or ectopic pregnancy)
2. Any part – spinal disease (fracture or tuberculous) with referred pain.
3. Upper abdomen – chest disease (pneumonia or pleurisy) with referred pain.
4. From where lower rib joins spine to genitalia or upper, inner thigh – ureteric colic (stones).

If the pain is constant 1. Where is the pain? What is the organ that is probably causing it? (See Figure 36.2.) (If the pain is all over, the peritoneum is affected) 2. What condition is probably affecting this organ? (See Figure 36.3.)

Transfer

Transfer urgently to Medical Officer if (but, first start treatment, see next page):

1. There is generalised peritonitis or blood in the peritoneal cavity. In both
   - *constant generalised pain*
   - *often vomiting and constipation*
   - *the abdomen is distended and does not move well on respiration*
   - *the abdomen is tender all over, often with guarding and rigidity*
   - *intestinal sounds are not present.*

   If peritonitis
   - *pulse fast, temperature raised, BP normal (later BP low and shock).*

   If bleeding
   - *pale, pulse fast, BP low (sometimes shock), usually no fever.*
2. Localised peritonitis (e.g. appendicitis)
   - *constant pain one part of the abdomen*
   - *abdomen does not move well over affected area and is tender over affected area, often with rebound tenderness and guarding*
   - *pulse fast*
   - *temperature raised*

   But you can treat liver abscess and hepatitis, or pelvic inflammatory disease, or splenic inflammation (not trauma), at the health centre.
3. Obstruction of intestine
   (a) *colicky abdominal pain*
   (b) *vomiting*
   (c) *constipation*
   (d) *abdomen*
   - *distended*
   - *no tenderness unless strangulation when tender over one area or over a hernia*
   - *intestinal (bowel) sounds increase when the pain comes.*
4. Ectopic pregnancy or severe 'Pelvic inflammatory disease'
   (a) *missed or late or irregular or heavy periods*, and
   (b) *lower abdominal pain*, and
   (c) *vaginal bleeding or discharge* and
   (d) *uterus enlarged and also tender* or
   - *a mass or tenderness next to the uterus* or
   - *tenderness of all the abdomen often with guarding and rigidity and no intestinal sounds* and

   (e) *pulse fast, BP low, pallor, normal temperature – if there is bleeding (ectopic, miscarriage, antepartum haemorrhage)* or
   - *pulse fast and temperature raised – if there is infection (septic abortion, pelvic inflammatory disease and sometimes ectopic pregnancy).*
5. Antepartum haemorrhage.
   (See an obstetrics book.)
6. Acute retention of urine that you cannot cure with catheterisation of bladder and treatment of urinary infection.
7. Ureteric colic (non-urgent).

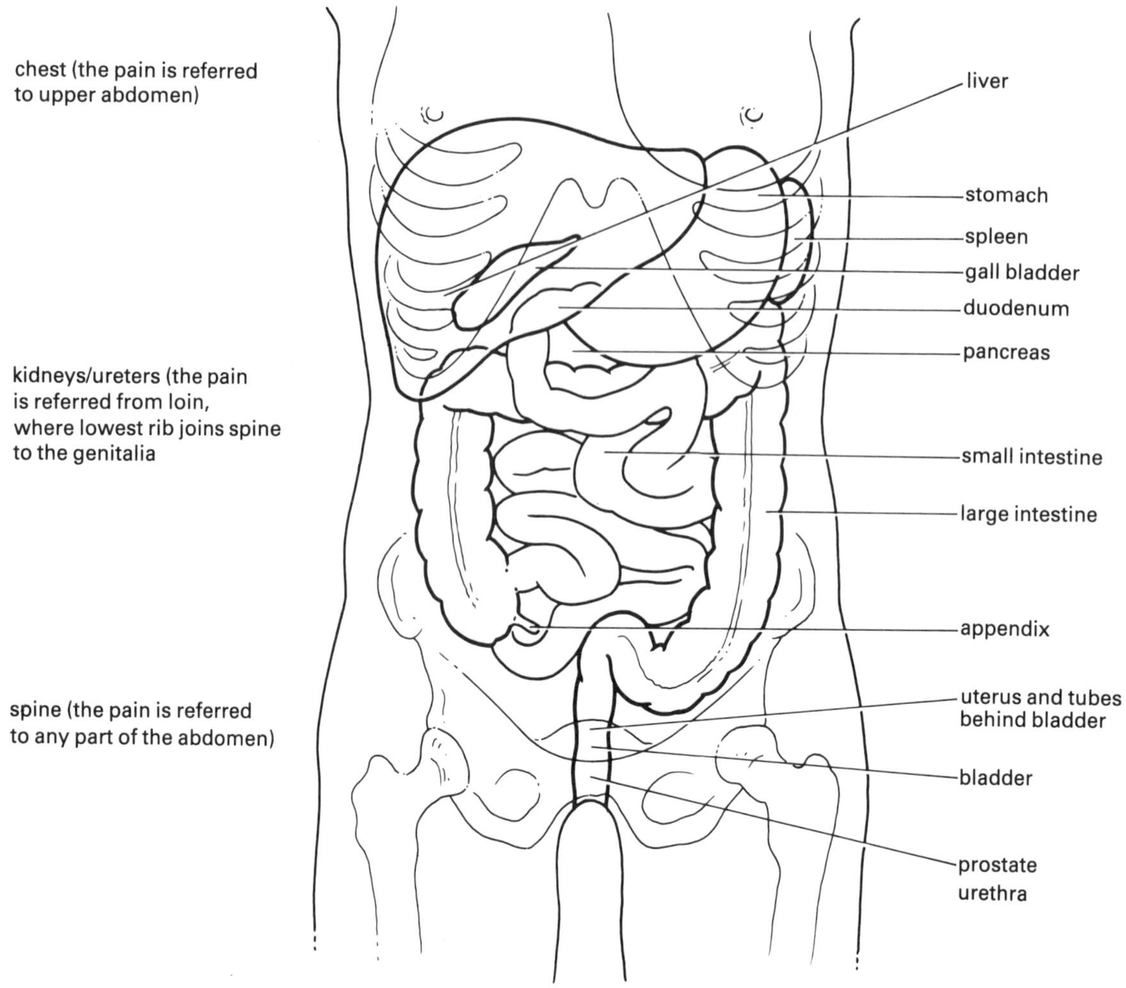

chest (the pain is referred to upper abdomen)

kidneys/ureters (the pain is referred from loin, where lowest rib joins spine to the genitalia

spine (the pain is referred to any part of the abdomen)

liver

stomach

spleen

gall bladder

duodenum

pancreas

small intestine

large intestine

appendix

uterus and tubes behind bladder

bladder

prostate

urethra

Figure 36.2 The position of organs which can cause abdominal pain.

Acute 'surgical' abdomen

(Peritonitis, bleeding into peritoneum, obstruction of the intestine)

1. The patient must not eat or drink.
2. Start an IV drip.
   - Give IV fluids as necessary.
   - If there is shock – see Chapter 27 page 378.
   - If bleeding into the peritoneum is probable (you suspect it from the history, examination, progressive pallor, rising pulse, etc. in absence of evidence of severe infection) – see Chapter 27 page 379 and arrange emergency transfer for urgent blood transfusion.
   - If there is dehydration – see Chapter 23 page 285.
   - If only maintenance fluids are needed $\frac{1}{5}$ normal saline in 4% dextrose 1 litre each 8–12 hours.
   - If you do not know if the patient is taking enough fluid and patient cannot pass urine, insert an indwelling urethral catheter and measure the urine passed every hour (it should be > 30 ml/hour). Increase the IV fluids until the urine passed is > 30 ml/hour.
3. Give chloramphenicol, unless infection is not probable.
   - Give chloramphenicol 2 g immediately and then 1 g every 6 hours.
   - Give by IVI if there is shock or a drip running; and by IMI to other cases.
4. Give an antimalarial drug by injection as indicated (see Chapter 13 page 61).

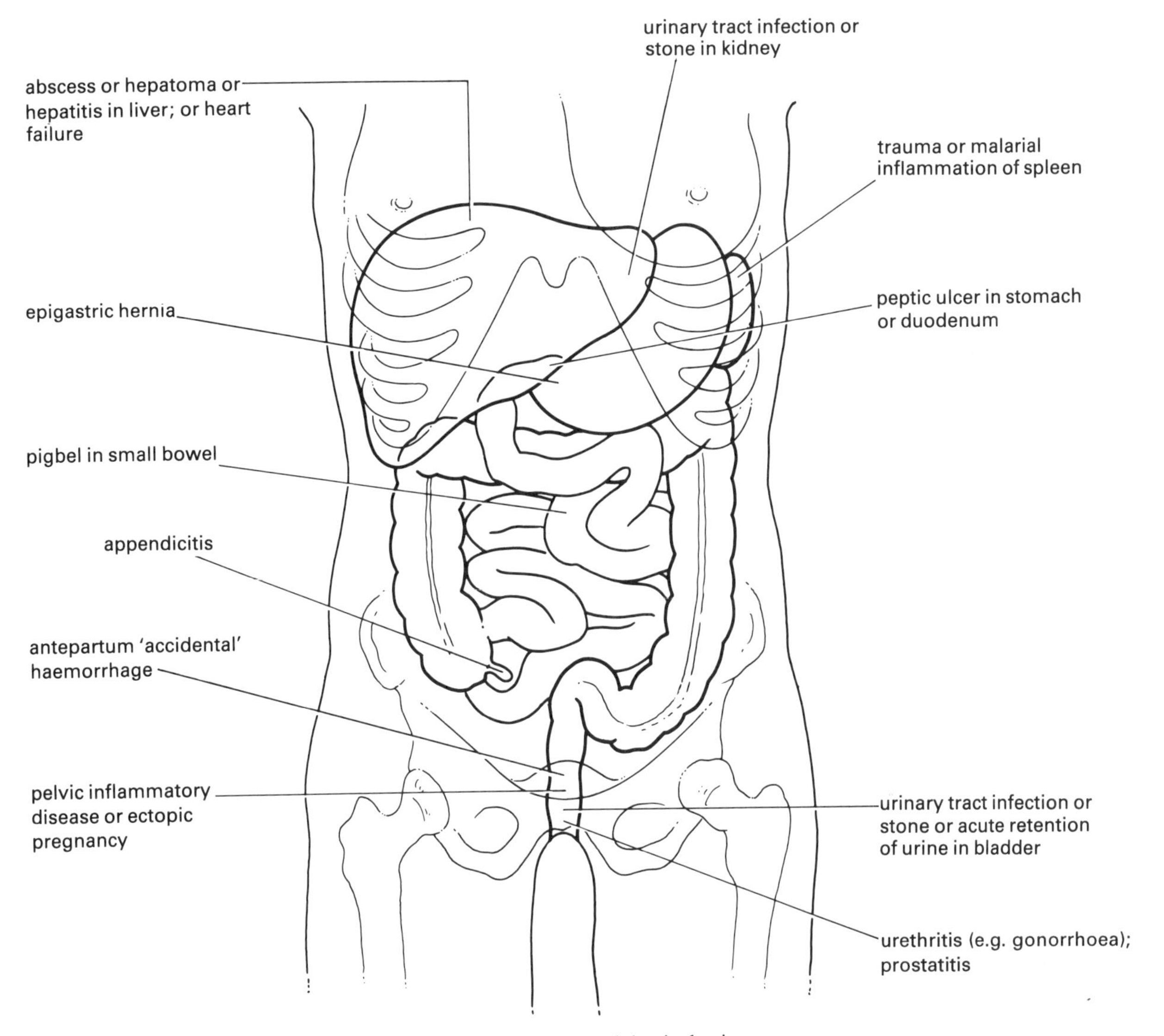

Figure 36.3 Common conditions of organs which cause constant abdominal pain.

5. Do intragastric suction if there is evidence of intestinal obstruction (repeated vomiting and distension and colic) or paralysis (repeated vomiting and distension).
   - Put a tube through the nose into the stomach.
   - Aspirate (suck out) all the fluid and gas possible, immediately and every hour.
   - Leave the end of the tube open, and hang it over the side of the bed, lower than the patient. Fluid will drain from it.
   - Check the volume of all the fluid which comes out of the tube, and is vomited.
6. Treat the underlying condition.
   - Abdominal surgery will almost always be necessary. Transfer to a Medical Officer urgently for the necessary surgery.
   - In enteritis necroticans (pigbel) and a few other conditions, the above treatment may be enough.
7. Treat any other conditions present, or any complications that develop, in the usual ways.
8. Transfer the patient urgently (emergency) to a Medical Officer at a hospital. First get the patient's written permission for any tests, treatment or surgery which may be necessary.
9. Give analgesics unless a Medical Office can see the patient almost immediately. (If so, do not give

analgesics because they may make the tenderness and signs in the abdomen less.)
Give IM pethidine

- 75 mg to a small adult (< 50 kg)
- 100 mg to a large adult (> 50 kg)

Abdominal tenderness – guarding – rigidity

You discover abdominal tenderness, guarding and rigidity during palpation of the abdomen.

> Palpate the abdomen to discover three things.
> 1. Tenderness. If it is present, where is it? Also, are rebound tenderness and guarding and rigidity present?
> 2. Are normal organs enlarged? – liver, spleen, uterus and bladder.
> 3. Are there masses or lumps in other places including hernia and lymph glands
>
> Do palpation only *after* inspection

Palpate first for tenderness – guarding– rigidity like this:

1. Be gentle. If you hurt the patient with your first palpation, the patient may not relax again. The examination will then be difficult.
2. First move the *palm* of your hand gently over the whole abdomen. This helps the patient to relax. Also you can often find an area of tenderness by feeling the patient's abdominal wall muscles contract (and seeing his eyes or face muscles also contract) when your hand moves over the tender area.
3. Then palpate with the *palm* of your hand held flat and not the tips of the fingers (Figures 36.4, 36.5 and 36.6). Again, look at the patient's face and feel the abdominal muscles contract to find tender parts.
   Palpate carefully all over the abdomen. Do not forget the loins (kidney area at the back), or any other part.
   Start in a place which is probably normal. Palpate a place you suspect is abnormal last.
4. If you do not find any tenderness with 2 and 3, then palpate more deeply. Again, palpate all areas of the abdomen.
5. If it is difficult to decide exactly where the most tender place is, you can do a gentle 'one finger palpation' in the place where you found the tenderness. If you look at the patient's face, feel the abdominal muscles contract and ask the patient where it hurts most, you can usually decide which is the most tender place with 'one finger palpation' (Figure 36.7).

Causes of abdominal tenderness – guarding – rigidity

Inflammation, swelling or stretching of an organ or of the peritoneum causes *tenderness* on palpation over the organ or periteoneum. If the condition is mild, tenderness may be the only sign that you find.

You can find *rebound tenderness* if you quickly remove the palpating hand (which is pressing firmly on the abdomen) from the abdomen. The release of the pressure on the contents of the abdomen causes movement and, therefore, pain over the inflamed or stretched organ or peritoneum (e.g. in appendicitis, if you suddenly lift your hand off the abdomen during palpation of the left iliac fossa, the patient will feel pain in the right iliac fossa, where the inflamed appendix is).

If the inflammation or swelling or stretching of the organ or peritoneum is more severe and acute then *involuntary guarding* may occur. When you do the palpation, the overlying muscles contract. This stops the palpation putting more pressure on the affected organ or peritoneum and causing more pain. The patient cannot completely stop this muscle contraction, even if you help him to relax (e.g. by talking to him) or he tries himself. (This is different from voluntary guarding which is often caused by worry, and goes if the patient does not think about his abdomen when you palpate it.)

Rigidity occurs if the inflammation, swelling or stretching of the organ or the peritoneum is even more severe and acute. The muscles do not relax at any time.

Localised tenderness – guarding – rigidity occur over the affected organ or peritoneum. The exact place of this tenderness usually shows which organ is affected, see Figure 36.8 (e.g. right iliac fossa, appendix, appendicitis; epigastrium, stomach/duodenum, peptic ulcer).

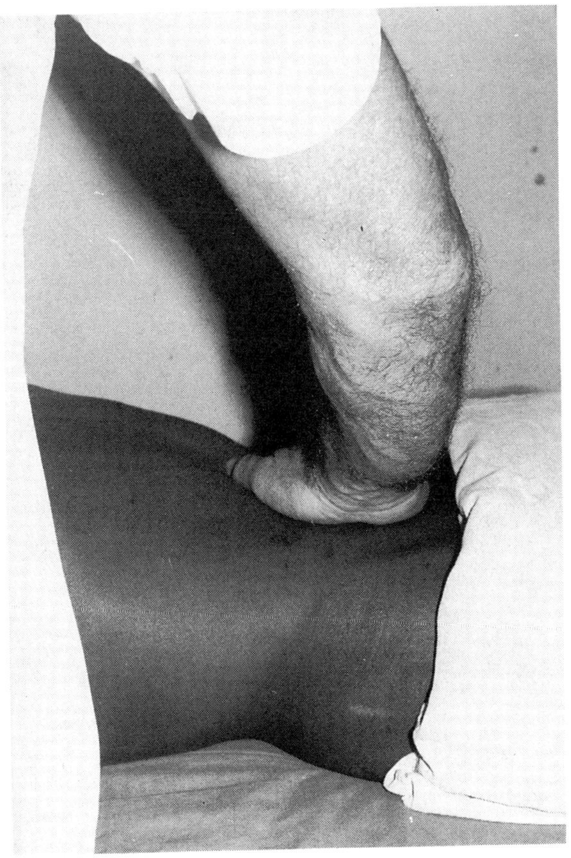

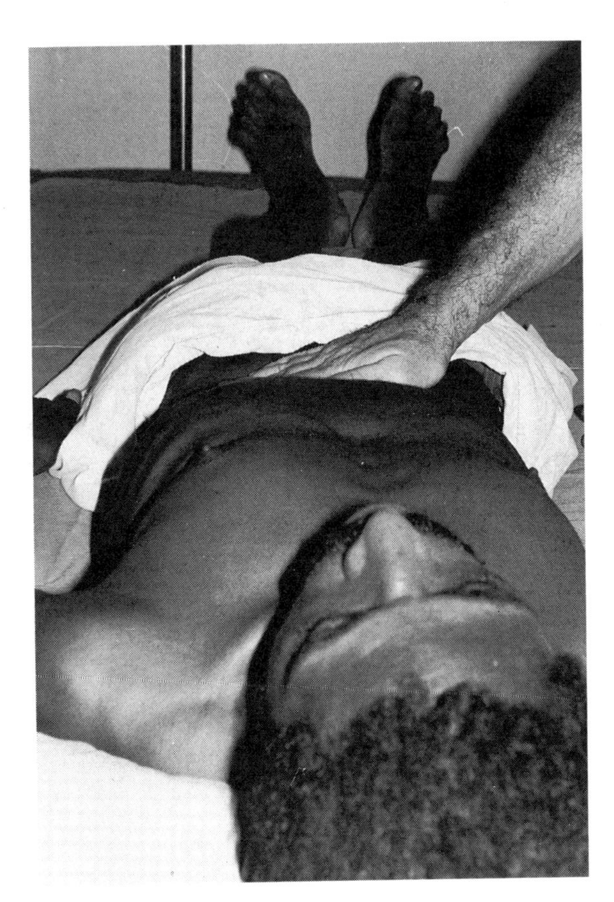

Figure 36.4 and 36.5 The proper way to palpate an abdomen, with the palm of the hand held flat. Do not bend the fingers, or use the tips of the fingers.

Abdominal mass

To find out what an abdominal mass is, you must decide:

1. Where is the mass? *or*
   In which organ or structure is the mass?
2. What type is the mass? *or*
   Is this mass congenital or traumatic or inflammatory or neoplastic or degenerative, etc. (see Chapter 4 pages 11–13)?

A full history and examination is necessary. A pelvic examination 'PR' and/or 'PV' is often also necessary.

It is also usually necessary to:

- test the urine for protein, pus, blood and bile,
- look at the stools,
- look at any vomit, and
- look at any vaginal discharge.

Where is the mass?

Think of all the structures and organs in the area which could be affected and could contain the mass.

Start at the skin on the anterior (front) of the abdominal wall, and think of all of the organs under it to the skin on the posterior (back) abdominal wall. See Figure 36.8.

Remember that if the patient contracts his anterior abdominal muscles (e.g. by lifting his head when he is lying on his back), any mass that you can still feel must be anterior to (in front of) the muscles. You cannot easily feel masses behind the hard contracted muscles.

If you think that a certain organ probably contains the mass, then look for other signs in history, examination and tests to show if the organ has abnormal function and disease, or not: e.g. if you think the mass is in the pelvic colon, then ask carefully about bowel colic, constipation or diarrhoea, blood in the

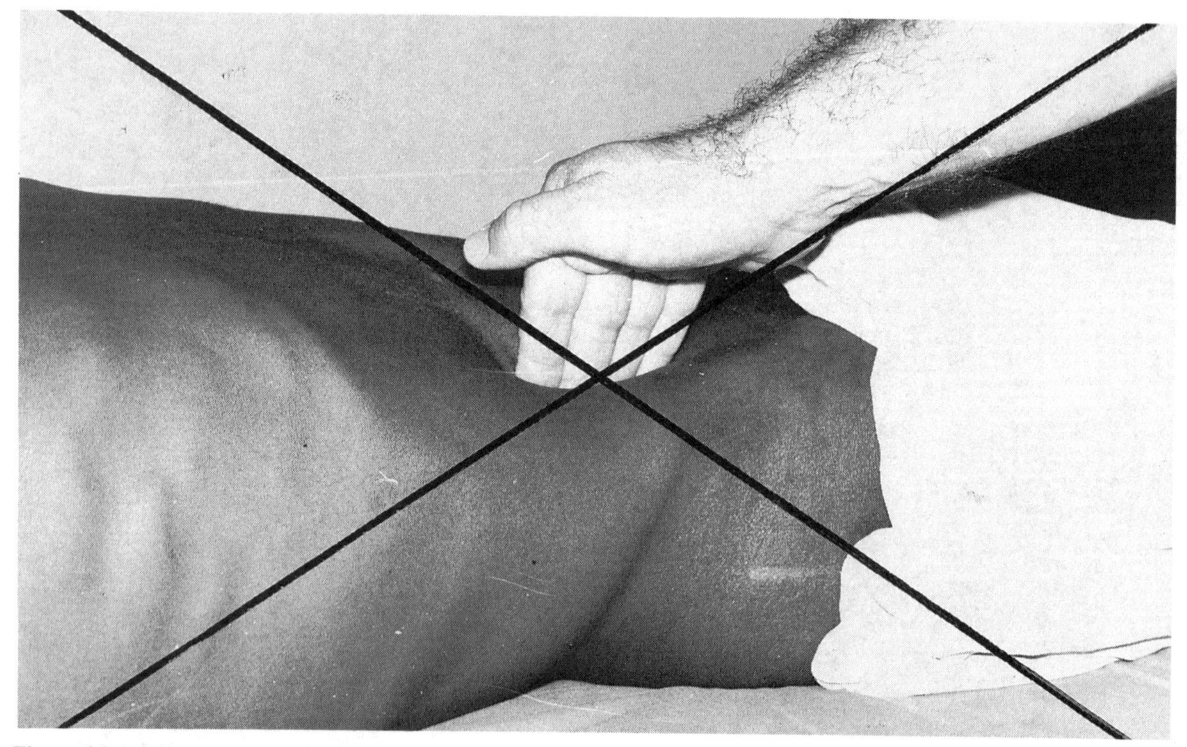

Figure 36.6 The wrong way to palpate an abdomen. *Use the palm of the hand.* DO NOT USE THE TIPS OF THE FINGERS LIKE THIS.

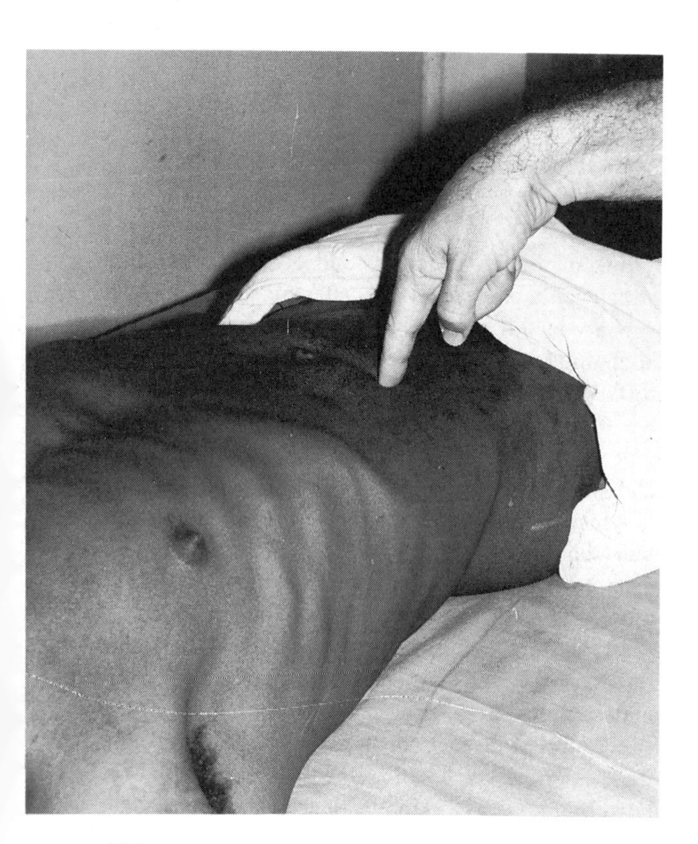

stool, weight loss, etc.; examine for weight loss; do a careful rectal examination to try to feel if the mass is in the bowel wall; and carefully look at the stool for blood.

What type is the mass?

The mass may be congenital or traumatic or inflammatory or neoplastic or degenerative etc. in any of the organs in that area.

Some types of mass are more probable in some organs than in others (e.g. the spleen is probably enlarged by malarial inflammation or leishmaniasis or lymphomatous cancers or blood disease – other types of mass such as congenital or degenerative are not probable).

For inflammatory masses, see in Chapter 3 page 9. For neoplastic masses, see Chapter 3 page 10 and below.

Figure 36.7 One finger palpation. Only do this when you have found a tender place with normal palpation, but you cannot decide which is the most tender place. Press the point of one finger gently onto different parts of the tender place like this, until you find the most tender area.

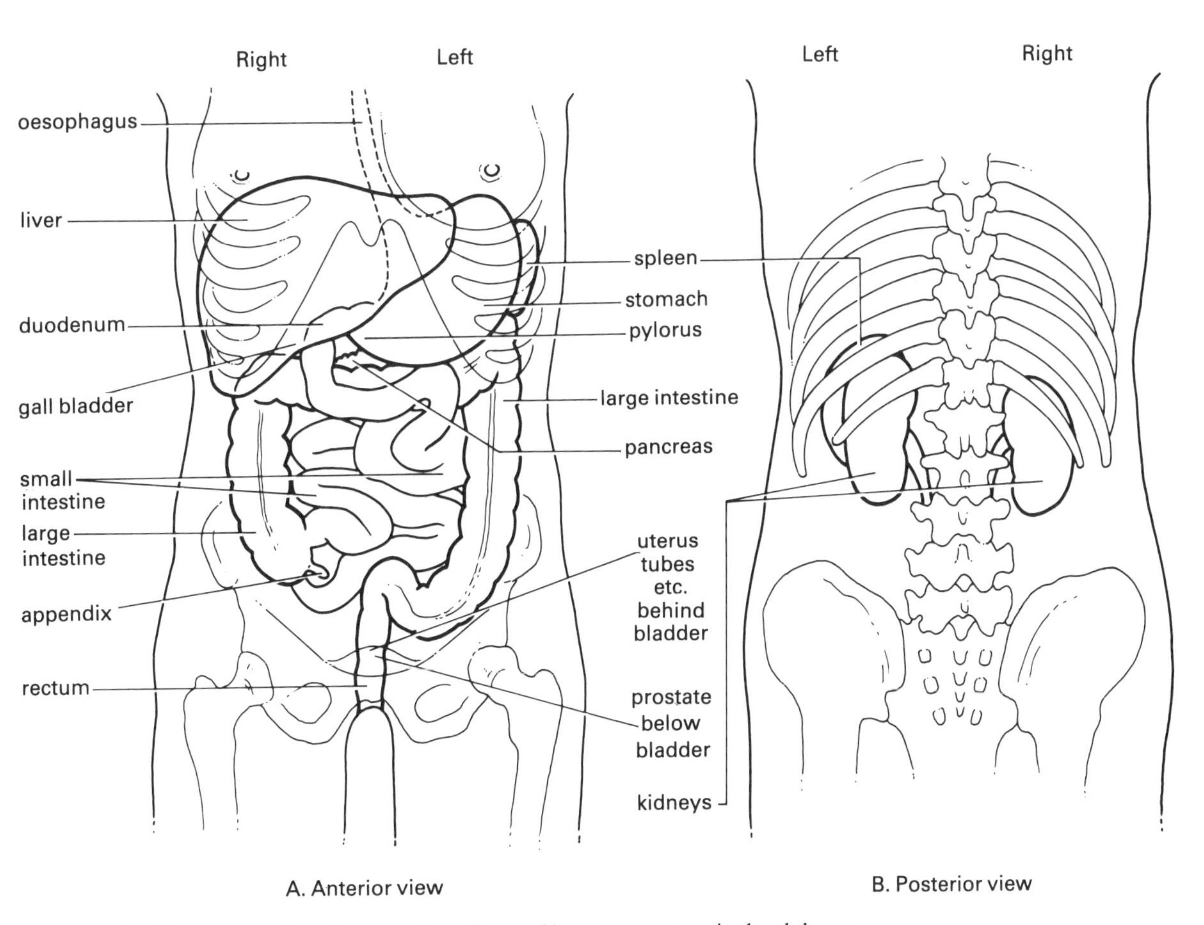

Figure 36.8 Diagrams to show the normal positions of important organs in the abdomen.

You can find other signs of the type of mass in history, examination and tests, e.g. fever, fast pulse, etc. if it is an inflammatory mass; or weight loss, enlarged hard fixed lymph nodes etc. if it is a neoplastic mass.

Common causes of abdominal masses

> You can find the causes of most masses if you answer these two questions:
> 1. Where is the mass or in which organ or structure is the mass? and
> 2. What type is the mass? and then look for
>   - other signs of disease in the suspected organ, and
>   - other signs of the nature of the pathological process suspected.

Common causes of abdominal masses include:

1. *Generalised enlargement* of:
   - liver
   - spleen
   - uterus
   - bladder
   - kidney
   - lymph glands on posterior abdominal wall
2. *Inflammatory masses* (e.g. abscesses) of:
   - any of the organs in 1 (above)
   - part of the gastrointestinal tract, or
   - the peritoneum
3. *Neoplastic masses* of:
   - any of the organs in 1 (above)
   - part of the gastrointestinal tract, or
   - the peritoneum

Especially common causes of masses in the abdomen include:

1. *In the right iliac fossa*
   - appendicitis/appendix abscess

- amoeboma of the intestine
- cancer of the intestine
- tuberculosis of the intestine

2. *In the left iliac fossa*
   - amoeboma of the intestine
   - schistosomiasis of the intestine
   - cancer of the intestine
   - diverticulitis/diverticular diseases
3. *In the lower abdomen*
   - distended bladder
   - pregnant uterus
   - ectopic pregnancy
   - pelvic abscess
   - cancer of the ovary or uterus
4. *In the left upper abdomen*
   - spleen (malaria, hyperreactive splenomegaly syndrome, visceral leishmaniasis, trypanosomiasis, schistosomiasis, lymphoma, thalassaemia, sickle cell anaemia and other blood disorders, subcapsular rupture of the spleen.
   - kidney tumour or infection (e.g. tuberculosis; or swelling caused by a blocked ureter)
5. *In the right upper abdomen*
   - liver (amoebic abscess, hepatoma)
   - kidney tumour or infection (e.g. tuberculosis; or swelling caused by a blocked ureter)
6. *In the epigastrium*
   - cancer of the stomach
   - liver (amoebic abscess, hepatoma, secondary cancer, leishmaniasis, trypanosomiasis; tuberculosis but also sometimes a normal large left lobe of the spleen.)

You may mistake normal structures for pathological masses (see Figure 36.9).

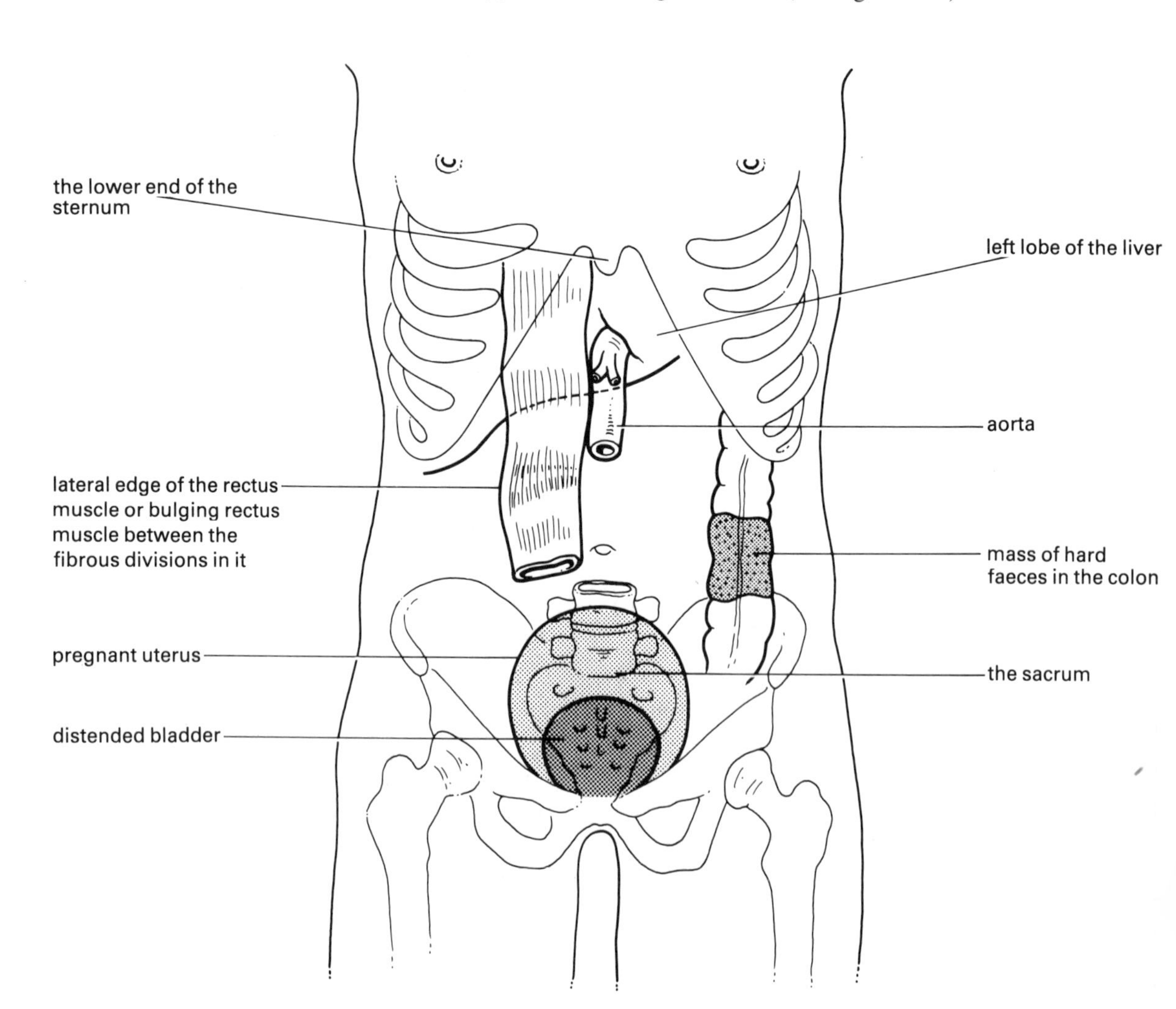

Figure 36.9 Normal structures which you may mistake for pathological masses.

Generalised abdominal swelling

Causes of swelling of the whole abdomen include five groups of conditions:

1. A solid mass inside the abdomen
   (a) *Generalised enlargement of any organ*, especially:
   - the liver
   - the spleen
   - the uterus (or ovary or tubes)
   - the bladder
   - the kidney, or
   - the lymph glands on the posterior abdominal wall

   (b) *Any large inflammatory mass* of:
   - any of the above organs, or
   - part of gastrointestinal tract, or
   - the peritoneum

   (c) *Any large neoplastic mass* of:
   - any of the above organs, or
   - part of the gastrointestinal tract, or
   - the peritoneum

2. Fluid inside the abdomen (see this page)
   (a) *Fluid in the peritoneal cavity* (ascites, blood or pus)
   Ascites (clear fluid)
   - cirrhosis of liver
   - schistosomiasis
   - heart failure
   - nephrotic syndrome
   - kwashiorkor
   - tuberculous peritonitis
   - cancer of peritoneum

   Blood
   - bleeding ectopic pregnancy
   - ruptured spleen, liver or other organ
   - tuberculous peritonitis
   - cancer of the peritoneum

   Pus
   - peritonitis

   (b) *Fluid in an ovarian cyst*

3. Gas and fluid in the intestines
   - Obstruction of the intestines
   - Paralytic ileus
   - Enteritis necroticans ('pigbel')
   - Peritonitis

4. Fat

5. Abdominal wall swellings
   - Hernia
   - Lipoma
   - Cellulitis

Inguinal swellings

Causes of inguinal swellings include:

- hernia (see a surgery book),
- lymph gland enlargement (see Chapter 22 pages 263–5)
- inflammation – cellulitis, abscess, etc., and
- traumatic swelling.

'Shifting dullness'

Shifting dullness is a sign which shows that *fluid (water or blood or pus)* is *in the peritoneal cavity.*

For *causes* of fluid (ascites, blood and pus) in the peritoneal cavity, see causes of 'Generalised abdominal swelling' (above).

Test for shifting dullness in all cases when the *abdomen is distended* or when *ascites or blood or pus* in the peritoneal cavity is possible.

The patient lies on his back, facing up. Percuss the abdomen as in Figure 36.10. The abdomen is resonant (hollow) on top and dull on both sides, as the gas in the intestine floats that part of the intestine to the top and the fluid runs down on both sides.

Find the place where resonance changes to dullness and mark it with a pen or chalk (see Figure 36.10).

In Figure 36.11A the patient is lying on his back facing up. The place where dullness changed to resonance is marked with an unbroken chalk line. In Figure 36.11B the patient is lying on his side. Fluid from the other side of the abdomen has run down to join fluid on this side of the abdomen. The new place where dullness changed to resonance is marked with a dotted chalk line. The 'dullness' has 'shifted' (moved) up. The patient has fluid in the abdomen.

The patient then rolls on to the other side. The dullness will then move to the other side of the abdomen. The places where dullness was marked will now be resonant. The dullness will now be in the area posterior (behind) the line on the other side of the patient, and will also shift closer to the umbilicus.

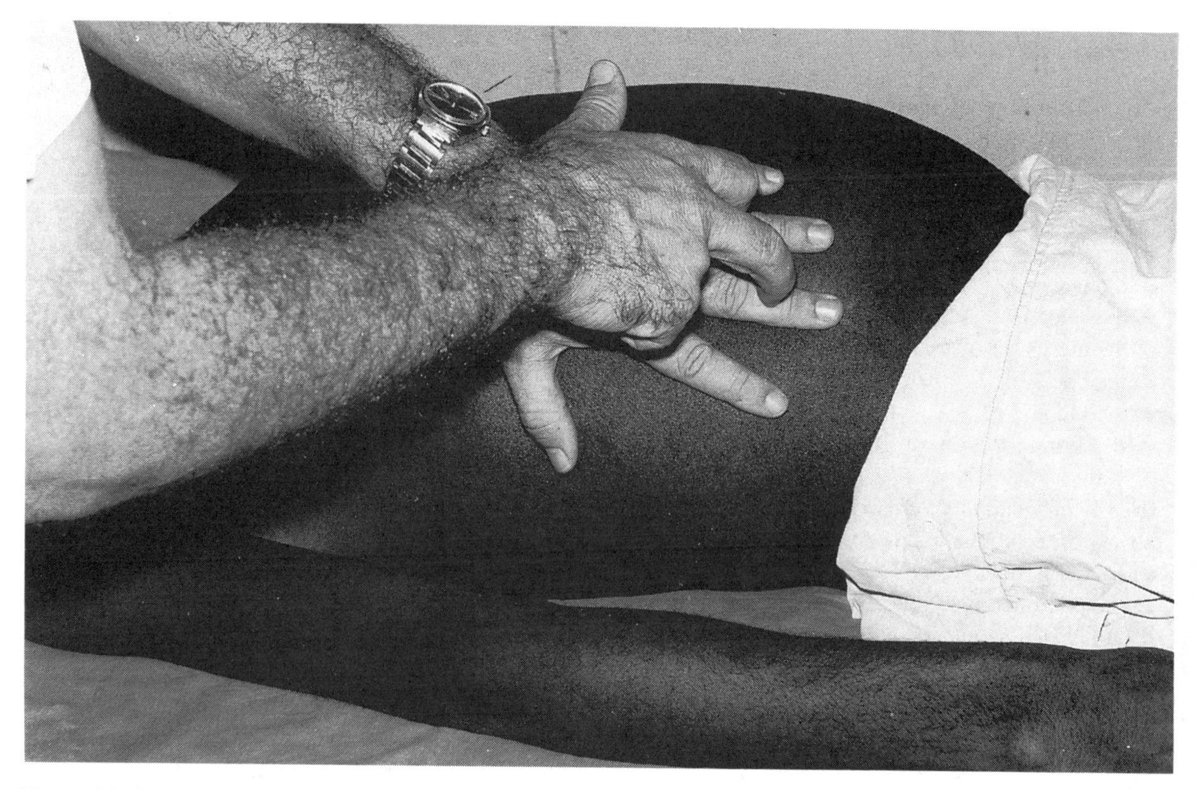

Figure 36.10 The method of percussion of the abdomen for fluid. Note that the finger on the abdomen is kept parallel to the patient's bed.

> Note that shifting dullness only means that fluid is present in the peritoneal cavity. It does not diagnose what type of fluid is present in the peritoneal cavity. Use other symptoms and signs and tests to find out what type of fluid is causing the shifting dullness.

The main differential diagnosis is an ovarian cyst (Figure 36.12).

Bowel sounds

Intestinal or bowel sounds may be:

- normal, or
- increased, or
- decreased or absent.

Intestinal sounds are increased when the patient feels colic, when there is:

- obstruction of the intestine or
- gastroenteritis.

Intestinal sounds are decreased or absent if there is:

1. pus in the peritoneal cavity (peritonitis from any cause), or
2. blood in the peritoneal cavity (e.g. bleeding ectopic pregnancy or ruptured spleen or other organ), or
3. paralytic ileus.

Listen for at least two minutes (10 minutes if possible), before you decide that bowel sounds are reduced or absent.

Figure 36.11 A and B (below) These figures show how to find if there is fluid in the abdomen (see text for details).

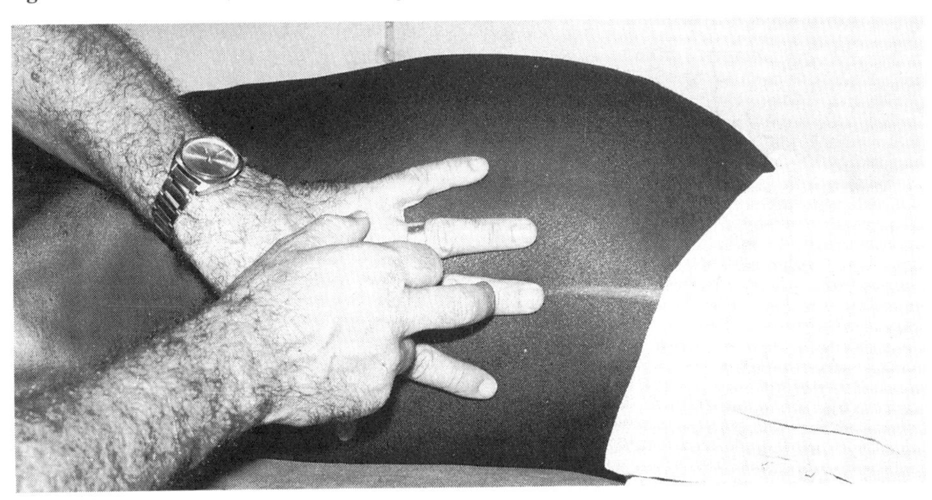

B

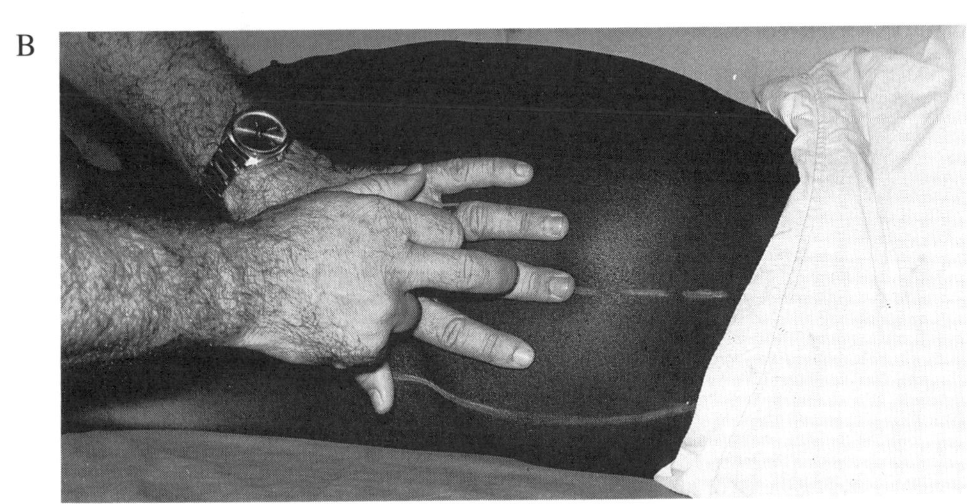

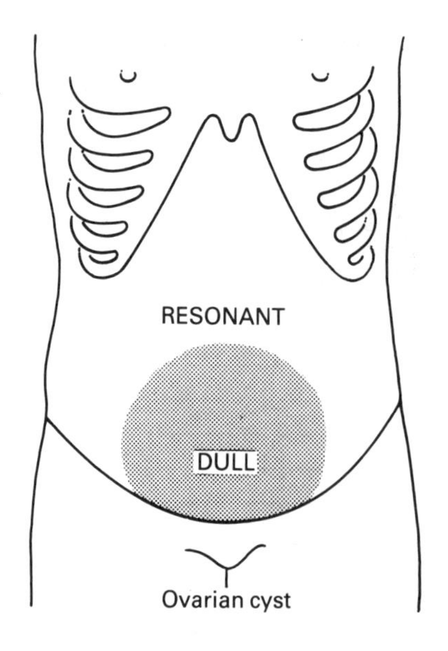

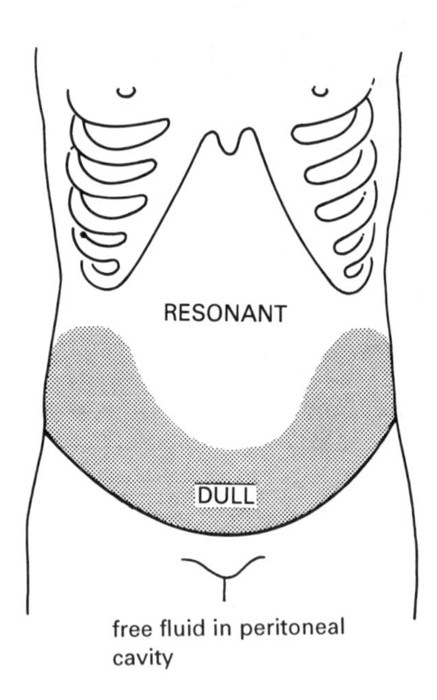

Figure 36.12 Diagrams to show one way of diagnosing an ovarian cyst or fluid in the peritoneal cavity. The patient is lying on her back facing up.

37

Emergency Resuscitation

Inhaled foreign body

If the foreign body is in the larynx or trachea, it will cause obstruction of the airway which may be complete or not complete.

If the obstruction is complete the patient usually makes violent breathing movements, with indrawing of the ribs; cyanosis and death quickly occur. Sometimes complete obstruction causes only sudden unexpected unconsciousness and no breathing and then death.

If the obstruction is not complete, there is severe shortness of breath, stridor and indrawing of the ribs on breathing in.

Obstruction of the larynx or trachea may occur when the patient is eating ('food choking'). Suspect it in every case of respiratory distress or loss of consciousness which occurs during eating. It is also common if the patient had a foreign body in his mouth or if he was drunk. It is more common in patients with chronic bronchitis.

If you suspect obstruction, act immediately.

If the patient cannot get the foreign body out by coughing, then you should try to get it out by bending the person over and hitting them hard on the back, between the shoulder blades, with the heel of your hand.

If the patient is small, you can lift him up by the waist leaving his chest and head hanging down, and then hit him very hard on his back (between his shoulder blades) with the heel of your hand. This will force some air out of the lungs and should expel the foreign body.

If the person is unconscious check that the airway is open (see page 504), roll the person onto their side and slap them on the back as described above.

Only if hitting on the back does not work should you try the *abdominal thrust* method as follows.

If the patient is standing or sitting, stand behind the patient and put your arms round his upper abdomen. Make a fist of one of your hands and hold this fist with the other hand. Put the fist on the patient's anterior abdominal wall between the umbilicus and the ribs. Then pull up and in with the arms quickly and strongly towards the back and chest of the patient (see Figure 37.1). Repeat two or three times, if necessary. This is not just squeezing the patient – it is like

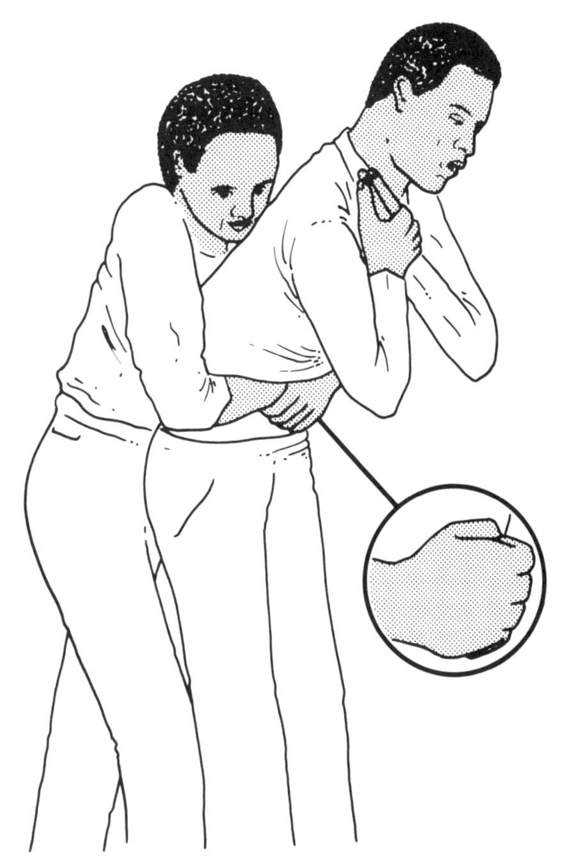

Figure 37.1 The abdominal thrust method of forcing a foreign body out of the trachea or larynx.

a punch; but with the fist starting on the abdominal wall and helped by the other hand. This should force air out of the lungs through the trachea and the larynx and expel (push out) the foreign body (see Figure 37.1).

If the patient is unconscious turn the person onto his back, make sure the airway is open and do the abdominal thrust downward using the heel of one hand with the other hand on top of it.

If these methods do not work, you can sometimes get the foreign body out of the throat, if you push your fingers down deep into the back of the patient's throat and pull out what is there.

Artificial ventilation (artificial 'respiration'), heart stimulation and external cardiac (heart) massage

Artificial ventilation is necessary if the patient cannot breathe enough.

This is done only when the patient is:

1. unconsciousness, *and*
2. not breathing or breathing with only a few breaths (even if deep).

Causes include:

- near drowning,
- paralysis from snake bite,
- an unconscious patient whose airway becomes blocked,
- very deep unconsciousness (especially after a drug overdose),
- sometimes after anaesthetics or operations,
- cardiac arrest (stopping of heart), and
- others.

Heart stimulation and possible external massage is necessary if the heart has stopped.

This is done only when the patient is unconscious *and* the pulse is absent.

Causes include:

- electrocution,
- reaction to drugs,
- shock that is not treated,
- low oxygen from any cause,
- breathing stops and no one gives artificial ventilation,
- myocardial infarction (heart attack),
- pulmonary embolus, and
- others.

Do artificial ventilation and heart stimulation or external cardiac massage *only if the patient may recover and return to normal life.* The underlying condition must be treatable. The patient must have collapsed suddenly or unexpectedly collapsed. Do not do these things if the patient is slowly getting worse, even with all possible treatment.

> *If* the patient is unconscious and you cannot feel a pulse (even if there is some breathing)
> or
> *if* the patient is unconscious and not breathing or is breathing with only a few breaths (even if you can feel a pulse)
> *then* emergency resuscitation is necessary. You must start artificial ventilation and, if necessary, heart stimulation or external cardiac massage within 3 minutes.
> If you do not do this, the patient will die or have severe brain damage from which he cannot recover.

Artificial ventilation of the lungs

Clear the airway

Extend the head (or move the head back on the top of the neck). Hold the back of the neck with one hand and push the top of the head back with the other hand. This will bend the head back on the top of the neck as far as possible.

Push the angle of the jaw forward from behind *or* pull the jaw forward from under the front of the jaw. This positioning will stop the tongue from blocking the airway (see Figure 37.2).

Extract (get out) anything from the mouth or throat which could block and airway. Use your fingers (and, if necessary, a cloth).

Suck out the airway if you have a sucker (but do not leave the patient unattended while you find one).

Mouth-to-mouth ventilation

See pages 507–8 about 'barrier methods' to protect the health worker from infection from the patient.

- Separate the patient's lips.
- Hold the patient's nostrils together.
- Take a deep breath.

- Open your mouth widely (Figure 37.3).
- Seal your lips around the patient's mouth.
- Blow your breath into the patient's lungs.
- Look to see if the patient's chest rises as you blow air into the patient's lungs.
- Then remove your mouth from the patient's mouth.
- Look to see if the patient's chest falls when you stop blowing air into the patient's chest (Figure 37.4).

If the chest does not rise and fall check that

- the head is extended,
- the jaw is well forward, and
- the airway is not blocked by foreign bodies, and try the mouth-to-mouth ventilation again.

If the chest still does not rise and fall, turn the patient onto his side and hit the patient *hard* on the back between the shoulder blades with the side of your fist. This will force air in the lungs through the

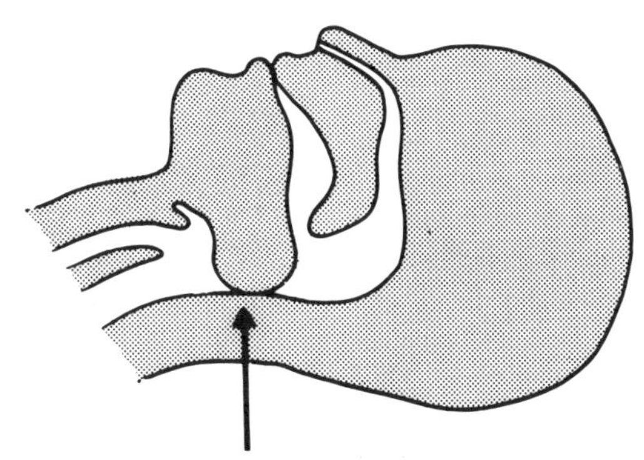

A The tongue is blocking the throat of an unconscious patient. Compare with B tongue

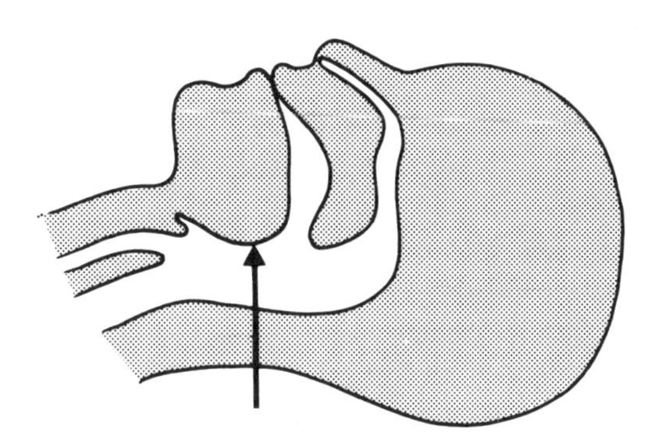

B Normal airway in a conscious patient

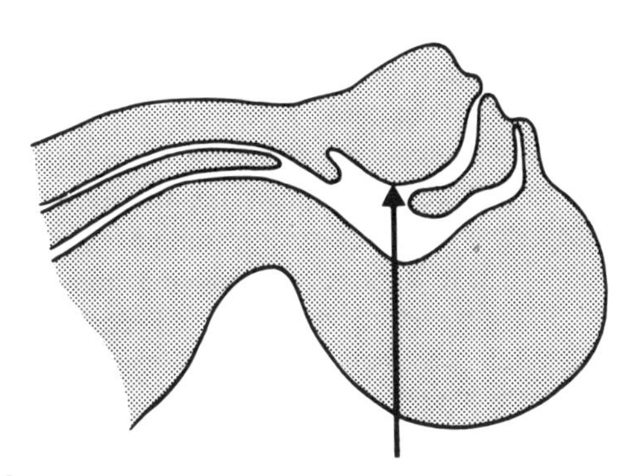

C The head extended and the jaw forward. In this position the tongue does not block the throat; the air passages are not obstructed, even in an unconscious patient

Figure 37.2 A, B and C. Diagrams to show how to stop the tongue blocking the airway of an unconscious person.

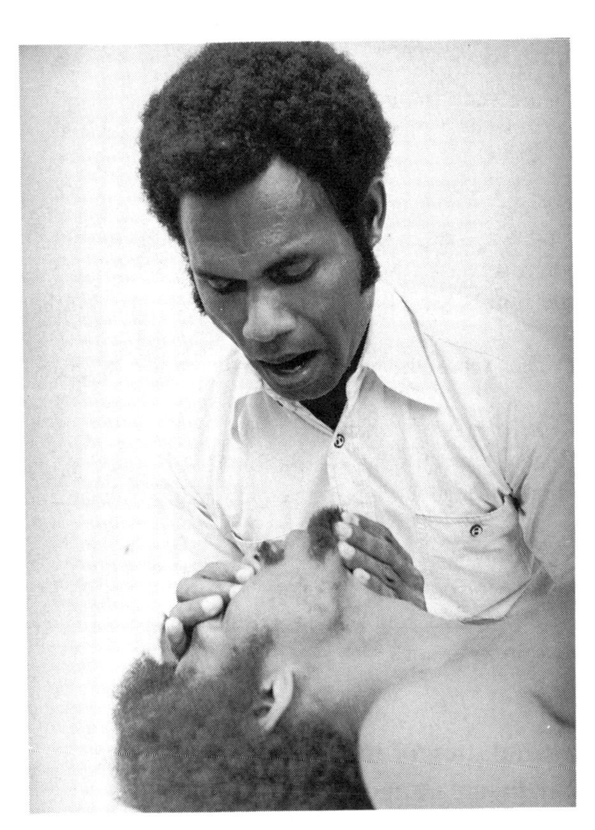

Figure 37.3 Patient ready for artificial ventilation. Note (1) airway cleared, (2) head extended, (3) jaw held forward, (4) nostrils held, (5) mouth open. It is safer now to also use a face shield. See Figures 37.7 and 37.8.

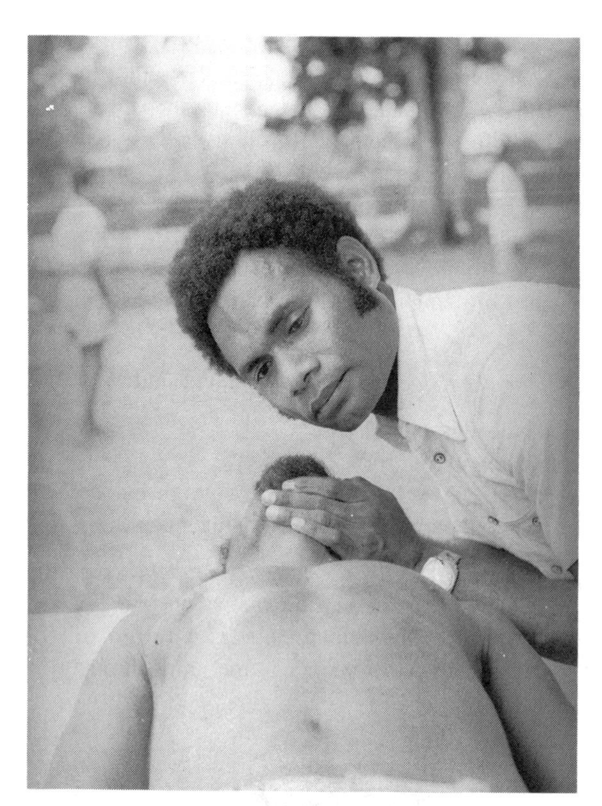

Figure 37.4 Health worker looking to see if the chest falls after he stopped blowing his breath into the patient.

airway and expel (push out) any foreign bodies in the lower airway, which are blocking the air going into the lungs. (See Figure 37.1 page 503 for another method.)

Then repeat the mouth-to-mouth ventilation again.

Continue artificial ventilation

Repeat the artificial ventilation 15–20 times every minute, i.e. about 3–4 seconds for each breath (in and out).

Check for cardiac arrest

After 4 breaths stop and check if the patient has a cardiac arrest or not.

Stimulation of the heart and external cardiac massage

> Feel for the pulse. If the patient is unconscious *and* has no pulse, the heart has stopped.

Stimulate the heart

Give a single hard quick blow with the side of the fist to the middle of the patient's sternum over the heart. This may start the heart.

Continue artificial ventilation for another 4 breaths.

Then check the pulse again. If the patient's heart is still stopped, hit the sternum again, 3–4 times in 3–4 seconds; and then give 4 breaths of artificial ventilation. Check the pulse again. If the patient's heart is still stopped, repeat all this 3–4 times.

If you can transfer the patient to a Medical Officer or a hospital *within minutes* (or less than 1 hour) and there are staff at the hospital who can do artificial ventilation and external cardiac massage, then start external cardiac massage, if you cannot start the heart as above. External cardiac massage is rarely successful in a health centre because you need special drugs and equipment to treat the patient.

Even if you do not do the external cardiac massage, continue the artificial ventilation because you may not have felt a weak pulse.

External cardiac massage

Put the patient on a hard surface, flat on his back.

Kneel beside the patient.

Put the heel of one hand on the lower part of the sternum, and put the heel of the other hand on top of the first hand (Figure 37.5).

Hold your arms straight and move backwards and forwards, using the body weight to push the sternum in, towards the backbone. (Do not lift the hand off the sternum.) Push the sternum down 3–5 cm (1–2 inches). This is one chest compression. You need about 20–30 kg of pressure in an adult. Do this at a rate of about 70 times a minute.

If two of you are giving artificial ventilation, one person does 5 chest compressions and the other person then does 1 chest inflation (mouth-to-mouth respiration). These 5 compressions and 1 inflation are 1 cycle. Keep repeating the cycle. Check for a pulse after 1 minute and then every 3 minutes.

If no one else is there to help you, give 15 chest compressions then 2 chest inflations (1 cycle) and repeat until someone comes to help. Check for a pulse after 1 minute (4 cycles) and then every 3 minutes (12 cycles).

Continue artificial ventilation until the patient

1. can breathe properly for himself, *or*
2. has been transferred to a Medical Officer, *or*
3. for more than 30 minutes the patient

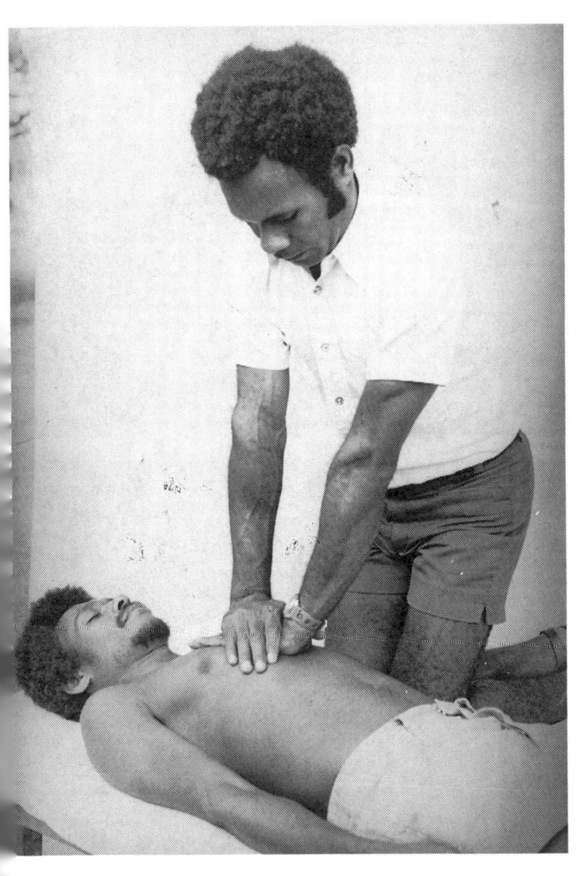

Figure 37.5 A health worker giving external cardiac massage. Note that the elbows are straight and that he uses the weight of his body to push down the sternum as he moves backwards and forwards (He is not pushing the sternum down by bending and straightening his elbows.)

- has not tried to take a breath himself, and
- has had no pulse without ECM, and
- has widely dilated pupils, and
- is obviously dead.

Continue external cardiac massage until the patient

1. has good pulse and BP himself *or*
2. has been transferred to a Medical Officer *or*
3. for more than 30 minutes
   - has had no pulse without ECM, and
   - has widely dilated pupils, and
   - is obviously dead.

Barrier methods to try to prevent cross-inflection during mouth-to-mouth ventilation

Special devices have been produced to try to reduce the risk of infection of the health worker by HIV and HBV (and tuberculosis and other) organisms from infected patients.

The risk of infection is very small unless the patient has blood on his face or in his mouth and the health worker has a cut or sore on his lips or mouth. There is also as yet no published scientific evidence that these devices do protect the health worker. However, these devices should give some protection and if possible should be used.

It is important that you find out from your Health Department what the risks are in your country, what special precautions should be taken and what are you to do about a device for mouth-to-mouth ventilation. If you are to use a device, then you must make sure you are trained how to use it correctly and always have one with you so that you can use it in an emergency.

Face masks (Figure 37.6) are probably the safest for the health worker; but are expensive, difficult to carry and difficult to use correctly.

A face shield (Figures 37.7 and 37.8) has a plastic sheet, which covers the patient's nose and mouth, and

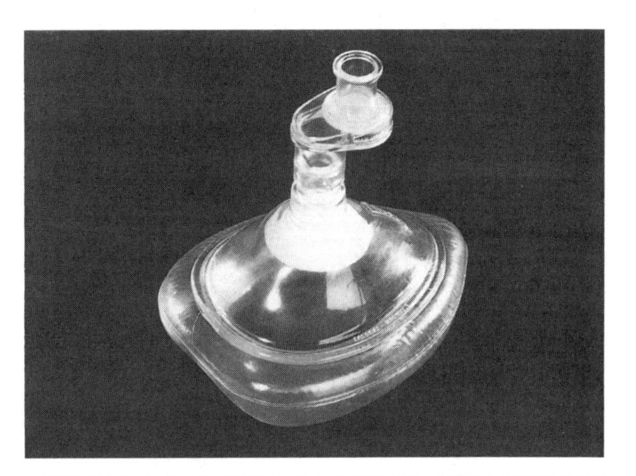

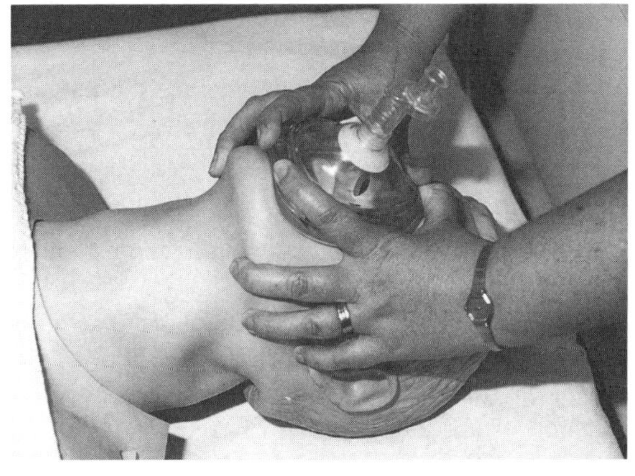

Figure 37.6 A and B. A typical face mask with valve (Laerdal Pocket Mask).

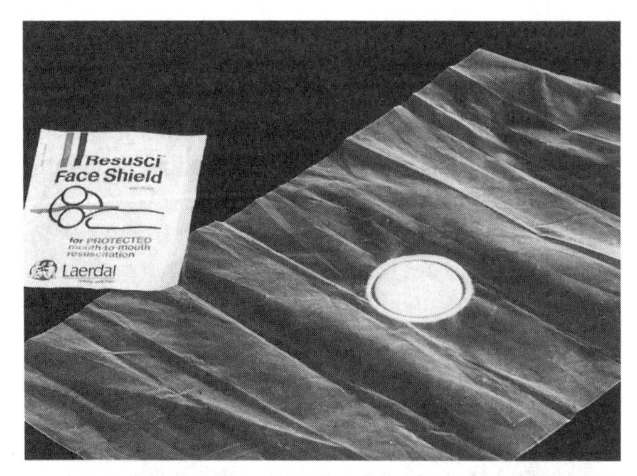

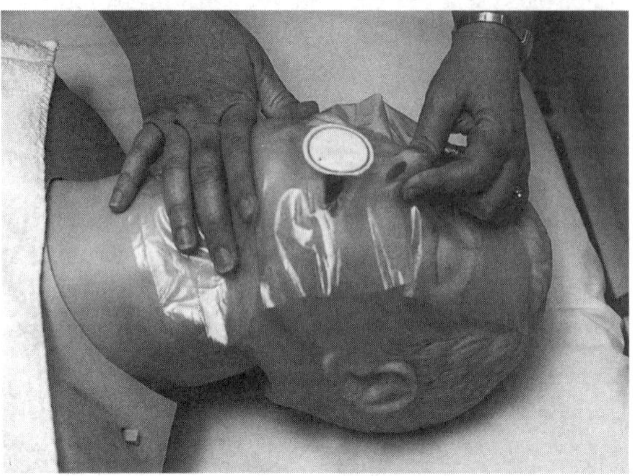

Figure 37.7 A and B. A typical face shield with filter (Laerdal Face Shield).

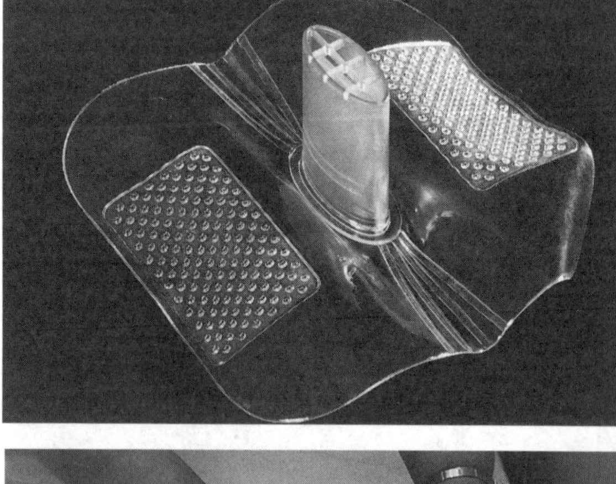

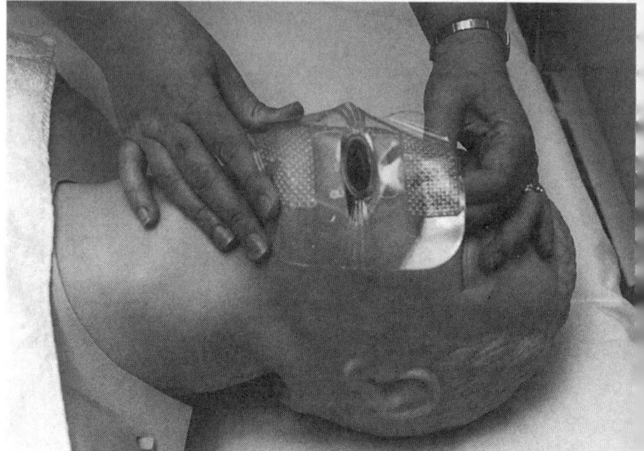

Figure 37.8 A and B. A typical face shield with valve (CPR Microshield).

has a central filter or valve, which goes over the patient's mouth, through which the health worker blows.

Near drowning

Start resuscitation immediately you see the patient, even before he is brought out of the water.

Resuscitation includes:

1. Clear the airway (see page 504).
2. Give mouth-to-mouth ventilation, if the patient is not breathing properly (see page 504).
3. Stimulate the heart and give external cardiac massage, if the heart has stopped (see page 506).
4. Change from mouth-to-mouth ventilation to ventilation with a self-inflatable bag (e.g. an Air Viva or Ambu-Bag) and oxygen as soon as possible.
5. Make sure the patient's temperature is not low. If rectal temperature is 35°C or less, warm the patient with heated blankets or by other means. Keep all near-drowned patients warm with a temperature of about 37°C.
6. If all this does not cause return of normal respiratio and heart beat, and if the patient is still alive, and i you can continue resuscitation while you transfe the patient to a hospital or Medical Officer's care then continue resuscitation and arrange urgen (emergency) transfer.
7. If these things are not successful, and if the patien is not starting to recover within 1 hour, then sto the treatment.
8. If the patient's breathing and circulation d improve, then treat like this:

   (a) Give intranasal oxygen 2 litres/minute fo some hours.

   (b) If the patient nearly drowned in sal water and becomes shocked, treat with plasm volume expander as in shock (see Chapter 2 page 379).

(c) Check the urine output carefully. If there is no urine output or only a little red or brown urine with protein in it, start treatment for acute kidney failure (see Chapter 26 page 363) and arrange urgent (emergency) transfer to hospital.
(d) Give antibiotics as if the patient had pneumonia (see Chapter 20 pages 218–22).
(e) Do not discharge the patient for at least 24 hours. Sometimes complications and death occur hours after the patient seems to have recovered.

Emergency laryngostomy

If complete block of the upper airway occurs (e.g. increasing stridor, insuction and rib retraction, the pulse gets faster, the patient develops cyanosis and is extremely distressed or unconscious), then immediately do the following as the patient will otherwise soon die. Push large-bore cannulas or needles through the cricothyroid membrane into the trachea. If this does not allow the patient to breathe well enough, do an emergency laryngostomy. See below for method of doing both.

The patient is laid on his back facing straight upwards. The patient's *head is extended* (head tipped right back) and *held in the midline* (i.e. facing straight up if the body is facing straight up). *These **two** things are **very** important.* Do not start the operation until these two things are done.

Feel for the bottom part of the thyroid cartilage. The thyroid cartilage is the large hard lump, often somewhat pointed at the top, in the middle of the front of the neck, which can be seen to move up then down during swallowing (Adam's apple). Below this, at the top of the trachea, the cricoid cartilage can be felt. The cricoid cartilage is the next hard piece of tissue felt going across the neck straight under the thyroid cartilage. Between the thyroid and cricoid cartilages is a hallow – the cricothyroid membrane.

Push one or two 13-gauge needles or four or more of the largest available needles through the membrane, pointing them backwards and downwards. If air can go through all, then oxygen may be run in through *one* of the needles. Artificial ventilation could be given by blocking the other needles with the fingers until the oxygen going in fills the lungs, and then taking the fingers off the needles to allow expiration.

If the patient is still not able to breathe or is not ventilated enough, do an emergency laryngostomy as follows. However, laryngostomy is:

1. used only in cases of desperate emergency (patient stopped breathing or about to stop breathing),
2. only temporary,
3. suitable for use in adults only.

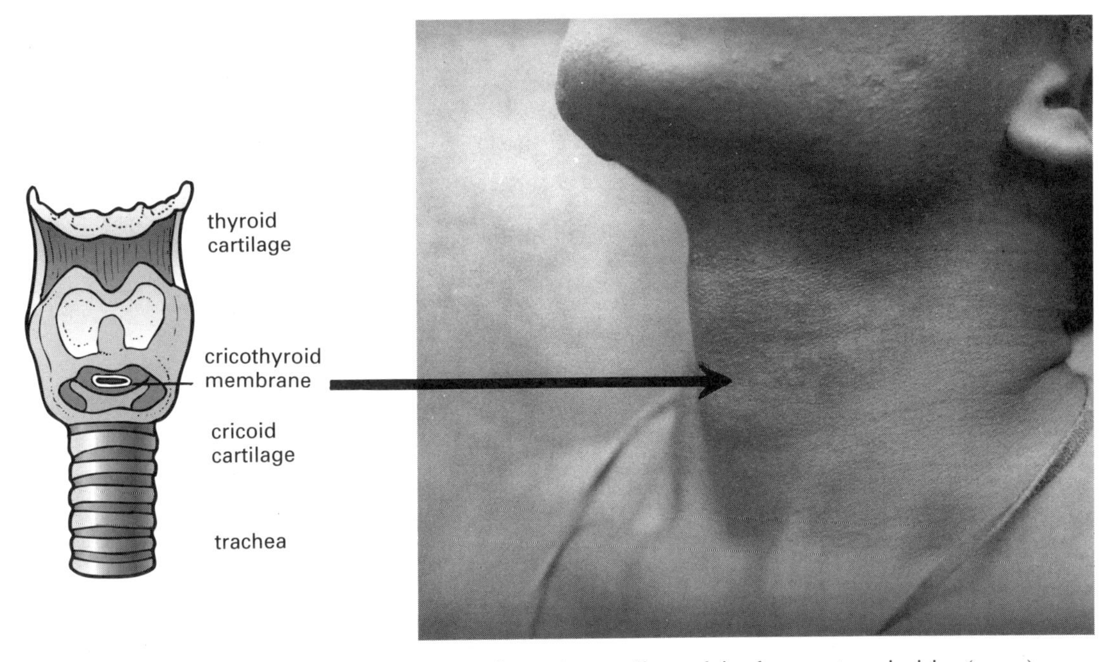

Figure 37.9 Diagram and photograph showing the place for putting needles or doing laryngostomy incision (arrow) through the cricothyroid membrane.

Put on glasses or goggles and a waterproof mask as blood will be sprayed into the air and sucked into the lungs with each breath.

If there is time, make a transverse incision about 2 cm (1 inch) long across the neck in this area. If there is time, use local anaesthetic and clamp and tie any bleeding points.

Then, with or without the above incision, either a pair of closed pointed scissors or the cutting end of a scalpel is pushed downwards and backwards as close to the upper border of the cricoid cartilage as possible. Either will easily go through the cricothyroid membrane into the lower larynx and upper trachea.

Then turn the instrument (and open the blades if it is a pair of scissors). Turning the instrument will open a hole between the larynx and trachea and the air outside. The patient will then be able to breathe through this hole.

If possible, put a short wide-bore tube through the hole. Use the cut-off end of a 20 or 10 ml disposable syringe barrel; or test tube with the bottom end broken off (put the top end with the flange or widened part into the hole); or a piece of pipe, tube, or hard plastic or rubber hose. Have the tube as short as possible, e.g. 3–5 cm (1–2 inches). Pull out the scissors or the knife when the tube is in place. The membrane will close on the tube and will keep a lot of the blood out of the trachea as the blood comes mostly from outside the membrane.

An oxygen tube can be put through the opening into the trachea. The trachea can be sucked out with a soft catheter on a sucker.

If the patient does not immediately start to breathe, artificial ventilation can be given by blowing into the tube.

The bleeding vessels can then be clamped with artery forceps and tied off.

Stick the tube firmly with plaster so that it cannot fall into the trachea or out of the hole in the larynx.

The patient is then transferred urgently (emergency) to Medical Officer care for further treatment and probably proper tracheostomy.

Appendix

Incubation Periods

Incubation periods can be misleading in areas where diseases are endemic. In practice in such areas it is probably sufficient to remember whether the incubation period is of long, medium or short duration.

Malaria
The incubation period in man (from the bite of an infected mosquito until the start of symptoms and signs of malaria) is usually about 2 weeks. However, it is often much longer. It cannot be shorter than 8 days.

Leprosy
The incubation period is usually 2–4 years; but it can be shorter or very much longer at times.

Measles
The incubation period is 1–2 weeks.

German measles
The incubation period is 2–3 weeks.

Chicken pox
The incubation period is 2–3 weeks.

Mumps
The incubation period is 2–3 weeks.

Leptospirosis
The incubation period varies from 1 to 3 weeks.

Plague
The incubation period is usually less than a week.

Typhus
The incubation period is 1–2 weeks.

Yellow fever
The incubation period is 3–6 days.

Typhoid
The incubation period is from 3 to 60 days, but usually about 10 days.

Gonorrhoea
The incubation period is usually less than 1 week, but can be longer.

Syphilis
The incubation period is about 3 weeks until primary syphilis develops (it can be 10–90 days)

Chancroid
The incubation period is 2–5 days.

Cholera
The incubation period is from a few hours to 5 days.

Acute viral hepatitis
The incubation period is 2 to 6 weeks for hepatitis A and between 6 weeks and 6 months for hepatitis B.

Tetanus
The incubation period is usually about 2 weeks; but it can be much longer or shorter.

References

Publications of particular value for health workers include the following:

Crofton, J., Horne, N. and Miller, F. (1998, or latest edition) *Clinical Tuberculosis*. London, Macmillan Education.

Edwards, C.R.W. *et al.* (1995 or latest edition) *Davidson's Principles and Practice of Medicine*, 17th edn. Edinburgh, Churchill Livingstone, 1203 pp. (low-priced edition available).

Harries, A.D. and Maher, D. (1996, or latest edition) *TB/HIV A Clinical Manual*. Geneva, WHO.

Holmes, W. (1993 or latest edition) *HIV Infection – Virology and Transmission* (for the Asia and Pacific Region). (Tape/Slide set) London, TALC.

Holmes, W. and Savage, F. (1989 or latest edition) *HIV Infection – Clinical Manifestations*. (Tape/slide set) London, TALC.

Holmes, W. and Savage, F. (1993 or latest edition) *HIV Infection – Clinical Manifestations in Asia*. (Tape/slide set) London, TALC.

Holmes, W. and Savage, F. (1989 or latest edition) *HIV Infection – Virology and Transmission* (in Africa). (Tape/Slide set) London, TALC.

Holmes, W., and Savage, F. and Hubley, J. (1989 or latest edition) *HIV Infection – Prevention and Counselling*. (Tape/Slide set) London, TALC.

Hubley, J. Makhumula, P. and Wynendaele, B. (1995 or latest edition) *Peer Group Education in AIDS and STD Programmes*. (Tape/Slide set) London, TALC.

Latif, A. and Murtagh, K. (1990 or latest edition) *Sexually Transmitted Diseases*. (Tape/Slide set) London, TALC.

Lawrence, D.R., Bennett, P.N. and Brown, M.Y. (1997 or latest edition) *Clinical Pharmacology*, 8th edn. Edinburgh, Churchill Livingstone (low-priced edition available).

Munro, J. and Edwards, C. (1995 or latest edition) *MacLeod's Clinical Examination*, 9th edn. Edinburgh, Churchill Livingstone. (low-priced edition available).

von Massow, Fr., Ndele, J.K. and Korte, K. (1997) *Guidelines to Rational Drug Use*. London, Macmillan Education.

Publications of particular value for Medical Officers in adult internal medicine in the tropics include:

Bell, D.R. (1995 or latest edition) *Lecture Notes on Tropical Medicine*, 4th (or latest) edition. Oxford, Blackwell Science.

Beneson, (ed.) (1995, or latest edition) *Control of Communicable Diseases Manual*, 16th (or latest) edition. Washington DC, American Public Health Association.

Cook, G.C. (ed.) (1996, or latest edition) *Manson's Tropical Diseases*, 20th (or latest) edition. London, W.B. Saunders.

Harries, A.D. and Maher, D. (1996, or latest edition). *TB/HIV A Clinical Manual*. Geneva, WHO.

WHO (1997) *Tropical Disease Research Progress 1995–1996*. Geneva, WHO.

Index

Numbers underlined refer to figures; *underlined italics* refer to tables.